→ dr. T.G.H. Davies

Graham —

For your reference:
See 1982 Clinical
Update, Page 198-205.

Tony Volpe

A Textbook of Preventive Dentistry

Second Edition

RICHARD E. STALLARD, D.D.S., Ph.D.

Adjunct Professor, School of Public Health, University of Minnesota,
Minneapolis, Minnesota
Active Staff, Fairview Hospital and St. Mary's Hospital
Minneapolis, Minnesota

1982

W. B. SAUNDERS COMPANY

Philadelphia   London   Toronto   Mexico City   Rio de Janeiro   Sydney   Tokyo

W. B. Saunders Company: West Washington Square
Philadelphia, PA   19105

1 St. Anne's Road
Eastbourne, East Sussex BN21 3UN, England

1 Goldthorne Avenue
Toronto, Ontario M8Z 5T9, Canada

Apartado 26370 — Cedro 512
Mexico 4, D.F., Mexico

Rua Coronel Cabrita, 8
Sao Cristovao Caixa Postal 21176
Rio de Janeiro, Brazil

9 Waltham Street
Artarmon, N.S.W. 2064, Australia

Ichibancho, Central Bldg., 22-1 Ichibancho
Chiyoda-Ku, Tokyo 102, Japan

Library of Congress Cataloging in Publication Data

Main entry under title:

A Textbook of preventive dentistry.

Includes bibliographies and index.

1. Preventive dentistry.   I. Stallard, Richard E. [DNLM:
   1. Oral health.   2. Preventive dentistry. WU 113 T355]

RK60.7.T49 1982   617.6'01   81–51074

ISBN 0–7216–8550–1   AACR2

A Textbook of Preventive Dentistry   ISBN   0-7216-8550-1

Last digit is the print number: 9   8   7   6   5   4   3   2   1

Contributors

R. ANTHONY ADAMS, B.D.S., M.S., Certificate in Periodontics

Assistant Professor, University of Mississippi School of Dentistry, Department of Periodontics; Staff Member, University of Mississippi Medical Center, Jackson, Mississippi.
Oral Hygiene Techniques and Home Care (with Wallace V. Mann).

M. BASHAR BAKDASH, D.D.S., M.P.H., M.S.D.

Associate Professor, Department of Periodontology, School of Dentistry, and Associate Professor, Dental Public Health Program, School of Public Health, University of Minnesota, Minneapolis, Minnesota.
Education and Motivation of the Dentist and Patient in Preventive Dentistry (with Hussein A. Zaki).

THOMAS K. BARBER, D.D.S., M.S.

Associate Dean and Professor of Pediatric Dentistry, School of Dentistry, University of California–Los Angeles, California.
Preventive Orthodontics (with L. S. Luke).

THEODORE E. BOLDEN, D.D.S., Ph.D., LL.D. (Hon.)

Professor, Department of General and Oral Pathology, CMDNJ—New Jersey Dental School, Newark, New Jersey. Consultant, Veterans Administration Hospitals in Tuskegee, Alabama, and Brooklyn, New York.
Epidemiology of and Factors Related to Oral Cancer. The Prevention and Detection of Oral Cancer.

SIDNEY B. FINN, D.M.D., M.S.

Late Professor Emeritus of Dentistry, University of Alabama School of Dentistry, Birmingham, Alabama.
The Epidemiology of Dental Caries.

RALPH A. HEISER, D.D.S., Ph.D.

Chairman, Board of Directors, Minndent Associates, Incorporated, Edina, Minnesota.
Marketing Preventive Dentistry (with Richard E. Stallard and Kären Hess).

KÄREN HESS, Ph.D.

Director, Innovative Programming Systems, Inc., Minneapolis, Minnesota.
Marketing Preventive Dentistry (with Ralph A. Heiser and Richard E. Stallard).

HERSCHEL S. HOROWITZ, D.D.S., M.P.H.

Chief, Community Programs Section, National Caries Program, National Institute of Dental Research, National Institutes of Health, Bethesda, Maryland. *Water Fluoridation and Other Methods for Delivering Systemic Fluoride.*

ROBERT G. JONES, D.D.S.

President, Oral Health Products, Inc., Tulsa, Oklahoma. *Introduction to Preventive Dentistry.*

LARRY S. LUKE, D.D.S., M.S.

Clinical Professor and Chairman, Section of Pediatric Dentistry, School of Dentistry, University of California–Los Angeles, California. *Preventive Orthodontics (with Thomas K. Barber).*

WALLACE V. MANN, D.M.D., M.S.

Professor of Periodontics, School of Dentistry, University of Mississippi. Attending Staff, University Hospital, University of Mississippi Medical Center, Jackson, Mississippi. *Oral Hygiene Techniques and Home Care (with R. Anthony Adams).*

JUAN M. NAVIA, Ph.D.

Professor of Nutrition Science, Professor of Oral Biology, and Professor of Public Health, Schools of Dentistry and Public Health, and Senior Scientist, Institute for Dental Research, University of Alabama, Birmingham, Alabama. *Nutrition in Oral Health and Disease.*

C. H. PAMEIJER, D.M.D., M.Sc.D., D.Sc.

Professor of Prosthodontics and Biomaterials and Chairman, Division of Biomaterials, Henry M. Goldman School of Graduate Dentistry, Boston University Medical Center, Boston, Massachusetts. *The Composite Resin: A Preventive Operative Procedure.*

CHARLES F. SCHACHTELE, M.S., Ph.D.

Professor of Dentistry, School of Dentistry, and Professor of Microbiology, Medical School, University of Minnesota, Minneapolis, Minnesota. *Dental Caries: Prevention and Control.*

LEONARD SHAPIRO, D.M.D., M.S.

Associate Professor of Oral Biology and Associate Professor of Periodontology, Henry M. Goldman School of Graduate Dentistry, Boston University Medical Center. Active Staff, Goddard Memorial Hospital, Stoughton, Massachusetts; Jordan Hospital, Plymouth, Massachusetts; Notre Dame Hospital, Central Falls, Rhode Island. Courtesy Staff, University Hospital, Boston, Massachusetts. *Etiology of Periodontal Disease (with Richard E. Stallard). Periodontal Disease: Prevention and Control.*

JAMES H. SHAW, Ph.D.

Professor of Nutrition, Harvard School of Dental Medicine, Boston, Massachusetts. *Etiology of Dental Caries.*

RICHARD J. SIMONSEN, D.D.S., M.S.

Associate Professor and Director of Research, Department of Operative Dentistry, New York University College of Dentistry, New York, New York.
Pit and Fissure Sealant. The Acid Etch Technique and Preventive Resin Restoration.

ANTHONY R. VOLPE, D.D.S., M.S.

Director, Clinical Investigations, Colgate-Palmolive Company Research Center, Piscataway, New Jersey. Clinical Associate Professor, Department of Pharmacology, Fairleigh-Dickinson University School of Dentistry, Hackensack, New Jersey.
Dentifrices and Mouth Rinses.

ARTHUR H. WUEHRMANN, D.M.D., A.B.

Professor of Dentistry (retired), University of Alabama, Birmingham, Alabama.
Preventive Dental Radiology.

HUSSEIN A. ZAKI, B.Ch.D., M.P.H., M.S.D.

Clinical Associate Professor, Department of Periodontology, School of Dentistry, University of Minnesota, Minneapolis, Minnesota.
Education and Motivation of the Dentist and Patient in Preventive Dentistry (with M. Bashar Bakdash).

Preface
to the Second Edition

Tremendous changes have occurred in the dental profession in general and preventive dentistry in particular since the conception of the first edition of this text. These have been brought about by both technological advances and economic readjustments that have resulted in alterations in the mode of practice, increased third party insurance plans, capitation dentistry, retail dentistry, and a reassignment of values by patients concerning prevention. These factors combined with the inflationary spiral and the current economic downturn bring home some of the predictions made by Dr. Robert Caldwell in the paper presented at the Eastman Dental Center over 10 years ago. At that time the wheels were already turning in the area of capitation grants for dental schools to increase the number of dentists to meet the perceived need for dental care without consideration of demand and other factors that have come to play in the late 1970s and early 1980s. Dr. Caldwell correctly prophesied that we would need fewer dentists in the future as the total effect of preventive dental measures—particularly communal water fluoridation, stabilization of population growth, and the increased productivity of the individual dentists through expanded-duty dental auxiliaries—was felt.

During this period of rapid increase in number of dental care providers, little if any effort has been devoted to changing the attitudes of the public and thereby increasing the demand for dental care. With the increase in consumerism and other pressures it is now apparent that dentists must change their philosophy from one of "selling" their services to one of "marketing" their services. Preventive dentistry is ideal for this approach, as preventive dental procedures, if marketed properly, fulfill a perceived need in the patient's mind and effectively control the cost of dentistry.

All the factors currently affecting dentistry throughout the world should not be looked upon as prophesies of gloom and doom for our profession but rather as challenges that if met properly through preventive dentistry will lead to a bright future for all members of our profession.

R.E.S.

Preface
to the First Edition

This text on preventive dentistry is intended to provide a base on which current concepts can be utilized by those members of the dental profession dedicated to the preservation of the natural dentition. Each subject unit is treated in detail and is in turn linked to the other units to provide a total picture of prevention as it can be practiced today. Both clinical and research data are included upon which sound judgment can be made. Additional reading lists accompany each chapter for those who desire to expand their knowledge in a given area.

I am indebted to all of the contributors to this text for their patience and understanding during the protracted period of preparation resulting, ultimately, in publication. Chapters have been updated and additional references added to include the most current materials available in all areas. I am also indebted to the staff at Saunders for their cooperation and utmost care in preparing the material. Special appreciation is extended to Mrs. Pamela Phillips for her secretarial assistance.

My thanks and appreciation are extended to Mrs. Marge Caldwell for her encouragement, initially to her late husband and finally to me, during all phases of preparation of this book. I am especially grateful to my wife, Jaxon, for her continuing support.

RICHARD E. STALLARD
Minneapolis, Minnesota

Contents

Chapter 10

DENTIFRICES AND MOUTH RINSES 170

Anthony R. Volpe

PART I–DENTIFRICES.. 170
Relationship of Dentifrices to a Preventive Dentistry Program 170
Definition and Functions of a Dentifrice... 170
Ingredients and Composition of Dentifrices 171
Therapeutic (Drug-Containing) Dentifrices... 179
Dentifrices for Periodontal Disease.. 189
Dentifrices for Hypersensitive Teeth 190
Dentifrices with Specialized Functions 190
Dentifrices and the Oral Tissues 190
Current Trends in Dentifrices.. 192

PART II–MOUTH RINSES 191
Definition of a Mouth Rinse.. 192
Composition of Mouth Rinses 192
Functions of a Mouth Rinse 193
Future Trends in Mouth Rinses 197
Fluoride Dentifrices and Mouth Rinses in a Fluoridated Water Area 198
Adult Use of Fluoride Dentifrices and Mouth Rinses 198

PART III–1982 CLINICAL FLUORIDE UPDATE 198

Chapter 11

ORAL HYGIENE TECHNIQUES AND HOME CARE.. 217

R. Anthony Adams and Wallace V. Mann

The Relationship of Oral Hygiene to Caries and Peridontal Disease....................... 218
The Role of Home Care in Caries Prevention.. 219
The Relationship Between Oral Hygiene and Periodontal Disease 220
The Preventive Equipment... 223
Plaque Detection and Disclosing Agents 224
Toothbrush.. 227
The Auxiliary Aids in Oral Hygiene... 235
Chemotherapeutic Agents in Home Care 237

Chapter 12

DENTAL CARIES: PREVENTION AND CONTROL.. 241

Charles F. Schachtele

Combating Cariogenic Bacteria.. 241
Diet Modification 249
Protecting the Teeth.. 252
Sealants.. 253

Chapter 13

PERIODONTAL DISEASE: PREVENTION AND CONTROL.................................... 255

Leonard Shapiro

Plaque Control Programs 256
Chemical and Chemotherapeutic Plaque Control.. 259
Patient Recall 261

Chapter 14

PREVENTIVE DENTAL RADIOLOGY 262

Arthur H. Wuehrmann

General Considerations 263
Radiation Reduction Methods in the Dental Office.. 264
Diagnostic Yield in Relation to Technique and Interpretation 272

CHAPTER ONE

Introduction to Preventive Dentistry

Robert G. Jones, D.D.S.

DISCOVERY OF THE MICROSCOPE

Some three hundred years ago, Antony Van Leeuwenhoek ground a dual convex lens and scraped some material from the mouth of an 8-year-old boy. Thus he viewed for the first time the bacterial world that occupies the oral cavity.

In a short twenty years, the scientists of the day stated that the microscope had outlived its usefulness. This ridicule by so-called scientific authorities who were venting their egotism and greed has caused most medical discoveries to lie dormant for years and even centuries.

Antony Van Leeuwenhoek has generally been credited with inventing the microscope. He did not invent it, but he improved it. He found that a single lens was much better than the compound lens microscopes that were generally in use. He was not trained in any scientific way, but he made his own microscopes. Having no education or background, his work was ridiculed by the so-called scientific establishment.

Today, he is looked on as the father of bacteriology and protozoology, but why have three centuries come and gone before his work was used to rid humanity of the diseases that have plagued us?

THE MICROSCOPIC WORLD OF MAN

The microscopic world that Leeuwenhoek discovered in its natural living motile state was destroyed by the compound microscope and the necessity to stain and kill the organisms. It was not until the fourth decade of this century that a German by the name of Cerni invented the phase contrast microscope, which allowed the observation of the microscopic world in its natural living state. Yet today, most pathologists are not using it, simply because they were not trained in its use.

The human body is a wonderful creation and was obviously meant to survive indefinitely. The microscopic organisms surrounding us were not created to bring disease to man but are used in the cycle of life, and man lived in harmony with them for centuries, oblivious of their existence.

RESISTANCE TO DISEASE

The human body was created with two methods of surviving in the environment. The first is passive resistance. As generations lived and died, the body reacted to the environment and remained healthy. This gradually acquired resistance was inherited through genes, and evidence seems to indicate that breast feeding is one of the methods that nature used. The second is active resistance, which comes into play when a disease-producing substance or organism is introduced into the body. The body reacts by producing antibodies that either destroy or nullify the effects of the toxic substance or organisms.

DISEASE

Pathologic disease is caused in three distinct ways, the body normally having a

1

resistance level that keeps it healthy in its environment. This is the natural law, and it must be violated for a disease to occur.

The first way in which an organism may have a chance to infect the body occurs when there is a lowering of resistance caused by violating the natural laws of nutrition, exercise, breast feeding, and environmental protection from heat, cold, and moisture. When the effect of disobeying one or more natural laws lowers the resistance to the point that man cannot live in the normal environment that surrounds him, then disease is produced. The second means by which disease is produced occurs when man changes his environment so that toxic substances or organisms are introduced into the body in such quantities that the normal resistance level is unable to control it. Disease can also be produced in a third way: by being carried to a culture that has never had the disease and who have no built-in resistance to it. A perfect example of this was the great plagues that ravaged humanity when means of traveling great distances were devised.

The Plains Indians of America are also a good example of disease spreading to a non-immune culture. They were not defeated by the U.S. Cavalry but by respiratory disease that was unknown in their culture. Thus they had no resistance to it and the White Death (tuberculosis) decimated them.

ROLE OF CIVILIZATION

So-called civilization is responsible for a great amount of the disease found throughout the world. Investigation of primitive people living in the world today, untouched by civilization, shows that they are totally free of many of the diseases that plague civilized man, and any attempt to civilize them, no matter how well intended (such as through missionaries), usually brings some of the diseases of civilization to them.

Teeth are the most indestructible part of the human body when exposed to the environment. Paleontology is almost entirely a study of teeth, because they are the only remaining thing left after being exposed to the environment for centuries. But civilization, through its ignorance of natural laws,

has devised ways of destroying them during the normal span of a lifetime.

ACQUISITION OF KNOWLEDGE

The profession of dentistry was born when dental disease became prevalent enough that one man started giving it some of his time and thought, and thus the search for knowledge of dental disease was started. Knowledge is acquired in three distinct stages. There is the stage of ignorance with awareness that the problem exists, and there is a search for answers with anything that can be devised. Thus witch doctors, soothsayers, and "gods" were all called upon to free man from the problems that plagued him. This gradually brings him to the scientific stage, which is the organized accumulation of knowledge on a particular subject. Usually this results in a man-made method of treating the disease or surgically removing the diseased part. Unfortunately, greed and egotism are fed in this stage, and practitioners of the art will do almost anything to discredit any attempt at elevating it to the next stage.

The final stage comes when man recognizes the natural laws that have been violated and disseminates the information so that anyone wanting to escape the disease can do so.

A perfect example of these stages can be found in the form of childhood diseases such as typhoid fever, which was fatal to so many young children in the first three decades of this century. The ignorant stage was when anything and everything was done. If the temperature went up, they tried to lower it. If the temperature went down, they tried to raise it. The same attempts were made with hot and cold foods. Then drugs were used that would accomplish this, and finally it was left up to the "gods."

The scientific stage came into being when it was found that one could give the patient an attenuated dose of the disease, and then his body would build antibodies that would protect it when he was exposed to a lethal dose.

The final stage came when it was discovered that the water supplies were stored unnaturally and that the typhoid bacillus was growing in numbers that exceeded the level of resistance in the body. Thus, sanitation laws were written and implemented, and typhoid fever is unknown and unseen by physicians today in the countries that have adopted these sanitation methods. This disease is still taking the lives of children in countries that violate these natural laws in ignorance.

DENTAL DISEASE

Dental disease is no different from those just mentioned, and it occurs because of a violation of natural laws.

Periodontal disease is such a slow process that it was accepted as a normal result of aging. Thus it was neglected during the state of ignorance. The first stage of gingivitis, which results in painful and bleeding gums, was not recognized as periodontal disease. Various medicaments were used in an attempt to alleviate the symptoms.

The man-made scientific stage began when dentists observed that calculus and pockets formed, thus gradually loosening the teeth. Calculus was named as the culprit, and the pockets were eliminated surgically. Although this did nothing to stop the disease, it was largely taught and practiced until a few years ago.

The final stage came when it was recognized that we have weakened our resistance to the point that we cannot live with the normal bacterial flora found in mouths throughout the world. Primitive natives have been found to have this same bacterial flora, but the natural resistance they have is such that these organisms are nondestructive. Civilized man has lost that resistance. He cannot correct this, since it is now known that the disease is caused by absorption of the waste products produced by the bacterial flora found in the zoogleal mass adhering to the teeth. The only alternative left to man is to remove or disrupt the zoogleal mass at intervals and prevent the absorption of the toxic waste products, thus preventing the progress of the disease.

Knowledge of dental caries has followed the stages mentioned, but because caries is visible when holes appear in the teeth, it was recognized earlier. Man, in his ignorance, tried every kind of cure, such as painting them with herbal stains, medicaments, and bitter drugs. When these approaches did not work, he turned to witch doctors and the "gods."

The scientific or man-made solution came when man surgically removed the diseased part and attempted to restore it to function by filling it with various metals or other materials. This did nothing to stop the onslaught of the disease, and ultimately, the teeth were removed and replaced by artificial ones. Full dentures were the result. In his ignorance, the dentist told patients that some people have soft teeth or that it is hereditary, and there was nothing that could be done about it.

The final stage has been brought about by the observation that caries occurs when products such as refined sugar are introduced into the mouth, and the waste products produced when they are ingested by the bacterial flora cause a dissolution of the tooth structure. Most natural sugars that occur in nature are not degradable to caries-producing waste products. The worst offender seems to be refined sugar produced from sugar cane or other products. When ingested, the bacterial flora of the mouth act upon it and produce waste products that bring about the dissolution of the tooth structure.

This has left civilized man with two solutions for escaping dental caries. One, he can eliminate cariogenic products from his diet. This is the way that primitive natives escape dental caries. He can also escape it by oral hygiene that removes or disrupts the accumulation of waste products on the surface of the teeth before the destructive process occurs.

This is the state and stage of dental knowledge to date, and it is the truth as we know it now. This does not mean it will be the ultimate truth, but it is all we have to go with now.

THE GOAL OF DENTISTRY

The supreme goal of the dental profession should be to eliminate the need for its own existence. To do this, we must correct some dental definitions that were made in ignorance in the so-called scientific stage. Dental caries is not a cavity in a tooth. It is a symptom of long-standing disease. Dental caries is a bacterial-chemical reaction that takes place on the surface of a healthy tooth and, if left undisturbed long enough, will produce the cavity.

Periodontal disease is not a pocket measured with a probe. This is a symptom of long-standing periodontal disease. Periodontal disease is an inflammatory reaction that occurs when the waste products of the normal bacterial flora found in the mouth are absorbed by the mucous membrane at the gingival crevice. The pocket is formed by the natural protective reaction of the gingival attachment mechanism to maintain its integrity and prevent a bacterial invasion into the body.

These are the definitions we are going to retrain ourselves to use when we attempt to free our patients from these diseases. Otherwise, we will continue to run "filling stations" as we have been taught to do.

GREAT MEDICAL DISCOVERIES

Who and what kind of men have given the world its great medical discoveries? Is there a common denominator that can be found? I believe there is, after sitting at the feet of Leeuwenhoek through the writings of his contemporaries and historians that followed him. They found that on examining and using his microscope they did not see the things he did. Could it be that they were blind to what was before their eyes, blinded by the vanity and greed of experts? We look with our eyes, but we see with our minds.

Could it be that these experts refused to see things with their minds because if they did see it, it would demonstrate the ignorance they had been teaching and promulgating in the past, thus taking a blow to their vanity that they could not accept?

The final conclusion that the many people who have studied Leeuwenhoek's life and work came to was that he had a different way of observing what he saw than they did. I believe that this was the ultimate truth about him. But I believe the reason he had a

"different way of observing what he saw" was that he was not blinded by vanity or greed. He never accepted any honor or money for what he did. When asked about his work, he pleaded ignorance and lack of education, and was only concerned with observing the natural world in its true state.

I have been privileged to sit at the feet of and learn from two men who contributed more to the cause of human health in this century than any other men.

Sir Alexander Fleming, a Scottish bacteriologist, gave the world penicillin in 1929, but he was ridiculed and scorned by the so-called scientific world, and because of their antagonism, penicillin was not accepted and used until 10 or 15 years later. It weighed very heavily on him that so many humans suffered and died during this time.

When I asked about his discovery of penicillin, he stated that *Penicillium notatum* was the mold responsible for ruining more bacterial experiments than any other cause, and he was taught to throw them out and start over. This he did for many years until one day he got tired of it and decided to observe this green mold that was such a nuisance. When he did, he observed that the pathologic organisms that he was trying to grow gave it a wide berth. Thus he gave the world penicillin, because he, like Leeuwenhoek "observed what he saw in a different way from other men." He was continually amazed that the thousands of men who had observed this phenomena before him had not seen the same thing.

Dr. Charles C. Bass, the youngest man ever to serve as dean of a medical school, was appointed to that position at Tulane. Hookworm was a disease that was endemic throughout the south. The childhood diseases of typhoid fever, whooping cough, and diphtheria were exacting a deadly toll in human life. He loved to hunt quail as a boy growing up in Mississippi, and looked on their rapid disappearance as not only a loss of personal pleasure, but a loss to humanity and nature. The Tulane Dental School was also under his jurisdiction, and the continual removal and replacement of teeth appalled him.

These phenomena were unacceptable to him, and he refused to believe the experts as to their cause. He saw the lack of results in their efforts to alleviate them. He promptly went back east and studied the microscope and its use. Then he carried the first one west of the Mississippi River.

He then carefully used it to "observe these phenomena in a different way." As a result, he wiped out hookworm in the south. He wrote the sanitation laws for New Orleans, and they were copied all over the world, thus stamping out the many childhood diseases. He wrote a book on the diseases of quail in an effort to preserve them. He was unable to get anyone in the dental school interested in preserving the natural dentition, so he promptly closed it.

He then turned his microscope on dental disease, and in 1943, he published an article simply stating that both caries and periodontal disease were caused by the waste products of the bacterial flora found in the zoogleal mass on the surfaces of teeth. He then proceeded to write down the optimum characteristics of a toothbrush and dental floss that would most effectively remove them and demonstrated the methods of how a toothbrush and floss should be used.

His work was met with antagonism and ridicule by the dental profession, and experts of the day continued to write books and teach that calculus, food impaction, and architecture were the causative agents. This nonsense was taught to me in dental school.

A CHALLENGE TO THE DENTAL PROFESSION

In the following chapters of this book you will be exposed to the latest accumulated knowledge of how and why dental disease occurs. It is my hope that some of you will be stimulated to use and add to that knowledge and thus bring dentistry closer to its supreme goal — to remove the necessity for its own existence.

The men that I have mentioned here, along with the other men throughout the centuries that have made medical discoveries, are now referred to as great men. But after studying and learning of their lives and work, I am convinced that there are no great men. Humanity has great problems, and ordinary men who are willing to "observe them in a different way" solve them. Thus the greatness of the problems rubs off on them.

The problems faced by humanity today involve every field of human endeavor. It is my hope that one or more of the men and women who read this book will look at the world around them, see these problems, then take off the blinding glasses of ego and greed, and "observe them in a different way."

CHAPTER TWO

Education and Motivation of the Dentist and Patient in Preventive Dentistry

Hussein A. Zaki, B.Ch.D., M.P.H., M.S.D.
M. Bashar Bakdash, D.D.S., M.P.H., M.S.D.

The treatment of teeth by extraction and restorative dentistry without the active sharing of the responsibility for protecting the dental health of the community should not be the philosophy of dental education, and it is a particular interest of this text to explore the preventive aspects of all phases of dentistry. One has simply to examine the statistics relevant to the incidence and prevalence of dental disease to visualize the magnitude of the problem that faces the dental profession today. Prevention, not therapy, is today's problem and hopefully tomorrow's answer.

Oral hygiene procedures and techniques are in reality the substantiating force in preventive dentistry. Their objectives are to attain and maintain the health of the oral tissues. These procedures are the most effective way known for the prevention of oral disease.[1-3] It has been reported[4] that only 5 per cent of 2,000 adult respondents believed that brushing protects the gingiva. In another survey,[5] it was shown that 9 per cent of the 3,000 young adult and adult participants stated that the main reason for cleaning their teeth was to improve their periodontal health. It is believed that a great deal of periodontal disease can be attributed to this lack of awareness and instruction in the area of oral hygiene. From previous studies[6, 7, 8] it is obvious that most dental diseases can be controlled and "prevented" through a comprehensive prevention program and through an effective dental health education program for the public. Education, therefore, should be the foundation for a sound preventive program.

Organized dental education has changed tremendously since the first dental school was organized in the United States in 1840. Unfortunately, the changes have been fostered by an overwhelming desire to produce technically competent individuals who are capable of handling the ravages of dental diseases, with particular emphasis on dental caries. The end result is that dentists have been entering practice with the concept that the bulk of their work is reparative, and they will probably continue with this concept for years to come.

In dental education throughout the world, training is concentrated on skills and knowledge with little emphasis directed toward attitudes and concepts. Prevention first and foremost requires the right attitude and philosophy of practice. Conviction, ideals, and enthusiasm are essential to the support of an effective preventive program. It is the obligation of dental educators to see that dental students are constantly stimulated and motivated to develop a strict preventive philosophy that hopefully will grow with them as they practice. The dental students of today, as they assume their responsibilities as practicing dentists, must be accountable for increasing dental public health awareness and for promoting a sound preventive program.

Several research studies have indicated that one of the central problems in preventive dentistry is in motivating the public to take the necessary action for continuous care of their own mouths. However, an important point often forgotten and not seriously investigated is the motivation of the dentist. It is logical that if the dentist lacks the conviction, ideals and enthusiasm necessary to support him in developing a preventive program, this program will be ineffective. The dental student of today can be the catalyst for initiating an increased oral awareness and public cooperation. In order for dental students to motivate patients and the public toward prevention, they must exhibit positive preventive dentistry attitudes by personally practicing all of the available preventive means. The problem we are facing in preventing oral diseases is one of teaching methods as they relate to the dental student. Although the technical aspects of oral hygiene may be recognized, the important question remaining is, How well do our instructions affect the student's attitude and behavior toward his own oral health?

In an attempt to evaluate the present status of the effectiveness of preventive periodontal education, a study was carried out at the University of Minnesota.[9] The study population consisted of approximately 400 dental students distributed equally among freshmen, sophomores, juniors and seniors. The students were evaluated in three areas. First, a clinical examination was conducted to evaluate the degree of oral cleanliness utilizing Greene-Vermillion's Oral Hygiene Index Simplified. Second, after the initial clinical examination, each student was given a 20-item questionnaire, which was developed to record existing "attitudes" and behavior patterns regarding different aspects of oral hygiene. This questionnaire provided a general assessment and an overall picture of the commonly used practices in dental care.

A scoring method was devised to give a numerical value to the responses obtained. Only those questions that reflected the student's oral hygiene procedures were considered. A score of 100 was the highest obtainable. Third, in order to assess the student's knowledge regarding preventive periodontal care, a final examination was given. Again, 100 points was the maximum score.

The means and standard deviations of scores of the Debris Index Simplified (DI-S), the Calculus Index Simplified (CI-S), the Oral Hygiene Index Simplified (OHI-S), the questionnaire and the test are shown in Table 2-1. They are arranged according to class.

The DI-S, CI-S and OHI-S scores remained stable for all classes. However, the scores were slightly lower for the sophomore class and slightly higher for the seniors. The lowest mean test score was 67.3, calculated for the freshman class, while the highest was 86.4, assigned to the sophomores. The mean test score for the junior class decreased slightly to 83.8 and was followed by a considerable drop to 74.5 for the seniors.

The mean questionnaire score for the

TABLE 2-1 MEANS AND STANDARD DEVIATIONS OF DI-S, CI-S, OHI-S, TEST AND QUESTIONNAIRE SCORES, ACCORDING TO THE DIFFERENT CLASSES OF DENTAL STUDENTS AND FOR THE GROUP AS A WHOLE

DENTAL CLASSES	NUMBERS	TYPE OF SCORES									
		DI-S		CI-S		OHI-S		TEST		QUESTIONNAIRE	
		Mean	S.D.	Mean	S.D.	Mean	S.D.	Mean	S.D.	Mean	S.D.
Freshmen	104	.77	.44	.32	.25	1.09	.60	67.3	10.1	73.0	9.2
Sophomores	106	.69	.31	.29	.27	.98	.46	86.4	7.2	72.6	7.4
Juniors	93	.77	.34	.32	.24	1.09	.49	83.8	7.9	72.0	8.2
Seniors	88	.80	.45	.38	.26	1.18	.61	74.5	10.6	74.6	11.3
Total	391	.75	.38	.33	.26	1.08	.54	78.0	11.9	73.0	9.1

whole student body was 73. The scores fluctuated slightly but were essentially the same for the four classes. The senior class, however, had the highest mean score, 74.6.

In order to obtain a better understanding of the relationship of these means, an analysis of variance technique was applied. Differences between DI-S, CI-S, OHI-S and questionnaire scores were not statistically significant. The differences between the class means of the test scores, however, were highly significant (P < 0.01).

Additional insight into the oral hygiene levels of the different classes was gained by classifying the students into five groups according to their degree of oral cleanliness: excellent, good, fair, poor and very poor. The criteria for this classification were based upon the number of teeth covered by plaque. Students with no plaque present were categorized as excellent. Such students would have a DI-S score of zero. A student with plaque present on one or two teeth was assigned to a "good" category. Fair oral cleanliness meant three or four teeth covered by plaque. Poor oral cleanliness meant five or six teeth covered by plaque, and a DI-S score of more than one was indicative of very poor oral hygiene. Since the number of students with "excellent" oral hygiene was small (three freshmen, two sophomores, two juniors, and two seniors), the good and excellent categories were combined.

A chi-square test was applied to this data to determine whether a significant difference in oral cleanliness existed between the four dental school classes. The chi-square test is highly significant at the P ≤ .005 level. The sophomores contributed fewer students to the "very poor oral cleanliness" category than expected, whereas the seniors contributed more than expected.

Information on frequency of toothbrushing was taken from the questionnaire. In order to verify the students' claims about toothbrushing, the means of DI-S, CI-S and OHI-S were grouped and examined according to the frequency of brushing, irrespective of class. As the frequency of toothbrushing increased, the scores of DI-S and OHI-S decreased. This negative relation is what one would expect. A similar relation can be seen between CI-S and frequency of brushing. A slight difference exists, however, between those who brush three times per day and those who brush two times per day. The analysis of variance technique that was applied disclosed a significant difference at the .01 level for the DI-S, CI-S, and OHI-S.

In reviewing the dental literature regarding dental health education and patient motivation it can be seen that many surveys have indicated a remarkable improvement in oral cleanliness associated with oral hygiene instruction even when comparatively little time was spent in instruction. In the case of dental students with an educational program of four years, however, the results do not appear consistent and are not proportional. The data, for example, suggest essentially no change in the level of oral hygiene maintained by students as they progressed through the four year dental curriculum. In addition, the fact that toothbrushing alone does not remove the plaque sheltered in the interproximal space does not seem to impress the students. Fifty-six per cent of the students in the study used the toothbrush as the only method to clean their mouths. Only 77 students, or 19 per cent, stated that they floss daily. This lack of behavioral change existed even though the students were giving their patients toothbrushing and flossing instruction.

This study dramatically demonstrates the need for specific oral hygiene instructions to dental students. An effective program must help a student improve his attitudes, as well as contribute to his acquisition and development of oral hygiene skills. It is important from the viewpoint of increasing the effectiveness of oral hygiene practices in the student's own mouth, and it is equally if not more important from the viewpoint of preparing the student to assume the responsibility for teaching and motivating patients in the oral hygiene procedures.

One investigation published in 1979 was designed to provide further insight into the relationships between a number of personal and academic variables and the oral hygiene status of dental students.[10] The study population consisted of 127 dental students from the School of Dentistry, University of Minnesota. All subjects were enrolled in various courses offered by the Department of Periodontology during the academic years 1975–1976 (second year) and 1976–1977 (third year).

The oral hygiene status of each student was determined during the first week of their second year without the students' prior knowledge by utilizing the Plaque Control Record.[11]

In addition to the assessment of oral hygiene status, a total of thirteen personal, pre-dental and dental academic variables were obtained and recorded for each student. Personal data included age and sex, while pre-dental academic variables included years in college, college grade point average, and the academic and manual portions of the dental aptitude test scores. Dental academic variables consisted of the first year dental grade point average and the total points achieved in each of the five didactic periodontal courses that included Periodontology I through Periodontology V.

The overall mean plaque score was 46.7 per cent. Only 18.8 per cent of the students had excellent and good oral hygiene, while 63 per cent of them had poor or very poor oral hygiene. An analysis of the variance for the mean of each of the eleven variables as classified by oral hygiene status was performed. In general, students with better oral hygiene tended to achieve significantly higher test scores than those students with less favorable oral hygiene in at least seven of the stated academic variables (Table 2–2).

The dentist's failure to stress effective preventive dental health services and to teach his patients effective oral hygiene has been demonstrated. Data published by The American Dental Association[12] indicates that less than 20 per cent of patients receiving care in dental offices were given oral hygiene instruction. Furthermore, it has been stated[4] that only 18 per cent of patients who see a dentist regularly receive thorough routine dental prophylaxis.

Although the dentist should assume prime responsibility for patient education, it is evident that the enormity of the task requires that implementation be delegated to others on the dental health team. Consider-

ing the present status of auxiliaries in dentistry and the Dental Practice Acts, it appears that the oral hygiene and preventive periodontal responsibilities can be assigned to the dental hygienist. Changes to permit expanded duties for the dental assistant will bring a tremendous influx of qualified personnel to the preventive dentistry program.

Dental hygiene education is already directed toward promoting oral health. There exist many programs that place special emphasis on patient education. When dental hygiene was recommended as a formal educational program by Dr. Fones in 1913, he suggested that dental hygienists be trained and employed mainly in schools to provide preventive treatment for children. In addition, research studies have reported that students in the social sciences tend to care more for people than do students in the physical or biological sciences. In this regard, dental hygienists may benefit from the inclusion of social science courses in the dental hygiene curriculum, since they may serve to strengthen their role in providing preventive dental health service.

In light of this feeling for the importance of dental auxiliaries in providing oral hygiene and preventive periodontal instruction, an evaluation similar to the one done with dental students was undertaken to analyze the effectiveness of preventive periodontal education in the dental hygiene curriculum.[13] The study was expanded to include evaluation one year after graduation for possible changes in attitudes. The final modification was a questionnaire developed to record information regarding different aspects of clinical practice. The questionnaire was administered to the students before graduation and again after one year of practice.

The study population included 42 first-year and 38 second-year dental hygiene students. The means and standard deviations of scores of DI-S, CI-S, OHI-S, test, and questionnaire are listed in Table 2–3. The results are arranged according to the different classes and for the entire group.

The mean OHI-S for the freshmen was 1.01, markedly higher than that for the seniors. The mean test score for the freshmen

TABLE 2-2 ANALYSIS OF THE VARIANCE FOR THE MEANS OF THE STATED ACADEMIC VARIABLES AND ORAL HYGIENE STATUS OF STUDENTS*

Oral Hygiene Status	Years in College	Pre-dent. G.P.A.	DAT-A	DAT-M	First Year G.P.A.	Second Year G.P.A.	Perio I	Perio II	Perio III	Perio IV	Perio V
						ACADEMIC VARIABLES					
Excellent	3.67	3.59	5.67	5.00	3.44	3.33	34.67	63.00	81.33	41.67	24.33
Good	4.14	3.33	5.05	5.48	3.15	3.05	32.90	57.52	78.52	39.38	23.95
Fair	3.74	3.42	4.91	5.13	3.00	3.00	31.70	58.70	80.13	39.83	24.43
Poor	3.98	3.14	4.93	5.70	2.75	2.73	31.33	55.38	75.93	36.35	23.84
Very poor	4.00	2.25	5.08	5.38	2.86	2.82	30.46	57.24	77.59	38.35	23.73
Total	3.96	3.27	5.01	5.45	2.91	2.87	31.48	57.06	77.73	38.19	23.94
Within mean square	0.907	3.088	1.041	2.063	0.303	0.162	8.852	24.598	28.330	12.976	4.495
F-test†	0.59	4.69	0.48	0.70	2.905	4.06	3.21	3.005	2.865	5.285	0.455
Probability	n.s.	p = .0015	n.s.	n.s.	p = .0245	p = .0040	p = .0152	p = .0210	p = .0261	p = .0006	n.s.

*Bakdash, M. B., and Proshek, J. M.: Oral hygiene status of dental students as related to their personal and academic profiles. J. Periodont. Res. 14:438–443, 1979.
†Bet. categories (df = 4.122)

TABLE 2–3 MEANS AND STANDARD DEVIATIONS OF DI-S, CI-S, OHI-S, TEST AND QUESTIONNAIRE SCORES, ACCORDING TO THE DIFFERENT CLASSES OF DENTAL HYGIENE STUDENTS AND FOR THE GROUP AS A WHOLE

DENTAL HYGIENE CLASS	NUMBERS	TYPES OF SCORES									
		DI-S		CI-S		OHI-S		TEST		QUESTIONNAIRE	
		Mean	S.D.	Mean	S.D.	Mean	S.D.	Mean	S.D.	Mean	S.D.
Freshmen	42	.73	.40	.28	.20	1.01	.51	76.60	9.0	81.60	5.7
Seniors	38	.49	.30	.18	.15	.67	.39	85.20	6.5	84.2	6.3
Total	80	.61	.37	.23	.18	.84	.48	80.9	7.8	82.9	6.0

class was 76.60 and increased to 85.20 for the seniors. The mean questionnaire score for the total student body was 82.9. The scores fluctuated slightly but were essentially the same for both classes, with the seniors scoring somewhat higher.

In order to clarify the differences between the means of these variables, the data were statistically analyzed. The differences between DI-S, OHI-S, and test scores were statistically significant at the 0.01 level. The differences, however, between questionnaire scores were not statistically significant.

Table 2–4 indicates that there is a trend for dental hygiene graduates to move to larger cities. It is evident that the percentage of dental hygienists intending to practice in a city population ranging from 100,000 to 250,000 decreased markedly from 26 per cent to 7 per cent, while the percentage who intended to practice in a city with a population of over 500,000 increased from 27 per cent to 43 per cent. It is interesting to note that the percentage in the smallest communities remained the same.

The number of years senior students predicted, before graduation, that they would practice full-time is illustrated in Table 2–5. The table also demonstrates how these predictions changed after only one year of practice. Thirteen per cent of the senior class stated that they would practice only two years. However, during the first year 42 per cent had already left full-time practice. It is interesting to speculate whether the reason for such large-scale abandonment of full-time practice resulted from disillusionment with the dental hygienists' role or from largely personal reasons, such as marriage.

The dental hygienists' visualization of the nature of their profession before gradua-

tion and then after one year of practice is shown in Table 2–6. Before graduation 90 per cent of the students indicated that they wanted to practice prevention. After one year of practice, however, only 61 per cent indicated that their practice was oriented toward prevention. This group stated that they treated 10 patients per day. In contrast, 39 per cent indicated that their practice was now therapeutic; this group treated an average of 12 patients per day. The number of patients in either category is a heavy work load for even the most efficient dental hygienist. It was also noted on the questionnaire that many of those who still visualized dental hygiene as preventive in nature admitted that they were unable to practice in that manner because of the office environment.

It is apparent, on the basis of substantial differences in both test scores and oral cleanliness, that the dental hygiene education program is effective in teaching preventive care. The hygienists, however, do not or cannot fully utilize this educational knowledge and skill in preventive dental programs for the public. Before graduation the majority of dental hygiene students strongly believed in stressing preventive dental care and oral hygiene in their practices. In practice

TABLE 2–4 TENDENCY OF DENTAL HYGIENE GRADUATES TO MOVE TOWARD LARGER CITIES

CITY SIZE	PERCENTAGE	
	Before Graduation	After One Year of Practice
Under 100,000	27	27
100,000–250,000	26	7
250,000–500,000	20	23
Over 500,000	27	43
Total	100	100

TABLE 2–5 PREDICTION AS TO LENGTH OF TIME IN FULL-TIME DENTAL HYGIENE PRACTICE

YEARS	PERCENTAGE Before Graduation	After One Year of Practice
		42% have already left full-time practice
One	0	5
Two	13	25
Three	20	5
Four	7	3
Five	42	6
More than five	18	14
Total	100	100

they were unable to do so. This is most likely a reflection of the attitudes prevalent in the dental practices in which they were located.

It is very surprising to note that numerous reports have indicated that a large percentage of the nation's dentists do not employ hygienists, and that once hired, 90 per cent of their time is spent on performing prophylaxis. Obviously, the hygienist is not given sufficient time to adequately educate the patient in home care procedures.

Millions of people who suffer from dental caries and periodontal disease cannot be treated because of economic and other barriers. Taking into consideration the gravity of the disease problem, it becomes evident that prevention is the logical solution. It is important, therefore, to develop a comprehensive and efficient program for patient education. An initial step is to fully realize the importance of the job that the hygienist can perform. She can make a major contribution to

TABLE 2–6 VISUALIZATION OF THE NATURE OF DENTAL HYGIENE PRACTICE

TYPE OF PRACTICE	PERCENTAGE Before Graduation	After One Year of Practice	Mean Number of Patients Seen Daily
Preventive	90	61	10.3
Therapeutic	10	39	12.3
Total	100	100	

the prevention and control of dental disease in the general practice of dentistry. However, until there are basic changes in the dentists' attitudes about oral hygiene and prevention and until these changes are reflected in their concept of practice, dental hygienists or any other auxiliaries will not be effectively utilized as teachers in preventive programs.

A fundamental question in the evaluation of preventive dental education concerns the outcome of the learning process. The student evaluation raised serious questions about the methods of education. Obviously participation in a complete dental curriculum, in and of itself, is not the answer. It is encouraging, however, to note the favorable results of a similar evaluation in the dental hygiene program. Although it too can be improved upon, it is apparent that effective methods for teaching the philosophy and practice of prevention are available.

In addition, there is evidence that new, effective methods of teaching preventive dentistry can be incorporated into our undergraduate curriculum. Educators, administrators and others are speaking out for prevention. In light of this, it is difficult to explain why dental students still spend over 70 per cent of their time in the dental school learning to repair and replace teeth. We are desperately asking for prevention, yet we remain actively engaged and oriented toward technical dentistry.

It is obvious that a problem of major proportion exists in the delivery of preventive dental care. Identification of the problem is only the first step. It must be followed by correction with available resources. The next step is application of the preventive procedures as an effective modality in the dental practice.

Motivating patients to carry out daily home care sounds deceivingly simple. It is not. Dispensing oral hygiene aids and agents is often used as the only means for motivation, but much more is needed.

A conceptual model was described that functions to educate and motivate patients.[14] The model consists of a sequence that may be likened to fitting various pieces of a puzzle together (Fig. 2–1). The conceptual model is composed of four separate but sequential

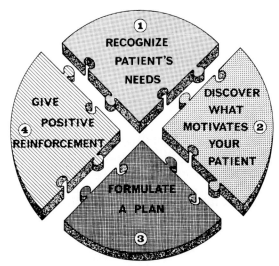

Figure 2–1 Conceptual model for patient motivation and education. The model is composed of four separate, sequential parts. Each part of this model defines the various motivational and educational processes necessary for long-lasting oral health.

parts that are necessary to achieve patient motivation and education. In other words, effective and long-lasting motivational and educational effects can only be achieved when all parts of the model have been fit together in their proper sequence (Fig. 2–2). The first part of the model deals with recognition of the patient's needs. Gaining some fundamental understanding of the patient's

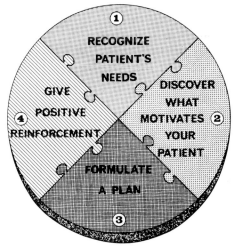

Figure 2–2 Conceptual model for patient motivation and education. Successful motivation and long-term oral health can be achieved when all parts of the model are fitted together in a puzzle-like sequence.

goals is essential. The second part deals with discovering what motivates a given patient. The third part deals with formulating and carrying out a plan to meet the needs of a given patient. Finally, the fourth part deals with follow-up and positive reinforcement. These steps may be used by the dentist as well as his team.

Recognizing the patient's immediate needs is the essential first step of the model's sequence. Asking a few pertinent questions of the patient regarding his dental problem or why he is seeking treatment is very useful. This may well uncover certain positive and negative influential conditions. The dentist and his team should recognize the patient's perception of his urgent needs. Immediate problems should be treated first. Some examples are the relief of pain or the improvement of one's appearance by temporarily restoring a broken front tooth or fabricating a temporary partial denture to improve chewing efficiency. This immediate intervention can serve to promote respect and trust between the patient and the dental team. The establishment of trust is necessary to the success of the other steps of the model.

The second part of this conceptual model is to discover what motivates a given patient. Such a task is time-consuming. However, this time is well spent. The process usually starts with the first contact with the patient. Verbal as well as non-verbal communication is of value in establishing baseline information. By assessing the patient's initial behavior through interview and observation, the dentist and his team will be better prepared to:

1. Recognize the emotional aspects that determine the patient's behavior.
2. Recognize the socioeconomic aspects that have contributed to the patient's attitudes, motives, and values.
3. Identify the patient's perception of dental problems, knowledge, and misconceptions.
4. Identify routines and current practices, using direct and non-threatening questions.
5. Identify oral health states.
6. Determine the interests of the patient.

Being courteous, gentle, tactful, and honest are important in establishing a relationship of trust between the patient and the dental team. Such a relationship is fundamental to the fruitful pursuit of knowledge about those factors that motivate the patient.

Motivating factors are numerous and vary from individual to individual and from time to time. However, the following are some of the motivating factors: pain, function, esthetics, approval of self, family pressure, social pressures, status-seeking, and fear.

Pain is the motivating factor that must be eliminated immediately. An attempt must be made later to discover the reason(s) for the patient's delay in seeking dental therapy. Patients usually state that such a delay was caused by cost, fear, or lack of time.

Inadequate or decreased function can be a motivational factor. Association of dental needs with the desire to satisfy the appetite and the pleasure derived from the ability to eat all foods can be a major motivating factor for certain individuals.

Esthetics, whether prompted by personal or social standards, also can be a motivational factor. A patient's deep concern for his facial appearance can be important in determining his acceptance of dental esthetically related therapy. Most psychologists agree that narcissism (self-love) is existent to some degree in almost every individual. A patient who visits the dentist on his own initiative is one who, when guided properly, becomes a stable part of the dentist's practice.

In certain cases, a patient seeks dental help only after considerable family prodding and pressure. This family pressure is probably because of ethnic, cultural, and social factors. For instance, some families believe that they are expected to visit the dentist regularly because they place high value on their appearance. In other families, teeth are not as important, so these people may not go to the dentist even though they may risk losing their teeth.

Advanced dental caries and periodontal disease may cause "bad breath." The resulting social pressure may sooner or later drive the affected person to seek the dentist's help. A patient who is extremely sensitive about the bad odor wants this problem to be eliminated and usually accepts the suggested therapy and preventive measures.

Finally, status seekers as well as success achievers are often highly motivated to be successful in business and in their social lives. This discovery can be used to motivate them.

Instructions in home care should be given in several increments. Present one procedure at a time. Through questions, the dentist should stimulate the patient to discuss the procedure, so that it is reinforced in his mind. Attempting to introduce all necessary home care procedures at one visit can lead to failure. Also, one must remember that home care aids and agents should be kept to a basic minimum. The patient must come to understand that he should depend upon his therapist *only* for tasks that he cannot do for himself. In other words, daily oral hygiene procedures are his personal responsibility, and the therapist cannot assume responsibility for the patient's part of the treatment.

The use of various educational materials, such as printed pamphlets,[14] filmstrips, slides and tapes, and programmed self-instruction are recommended. However, frequent personal contacts and reinforcement are vital in any preventive program.

Since every individual patient has his own behavioral attitude, habits and manual dexterity, some are able to learn more quickly than others. However, an average patient usually requires three to five sessions of instruction to achieve a significant improvement in oral hygiene level.

The fourth and last part of the conceptual model is the follow-up process. Success with an individual patient is possible if the dentist and his team take the time and energy to reach the patient. The amount of time and effort required is considerable. However, it is rewarding. Motivation is a continuing process in which frequent contact and positive reinforcement are important if the patient is to maintain the new preventive habits. Although there is no magic formula for long-term motivational success, presently available knowledge suggests that the approach should fit into the following framework:

Established rapport with the patient. Without good rapport and mutual trust between the patient, the dentist, and his team very little can be accomplished. Assertiveness in communication is essential and can make the difference between a confused and a convinced patient.

Continue to evaluate every patient in terms of possible motivational incentives. Being a good listener is indispensable. Encourage the patient to talk about himself and to express his views on the subject of oral health and prevention. This helps to reveal preconceived or prejudiced ideas that the patient may have.

Use a variety of motivational techniques. Such techniques should be based on the empirical assessment of each patient's need. Again, this depends to a large extent on establishing good communication and knowing the various motivational incentives of a given patient.

Reinforce previously given instruction. This can be carried out during the active phase of therapy as well as during the recall visits. The utilization of appropriate motivational techniques and the most effective home care aids and agents helps the patient to achieve long-term success. Positive reinforcement in terms of encouragement and compliments is one of the simplest ways to develop self-confidence in a patient.

The dentist and his staff must be absolutely convinced of the value of preventive dentistry not only in principle but also in daily clinical practice as well. A patient is not apt to be convinced and well motivated when his dentist or dental team are not "tuned in" to increasing the patient's knowledge or are not convinced of the role and value of prevention in today's dental practice.

Moreover, we should not expect to motivate a patient when a closet or a hallway in a dental office is used for patient education. This non-verbal de-emphasis and disinterest is communicated by the dentist and his team and is often observed by the patient. On the other hand, having a prime and well-organized area for patient education demonstrates to the patient the value and importance of this part of his dental care and should have a positive motivational impact.

The success of this conceptual model is based on the dental team approach. Thus, dental team interrelationships must be established. It is worth remembering that better interpersonal relationships between patients and the dental team can enhance the dentist's prestige in his community and augment referrals, which will result in the constant growth of his dental practice.

The conceptual model presented can be utilized in the development of a successful oral hygiene program. The following is a suggested method of presentation:

FIRST SESSION

The session is devoted primarily to exploring learning objectives, methods of operation and importance of the subject. This procedure is intended to make the situation meaningful to the learner.

The patient is given a disclosing agent and the presence of plaque is recorded (Fig. 2–3), utilizing the criteria and methods outlined in Figures 2–4 and 2–5. The patient is then asked to demonstrate his brushing and flossing movements, under supervision, in his own mouth. If shown to be inadequate, the movements are corrected. In this way the patient is given a clear idea of what is to be accomplished in order to solve the problem.

SECOND SESSION

This session is primarily for reinforcement. It should be conducted approximately three weeks after the first session. The utilization of the Sulcular Bleeding Index and the Plaque Control Record allows the patient to visualize his own progress (see Fig. 2–3). It should be noted that the use of the plaque score shows the patient improvement that he made in terms of plaque removal. The bleeding index demonstrates to him the outcome of oral hygiene in terms of improved gingival health (see Figs. 2–4 and 2–5).

Additional oral hygiene instruction is provided, when needed, to eliminate undesirable responses and to focus the patient's attention on the relevant aspects of his task. Further attempts are made to correct the

Name _____   Chart Number _____

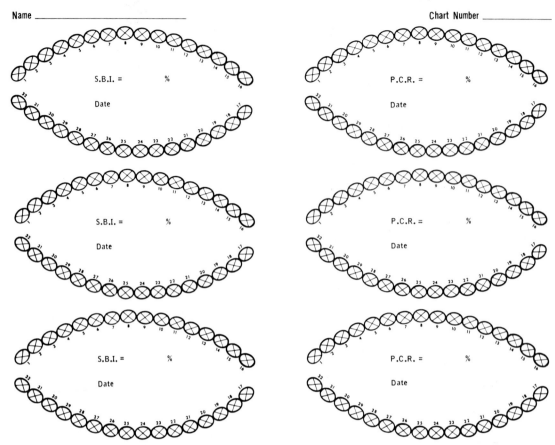

Figure 2–3 Patient's Sulcular Bleeding Index (SBI) and Plaque Control Record (PCR) progress sheet. (Adapted from O'Leary, T. J., Drake, R. B., and Naylor, J. E.: The plaque control record. J. Periodontol. 43:38, 1972; reprinted with permission from Bakdash, M. B.: A clinical model for monitoring patients' oral hygiene performance. Northwest Dentistry 60:77–83, 1981.)

toothbrushing technique. Whenever possible, reinforcement is given by informing the patient about how well he is doing.

THIRD SESSION

The third session is one of evaluation, although additional instruction is provided when necessary. This session is conducted two months after the start of the program. The Sulcular Bleeding Index and the Plaque Control Record are again used to evaluate the levels of improvement in gingival health and oral cleanliness.

Although it has been shown in many studies that the three-session model system is most ideal for reinforcement in establishing changes in patient behavior, this is not always practical in the routine dental prac-

tice. For patients who require additional dental therapy beyond routine dental health maintenance, the reinforcement sessions can be built into their appointments resulting in marked alterations in behavior patterns. To overcome the problem of the single visit, if the patient does not require additional dental care, preventive dental education for the family unit is ideal. Reinforcement then occurs at home by parents and siblings.

As part of the patient's permanent dental record, progress in dental health maintenance must be recorded (see Fig. 2–3).

Only through a total commitment and effort on the part of the dentist, dental hygienists, dental assistant, patient, and family unit can a preventive dental program achieve the maximum effectiveness reported in the literature.

SCHOOL OF DENTISTRY, UNIVERSITY OF MINNESOTA

KEY FOR THE USE OF THE SULCULAR BLEEDING INDEX AND THE PLAQUE CONTROL RECORD

I. The SULCULAR BLEEDING INDEX (S.B.I.)*

1. Obtain patient's S.B.I. and P.C.R. progress sheet.
2. Cross out all missing teeth.
3. Without drying or cleaning the gingiva to be examined, gently probe around the entire circumference of each tooth. Using a "gentle" force, the periodontal probe is carefully inserted into each sulcus, until slight resistance is encountered. The probe tip is then moved laterally back and forth.
4. Probe the upper right quadrant first and then go back to examine the first tooth probed until the last tooth in that quadrant is examined and then record the areas where bleeding has occurred. Repeat the same procedure in the other three remaining quadrants.
5. The S.B.I. score can be easily determined from the chart on the reverse side of this sheet. By knowing the total number of teeth present and sulci available for scoring (top horizontal line of the chart), count the total number of bleeding sulci. Read down the vertical line. The intersection of the two will give you the S.B.I. score.

II. THE PLAQUE CONTROL RECORD (P.C.R.)**

1. Cross out all missing teeth. However, pontic(s) of fixed bridge(s) should be considered as teeth and should be scored in a similar manner to that of natural teeth.
2. Have the patient rinse vigorously with water to dislodge and remove any loose food debris from the mouth.
3. Apply the disclosing agent to all teeth, being sure that the dento-gingival junctions are covered.
4. Next, have the patient take a mouthful of water and rinse vigorously for 15 seconds.
5. Starting on the most posterior teeth in the upper right quadrant and ending on the last tooth in the lower right quadrant, check every stained tooth surface (distal, mesial, facial and lingual) in contact with the gingival margin and record the presence of plaque in the appropriate spaces.
6. The P.C.R. score can be calculated in a similar manner to that of the S.B.I.

---

*Muhlemann, H. R. and Son, S.: Gingival sulcus bleeding—a leading symptom in initial gingivitis. Helv. Odont. Acta, 15:107-113, 1971.
**O'Leary, T. J., Drake, R. B. and Naylor, J. E.: The plaque control record. J. Periodontol. 43:38, 1972.

Bakdash '80

Figure 2–4   Key for the use of the Sulcular Bleeding Index and Plaque Control Record shown in Figure 2–3.

Number of Teeth/Total Number of Surfaces

Left vertical axis: Total Number of Surfaces with Bleeding/Plaque
Right vertical axis: Total Number of Surfaces with Bleeding/Plaque

Surfaces w/ B/P (left)	32/128	31/124	30/120	29/116	28/112	27/108	26/104	25/100	24/96	23/92	22/88	21/84	Surfaces w/ B/P (right)
1	1	1	1	1	1	1	1	1	1	1	1	1	
4	3	3	3	2	4	4	4	4	4	4	5	5	
7	5	5	6	6	6	6	7	7	7	8	8	8	
10	8	8	8	9	9	9	10	10	10	11	11	12	
13	10	10	11	11	12	12	13	13	14	14	15	16	
16	13	13	13	14	14	15	15	16	17	17	18	19	
19	15	15	16	16	17	18	18	19	20	21	22	23	
22	16	18	18	19	20	20	21	22	23	24	25	26	
25	20	20	21	22	22	23	24	25	26	27	28	30	
28	22	23	23	24	25	26	27	28	29	30	32	34	
31	24	25	26	27	28	29	30	31	32	34	35	37	
34	27	27	28	29	30	31	33	34	35	37	39	40	
37	29	30	31	32	33	34	36	37	39	40	42	44	
40	31	32	33	34	36	37	38	40	42	43	45	48	
43	34	35	36	37	38	40	41	43	45	47	49	51	
46	39	37	38	40	41	43	44	46	48	50	52	55	
49	38	40	41	42	44	45	47	49	51	53	56	58	
52	41	42	43	45	46	48	50	52	54	57	59	62	
55	43	44	46	47	49	51	53	55	57	60	63	65	
58	45	47	48	50	52	54	56	58	60	63	66	69	
61	48	49	51	53	54	56	59	61	64	66	69	73	
64	50	52	53	55	57	59	62	64	67	70	73	76	
67	52	54	56	58	60	62	64	67	70	73	76	80	
70	55	56	58	60	63	65	67	70	73	76	80	83	
73	57	59	61	63	65	68	70	73	76	79	83	87	
76	59	61	63	66	68	70	73	76	79	83	86	90	
79	62	64	66	68	71	73	76	79	82	86	90	94	
82	64	66	68	71	73	76	79	82	85	89	93	98	
85	66	69	71	73	76	79	82	85	89	92	97		
88	69	71	73	76	79	81	85	88	92	96	100		
91	71	73	76	78	81	84	88	91	95	99		99	79
94	72	76	78	81	84	87	90	94	98		100	95	78
97	76	78	81	84	87	90	93	97			96	91	73
100	78	81	83	86	89	93	96	100		97	92	86	70
103	80	83	86	89	92	95	99		99	93	88	84	67
106	83	85	88	91	95	98		100	94	89	84	80	64
109	85	88	91	94	97			95	90	85	80	76	61
112	88	90	93	97	100		97	91	85	81	76	73	58
115	89	93	96	99		98	92	86	81	76	72	69	55
118	92	95	98		100	93	87	81	76	72	68	65	52
121	95	98			94	88	82	77	72	68	64	61	49
124	97	100		96	88	82	77	72	68	64	61	58	46
128	100		98	90	83	77	72	67	63	60	57	54	43
		100	91	83	77	71	67	63	59	56	53	50	40
		93	84	77	71	66	62	58	54	51	49	46	37
	94	85	77	71	65	60	55	53	50	47	45	43	34
	86	78	70	65	60	55	52	48	46	43	41	39	31
	78	70	64	58	54	50	47	44	41	39	37	35	28
	69	63	57	52	48	45	42	39	37	35	33	31	25
	61	55	50	46	42	39	37	34	32	31	29	28	22
	53	48	43	40	37	34	32	30	28	26	25	24	19
	44	40	36	33	29	27	25	24	21	21	20		16
	36	33	30	27	25	23	22	20	19	18	17	16	13
	28	25	23	21	19	18	17	16	15	14	13	13	10
	19	18	16	15	13	13	12	11	10	10	9	9	7
	11	10	9	8	8	7	7	6	6	6	5	5	4
	3	3	2	2	2	2	2	2	1	1	1	1	1
(bottom headers)	9/36	10/40	11/44	12/48	13/52	14/56	15/60	16/64	17/68	18/72	19/76	20/80	

Number of Teeth/Total Number of Surfaces

Figure 2–5 The Sulcular Bleeding Index and the Plaque Control Record chart that is used to determine the SBI and PCR scores. (Reprinted with permission from Bakdash, M. B.: A clinical model for monitoring patients' oral hygiene performance. Northwest Dentistry 60:77–83, 1981.)

REFERENCES

1. Lobene, R. R.: The evaluation of oral hygiene in preventive dentistry. J. Mass. Dent. Soc. *15*:1–7, 1966.
2. Brandtzaeg, P.: The significance of oral hygiene in the prevention of dental diseases. Odont. Tidskrift *72*:460–486, 1964.
3. Morch, T., and Waerhaug, J.: Quantitative evaluation of the effect of toothbrushing and toothpicking. J. Periodontol. *27*:183–190, 1958.
4. Linn, E. L.: Oral hygiene and periodontal disease: Implication for dental health programs. J. Am. Dent. Assoc. *71*:39–42, 1965.
5. Bakdash, M. B., and Keenan, K. M.: Dental knowledge, attitude and habits of Minnesotans. Unpublished data, 1978.
6. Stanmeyer, W. R.: A measure of tissue response to frequency of toothbrushing. J. Periodontol. *28*:17–22, 1957.
7. Lovdal, A., Arno, A., Schei, O., and Waerhaug, J.: Combined effect of subgingival scaling and controlled oral hygiene on the incidence of gingivitis. Acta Odont. Scand. *19*:537–555, 1961.
8. Arnim, S. S.: An effective program of oral hygiene for the arrestment of dental caries and the control of periodontal disease. J. South. Calif. Dent. Hyg. Assoc. *35*:264–280, 1967.
9. Zaki, H. A., and Stallard, R. E.: An evaluation of the effectiveness of preventive periodontal education. J. Periodont. Res. (Suppl. 3), 1969.
10. Bakdash, M. B., and Proshek, J. M.: Oral hygiene status of dental students as related to their personal and academic profiles. J. Periodont. Res. *14*:438–443, 1979.
11. O'Leary, T. J., Drake, R. B., and Naylor, J. E.: The plaque control record. J. Periodontol. *43*:38, 1972.
12. Bureau of Dental Health Education and Bureau of Economic Research and Statistics of the American Dental Association: Surveys of family toothbrushing practice. J. Amer. Dent. Assoc. *72*:1489–1491, 1966.
13. Zaki, H. A., and Stallard, R. E.: The role of the dental hygienist in preventive periodontics. J. Periodontol. *42*:233–236, 1971.
14. Bakdash, M. B.: Patient motivation and education: A conceptual model. J. Clin. Prev. Dent. *1*:10–14, 1979.
15. Zaki, H. A., and Bandt, C. L.: The effective use of a self-teaching oral hygiene manual. J. Periodontol. *45*:491–495, 1974.

ADDITIONAL REFERENCES

Adams, F., Drucker, H., and Stewart, R.: Report on the periodontal disease detection center. Periodontal Abstr. *17*:105–110, 1969.
Bakdash, M. B.: An introduction to preventive dentistry and personal oral care: A program for first year dental students. School of Dentistry, University of Minnesota, 1976.
Binnie, W. H., Forest, J. O., and Wright, B. A.: Survey of the oral health status of dentists. Dent. Pract. *2*:1–2, 1970.
El-Mostehy, M. R., Zaki, H. A., and Stallard, R. E.: The dental student's attitude toward the professions as reflected in his oral cavity. Egypt. Dent. J. *15*:104–109, 1969.
Field, H. M., and Lainson, P. A.: Gingival, plaque health assessment program for incoming dental students. J. Dent. Res. *57*:(Special Issue A) Abs. no. 1116, 1978.
Greene, J. C., and Vermillion, J. R.: The simplified oral hygiene index. J. Am. Dent. Assoc. *68*:7–13, 1964.
Hix, J. O., and O'Leary, T. J.: The relationship between cemental caries, oral hygiene status and fermentable carbohydrate intake. J. Periodontol. *47*:398–404, 1976.
Kelley, J. E., Van Kirk, L. E., Jr., and Garst, C. C.: Oral hygiene in adults. Vital and Health Statistics, U.S. Public Health Service. Series 11, No. 16, June, 1966.
Lang, N. P., Cumming, B. R., and Loe, H. A.: Oral hygiene and gingival health in Danish dental students and faculty. Community Dent. Oral Epidemiol. *5*:237–242, 1977.
Meister, F., Jr., Davies, E. E., Lommel, T. J., and Edmundo, B. N.: Survey of the oral hygiene and periodontal health status of freshman dental students. J. Prev. Dent. *5*:21–28, 1978.
Moore, D. S.: Preventive dentistry in action in a dental college. J. Dent. Educ. *40*:349–354, 1976.
Muhlemann, H. R., and Son, S.: Gingival sulcus bleeding — a leading symptom in initial gingivitis. Helv. Odontol. Acta *15*:107–113, 1971.
Polgar, R. L., Kaslick, R. S., Giddon, D. B., and Chasens, A. I.: Plaque, gingivitis and dental aptitude test scores of dental students. J. Periodontol. *47*:79–81, 1976.
Wade, A. B.: Report on periodontal awareness. Periodont. Abstr. *20*:4–10, 1976.

CHAPTER THREE
The Epidemiology of Dental Caries

Sidney B. Finn, D.M.D., M.S.

Throughout his evolutionary advancement, man has been subjected to a constantly changing environment. Some of these alterations have proved beneficial, others detrimental to his well-being. Among those environmental problems with which man has been unable to cope completely is an increased susceptibility to dental caries. In the United States of America, there are today approximately one billion carious teeth in need of being filled that cannot be cared for professionally for various reasons, such as economy, prevalence of the disease and a lack of complete preventive and corrective measures. In view of this situation, dental caries assumes the enormity of a major national disaster. Man, because of present living habits, is the only species susceptible to this disease in his normal environment, and present attempts at preventing its ravages fall short of approximating the caries freedom enjoyed by other animal species that are subsisting on their natural diet in a wild habitat.

The skulls of prehistoric human beings evidenced a slight susceptibility to dental caries and its sequelae. When man first learned to eat various tubers, grains, and berries and to enjoy the sweet taste of honey and other natural sugars, dental caries increased. Skulls found in France dating back 2500 years indicate that even at this early period, one per cent of the teeth were carious.

Primitive man probably ate his food unwashed. The dust on the food combined with the grit from the soft sandstone mortars used in grinding his grain abraded the occlusal surfaces of the teeth and obliterated the pits and fissures. By this means the surfaces were rendered free of dental caries, but the destruction of the normal spillways allowed for the interproximal impaction of food and the development of proximal lesions. Present civilization is characterized by a relatively high caries susceptibility on all tooth surfaces.

In contemporary man the occurrence of dental caries has become universal, affecting all ages and all races from all geographic areas of the world. Figure 3–1 depicts the broad distribution of this disease.

Because of the marked variation in methods of examination and reporting, considerable caution must be exercised in interpreting the data. An increase in dental caries directly correlates with the densely populated and highly industralized areas of the world. Easy access to commercially prepared foods with a concomitant change in dietary habits might account for this difference. However, the prevalence rates may vary in limited areas because of other geographic, genetic, and environmental factors that will be discussed in subsequent chapters.

Dental caries is progressive. A continuation of the same environmental conditions that induced the lesion will inevitably complete the destruction of the tooth unless the affected area becomes self-cleansing or unless preventive or corrective treatments are employed.

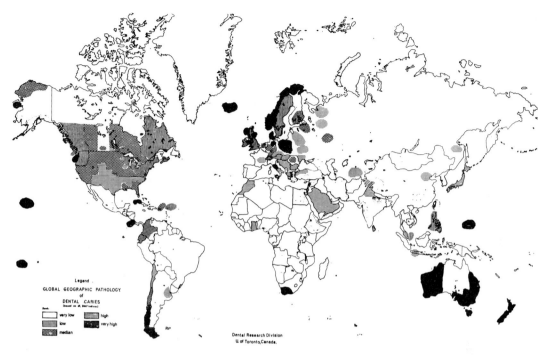

Figure 3–1 Caries distribution throughout the world. (From McPhail and Grainger: A mapping procedure for the geographic pathology of dental caries. Int. Dent. J. *19*:380, 1969.)

PERMANENT TOOTH INDICES

A comprehensible index to express dental caries experience either of an individual or a population needs to be developed so that all surveys and clinical trials can be universally understood and evaluated on a common basis. Progress is being made toward establishing comparable examination techniques and data compilations.

The index most widely accepted for compiling data for the permanent teeth is based on the number of decayed, missing and filled teeth (DMFT) or surfaces (DMFS) either per individual, per hundred erupted teeth or per thousand erupted surfaces. The missing teeth and surfaces are sometimes excluded from the index (DFT) and (DFS) when the reason for extraction of the teeth is difficult to establish, as with older individuals in whom periodontal disease is a common cause of tooth loss. Another index is based on the number of (DMF) teeth or surfaces as calculated on the basis of a full complement of teeth and surfaces. An index of this type would compensate for age and sex differences. Determining the number of

surfaces that were originally carious in a missing tooth presents a problem and affects the reliability of the DMFS index. There are other types of indices, which, because of their infrequent use, are not included in this chapter.

PRIMARY TOOTH INDICES

During the period of changing dentition, it is not possible to make a reliable determination as to whether teeth have been lost because of exfoliation or through extraction. This makes it unsatisfactory to use the same indices that are used for the permanent teeth. Indices for the primary dentition generally employ the terms decayed, indicated for extraction, and filled (def) teeth and surfaces, or decayed and filled (df) teeth and surfaces. Because of the exfoliation factor, the def index is not completely reliable for children over five years of age. An index that counts only the primary cuspid and molar teeth would be reliable until approximately nine years of age, since these teeth are generally lost physiologically, beginning at this age. An index of only df teeth and surfaces ignores missing teeth and would be accurate only if the teeth were lost because of exfoliation and were known to have been caries-free.

The RID index, based on the caries experience of the individual, is calculated from the number of teeth and surfaces present in the mouth. Although not as widely used as the def index, it has several advantages in that the index can be used for the primary, mixed, and permanent dentitions and considers only the teeth that are present in the oral cavity. As one gathers from the discussion, there is no perfect index but a few are adequate within expressed limits.

EXAMINATION TECHNIQUES

Examination techniques vary depending upon the goals of the individual study. Competent epidemiological surveys reporting dental caries prevalence should include the use of sharp explorers and mirrors under good light. For limited short-term studies, where testing the efficacy of a preventive agent is the objective, the importance of detecting all lesions as early as possible is critical. In this type of study, radiographs are desirable and perhaps essential, especially if the major inhibition occurs on the proximal surfaces. However, because of the harmful effects of radiation, caution must be employed to limit the amount of radiation received by the subjects, and the advantages to be gained must be weighed against the essentiality of the additional information.

Surveys concerned only with the number of missing teeth require less critical precision than those used in detecting caries, since there is only a need for tooth identification.

Figure 3–2 illustrates the number of proximal lesions detected in the Evanston Water Fluoridation Study by direct observation and by radiography. These figures indicate that over 64 per cent of the lesions were found by x-ray.

Other Considerations

Such factors as the type of population from which the sample is drawn, the sample size, the elimination of bias and the statistical treatment of data are important to the relevance and reliability of any data presented. Since the dental caries prevalence from community to community or from area to area may vary, it should be clearly understood that the information provided by a study applies specifically to that area studied and only relatively to all communities or areas either in the United States or throughout the world.

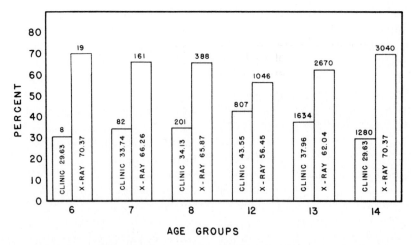

Figure 3–2 Comparison of the number of carious lesions found on proximal surfaces of permanent teeth by direct observation and by radiographic examination. (From Blayney, J. R. and Hill, I. N.: Fluorine and dental caries. J. Am. Dent. Assoc. 74:223, 1967.)

DENTAL CARIES IN THE PRIMARY DENTITION

Primary teeth, subject to attack at a very early age, may become carious prior to the eruption of the completed deciduous dentition. Dental caries attack in these teeth is progressive and, until all teeth are exfoliated by 11 to 12 years of age, can create a serious problem in the proper functioning of the masticatory apparatus.

A number of studies have reported positive correlations between the caries experience in the primary teeth and those of the permanent dentition. However, this is not always substantiated and must be qualified. Though the primary dentitions of the children in India and Ceylon develop rampant caries, the permanent teeth are relatively caries-free. Governed to some extent by prenatal and early postnatal environmental factors, this host resistance may account for the susceptibility of the primary teeth and yet have little influence over the permanent dentition.

Since exfoliation of the primary teeth commences at five years of age, surveys of the complete primary dentition must be done on infants and preschool children. There is difficulty in assembling large population groups of preschool children. Therefore, the number of surveys made with this age group has been limited and the number of individuals in each study relatively small. This may account for some of the wide variation in reported findings.

In the midwest, a clinical and radiographic study conducted in a fluoride-free area disclosed that in a group of children under two years of age, there were already 1.5 def teeth per child. The prevalence rate rose rapidly, and by three years of age there were over four def teeth per child, as shown in Figure 3–3.

The number of def surfaces rose more precipitously than the number of involved teeth, from 1.7 at 21 months of age to 6.1 at 37 months, because of the enlargement of existing cavities and the development of new lesions on teeth already cariously involved.

It is of striking importance that the number affected with def teeth rose from 10.3 per cent in children less than two years

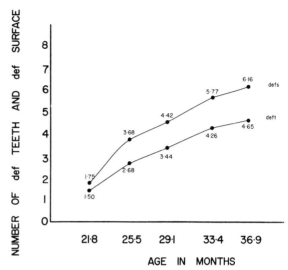

Figure 3–3 Caries experience in the primary teeth in infants and preschool children. (From Hennon, D. K., Stookey, G. K. and Muhler, J. C.: Prevalence and distribution of dental caries in preschool children. J. Am. Dent. Assoc. 79:1405, 1969.)

of age to 75 per cent in children five years of age (Fig. 3–4).

There appears to be no significant difference between sexes concerning caries in the primary dentition, although there is a definite variation between sexes at any specific age in caries experience in the permanent dentition.

Each tooth in both dentitions has a caries susceptibility that is related to the

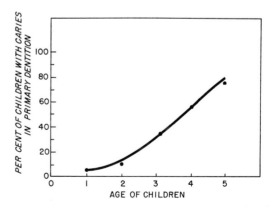

Figure 3–4 Per cent of infants and preschool children with caries experience in the primary dentition. (From Finn, S. B.: Prevalence of dental caries. *In* Toverud and coworkers: A Survey of the Literature of Dental Caries. Washington, D. C., National Academy of Sciences–National Research Council, 1952, pp. 117–173.)

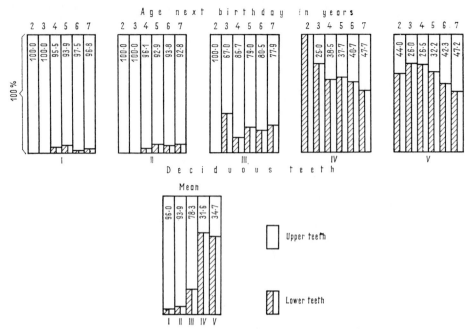

Figure 3–5 Comparison of caries prevalence in the maxillary and mandibular primary teeth. (From Toth, K.: The Epidemiology of Dental Caries in Hungary. Budapest, Akademiai Kiado, 1970.)

other teeth of the complete dentition. On any individual tooth, there may be different reasons why a carious attack might favor one surface over another. Developmental pits and fissures may foretell the early development of occlusal caries, but other morphologic differences such as the size of the contact area between adjacent teeth or the amount of space between teeth might govern the rate of development of proximal caries. Because of the variation of interproximal contact, the surfaces of approximal teeth have a more similar caries experience than the mesial and distal surfaces of either tooth. Proximal surfaces, before there is a tooth in juxtaposition, usually have remained caries-free until the tooth approximating this surface erupts. The presence of an apposing tooth appears to have little effect on the development of occlusal caries.

The lower second molars are the most susceptible teeth in the primary dentition because of the length of the fissures and the broad extent of both proximal contacts. In general the lower incisors are the most resistant, accounting for only about 10 per cent of the total caries experience. The lower molars, being about twice as susceptible as the upper molars, account for about 52 per cent of the

total caries experience. If an infant has a caries-free lower dentition, there is a strong implication that the upper dentition will also be decay-free. There are certain exceptions to this observation as exemplified by the early and rampant carious breakdown of the upper anterior teeth seen in nocturnal bottle-feeders given milk sweetened with sugar. Figure 3–5 compares the relative susceptibility of the maxillary and mandibular primary teeth from two through seven years of age. The lower anterior primary teeth at all ages have lower caries scores in contrast to the molar teeth.

DENTAL CARIES IN THE PERMANENT DENTITION

Dental caries experience involving the mixed and permanent dentitions has been surveyed in numerous studies that have included individuals of all ages. The onset, progression and eventual fate of these teeth has been recognized as one of the major public health problems involving present-day man. As early as 14 years of age, 97 per cent of the children have evidenced caries in the permanent teeth, as indicated in Figure 3–6.

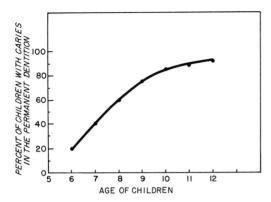

Figure 3–6 The per cent of children with caries experience in the permanent teeth according to age. (From Finn, S. B.: Prevalence of dental caries. *In* Toverud and coworkers: A Survey of the Literature of Dental Caries. Washington, D. C., National Academy of Sciences–National Research Council, 1952, pp. 117–173.)

Since the first permanent molars erupt between five and six years of age, at which time 20 per cent of the children have experienced dental decay, this clearly demonstrates the vulnerability of these teeth to attack.

The number of DMF teeth rises sharply from 0.4 at six years of age to 8.33 at 14 years of age. The yearly increment, approximating .75 of a new tooth per year, involves approximately two surfaces per year. Despite the parallelism between the number of carious surfaces and that on DMF teeth for the chronological period indicated in Figure 3–7, there is an abrupt rise in the number of surfaces attacked. This situation is attributable to the development of new carious surfaces on previously decayed teeth and to increase in the size of some existing lesions, so that these lesions extend to other surfaces.

Although at six years of age there is an average of less than one DMF tooth per child, the rate rises to over five DMF teeth with nearly eight DMF surfaces at about 12 years of age.

Dental caries appears to develop bilaterally; more cavities occur on homologous teeth and surfaces than occur unilaterally. As in the primary dentition, each tooth or each pair of homologous teeth has its specific susceptibility to dental caries. When dental caries is reduced by preventive measures,

teeth remain caries-free according to a decreasing order based on original susceptibility; that is, the teeth that are more resistant to the caries attack are the first to remain caries-free. This may possibly explain the observation that currently used caries-preventive agents appear to be more effective on the proximal surfaces than on the occlusal surfaces.

Figure 3–8 shows the percentage of caries experience contributed by each tooth to the total for each child at 7, 9, 11, and 13 years of age.

At seven, nine and 11 years of age the mandibular first molars contribute more than half of the total caries experience, with the maxillary molars contributing approximately 40 per cent. At 11 years of age all other teeth contribute approximately 10 per cent of the total caries experience.

Dental caries increases in a straightline progression through the teen ages and then levels off as the teeth mature and are consequently less susceptible to attack, and as the number of available susceptible surfaces is reduced by previous carious involvement.

On the molars, pit and fissure areas of the occlusal surfaces usually become carious

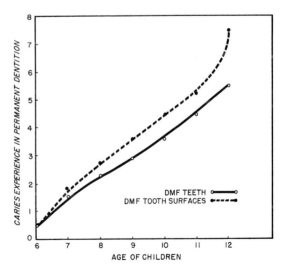

Figure 3–7 DMF teeth and DMF tooth surfaces in the permanent dentition of 6- to 12-year-old children. (From Finn, S. B.: Prevalence of dental caries. *In* Toverud and coworkers: A Survey of the Literature of Dental Caries. Washington, D. C., National Academy of Sciences–National Research Council, 1952, pp. 117–173.)

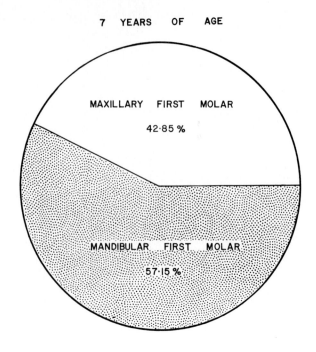

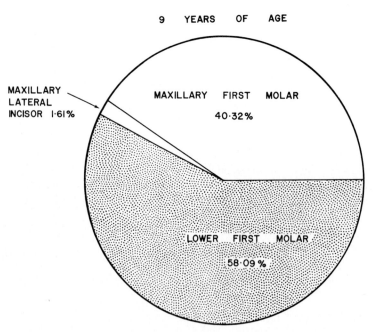

Figure 3–8 Contributions of homologous permanent tooth pairs to the total caries experience in the permanent dentition (155 children).

Illustration continued on opposite page

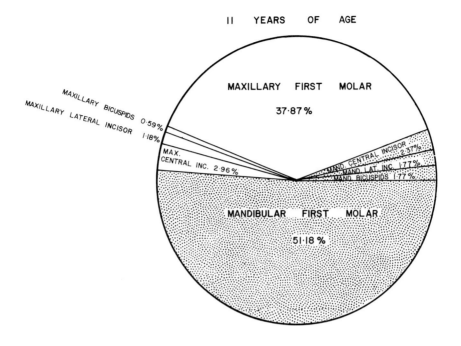

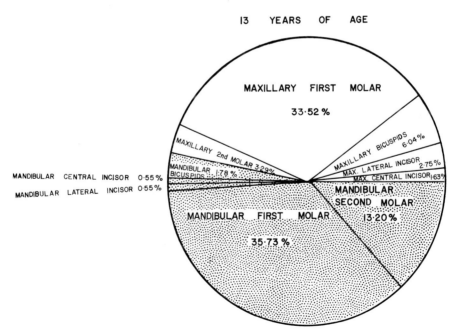

Figure 3–8 *Continued*

earlier than the proximal and other smooth-surface areas. Cervical caries is generally the last to develop on the enamel. Root caries develops after gingival recession and is principally a disease of adulthood or old age. Occlusal caries is dependent upon the existence of pits and fissures (original faults of development) and to the steepness of the cusps. Where such faults are nonexistent, especially in the bicuspids, proximal lesions quite commonly occur earlier than those in the occlusal surfaces.

The most susceptible tooth surface in the permanent dentition is the occlusal surface of the mandibular first permanent molar, which may possess a fissure transversing practically the entire mesiodistal diameter of the tooth and by gravity invites impaction of food and debris. The maxillary molars possess a well-defined transverse ridge that divides this surface into two smaller pits. Pits are also present on the buccal surfaces of the lower molars and the lingual surfaces of the upper molars. Cavities appear earlier in these faults than in cervical areas on these same surfaces.

Caries Progression

The length of time required for the development of a carious lesion bears an important relation to preventive treatment. Investigators recognize that some lesions never progress beyond the incipient stage and that other identifiable lesions may become benign and progress very slowly. The time required for caries development is highly dependent upon the environment which exists at any particular period. Should this environment change to a less conducive one, because the surface becomes self-cleansing or for some other reason, the caries process may be completely arrested or there is a possibility that incipient lesions may remineralize.

In the United States, children in nonfluoride areas average about 0.75 new lesions a year. Occlusal caries may take from less than three to 48 months for development into recognizable cavitation. In one reported study, 28 per cent of this type of caries

progressed beyond the incipient stage in less than six months, but 53 per cent remained in a quiescent state for more than two years. With approximately a quarter of the lesions developing in less than six months, it would seem prudent to repeat office preventive treatments at intervals of not longer than six months in order to achieve maximum benefit.

Sex Differences

Between males and females of the same chronologic age, there is a statistically significant difference in caries prevalence. Girls, especially in adulthood, show a slightly higher prevalence than boys. This difference can be partially explained through the earlier eruption of the teeth in girls, which provides a longer period of exposure for the teeth to the oral environment. Perhaps morphologic differences existing between the teeth of males and females might also account for some of this difference.

HEREDITY AND DENTAL CARIES

Investigators have recognized genetic variations in dental caries prevalence based on two sources of evidence in humans: (1) family studies and (2) twin studies.

The data pertaining to family studies have been derived from information supplied by several investigators. In one study, parents with either low or high caries scores were compared with their siblings. The offspring had caries scores similar to their parents. If both parents had low caries scores, the offspring had low caries scores, and the reverse was equally true. If scores of the parents differed, the offspring had intermediate scores. Likewise, the caries-free children in another study had a close resemblance, in this respect, to their siblings.

In another study, caries-free inductees into military service had siblings and parents with significantly lower caries scores than the families of a control group of similar age inductees. It must be recognized, however, that a likeness in dietary and food preferences of members of the same family may account for some of the caries similarities between the inductee and his family.

In a number of twin studies, monozygotic and dizygotic twin pairs of like sex have been compared relative to caries experience. There was a greater concord between the monozygotic than between the dizygotic pairs and an even greater similarity between either type of twin pairs than between pairs of unrelated children of the same sex and age. The unrelated pairs of children, living in different households, may have received unlike diets. This may have accounted for the greater discrepancies that were noted between their caries experience and those of the pairs of twins who live in the same home. At any given age there was a greater similarity between the number of teeth that were erupted in the monozygotic than in the dizygotic twin pairs, which may explain to some extent why there were greater differences between the dental caries experience in the dizygotic than in the monozygotic twin pairs.

No correlation has been established between the caries experience of an individual and the ages of his parents, the number of children in his family or the relative position of the individual in his family.

Racial Differences

A number of studies indicate that Negroes of comparable sex and age have a lower caries score than Caucasians. It has not yet been determined whether this difference is a reflection of other dietary modifications, though a recent report suggests that this score does not arise from a difference in sugar consumption. In a Baltimore study, it was found that whites and blacks living under similar environmental conditions had comparable caries scores.

Socioeconomic Status and Dental Caries

There is ample evidence that an inverse relationship exists between socioeconomic level and dental caries experience in the primary dentition. Such a relationship in the permanent dentition has not been clearly established. The difference, if any, is small.

Geographic Variation

There are recognizable geographic variations in dental caries experience in different areas of the United States and throughout the world. In the United States the northeastern region has the highest and the south central region the lowest prevalence caries scores. Intermediate prevalence rates prevail over most of the midwest, the far west and southeastern coastal areas.

Investigators have pointed out the relationship between depleted soil areas and caries prevalence. Similar comparisons have been made in respect to abundance of sunshine, higher temperatures, hardness of water and greater distance from the sea coast. These factors are correlated with lower caries scores. The trace elements selenium, molybdenum, vanadium, and fluorine have been studied for their effect on caries. Selenium shows some direct correlation with caries resistance, but fluorine is the only element associated with an unequivocal caries reduction.

Further study will perhaps reveal other essential elements that can be associated with reduced dental caries experience.

DENTAL CARIES IN THE MILITARY

The dental caries status of young adult males has been derived mainly from examination of inductees into the armed services. Naval recruits numbering over 2,000 were found to have an average of 13.6 DF teeth and 22.5 DF surfaces. Of the 25.6 remaining teeth per individual (excluding third molars), approximately seven were carious and six restored. Of the total DF surfaces, 12.5 were carious and 10 restored.

It is a sad commentary on the dental treatment received by young adults to realize that there were more unfilled than restored teeth in this group.

In 1962, a National Health Survey conducted among the adult population of the United States revealed pertinent facts about

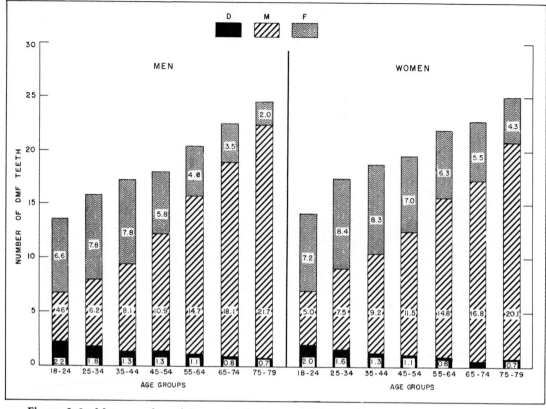

Figure 3–9 Mean number of decayed, missing, and filled teeth among dentulous men and women by age group. (From U.S. Department of Health, Education and Welfare Public Health Service: *Decayed, Missing, and Filled Teeth in Adults — United States — 1960–1962.* Public Health Service Publication No. 1000, Series 11, No. 23, Washington, D.C.: Superintendent of Documents, February, 1967.)

the unsatisfactory condition of the teeth or lack of teeth. With advancing age, the adult group exhibited a consistent increase to a total of approximately 25 DMF teeth.

There was a gradual decline in the number of DF teeth, since many of the teeth lost through periodontal disease were either carious or restored previous to their loss (Figure 3–9).

Considering all age, sex and racial groups, there were 17.9 DMF teeth per person: 1.4 decayed, 9.4 missing, and 7.0 filled. Of the total filled teeth, 90 per cent occurred in only half of the population. Half of the number of carious teeth occurred in one-tenth of the population. Females had higher DMF scores than males and whites higher than blacks. Although the number of edentulous individuals at 75 years of age increased to just under 60 per cent, the number

of edentulous persons did not alter the differential between race, sex and age.

CONCLUSION

The magnitude of the dental caries problem is well expressed by the statistics presented in this chapter. With the realization that the number of unfilled teeth in the United States approximates one billion, the enormity of the task of reducing this chronic situation becomes exceedingly important. It is only through an understanding of the problem that there is hope of arriving at a satisfactory solution.

REFERENCES

1. Adler, P.: Correlation between dental caries prevalences at different ages. Caries Res. 2:79, 1968.

2. American Dental Association: Proceedings of the conference on the clinical testing of cariostatic agents. October 14–16, 1968.

3. Backer-Dirks, O. B.: The distribution of caries resistance in relation to tooth surfaces. *In* Wolstenholme, G. E. W., and O'Connor, M. (eds.): Caries Resistant Teeth. Boston, Little, Brown and Company, 1965, pp. 66–85.

4. Baume, L. J.: Caries prevalence and caries intensity among 12,344 schoolchildren of French Polynesia. Arch. Oral Biol. *14*(2), February 1969.

5. Blayney, J. R., and Hill, I. N.: Fluorine and dental caries. J. Am. Dent. Assoc. *74*:223, 1967.

6. Dunning, J. M.: Incidence and distribution of dental caries in the United States. Dent. Clin. N. Amer. *6*:291, July, 1962.

7. Cohen, B., and Kramer, J. (eds.): Epidemiology of Dental Caries. *In* Scientific Foundations of Dentistry. London, Heinemann, 1976.

8. Finn, S. B.: Prevalence of dental caries. *In* Toverud and coworkers: A Survey of the Literature of Dental Caries. Washington, D.C., National Academy of Sciences — National Research Council, 1952, pp. 117–173.

9. Gisclard, L. F., and Lavergne, J.: Etude Odontologique de Quelques Sites de Préhistoire Récente. Actualités Odonto-Stomat *24*:391–406, 1970.

10. Glass, R. L., Becker, H. M., and Shiere, F. R.: Caries incidence in human primary teeth during the period of the mixed dentition. Arch. Oral Biol. *15*:1007, 1970.

11. Hennon, D. K., Stookey, G. K., and Muhler, J. C.: Prevalence and distribution of dental caries in preschool children. J. Am. Dent. Assoc. *79*:1405–1414, 1969.

12. Hill, I. N., Blayney, J. R., Zimmerman, S. O., and Johnson, D. E.: Deciduous teeth and future caries experience. J. Am. Dent. Assoc. *74*:430, 1967.

13. Jackson, D., and Burch, P. R. J.: Dental caries: Distribution, by age-group between homologous (right-left) mesial and distal surfaces of human permanent maxillary incisors. Arch. Oral Biol. *15*:1059, 1970.

14. Katz, S.: Socio-economic factors and dental caries frequency. J. Indiana State Dent. Assoc. *60*:57, 1967.

15. Knutson, J. W.: Epidemiological trend pattern of dental caries prevalence data. J. Am. Dent. Assoc. *57*:821, 1958.

16. Knutson, J. W., and Klein, H.: Studies of dental caries, Part IV: Tooth mortality in elementary school children, Public Health Rep. (Wash.) *58*:1701, 1938.

17. Littleton, N. W., Kakehashi, S., and Fitzgerald, R. J.: Study of differences in the occurrence of dental caries in Caucasian and Negro Children. J. Dent. Res. *49*:742, 1970.

18. Ludwig, T. G., and Bibby, B. G.: Geographic variations in the prevalence of dental caries in the United States of America. Caries Res. *3*:32, 1969.

19. Mandel, M.: Dental Caries. *American Scientist, 67*:680–688, 1979.

20. McCauley, H. B., and Frazier, T. M.: Dental caries and dental care needs in Baltimore school children (1955). J. Dent. Res. *36*:546, August, 1957.

21. McPhail, C. W. B., and Grainger, R. M.: A mapping procedure for the geographic pathology of dental caries. Int. Dent. J. *19*:380, 1969.

22. Miller, J., Hobson, P., and Gaskell, T. J.: The effect on the onset of human fissure caries of the early or late eruption of teeth and the presence of an opponent tooth. Arch. Oral Biol. *13*:661, 1968.

23. National Health Statistic Centre, Department of Health: Dental health status of the New Zealand population in late adolescence and young adulthood. Wellington, New Zealand, 1968.

24. Parfitt, G. J.: The speed of development of the carious cavity. Brit. Dent. J. *100*:204, 1956.

25. Porter, D. R., and Dudman, J. A.: Assessment of dental caries increments — I. Construction of the R.I.D. index. J. Dent. Res. *39*:1056, 1960.

26. Rosenzweig, K. A.: Tooth form as a distinguishing trait between sexes and human population. J. Dent. Res. *49*:1423, 1970.

27. Rovelstad, G. H., Irons, R. P., McGonnell, J. P., Hackman, R. C., and Collevecchio, E. J.: Survey of dental health of the naval recruit. I. Status of dental health. J. Am. Dent. Assoc. *58*:60, 1969.

28. Toth, K.: The Epidemiology of Dental Caries in Hungary, Budapest, Akademiai Kiado, 1970.

29. U.S. Department of Health, Education and Welfare Public Health Service: Decayed, Missing, and Filled Teeth in Adults — United States — 1960–1962. Public Health Service Publication No. 1000, Series 11, No. 23, Washington, D.C.: Superintendent of Documents, February, 1967.

30. Volker, J. F., and Caldwell, R. C.: The epidemiology of dental caries. *In* Finn, S. B. (ed.): Clinical Pedodontics. 3rd Ed. Philadelphia, W. B. Saunders Co. 1967, pp. 610–653.

31. Williams, E. J., Donnelly, C. J., and Fulton, J. T.: An appraisal of the necessity for radiographs in clinical trials of caries-inhibitory agents. J. Public Health *27*:54, 1967.

CHAPTER FOUR
Etiology of Dental Caries

James H. Shaw

The causes of dental caries can be grouped into three major categories: microbial agent(s), host and teeth, and general and local environment. In addition, numerous interrelationships exist among the various factors within and between these etiologic categories. In order for carious lesions to occur in human beings or experimental animals, three conditions representing these major categories must be met simultaneously: (1) caries-producing microorganisms must be present in the mouth and colonize the teeth in sufficient numbers, (2) the host and the teeth must be prone to develop carious lesions, and (3) foods with caries-producing potential must be consumed in a caries-conducive way. Unless all three parameters are fulfilled simultaneously (as indicated at the center of Figure 4–1 where the three circles interlock), carious lesions cannot occur.[1] Since dental caries is a chronic disease, these conditions must prevail for weeks, months, or years in order for tooth substance to be destroyed sufficiently for carious lesions to be evident clinically. Progression of the carious process is intermittent. There is active metabolism of the caries-producing microorganisms while food is available to them and relative or complete lack of metabolism in the absence of food.

The number of carious lesions and the rapidity of their progression are directly correlated to the composite pressure for caries initiation and development exerted by the various factors in the three categories. If the intensity of any one category is reduced

materially, the carious process is reduced. Thus, if the local environment in the mouth is altered by changing food choices and habits effectively, caries initiation and progression during that interval is reduced; the caries reduction will occur even though no direct change is made in the oral flora or in the ability of the teeth to resist caries attack. If the potential for caries production can be reduced simultaneously in two or three of these categories, the effects on the initiation and progression of carious lesions are additive.

In the formulation of a program for optimal caries prevention, it is important to know the point in the etiologic relationships at which each preventive method acts and to combine methods that act at different points. Ideally, for a maximally effective preventive program, each of the major categories should be addressed simultaneously and continuously by preventive procedures in order that the intensity of the microbial attack is reduced, the resistance of the host and the teeth to decay is increased, and the use of foods with caries-producing potential is decreased in amount and frequency by replacement with more desirable items. When this is pictured schematically as in Figure 4–1, the goal in the prevention of caries is to pull each of the circles away from the present center as far as possible in order that each category of etiologic factors contributes as little as possible to the caries attack. The objective of this chapter is to describe the etiology of dental caries precisely, but without all the possible

32

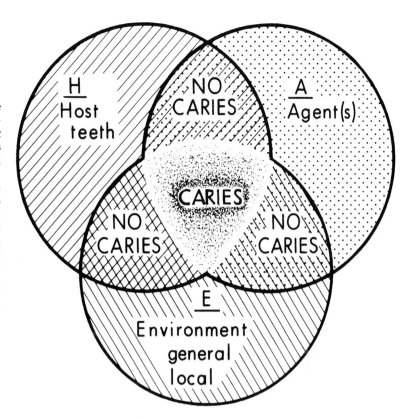

Figure 4–1 This scheme demonstrates the interrelationship between cariogenic agents (A), the host and his teeth (H), and the general and local environment (E). (Modified from Keyes, P. H., and Jordan, H. V.: Factors influencing the initiation, transmission, and inhibition of dental caries. *In* Sognnaes, R. F.: Mechanisms of Hard Tissue Destruction. Publication 75. Washington, D.C., American Association for the Advancement of Sciences, 1963, p. 764.)

minutiae, to permit the continued development and effective application of preventive measures.

MICROBIAL AGENTS

The mouth has a diverse resident microbial flora.[2] The humidity and temperature of the mouth and the passage of all nutrients needed by many types of microorganisms through it several times each day provide ideal circumstances for microbial colonization of various stable and relatively stable surfaces within the mouth. The normal inhabitants become established early in life, probably from the person or persons primarily responsible for care of the infant.[3, 4] They continually replenish themselves in the niches in which they have been able to establish themselves.

In addition to the common oral residents, a wide variety of other microorganisms may be isolated in small numbers from the mouths of a small percentage of the population at any time. The mouth is subjected to repetitious microbial contamination from air, food, fingers, and numerous other items that are placed in it. Most invaders fail to become established in competition with the normal residents and soon disappear from the scene.

The environment within the mouth varies widely in such different ecological niches as the enamel surfaces of the teeth, the root surfaces, deep carious lesions, the tongue, the gingival crevice between the gingiva and the tooth, and saliva.[2] As a result, wide variations in the species and distribution of microorganisms are observed from one niche to another. The flora also varies, even within a given niche. For example, the flora of plaque on smooth surfaces varies from one area in the mouth to another. Even within the plaque on a single tooth, sampling of minute areas reveals different distributions of microorganisms. The high hydrogen ion concentrations (low pH values) in carious lesions favor colonization and growth of aciduric organisms such as the lactobacilli. Likewise, the strict anaerobic conditions of the gingival crevice favor the *Bacteroides* species and *Veillonella* species.

Since saliva is swallowed as rapidly as it is secreted, microorganisms do not have sufficient time to reproduce in it; therefore, saliva does not have a truly resident or characteristic flora. Instead, the microorganisms in saliva have been dislodged from the numerous and varied oral surfaces. The microorganisms in saliva most closely represent the flora on the dorsum of the tongue, probably because of the latter's large surface area with its crypts and papillae and the relatively large microbial population per unit area. Since saliva bathes all oral surfaces and is the catchment basin for the microorganisms from all parts of the mouth, study of salivary flow is not profitable when trying to obtain a specific understanding of the microorganisms associated with the enamel surfaces, root surfaces, or early or deep carious lesions. The high concentration of *Lactobacillus acidophilus* in saliva of individuals with extensive caries and the sharp reduction in the number of these organisms when carious lesions are excavated and restored or when low carbohydrate diets are fed may be an indication that active carious lesions are reservoirs from which *L. acidophilus* are shed rather than an indictment of *L. acidophilus* as the single or one of several cariogenic microorganisms.

In order to form plaque and establish a carious lesion, appropriate microorganisms must be able to colonize, multiply, and metabolize on the enamel of the smooth buccal and lingual surfaces of the crowns, in the pits and fissures of the occlusal surfaces, in the approximal space between adjacent teeth and on their mesial and distal surfaces, or on the cementum of root surfaces that have been exposed by periodontal disease. Microbial colonization of the smooth buccal and lingual surfaces can be expected to be more difficult than in the pits and fissures of the occlusal surfaces or on the mesial or distal surfaces. Since the buccal and lingual surfaces are smooth and are rubbed by the tongue and the cheeks and bathed extensively by saliva, colonization has to be a relatively active and vigorous process. In contrast, microbial colonization of a pit or fissure or of a mesial or distal surface is more passive and undoubtedly is aided by mastication and the fact that the environment of such areas is relatively stagnant and inaccessible to saliva. The ability of the individual to cleanse the smooth surfaces mechanically is also much greater than the ability to remove all plaque and food debris from the approximal spaces or from the pits and fissures.

A thoroughly cleaned tooth surface remains free of microorganisms for a few minutes at most. The microbial population that colonizes a clean buccal or lingual surface is dependent upon the concentration of cells in its environment, the ratios among the various microorganisms in the bathing fluid, and the ability of the cells to adhere to, to become established on, and to proliferate on the surface. Of the numerous microorganisms that immediately adhere to a cleaned tooth surface, the majority are transients, and only a small percentage becomes established and colonizes that surface.

While numerous hypotheses have been formulated about the actual chemical reactions that destroy tooth substance, including proteolysis and chelation, the consensus is that the primary reaction is the slow and intermittent dissolution of hydroxyapatite by acid. The tiny percentage of organic matter in enamel, even though minutely dispersed throughout the structure in a membranous network, does not appear to pose any barrier to the dissolution of mineral in an acidic environment. As a carious lesion progresses into the dentin with its much higher organic concentration, primarily collagen, dissolution of hydroxyapatite by acid and proteolysis go hand in hand to produce the typical deep carious lesion.

Numerous oral microorganisms that colonize the smooth and approximal surfaces and the pits and fissures produce acid during their metabolism and are aciduric, that is, they are able to continue metabolism at low pH values. They metabolize particularly rapidly when carbohydrates are readily available in their surroundings. Two species of microorganisms have received special attention as potential caries-producing agents.

L. acidophilus for many years was considered the most likely caries-producing microorganism. Many studies were conducted to evaluate the role of this species in the causation of dental caries. Particular interest centered on its concentration in saliva during various dietary regimens and on correlations between salivary concentrations and the caries attack rate in the hope of having a valuable predictor of an individual's caries susceptibility. The latter goal never was achieved to the point of being widely accepted, although such tests are still used to some extent as a possible predictor of caries susceptibility or of clinically active carious lesions.

More recently, *Streptococcus mutans* has received special attention for various reasons.[5] This microorganism is either not present in the human oral cavity before teeth erupt or, at least, is not present in sufficient concentration to be detected by currently available methods. However, soon after the primary teeth erupt, *S. mutans* can be detected on tooth crowns.[4]

S. mutans is also of interest because it has the ability to form from sucrose an extracellular polymer of glucose, mutans, which aids the microorganism in adhering to the enamel surface and in establishing a stable relationship there.[5] This microorganism does not form a comparable polymer from other monosaccharides or disaccharides. This factor may be of special importance in the colonization of the smooth surfaces but is probably of lesser importance in pits and fissures or on approximal surfaces where microorganisms and food are more readily trapped and held in contact with tooth surfaces mechanically. This microorganism is also identifiable, although often at low concentrations, in most carious lesions that clinically appear to be active. It is not known whether one or two per cent of *S. mutans* in a lesion is a sufficient concentration to cause caries to progress in an area that would otherwise be inactive. Since sucrose, table sugar, is the most common sugar in the human dietary, the S. mutans-sucrose-mutans polymer relationship results in an appealing hypothesis that sucrose and *S. mutans* are the villains in human caries.[6]

The absolute demonstration of a specific microorganism as the causative agent of dental caries in man by complete fulfillment of Koch's postulates to identify the organism responsible for an infectious disease may be impossible because of the diverse organisms that are always present in the oral cavity and on the teeth. When germ-free rats are inoculated with cultures of single microorganisms, some strains of *S. mutans* isolated from human or animal carious lesions have been highly cariogenic.[5] However, several other species of microorganisms have also caused caries when mono-inoculated into germ-free rats, especially in the occlusal sulci that resemble human occlusal pits and fissures.[5]

In hamsters that do not harbor *S. mutans*, carious lesions occur when they are mono-inoculated with cariogenic strains of *S. mutans*.[5] Enamel lesions have also been produced in the hamster by some strains of *S. salivarius*. The molar teeth of the hamster have sharp cusps with broad intervening valleys. The carious lesions of the hamster molars more nearly resemble smooth surface lesions in man in whom microbial colonization may be much more difficult than in the occlusal sulci of the rat.

Filamentous organisms typical of the genus *Actinomyces* have been found at the advancing front of root surface lesions.[7] In studies with rats and hamsters *A. viscosus* and *A. naeslundii* caused extensive carious lesions of the root surfaces but had little or no adverse effect in the sulci and on the smooth surfaces.

It is certainly premature to accept *S. mutans* as the uniquely cariogenic microorganism in man despite the attractive findings pointing in that direction. Numerous oral microbiologists have been tending toward a broader evaluation of oral microorganisms in recent years than in the preceding decade. This is partly because of the fact that plaque and carious lesions routinely contain complex mixtures of microorganisms and rarely, if ever, contain as little as one or two species of microorganisms. While *L. acidophilus* does not have the ability to produce an extracellular polymer or to colonize smooth surfaces, high concentrations are normally present in well-established carious lesions. *L. acidophilus* and other acidogenic microorganisms in plaque and carious lesions may be capable of producing carious lesions by themselves, or they may be able to act synergistically with S. mutans in caries initiation.

In rodents in which the oral flora has been manipulated so that S. mutans is the sole or the predominant microorganism, some immunization procedures have reduced the incidence of carious lesions. The goal is to increase the secretory immunoglobulin A (sIgA) concentration in saliva so as to prevent or reduce the attachment of S. mutans to enamel surfaces or to inhibit the activity of the bacterially produced enzyme glucosyltransferase in the production of mutans from sucrose. These studies are of fundamental importance in the evaluation of the potential role of immunization for the manipulation of the secretory immunoglobulin in saliva as a possible means to alter oral disease. It is not known whether comparable immunization procedures may be effective in man, in whom the role of S. mutans in caries etiology is still uncertain. Nor is it known whether immunization will be safe in man because of the possibilities of disastrous cross-reactivity.

Avenues for caries prevention by reducing or altering the microbial agent(s):

1. Thorough oral hygiene augmented by frequent prophylaxis.

2. Sterilization of tooth surfaces by a bactericidal agent.

3. Use of short-term antibiotic treatment with an agent that has no medical significance.

4. Hydrolyze or inhibit the formation of extracellular polysaccharides such as mutans or otherwise interfere with microbial attachment to tooth surfaces.

5. Replacement of cariogenic agents with attenuated microorganisms of low caries-producing ability.

6. Immunization prior to establishment of the oral flora.

HOST AND TEETH

The factors influencing dental caries in the etiologic category associated with the host and his teeth may be divided into at least three segments: those related to the genetic constitution of the individual, those influenced by the physiologic status of the host, and those non-genetic factors associated with the development of the teeth.

Genetic Determinants

Experimental animals have been very helpful in the elaboration of many facets of the etiology of dental caries because they afford the opportunity of conducting more exactly controlled studies as well as trials that would be unethical in human populations. Wherever results of experiments with animal models and clinical experiments can be compared judiciously, the concordance of the results from the two lines of evidence is remarkable, as is typically the case for research on other human problems.

In rodents, the search for genetic determinants of caries activity strongly suggested that some strains tended to be more prone to develop carious lesions than other strains of the same species when offered the same diet and maintained under what appeared to be identical conditions. As more intensive studies were conducted and more information about the etiology of dental caries became available, the less prone or more "resistant" rodents tended to have different and less cariogenic oral flora or to eat less frequently than the rodents that were more prone to develop carious lesions. In other words, either the microbial or the oral environmental challenge in the more "resistant" rodents was less than in those more prone to develop carious lesions.

In human populations, the evidence for truly genetic determinants of caries proneness also appears to be relatively weak. Decades ago the striking difference between the lower dental caries prevalence in the people of the countries of the developing world and the higher prevalence in the nations of the industrialized world was thought to be possible evidence of genetically determined resistance among some races. Early evidence that did not support this premise was provided by a study of Eskimos in Alaska.[8] Those groups in areas remote from the influences of the colonizing and trading Europeans continued to have low dental caries prevalences. However, those to whom the sugars, refined flours, and confections of the "outside" world became available at trading posts soon had striking increases in dental caries. Similar information is now available for individuals who moved from a country with a low caries experience to an industrialized nation with a high caries experience. When these individuals adopted the dietary habits of their new homes, their caries experiences increased dramatically. Likewise, as the economic resources of some developing nations have increased, they have begun to adopt the use of sugars and various foods and confections of the more developed countries, and the caries experiences of these people have increased rapidly.

Another possible explanation for these increased caries activities could be infection of the low caries populations with cariogenic flora from contacts with individuals who have high caries experiences. There seems to be little support for this possibility. The sparse observations of individuals from areas with low caries experiences indicate that they are not devoid of the oral microorganisms believed to be associated with dental caries production, although the concentrations are lower than in individuals with high caries experiences.

Several investigators sought evidence for genetic determinants of dental caries susceptibility through the study of twins. In general, twins tend to have more similar dental caries experiences to each other than to their siblings. A possible explanation for this could be that their identical ages and more similar environments resulted in more similar situations of infection, diet, and instruction about health than siblings born a year or more apart could possibly have had. In one study, this time difference was reduced by comparing the caries prevalence on interproximal surfaces in mono- and dizygotic twins; it was found that the monozygotic twins of either sex had significantly more similar caries experiences than dizygotic twins of the same sex.[9]

It has been suggested that genetic influences are expressed in tooth structure and chemical composition and the morphology of the pits and fissures of the occlusal surfaces. If truly genetic influences on the caries susceptibility of human populations exist, they appear to be relatively weak and easily overwhelmed by cariogenic flora or oral environmental exposure to foods that have high caries potential and are frequently consumed.

Physiologic Determinants

Removal of some or all of the major salivary glands or ligation of their ducts in experimental animals causes tremendous increases in the initiation and rate of progression of carious lesions with the involvement of all surfaces. For example, in experimental animals surgical removal of the parotid, submaxillary, and sublingual glands causes approximately a 20-fold increase in caries activity above that for normal siblings fed the same cariogenic diet for the same interval.[10]

Likewise, in humans, the congenital absence of one or more major salivary glands or the loss of function caused by disease (such as Sjögren's disease), surgery, or radiotherapy results in major increases in dental caries incidence, which is presumably a result of the reduced salivary flow. For example, in a group of 10 males who received daily irradiation from a ^{60}cobalt source for six weeks and an average of 4,432 rads, the average volume of unstimulated whole saliva decreased from the pretreatment value of 0.722 ml/min to 0.036 ml/min.[11] With continued irradiation, it becomes virtually impossible to collect an unstimulated saliva sample.

The value of saliva can be attributed to at least the following characteristics:

1. The normal volume of about one liter per day washes and lubricates all oral surfaces routinely with augmented rates of flow during food consumption.

2. The carbonate buffer system in saliva neutralizes substantial amounts of acid without important reductions in pH.

3. Numerous organic compounds, including secretory immunoglobulin A and inorganic components, have the potential to be antimicrobial by various mechanisms.

Investigators have sought for more subtle differences in saliva composition, such as its viscosity or phosphorus content, to determine if such differences are related to dental caries experience in humans. As yet, no clear evidence of any relationships has been demonstrated.

One series of experiments in rats in which a borderline protein deficiency was imposed during lactation indicated that the caries activity of the offspring was strikingly increased.[12] It is possible that there was an adverse influence on the developing salivary glands so that the volume of saliva decreased and the protein concentration was altered.[13] Another possibility is that development of the immune system had been retarded.

As yet no comparable influence has been reported in human populations. In view of the high frequency of protein-calorie malnutrition among children of the developing countries where the dental caries experience is still low, is it possible that dental caries susceptibility might be very high but unexpressed because of a relatively non-cariogenic oral environment?

Saliva is the most obvious physiologic component of the oral milieu in which physiologic variations such as the rate of flow or the composition could influence the development of carious lesions. Probably much is yet to be learned about the relationship to dental caries of unrecognized variations in saliva that accompany disease or emotional disturbances. Indeed, genetic variations may be expressed in important ways in the saliva.

Developmental Influences on the Host

The best known example of an influence on the developing teeth is the ingestion of optimal amounts of fluoride because of the resulting increased concentrations of fluoride in enamel and dentin and the well-documented increased resistance to tooth decay. However, relatively early in the history of the science of experimental nutrition, other nutrients were shown to be related to the development of teeth. The classical studies of Wolbach and Howe in the 1920's demonstrated the need for an adequate amount of vitamin A to maintain the integrity of the ameloblasts and to enable them to form normal enamel,[14] and an adequate amount of vitamin C to maintain the integrity of the

odontoblasts and to form normal dentin at the optimal rate.[15] In the same era, Mellanby demonstrated the inadequate mineralization of the organic matrix of enamel and dentin during vitamin D deficiency, resulting in enamel hypoplasia in prolonged chronic deficiencies.[16] Other investigators demonstrated the adverse influence of calcium or phosphorus deficiencies and of grossly unbalanced calcium to phosphorus ratios on the mineralization of developing teeth. These deficiencies exerted on the developing dental structures the same influences that they exerted on comparable structures elsewhere in the body.

Nutrient deficiencies severe enough to cause the gross and histologic abnormalities produced in the animal model systems just described are not likely to occur in human populations, even in developing countries, except possibly in special circumstances, such as occurs in linear hypoplasia of the deciduous incisors.[17] Indeed, there is insufficient evidence to support even the possible role of inadequate mineralization of tooth structure resulting from vitamin D, calcium, or phosphorus inadequacy or imbalance as an agent in the etiology of dental caries. However, it is noteworthy that the dental caries experience in 12- to 14-year-old boys from the states along the Canadian border is about twice as high as the caries experience in the states along the southern border.[18] An obvious possible explanation is the longer hours of sunlight and the higher intensity of the light in the southern states with a possible influence on vitamin D formation in the skin and the overall vitamin D metabolism.

Other experimental models suggest that the dietary composition during tooth development may adversely influence not only the teeth but also the development and ultimate functional capability of organs such as the salivary glands as well as the quality of their secretions. Borderline protein deficiency during tooth development in rats results in delayed eruption, smaller teeth, and higher caries susceptibility.[12] In addition, the salivary glands of the protein-deprived rats are smaller and produce less saliva, which is altered in its protein composition, as mentioned in the preceding section.[13] The interwoven nature of the etiologic parameters of dental caries is particularly evident in such studies as those on the relationship of borderline protein deficiency to the development and maintenance of teeth in rats.

No clear relationship of protein-calorie malnutrition in children in developing countries to an increased susceptibility to dental caries has been demonstrated. In part, this may be because their overall dietary habits and the resulting oral environment are not conducive to high dental caries experience. Russell has drawn attention to a paradoxical situation observed in developing countries, that is, he found much higher dental caries experiences in the deciduous teeth than in the permanent teeth.[19] Sweeney and coworkers have pointed out the possibility that the particularly common occurrence of linear hypoplasia of the anterior teeth of those living in developing countries may be, at least in part, of nutritional origin, and that these areas are highly susceptible to carious lesions.[17] Also, carious lesions in these hypoplastic areas may explain, at least partly, the higher incidence of caries in the deciduous than in the permanent teeth that Russell described. Thus, the fact that numerous nutrients have been so clearly identified as necessary for normal tooth development is again an indication of the necessity for the use of a well-balanced, varied diet throughout tooth development.

FLUORIDE

Early in this century, a developmental abnormality resulting in teeth with mottled areas of varying colors was described in Italy among people emigrating from Naples to the United States.[20] Descriptions of similar abnormalities were provided in Colorado Springs in 1916 by McKay and Black, who recognized that the problem was related to the drinking water supply.[21] They also pointed out in their early studies that mottled teeth were more resistant to dental caries than normal teeth, although one would expect these teeth to be more susceptible to caries, based on the developmental abnormalities. In 1931, excessive fluoride during tooth development was identified as the cause of mottled enamel by several investigators; the Colorado Springs water supply contained about 2.5 ppm fluoride. The enamel abnormality was described thereafter as chronic endemic dental fluorosis. Primary attention was given to how to prevent aesthetically undesirable mottling, and the importance of McKay's observation about dental caries was not recognized until the late 1930's and early 1940's. Then Dean and coworkers observed a correlation between the levels of fluoride in the water supply and the dental caries experience of the children in four communities in west central Illinois where mottled enamel was not a problem.[22] These studies were then extended to include 7,257 children in the age range of 12 to 14 years old in 21 cities of four states (Fig. 4–2).[23] The optimal level of fluoride for that environmental region was 1.0 to 1.2 ppm, at which level the 12- to 14-year-old children who had grown up in the community had approximately 60 per cent less caries than in nearby communities where the fluoride concentration was 0.1 ppm or less. As demonstrated in this figure, a good dose response

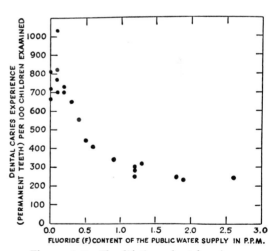

Figure 4–2 The lifetime dental caries experience for the permanent teeth of 7,257 children from 21 cities in four states is plotted against the fluoride content of the communal water supply. (From Dean, H. T., Arnold, F. A., Jr., and Elvove, E.: Domestic water and dental caries. V. Additional studies of the relation of fluoride domestic waters to dental caries experience in 4,425 white children, aged 12 to 14 years, of 13 cities in 4 states. U.S. Public Health Reports 57:1155–1179, 1942.)

was observed. The benefit was much higher for the anterior teeth than for the posterior teeth and for lesions occurring on the smooth buccal and lingual surfaces than in the pits and fissures of the occlusal surfaces. While most data on the benefits of fluoride during tooth development and dental caries experience are expressed in terms of the number of decayed, missing, and filled teeth per child, it is important to emphasize that the size of the individual carious lesion and the rate of its progression are also reduced. Tooth loss is also greatly reduced, especially for particularly vulnerable teeth such as the first permanent molar. The number of caries-free children in a community with optimal fluoride in the communal water is five to six times the number in a low fluoride community. These reductions in disease manifestation resulted in greatly reduced figures for the annual cost of delivery of total dental care to each child.

The fluoride-related reductions in dental caries experience have been shown to continue at least into middle age. While some of the benefit appears to be lost when individuals move from optimal fluoride areas after their teeth are fully formed, the benefit that is retained is still substantial, presumably because fluoride is incorporated at an optimal level into the mineral lattice throughout the tooth.

The observations of dental benefit from the optimal use of fluoride naturally contained in public water supplies not only in childhood but also in adult life led to intensive and extensive investigations of whether or not the ingestion of water containing 1.0 ppm fluoride throughout life in a temperate region was completely safe. The first concern was mottled enamel. The most sensitive cells in the body to the toxic manifestations of excess fluoride appear to be the ameloblasts; in the presence of excess fluoride, their function is altered, affecting the enamel formed during the period of excess. The severity of mottled enamel varies in relation to the degree of fluoride excess through a range from detectable only by the most careful clinical examination to grossly visible and aesthetically undesirable. Dean assigned grades from zero to four to denote the range from normal to severe and plotted both dental caries experience and degree of mottling against the fluoride concentration of communal water supplies, as shown in Figure 4–3.[24] The optimal dental caries benefit was obtained around 1.0 ppm fluoride in the drinking water whereas mottling did not become a problem until the fluoride concentration was in excess of 2.0 ppm.

Many studies in laboratory animals and in human subjects as well as epidemiologic surveys were conducted on various aspects of metabolism and disease entities. Studies

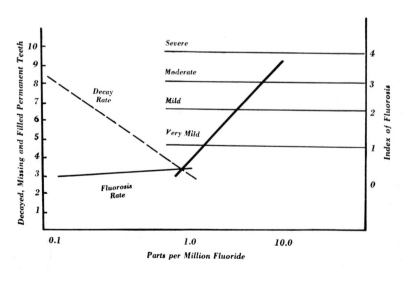

Figure 4–3 The relations between the number of decayed, missing, and filled teeth (dotted line) and the severity of chronic endemic dental fluorosis (solid line) are plotted against the fluoride concentration of the public water supply expressed on a logarithmic scale. (From Hodge, H. C., and Smith, F. A.: Some public health aspects of water fluoridation. *In* Shaw, J. H. (ed.): Fluoridation as a Public Health Measure. Washington, D.C., American Association for the Advancement of Science, 1954, p. 79. Copyright 1955 by the American Association for the Advancement of Science.)

continue to be conducted with increasing refinement on selected topics. The composite body of information has satisfied and continues to satisfy many national and international organizations who have evaluated the evidence.

Safety had been sufficiently demonstrated by 1945 that three trial communities, Newburgh, N. Y., Grand Rapids, Michigan, and Brantford, Ontario began to add sufficient fluoride in their water processing facilities to increase the fluoride concentration to 1.0 to 1.2 ppm. Figure 4–4 represents the decrease in dental caries experience among the children of Grand Rapids, Michigan after nine years of fluoridation.[25] For the permanent teeth of the children 5 to 11 years of age, the dental caries experience after nine years was remarkably similar to that in a typical community with fluoride naturally present in the drinking water. Likewise, their dental caries experience was strikingly different from children of the same ages in Grand Rapids before fluoridation was initiated. In the age group 5 to 11, all permanent teeth were formed during optimal fluoride ingestion. However, for the children 12 to 16 years of age, their dental caries experience lies

midway between the dental caries experience for pre-fluoridation Grand Rapids children and for children of the same ages from a natural fluoride community. The explanation for this difference between these two younger and older groups is related to the time when teeth are developing and erupt. The incisors and first permanent molars in the older groups of children were largely mineralized before fluoridation began, whereas their canines, premolars, and second permanent molars were mineralized after fluoridation was initiated. Thus, within the same mouths, the beneficial effect of fluoridation was shown: Pre-fluoridation, high caries teeth were adjacent to post-fluoridation, low caries teeth. This demonstration of the developmental influence of fluoride is important to stress. After 15 years of fluoridation, the caries experience in the older groups closely paralleled that of the natural fluoride controlled community. Undoubtedly, the local influence of fluoride in food, water, and saliva on the surface of erupting teeth is important; however, the incorporation of increased fluoride into the crystal lattice of enamel and dentin during development is essential for maximal ben-

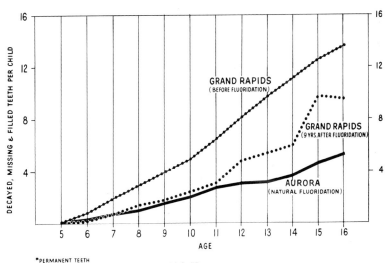

Figure 4–4 The numbers of decayed, missing, and filled permanent teeth of 5- to 16-year-old children are compared for Aurora, Illinois, where the water contains 1.2 ppm fluoride, for Grand Rapids before fluoridation of the public water supply was initiated, and for Grand Rapids nine years after fluoridation of the public water supply was begun. (From Arnold, F. A., Jr., Dean, H. T., Jay, P., and Knutson, J. W.: Effect of fluoridated public water supplies on dental caries prevalence. Tenth year of the Grand Rapids–Muskegon study. U.S. Public Health Reports 71:652–658, 1956.)

efits. The cost effectiveness of community water fluoridation is clearly higher than for any other dental preventive measure.

Fluoridation of public water supplies has been and continues to be accompanied by opposition from a small, vocal, and aggressive minority that becomes particularly evident in any community whenever fluoridation of a water supply is being considered. The opposition has varied in its emphasis from violation of individual rights to allegations of increased mongolism, allergy, or cancer. No amount of laboratory, clinical, or epidemiologic research has been adequate to satisfy the opponents. Possibly the most serious reason for concern about the scientific objectivity of the opponents of fluoridation is the statement by the most ardent of these that dental benefits of water fluoridation have not been satisfactorily demonstrated.

At present in the United States, about 110 million people (half of the population) live in communities where the water naturally contains about the correct amount of fluoride or the water is fluoridated at an optimal level. One half or more of the remaining Americans live in small communities or in rural areas with their own wells so that water fluoridation is not economically feasible or practical. In some rural communities, the water supply in consolidated schools is fluoridated. Since children are only present for about one third of any day and for only about one half of the days in any year, the level of fluoride in the water needs to be appreciably higher than in the water supply for the entire community, usually 4.5 ppm. Under these circumstances, reductions in dental caries experience have been reported in the neighborhood of 40 per cent. The cost per child is approximately ten-fold higher for school fluoridation than the per capita figure for community fluoridation.

An additional systemic route for provision of fluoride is by a pharmaceutical preparation provided daily from infancy until tooth development has ceased. This procedure is approximately as effective as water fluoridation when it is followed consistently. However, this prolonged use results in very low levels of compliance except in the most conscientious health-oriented families. This procedure is also much more expensive than water fluoridation because of the need to purchase a pharmaceutical preparation by prescription.

There are three non-systemic procedures to obtain the partial benefits of fluoride by applying it to the outer surfaces of erupted teeth and allowing it to be incorporated into the surface mineral. The use of fluoridated toothpaste is the least effective procedure and requires regular and thorough application by the individual. Application of a concentrated solution of fluoride to cleaned tooth surfaces by the dentist or hygienist under careful conditions annually or more frequently is intermediate in effectiveness and is the most expensive because of the professional time involved. Rinsing with a fluoride solution on a weekly basis under supervision in school is the most effective of the topical procedures for fluoride application and is intermediate in cost.

The exact mechanism for fluoride's action is not entirely understood. Incorporation of ingested fluoride into the crystal lattice of the mineral in enamel and dentin results in a partial replacement of the hydroxyl ions in hydroxyapatite by fluoride. As a result, the lattice dimensions are reduced slightly in size and the crystals are somewhat more perfect and slightly less acid-soluble. Mineralization appears to be favored in the presence of fluoride. Other hypotheses suggest that bacteria are less able to adhere to surfaces with elevated fluoride concentrations and that bacterial metabolism may be reduced by the presence of additional fluoride.

Avenues for prevention of dental caries that involve the host and the teeth:

1. Consume a well-balanced diet, with varied choices and good representation from all the food groups.

2. Provide adequate fluoride throughout the development of the teeth.

3. Use an appropriate combination of topical fluoride procedures: fluoride dentifrice, professionally applied fluoride solution or gel, or a fluoride rinse.

4. Seal the occlusal pits and fissures with an appropriate polymer.

ENVIRONMENT

Environmental relationships to dental caries can be divided into three general areas: The first is concerned with the impact of the general environment in the community in which the individual develops and lives, the second is related to the family environment, and the third is concerned with the oral environment and particularly the environment on and around the tooth surfaces.

Community Environment

Numerous components of the general environment influence the prevalence and severity of dental caries among the individuals who grow up and live in a community. Fluoride availability as described in the preceding section has undoubtedly the best known and most striking community-wide relationship to the dental caries incidence of a population. Although the optimal fluoride effect operates through systemic mechanisms during tooth development, fluoride is clearly an environmental variable. Inadequate fluoride in the communal water supply during tooth development because of inability or unwillingness to fluoridate results in a much higher caries incidence than in comparable populations where optimal amounts of fluoride are provided during tooth development.

Another example of the relationship between the community and dental caries concerns the generally lower dental caries experience in developing countries compared to the industrialized nations. The reasons for the lower caries experience in the developing countries probably include less food availability, resulting in little or no eating between meals; less use of sugar and sugar-containing foods; and the use of a greater percentage of relatively unrefined foods, including such items as unrefined salt, which often has an elevated fluoride concentration.

Various geographic variations have been reported. For instance, in the southern United States the dental caries experience, for reasons that are not adequately explained, is one half of that in the northern United States. Thus, the community where an individual lives determines in various ways — some explained, others uncertain — a general baseline in dental caries experience for the individual from which he or she may deviate for various reasons.

The degree of availability and type of professional dental care in the community is another environmental variable. In general, the easy availability of restorative care probably does not alter the total amount of dental caries but, rather, influences whether an early lesion is restored or is allowed to progress until the tooth is destroyed to the point at which it must be extracted. However, when professional care is provided on a preventive basis rather than simply for restorative purposes, the prevalence of dental caries can be materially reduced.

The kind and amount of teaching about oral health in the school system may also result in variations in dental caries experience. The potential is increased when appropriate teaching is accompanied by support in the breakfast and lunch programs, by restricted availability of vending machines with undesirable food choices, by improving the choices provided through the vending machines and by fluoride rinsing programs.

Familial Environment

Familial influences encompass a wide variety of parameters that include supervision and instruction by word and example about nutritional needs and how they can best be fulfilled not only to nourish the individual adequately for general health but also to maintain optimal oral health; concern about general and oral health and the level of education in this area; economic resources to purchase appropriate food and health care. The attitude within the family about undesirable between-meal snacks, the provision of a fluoride supplement in the absence of water fluoridation, oral hygiene, and periodic dental care probably is the single most important familial environmental factor in determining whether the individual is typical of or diverges from the general baseline of caries prevalence in his community.

Oral Environment

The quality and caries-producing capabilities of the oral environment are determined to a large extent by the dietary patterns encouraged by the community and family environments described in the preceding paragraphs and by peer group pressures. It is widely and justifiably thought that the oral environment and dental caries activity are closely linked to the frequency of usage and the duration in the mouth of sugar-containing foods, beverages, and confections. Evidence for this consensus does not come from any single conclusive source but from many evaluations that can be classified into five general types. They include the following:

1. The historical record. Dental caries occurred in antiquity, as evidenced by lesions in human skulls of ancient civilizations and by descriptions in early writings and paintings. However, the frequency and severity of tooth decay have increased dramatically from the relatively infrequent occurrence then to the almost universal occurrence in low-fluoride populations in the industrialized nations.

2. Variations in dental caries prevalence in contemporary populations. The prevalence of dental caries varies widely in different parts of the world (see Chapter 3). Populations in such developed countries as Western Europe, Scandinavia, Canada, Australia, New Zealand, and the United States have high caries prevalences compared to populations in the Near East, the Orient, and much of Africa. Individuals moving from low caries areas to high caries areas commonly experience major increases in caries, and their children are affected even more adversely.

Striking variations in dental caries prevalence occurred in brief intervals of time during major conflicts that changed dietary habits. In both World Wars I and II, dental caries prevalence in European countries decreased tremendously during the periods that sugar and refined flour availability was decreased dramatically.

3. Surveys of dietary habits. Many surveys have been conducted to compare the relationship of current dietary habits to lifetime dental caries experience or to the dental caries incidence during a finite period. Although variations occurred among these surveys, the weight of evidence clearly supports the position of a positive relationship between dental caries experience and the frequency and amount of consumption of sugar-containing food, beverages, and confections.

4. Clinical trials. The manipulation of the diet has been evaluated in two ways, either by seeking to modify dietary habits through counselling or by evaluating the influence of added amounts of sugar or confections to the diet in an experimental situation. When good patient compliance has been obtained as a result of counselling, reductions in the use of various sugar-containing products, particularly between meals, resulted in reduced dental caries incidences. In the numerous experiments in which sugar or confections were added to the regular dietary regimen, increases in dental caries occurred. A typical example of the latter experimental procedure was the five-year study at the Vipeholm mental institution in Sweden (Fig. 4–5).[26] Sugar in solution or in bread when consumed with the meals did not elicit any noticeable increase in caries activity above the baseline for the normal diet. However, chocolate, caramels, and toffees between meals caused major increases in dental caries that ceased when the between-meal supplements were deleted. Clinical trials of this nature probably could not be conducted for moral and ethical reasons in the United States and numerous other socially conscious countries today because the consensus is so strong that the influence of added sugar or candy is detrimental to oral health.

5. Evaluations with animal models. In many animal studies, dental caries has not occurred in the absence of some sugar in the experimental diet except in special circumstances. Carious lesions can be produced without dietary sugar when the major sali-

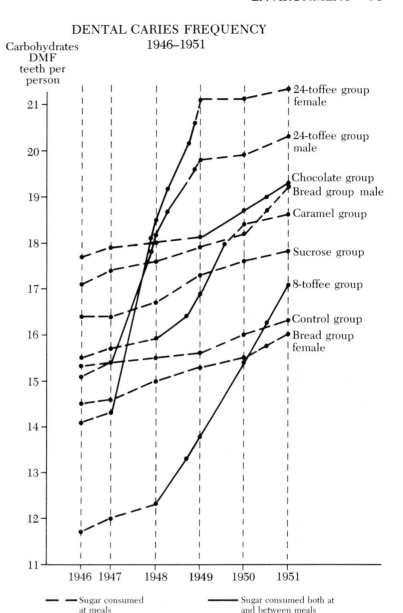

DENTAL CARIES FREQUENCY
1946–1951

Carbohydrates
DMF
teeth per
person

24-toffee group
female

24-toffee group
male

Chocolate group
Bread group male

Caramel group

Sucrose group

8-toffee group

Control group
Bread group
female

— — Sugar consumed
at meals

———— Sugar consumed both at
and between meals

Figure 4–5 The data from the Vipeholm study are presented for the period from 1946 to 1951 in terms of the number of decayed, missing, and filled teeth per person for the several groups where the individuals were consuming sugar in various forms and at various times. (From Gustafsson, B. E., Quensel, C. E., Lanke, L. S., Lundquist, C., Grahnén, H., Bonow, B. E., and Krasse, B.: The Vipeholm dental caries study. The effect of different levels of carbohydrate intake on caries activity in 436 individuals observed for five years. Acta Odontol. Scand. *11*:232–364, 1954.)

vary glands are removed or their ducts ligated or when particles containing starches of the appropriate size are forced into occlusal sulci during mastication.

From the above five types of evidence, the only reasonable conclusion is that the frequency of the presence of sugar and sugar-containing foods, beverages, and confections in the human oral cavity and particularly on the tooth surfaces and the duration of the presence of the sugar-containing materials are directly and causatively related to

dental caries activity. The absolute amount of sugars in the diet is not necessarily related to caries activity but as the amount of sugars increases, it is likely that the frequency and duration of exposure increases. While some individuals continue to protest that the above conclusion is not completely tenable, no satisfactory alternative to the vast body of information has been proposed.

In the absence or the infrequent presence of carbohydrates in the immediate oral environment, caries-producing microorganisms do not metabolize rapidly enough to reduce the pH at the plaque-tooth surface interface sufficiently often or long enough to demineralize tooth substance. However, when carbohydrates are available in the mouth in forms that diffuse into the plaque, the microorganisms metabolize rapidly and the pH decreases sufficiently to demineralize tooth substances. The pH does not return to a neutral resting value until those available carbohydrates have been metabolized and the resulting acids have been neutralized by the reaction with tooth minerals or by the buffers of saliva. In periods of microbial quiescence, remineralization of early lesions may occur as long as a framework remains in which mineral crystals can form.[27-29] Thus the development of an early carious lesion is the result of alternating processes of demineralization and remineralization so that the rate of progression of the lesion is dependent upon the balance between these processes. In view of the many food contacts per day in the typical American child, the likelihood is high for rapid progression of carious lesions.[30]

Sugars that are in solution or that dissolve readily from foods and confections have the greatest potential to penetrate the plaque and become available to the microorganisms. However, these readily dissolved forms are probably diluted relatively rapidly by saliva, and some of the acid produced from them is neutralized by the buffers in saliva. These sugar sources probably have a more transient influence on the pH in plaque than sugars and sugar-starch adherent mixtures in various foods and confections that adhere to tooth surfaces or are otherwise held in the mouth for prolonged periods. In these situations, not only the sugars are metabolized by the microorganisms but also the starch is hydrolyzed to some extent to glucose by the plentiful salivary amylase and becomes available for metabolism by plaque microorganisms. Various hard candies, lozenges, and gum also release their sugar relatively slowly so that the sugar is available for utilization by oral microorganisms for a long period. A given weight of sugar made slowly available can be expected to be more harmful than the same weight of sugar in solution

consumed in a brief interval. The frequency of eating potentially caries-producing food items coupled with the length of time that each item is in the mouth and on tooth surfaces are major determinants of how cariogenic the local environment will be.

Clearly, the preference for between-meal snacks is for fruits, vegetables, nuts, and cheese rather than for candy, cake, lozenges, soft drinks, and gum. The total amount of carbohydrate and even the total amount of sugars consumed in a given period of time are not nearly as important as the frequency of cariogenic food consumption and the length of time that food is in the mouth.

The question of whether sucrose is uniquely cariogenic in man is not wholly answerable. Many studies in experimental animals indicate that the mono- and disaccharides do not differ appreciably from each other in their caries-producing abilities. However, in assay situations in which caries production is uniquely attributable to *S. mutans* as the only or the overwhelming organism present and in which smooth surface lesions predominate, sucrose appears to be more cariogenic than the monosaccharides or other disaccharides. However, this finding has not been substantiated in animal assays or human populations where a mixed population of microorganisms was present or for lesions in the pits and fissures of the occlusal surfaces.

Sucrose is the predominant sugar in the human dietary and for that reason alone may be the principal contributor to dental caries. However, currently no evidence indicates that major replacement of sucrose by other mono- or disaccharides will reduce the incidence of dental caries to any striking degree in test situations in man. Once plaque has formed or a lesion has been initiated in a restricted area, its resident microorganisms, including *S. mutans,* are capable of metabolizing all available mono- and disaccharides.

Avenues for prevention of dental caries that involve the environment:

1. Fluoridate the public or school water supply. When this is not possible, provide a fluoride supplement daily throughout tooth development.

2. In the public school system and in the home, teach the value of the natural dentition and the methods of maintaining it. Support this instruction in the school by wise cafeteria menu planning and vending machine choices and by a fluoride rinse program. In the home, consistent examples of good oral hygiene, menu planning, and regular dental care should be carried out.

3. At the individual level, follow good oral hygiene practices of tooth brushing with a fluoride dentifrice and flossing with periodic use of a disclosing solution.

4. Maintain a low usage of those undesirable snacks that have the potential to be retained in the mouth and cause caries. Replace undesirable snacks with ones that are both more nutritious and less likely to be cariogenic.

INTERRELATIONSHIPS BETWEEN AND WITHIN THE THREE MAJOR PARAMETERS

As in any other chronic multifactorial disease, numerous interrelationships occur between the major categories (agent, host, and environment) responsible for the initiation and progression of carious lesions. The more conspicuous interrelationships have been pointed out in preceding sections. Two of these are particularly noteworthy. The metabolic activity of the cariogenic flora is highly dependent upon how long and how frequently suitable carbohydrates are present in the oral environment and, more particularly, the availability of the carbohydrates to the microorganisms in the plaque on tooth surfaces. The resistance of the tooth to caries attack and, thereby, the overall resistance of the host is highly dependent upon the amount of fluoride available for incorporation into tooth substance during development, which is determined by the fluoride in the communal water supply, in the school water supply, or in a pharmaceutical preparation provided by the parent. These interrelationships can be depicted in diagrams such as that shown in Figure 4–1.

In addition, many more elaborate schemes could be constructed to suggest numerous other kinds of relationships, some of which are well-established, such as the striking increases in caries activity with major reductions in salivary flow rates. Other relationships are less well recognized or are suspected rather than proven. The possibility that there are compounds with caries-inhibiting properties in some foods and confections is often proposed. As yet none of these compounds have been adequately identified or shown to vary enough from one product to another or to be strong enough inhibitors to be meaningful in clinical situations. This idea is not discussed here in detail, since it is in need of further exploration. However, an illustration of the complexity of such theories can be given with regard to foods and confections that are to be modified to reduce their sugar content and, at the same time, to maintain their consumer acceptability. Since none of the sugars have been shown to be distinctly different from sucrose in their potential to support the caries process, it is not adequate to replace sucrose in a product with some other sugar or with honey, raw sugar, or molasses. If the level of sweetness in the modified product is to be kept identical with the original product, then some other sweet compound of non-caloric value such as saccharin or cyclamate has to be introduced. If the caloric value of the new product is to be the same as the original product, the calories originally supplied by sugar must be replaced by starch, fat, or protein or by some combination of two or three of these major food components. Protein is less likely to be one of these replacements, since it is more expensive than the others. Any one of these substitutes for sugar automatically changes the flavor, the texture, the viscosity (in the case of fluids), the crispness or crunchiness (in the case of cookies or crackers), or the ability of the food to adhere to tooth surfaces or be retained in the mouth. All of these factors in one way or another may alter consumer acceptability or the potential to cause carious lesions quite apart from the change in sugar concentration.

The likelihood is high that numerous

important relationships among known and yet to be identified etiologic factors will be discovered. Some of these may be utilized in the development of new methods for the prevention of dental caries.

SUMMARY

Dental caries is a chronic, complex, multifactorial infectious disease with many interrelationships between the numerous etiologic factors. Decades may be required to discover all of the etiologic factors and interrelationships. However, from a preventive standpoint, sufficient knowledge is available that, if applied effectively, dental caries incidence could be reduced significantly in an entire population. The unknown etiologic factors in the development of dental caries should not prevent the application of preventive dental measures based on what is already known.

REFERENCES

1. Keyes, P. H., and Jordan, H. V.: Factors influencing the initiation, transmission, and inhibition of dental caries. In Sognnaes, R. F.: Mechanisms of Hard Tissue Destruction. Publication 75. Washington, DC, American Association for the Advancement of Science, 1963, p. 764.
2. Gibbons, R. J., and van Houte, J.: Oral bacterial ecology. In Shaw, J. H., et al. (eds.): Textbook of Oral Biology. Philadelphia, W. B. Saunders Co, 1978, p. 684.
3. Berkowitz, R. J., Jordan, H. V., and White, G.: The early establishment of *Streptococcus mutans* in the mouths of infants. Arch. Oral Biol. 20:171–174, 1975.
4. Berkowitz, R. J., and Jordan, H. V.: Similarity of bacteriocins of *Streptococcus mutans* from mother and infant. Arch. Oral Biol. 20:725–730, 1975.
5. Gibbons, R. J., and van Houte, J.: Bacteriology of dental caries. In Shaw, J. H., et al. (eds.): Textbook of Oral Biology. Philadelphia, W. B. Saunders Co., 1978, p. 975.
6. Newbrun, E.: Sucrose, the arch criminal of dental caries. Odont. Rev. 18:373–386, 1967.
7. Sumney, D. L., and Jordan, H. V.: Characterization of bacteria isolated from human root surface carious lesions. J. Dent. Res. 53:343–351, 1974.
8. Rosebury, T., and Waugh, L. M.: Dental caries among Eskimos of Kuskokwin area of Alaska. I. Clinical and bacteriologic findings. Am. J. Dis. Child 57:871–893, 1939.
9. Kent, R. L., Jr., and Moorrees, C. F. A.: Associations in interproximal caries prevalence from a longitudinal twin study. Abstract no. 526. Proceed-

ings of International Association for Dental Research, 1979.
10. Schwartz, A., and Shaw, J. H.: Studies on the effect of selective desalivation on the dental caries incidence of albino rats. J. Dent. Res. 34:239–247, 1955.
11. Shannon, I. L., Starcke, E. N., and Westcott, W. B.: Effect of radiotherapy on whole saliva flow. J. Dent. Res. 56:693, 1977.
12. Shaw, J. H., and Griffiths, D.: Dental abnormalities in rats attributable to protein deficiency during reproduction. J. Nutrition 80:123–141, 1963.
13. Menaker, L., and Navia, J. M.: Effect of undernutrition during the perinatal period on caries development in the rat. III. Effects of undernutrition on biochemical parameters in the developing submandibular salivary gland. J. Dent. Res. 52:688–691, 1973.
14. Wolbach, S. B., and Howe, P. R.: Tissue changes following deprivation of fat soluble A vitamin. J. Exp. Med. 42:753–777, 1925.
15. Wolbach, S. B., and Howe, P. R.: The effect of the scorbutic state upon the production and maintenance of intercellular substances. Proc. Soc. Exp. Biol. Med. 22:400–402, 1925.
16. Mellanby, M.: An experimental study of the influence of diet on teeth formation. Lancet 2:767–770, 1918.
17. Sweeney, E. A., Cabrera, J., Urrutia, J., and Mata, L.: Factors associated with linear hypoplasia of human deciduous incisors. J. Dent. Res., 48:1275–1279, 1969.
18. Mills, C. A.: Factors affecting the incidence of dental caries in population groups. J. Dent. Res. 16:417–430, 1937.
19. Russell, A. L.: World epidemiology and oral health. In Kreshover, S. J., and McClure, F. J. (eds.): Environmental Variables in Oral Disease. Publication no. 21, Washington, D.C., American Association for the Advancement of Science, 1966, p. 312.
20. Eager, J. M.: Denti di Chiaie (Chiaie teeth). US Public Health Reports 16:2576–2577, 1901.
21. McKay, F. S., and Black, G. V.: Mottled teeth: An endemic developmental imperfection of the teeth heretofore unknown in the literature of dentistry. Dental Cosmos 58:129–156, 1916.
22. Dean, H. T., et al.: Domestic water and dental caries, including certain epidemiological aspects of oral *L. acidophilus*. US Public Health Reports 54:862–888, 1939.
23. Dean, H. T., Arnold, F. A., Jr., Elvove, E.: Domestic water and dental caries. V. Additional studies of the relation of fluoride domestic waters to dental caries experience in 4,425 white children, aged 12 to 14 years of 13 cities in 4 states. US Public Health Reports 57:1155–1179, 1942.
24. Hodge, H. C., and Smith, F. A.: Some public health aspects of water fluoridation. In Shaw, J. H. (ed.): Fluoridation as a Public Health Measure. American Association for the Advancement of Science, Washington, DC, 1954, p. 79.
25. Arnold, F. A., Jr., Dean, H. T., Jay, P., and Knutson, J. W.: Effect of fluoridated public water supplies on dental caries prevalence. Tenth year of the Grand Rapids-Muskegon study. US Public Health Reports 71:652–658, 1956.
26. Gustafsson, B. E., et al.: The Vipeholm dental caries study. The effect of different levels of carbohydrate intake on caries activity in 436 individuals

observed for five years. Acta Odontol. Scand. 11:232–264, 1954.

27. Backer Dirks, O.: Posteruptive changes in dental enamel. J. Dent. Res. 45:503–511, 1966.
28. Silverstone, L. M.: Remineralization phenomena. Caries Res. 11:Suppl. 1, 59–84, 1977.
29. Moreno, E. C., and Zahradnik, R. T.: Demineralization and remineralization of dental enamel. J. Dent. Res. 58:896–903, 1979.
30. Shapiro, L. J., Bohmbach, D.: Eating habits force changes in marketing. In Advertising Age. October 30, 1978, p. 27.

ADDITIONAL REFERENCES

Adler, P., et al.: Fluorides and Human Health. Geneva, World Health Organization, 1970.
McClure, F. J.: Water Fluoridation. The Search and the Victory. Washington, DC, National Institute of Dental Research, National Institutes of Health, Supt. of Documents, U.S. Government Printing Office, 1970.
Newbrun, E.: Cariology. Baltimore, Williams & Wilkins Co., 1978.

CHAPTER FIVE
Epidemiology of Periodontal Disease

Richard E. Stallard, D.D.S., Ph.D

The significance of epidemiologic investigations into the occurrence of any disease is becoming increasingly important. The data assembled are not only of statistical curiosity, but also of great value in correlating etiologic factors with the disease to bring about successful therapeutic measures.

In the area of periodontal disease, it has been stated that the exact prevalence is unknown because of the lack of generally accepted epidemiologic tools with which to measure it; however, many reports have indicated a universal distribution of periodontal pathology in the world's population.[1-4] The apparent increase in periodontal disease is not caused entirely by an increase in the incidence of disease itself but rather is due to a better understanding by both the dental profession and the public of periodontal problems.

If maintenance of an efficient natural dentition throughout the life of the individual is a principal objective, then periodontal disease must rank with dental caries as a matter of immediate concern in the practice of dental public health. According to a United States H.E.W. study,[5] dental decay accounted for 41.4 per cent of required extractions, and periodontal disease for 38.3 per cent. It was found that the average need for extractions due to decay did not decline greatly with age, but the number of extractions due to periodontal disease increased markedly. The incidence of extraction resulting from periodontal disease in males over 35 and females over 40 years of age ranked higher than extraction because of caries at a ratio of 3:1.

It can be demonstrated that nearly every adult shows some deviation from the ideal condition of the periodontium. Gross deviation from normal was found to affect half the

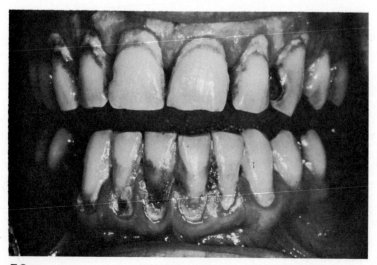

Figure 5–1 Clinical photograph of a 35-year-old male patient from the United States. The gross dental pathology appears to be a direct result of inadequate preventive measures and poor oral hygiene.

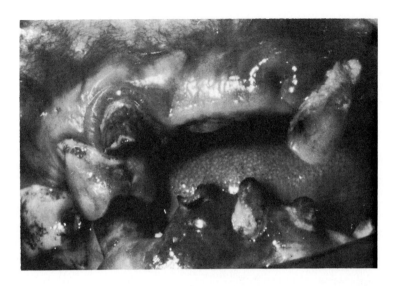

Figure 5–2 Clinical photograph of a 35-year-old male South Vietnamese patient. As in the case of Figure 5–1, a mutilated dentition already manifests itself by the age of 35. Possible genetic and environmental factors may account for the differences observed in the severity of the disease process. Dental plaque, however, has been implicated as the primary etiologic factor in both dental caries and periodontal disease, with the host factors acting only as modifying influences.

population over 70 years of age[6] despite the fact that many of the causative factors in periodontal disease are accessible, controllable, and correctable (Figs. 5–1 and 5–2).

MEASUREMENTS OF PERIODONTAL DISEASE

Periodontal disease is expressed clinically through a variety of signs and symptoms, including color changes in the gingival tissue, radiographic evidence of bone loss, and the presence of various etiologic factors such as the first pellicle formation, maturation of dental plaque, and, ultimately calcarious deposits. The significance of the individual factors in the disease process itself and also as measurements in the study of the epidemiology of periodontal disease must be analyzed individually and in totality.

Let us now examine in detail the current epidemiologic tools utilized in assessing the occurrence of periodontal disease. The present indexes are basically measurements of specific factors that in theory express the status of a group or population with respect to the disease. The fact that there are many indexes with a multitude of variations and modifications leads one to the realization that there is apparently no perfect index. Each investigator has selected various etiologic factors or symptoms that in his opinion most accurately reflect, clinically, the periodontal health of an individual. Inherent weaknesses, such as subjectivity, inadequate

methods, untrained examiners, or improperly weighted scoring systems, are built into every index. Many of the weaknesses have arisen because the various indexes were originally designed to evaluate specific problems but were subsequently used and modified for other evaluations.

One of the early attempts to assess periodontal disease quantitatively was the PMA Index.[7] Many other indexes designed specifically for large-scale epidemiologic investigations,[8] the evaluation of oral hygiene,[9] and other specific etiologic factors[10] followed. Additional attempts have been made to assess the relationships of etiologic factors to periodontal disease.[11, 12]

Crevicular fluid flow measurements also have become a widely used and accepted method of determining and evaluating inflammatory changes in gingival tissues in response to systemic and local factors[13, 14] and may be of value in assessing gingival health. In addition, bacterial and cytologic smears have been suggested as possible methods of evaluating gingival health.[15] Ultimately, in studying the health of gingival tissues, it is necessary that a biopsy be taken to assess the state of health; only by this method can one accurately determine the extent and type of inflammation present.

In evaluating dental indexes, it becomes apparent that the ideal index has probably not yet been developed. Confusion exists because of the disagreement among investigators regarding the clinical signs, the symptoms, and the etiologic factors related to periodontal disease. Our inability to agree on the primary etiologic factors and their control has resulted in the establishment of many indexes representative of investigators' particular interests and opinions. It would seem important that an index evaluating oral health be as sensitive in the individual evaluation as it is in group evaluations, particularly if it is used in clinical investigations. In this regard, it is essential to know the relation between individual clinical scores and the histologic status of gingival health. From this point of view, it is essential to assess the validity of the commonly used indexes and their components on an individual and population basis.

The various indexes and their respective components were investigated in a detailed study and compared to biopsy scores, which were considered to be the most accurate evaluation of gingival health.[16] As a method of predicting or evaluating gingival health,

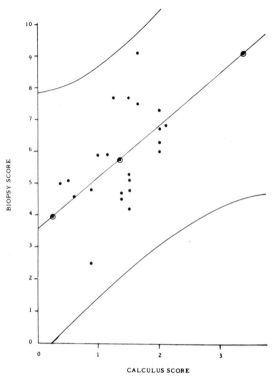

Figure 5–4   When accumulations of calculus are compared with biopsy scores, results are nearly identical with those for gingivitis. In both situations, a clinical symptom is scored and not a primary etiologic factor. (From Orban, J. E., Stallard, R. E., and Bandt, C. L.: An evaluation of indexes for periodontal health. J. Am. Dent. Assoc. *81*:683–687, 1970.)

the inflammatory condition (Fig. 5–3) and calculus scores (Fig. 5–4) were unreliable and inaccurate. Crevicular fluid flow measurements also proved to be only as accurate in predicting gingival health as were the calculus scores.

The relationships among oral hygiene, gingivitis, and periodontitis have been accepted for years. It is not surprising, therefore, to find a highly significant relationship between OHI-S scores and biopsy scores (r = 0.60 at the .01 level). This is a combination, however, of two possible etiologic factors: oral debris and calculus. From the data obtained, it is suggested that calculus has less influence on the combined scores than plaque measurements.[16] Gingivitis scores had the second highest correlation; however, the direct correlation with the biopsy scores is lost because etiologic factors and clinical symptoms are again combined.

The fact that plaque exerts a significant effect on tissue health (Fig. 5–5) is of great

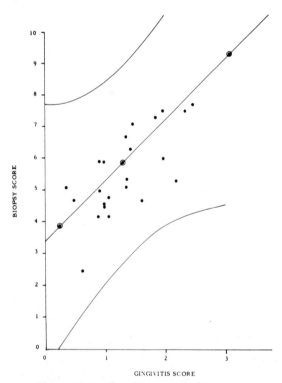

Figure 5–3   On this scatter diagram, a regression line and 95% prediction bands have been calculated for gingivitis versus biopsy scores depicting the degree of correlation. (From Orban, J. E., Stallard, R. E., and Bandt, C. L.: An evaluation of indexes for periodontal health. J. Am. Dent. Assoc. *81*:683–687, 1970.)

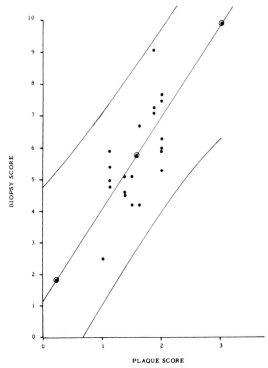

Figure 5–5 This scatter diagram, with its computed regression line, demonstrates clearly the nearly linear relationship between the quantity of dental plaque present and the inflammatory status of the tissue as revealed by a biopsy. (From Orban, J. E., Stallard, R. E., and Bandt, C. L.: An evaluation of indexes for periodontal health. J. Am. Dent. Assoc. 81:683–687, 1970.)

importance not only to the epidemiologist but to the clinician, as periodontal disease appears to be the result of local factors combined with systemic influences and host resistance. Thus the control, reduction, or elimination of plaque accumulations appears to be the most effective measure in rendering a preventive dental service, whether on a population or an individual basis.

GENETIC FACTORS

Epidemiologic studies on the relationship between genetic factors and periodontal disease have been meager. In patients with acatalasia, hypophosphatasia, or cyclic neutropenia, which are the result of single mutant genes, periodontal disease is a constant finding.[17] These genes exert their effects on periodontal structures in all environments and thereby illustrate that inborn characteristics can be extremely potent in producing periodontal pathology. However, these conditions are obviously rare and do not represent common periodontal disease, which is clearly caused by a multitude of factors. Nevertheless, it is equally apparent that these causative agents act on tissues that possess inborn potentials of reaction. Therefore, the contribution of hereditary factors in general must be considered in its relationship to other etiologic agents that act on the organism to produce the diseased state.

In a detailed review of the literature,[18] several major categories of genetic investigations of periodontal disease were enumerated, including family, twin, and racial studies. Numerous attempts have been made to detect in families genetic factors related to periodontal disease.[19, 20, 21] Unfortunately, the genetic tools that provide the most precise answers are also those that are most fastidious. Simple pedigree analysis can be rewarding but must be used for rare, clearly defined entities caused by single abnormal genes. It is certain that the common form of the disease is not caused by a single gene segregating within families. Family studies may provide confirmation if specific factors are examined, such as calculus formation.

Twin investigations have also been used to ascertain genetic influences in the production of periodontal disease.[21, 22] Identical twins have all of their genes in common, while in sibs and fraternal twins and in parents and children, half the genes are shared. More distant relatives are less valuable, since they share a quarter or less of the same genes.

The technique employed in twin studies involves ascertaining whether a trait is present in one twin and then deciding whether the other twin is affected and whether or not the condition is identical.

Of significance was a study carried out in 1958[23] on the occurrence of subgingival calculus. Analysis of 82 identical and 79 non-identical pairs of twins revealed a greater discordance and intra-pair variation among the fraternal twins, suggesting some genetic relationship in subgingival calculus formation.

RACIAL FACTORS

The importance of race and the tendency of various racial groups to exhibit different

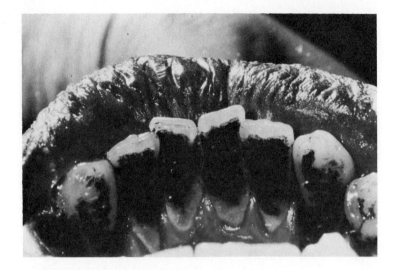

Figure 5–6 Clinical photograph of a patient from India demonstrating additional local environmental factors that may influence the sequence of events in the natural history of periodontal disease. Environmental factors must be weighed carefully before any conclusions are drawn regarding racial tendencies and periodontal disease.

incidences of periodontal disease have been discussed by many authors.[24, 25, 26] The differences between races in frequency of a condition such as periodontal disease suggest a genetic basis for the disease, provided it is not due to environmental factors such as food, various spices, materials chewed in a habitual manner, and oral hygiene practices. Nevertheless, detection of differences, whether they be genetic or environmental, suggests the need for further study (Fig. 5–6).

It is interesting to note the change in the incidence of various disease processes with transplanted ethnic groups. This holds true for periodontal disease as with other diseases, providing a strong indictment for environmental factors in the epidemiology of periodontal disease.

LOCAL FACTORS

In addition to the more common local environmental factors in the etiology of periodontal disease, a major concern that must be analyzed is malocclusion. Crowding and tipping of both anterior and posterior teeth with resultant malocclusion (Fig. 5–7) is an important epidemiologic factor in periodontal disease, which results in insufficient alveolar bone to resist the spread of gingival inflammation, difficulty in oral hygiene, and an imbalance in occlusal forces. Orthodontic treatment to correct such abnormalities may also have an effect on epidemiologic studies of these specific population groups.

It would appear that crowding is more likely associated with discrepancies in tooth size than with the eruptive pattern itself.

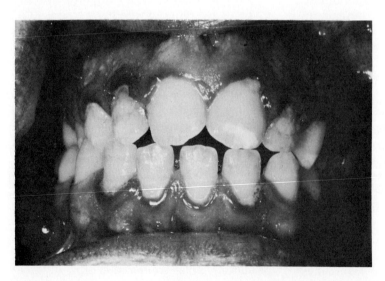

Figure 5–7 Clinical photograph of an adolescent demonstrating crowding and tipping of teeth. The tendency toward malalignment of teeth may be inherited. The neglect, as exemplified in poor oral hygiene, however, represents the most significant variable in production of the disease process.

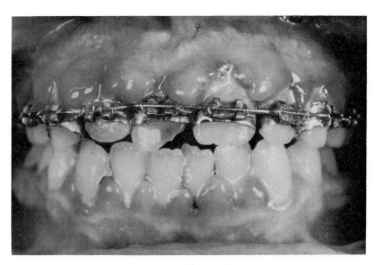

Figure 5–8 Periodontal pathology is readily apparent in both the maxillary and mandibular arches of this child. The severity of the disease, as observed clinically, is similar in both the banded and non-banded arch.

While third molars are often blamed for crowding in the incisor area, particularly mandibular, no direct evidence of a cause/effect relationship can be found. The third molars just happen to be forming and going through their eruptive phase at a time coincident with the beginning of crowding. In situations in which the third molars are congenitally missing or are extracted early, a similar degree of crowding occurs.

Orthodontic correction of malpositioned teeth may also act as a local etiologic factor, and therefore, these teeth are important in the epidemiology of periodontal disease. Gingival enlargement occurs frequently, particularly in the interdental area, with teeth that had been banded orthodontically. This appears to be the result of a combination of local irritation and difficulty in oral hygiene procedures and the fact that, as teeth are

moved together, excess gingival tissue develops in the interdental area. The use of direct bonded orthodontic techniques has reduced the first two factors, while the third obviously remains consistent. Normally, periodontitis does not occur in the child or adolescent patient except in situations in which there is a major alteration in the systemic resistance to the local environment. Long-term treatment can provide such a situation with a combination of increased local factors and an altered systemic reaction from the process of tooth movement itself (Figs. 5–8 and 5–9).

Occasionally during treatment, a rubber or plastic ligature will be improperly placed, which slowly works apically as a result of the conical shape of the tooth root. Isolated cases have also been identified in which a child wishing to mimic an older brother or sister

Figure 5–9 In these radiographs of the child seen in Figure 5–8, alveolar bone loss is occurring in the maxillary arch to a much greater degree than in the mandibular arch. Evidence of root resorption is also present, which seriously jeopardizes the long term periodontal health of these teeth by adversely affecting the crown root ratio.

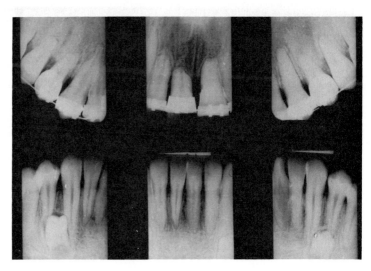

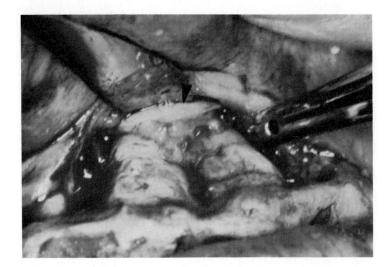

Figure 5–10 Advanced periodontal destruction can be seen in this clinical photograph in which an improperly placed rubber band has worked its way apically beneath the gingival tissue, destroying basically all the alveolar bone in its path.

has placed ligatures around his or her teeth, which have worked their way gingivally and become an etiologic factor in early severe destruction of alveolar bone (Fig. 5–10).

SYSTEMIC FACTORS

Numerous oral manifestations of systemic diseases associated with resorptive periodontal lesions must be considered in all epidemiologic investigations. Systemic disorders, such as sickle cell anemia, that occur primarily in one segment of the population have been associated with periodontal disease. Diabetes mellitus has also been directly linked with early onset and severity of periodontal disease. While the oral lesions seen in the diabetic patient are not diagnostic of diabetes, studies of biopsied tissue of diabetic patients reveals vascular changes similar to those seen in other tissues affected by the diabetic condition. Periodontal abscesses tend to be more prevalent in the diabetic patient, suggesting a decrease in the resistence to acute periodontal breakdown (Fig. 5–11).

Drug-induced systemic changes may also exaggerate periodontal breakdown. Since over 50 per cent of all cases of blood dyscrasias (neutropenias) are drug related, studies of various population groups who are more prone to develop the disease entities that require specific therapeutic agents over a long period of time produce skewed epidemiologic data when compared with other segments of the population. In addition to the blood dyscrasias and their charac-

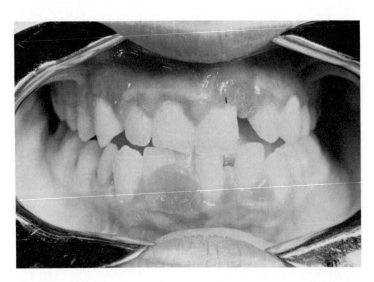

Figure 5–11 Acute multiple periodontal abscesses appear more often in the diabetic patient than in the general population.

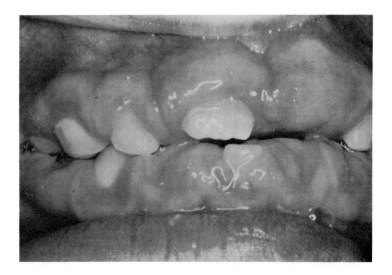

Figure 5–12 The gingival tissue has nearly overgrown the clinical crown of this patient receiving Dilantin in the treatment of a convulsive disorder.

teristic ulcerative destructive lesions, anticonvulsants, particularly diphenylhydantoin sodium (Dilantin), often result in hyperplastic gingival disease. The lesion begins characteristically within the interdental papilla and eventually involves all of the attached gingiva. Left unchecked, the tissue will grow until the teeth are nearly completely covered by the hyperplastic condition (Fig. 5–12). Interestingly, hyperplastic gingival tissue does not occur in patients who are edentulous.

Other systemic disorders, such as the Sturge-Weber syndrome (Fig. 5–13) and histiocytosis X (Fig. 5–14), also produce characteristic periodontal disease symptoms. Epidemiologic studies of institutionalized patients and those more prone to suffer from a specific systemic disease produce data that is characteristic of these specific populations, and this data may be compared epidemiologically with other population groups.

PSYCHOSOMATIC FACTORS

Studies of segments of the population suffering from various mental disturbances suggest an increase in the incidence of certain types of periodontal disease. The psychosomatic factors undoubtedly influence the incidence of periodontal disease through multi-factorial effects. These effects include the existence of abnormal oral hygiene habits, stress-related clenching or bruxism, nutritional factors, destructive mechanical oral habits, and other predisposing factors.

The tendency for patients with certain psychologic characteristics to develop acute

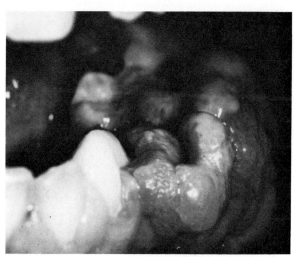

Figure 5–13 This patient is suffering from meningofacial angiomatosis, or Sturge-Weber syndrome, demonstrating the characteristic gingival hemangioma.

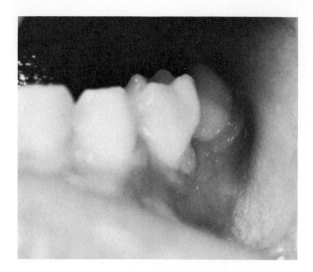

Figure 5-14 Advanced periodontal breakdown with root exposure on the primary molar is the result of a systemic factor in a child suffering from histiocytosis X.

necrotizing ulcerative gingivitis has been observed. The local etiologic factors are present in all patients, which tends to support the concept that altered local resistance is a result of psychosomatic factors. Utilization of the epidemiologic tools for the identification and classification of periodontal disease in specific groups can be applied effectively in studying patients with psychologic disorders. Patient management both from the clinical and etiologic points of view is extremely important in effecting a successful periodontal treatment regimen in these patients.

GOVERNMENTAL FACTORS

While one does not normally associate political and legislative actions in the category of epidemiologic factors in disease, their influence in dentistry is becoming increasingly important. The epidemiologic data on dental caries is changing rapidly in areas where mandatory fluoridation of municipal water supplies has been legislated. Unfortunately, in the case of periodontal disease, governmental and regulatory agencies have had a negative effect. In the majority of places where a national dental health program has been instituted, preventive periodontal procedures have been effectively eliminated through a policy of discriminatory fee schedules. Restorative dental procedures and, in particular, prosthetic procedures can be measured (both the need prior to treatment and the end result [Fig. 5–15] after treatment) and appropriate fees established. The end result is basically a "dead end" for the patient (Fig. 5–16) and produces a skewness in the dental disease curve that

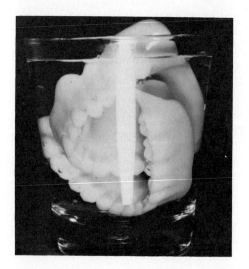

Figure 5–15 While fees can be attached to prosthetic dental appliances, this represents the "end of the road" for the patient and a total failure for the dental profession.

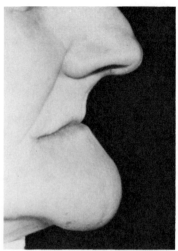

Figure 5–16 The lack of adequate preventive dental care is readily apparent in this 40-year-old female patient. Her dentures were in place when this photograph was taken; however, statistically, if the full upper and lower dentures are used as a measure of the success of a dental program, this represents one of dentistry's "successes."

results in abnormalities in epidemiologic studies of periodontal disease in these countries (Fig. 5–17). Under such systems, full upper and lower dentures become the ultimate measurement of the success of the national dental health program.

With cutbacks in federal funding in the

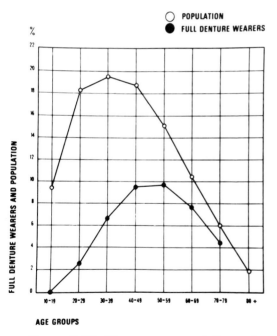

Figure 5–17 The success or failure of a national dental health program is readily apparent in this WHO diagram. The percentage of full denture wearers in the fourth decade is nearly one third, in the fifth decade over one half, and by the sixth decade in excess of two thirds of the entire population.

United States for medical assistance programs, similar changes within specific population groups are occurring that again produce abnormal results in epidemiologic studies of dental disease within these populations. As with national dental health programs, we are beginning to see the placement of dentures rather than periodontal treatment, since that is the only service for which the dentist will be paid in many instances. The elimination of large numbers of people from medical assistance effectively precludes the ability of a large proportion of these individuals from receiving even minimal dental care. This is reflected in the epidemiologic data collected from these segments of the population.

The ever increasing percentage of the private dental insurance market that is being taken over by health maintenance type organizations (for example, HMO) should have a positive effect on the segments of the population utilizing these systems. Any program based on a capitation fee basis rather than a fee-for-service indemnified basis will survive only if stringent preventive maintenance programs are instituted that effectively reduce the need for expensive restorative dental procedures.

CONCLUSION

While there is no universally accepted epidemiologic index to evaluate the incidence of periodontal disease, many investigators have established its enormity as a dental health problem. The definitive cause of periodontal disease is also not fully understood; however, it is accepted that there is an interplay of a multiplicity of etiologic factors. The human resource of trained personnel necessary for the administration of periodontal therapeutic procedures throughout the world is overwhelmed by the need; therefore, it is necessary to look increasingly to the primary prevention of oral disease as the ultimate answer in this costly area in national health.

REFERENCES

1. Maxcy, K. F., and Rosenau, M. J., eds.: Preventive medicine and public health. 9th Ed., Appleton-Century-Crofts, New York, 1965.
2. W.H.O. Technical Report Series, No. 207: Periodontal disease: Report of an expert committee on dental health. Int. Dent. J. *11*:544, 1961.
3. Marshall-Day, C. D., and Stephens, R. E.: Periodontal disease: Prevalence and incidence. J. Periodontol. *26*:185, 1955.
4. Littleton, N. W.: Dental caries and periodontal disease among Ethiopian civilians. Public Health Res. *78*:631, 1963.
5. U.S. Department of Health, Education and Welfare: Selected dental findings in adults by age, race and sex. Publication No. 1000, Series 11, No. 7, 1952.
6. U.S. Department of Health, Education and Welfare: Periodontal disease in adults. Publication No. 1000, Series 11, No. 12.
7. Schour, I., and Massler, M.: Prevalence of gingivitis in young adults. J. Dent. Res. *27*:733, 1948.
8. Ramfjord, S. P., and others: Epidemiological studies of periodontal diseases. Am. J. Public Health *58*:1713, 1968.
9. Greene, J. C., and Vermillion, J. R.: Oral hygiene index: A method for classifying oral hygiene status. J. Am. Dent. Assoc. *61*:172, 1960.
10. Volpe, A. R., Kupczak, L. J., and King, W. J.: In vivo calculus assessment III. Scoring technics, rate of calculus formation, partial mouth exams vs. full mouth exams and intraexaminer reproducibility. Periodontics *5*:184, 1967.
11. Lindhe, J., and Koch, G.: The effect of supervised oral hygiene on the gingiva of children. J. Periodont. Res. *1*:260, 1966.
12. Loe, H., and Silness, J.: Periodontal disease in pregnancy. Acta Odont. Scand. *21*:533, 1963.
13. Mann, W. V.: The correlation of gingivitis, pocket depth, and exudate from the gingival crevice. J. Periodontol. *34*:379, 1963.
14. Linhe, J., and Attstrom, R.: Gingival exudation during the menstrual cycle. J. Periodont. Res. *2*:194, 1967.
15. Egelberg, J., and Crowley, G.: The bacterial state of different regions within the clinically healthy gingival crevice. Acta Odontol. Scand. *21*:289, 1963.
16. Orban, J. E., Stallard, R. E., and Bandt, C. L.: An evaluation of indexes for periodontal health. J. Am. Dent. Assoc. *81*:683, 1970.

17. Gorlin, R. J., and Pindborg, J. J.: Syndromes of the head and neck. New York, McGraw-Hill Book Co., 1964.
18. Gorlin, R. J., Stallard, R. E., and Shapiro, B. L.: Genetics and periodontal disease. J. Periodontol. *38*:5, 1967.
19. Denney, R. E.: Heredity and its influence on the teeth. Dent. Cosmos *72*:596, 1930.
20. Roccia, B.: Krankheiten des Stoffwechsels und des endokrinen Systems bei der Ätiologie der Parodontose und der Paradentitiden. (Alveolaryphyorrhoe). Zahnaerztl. Rdsch., *49*:1057, 1940.
21. Korkhaus, G.: Über die erbliche Disposition zur Paradentose. Dtsch. Zahnaerztl. Z., *7*:441, 1952.
22. Noack, B.: Die Parodontoseätiologic im Lichte der Vererbung. Untersuchungen an erbverschiedenen und erbgleichen Zwillingspaaren. Osterr. Z. Stomatol. *38*:267–278, 369–377, 395, 1940.
23. Reiser, H. E., and Vogel, F.: Über die Erblichkeit der Zahnsteinbildung beim Menschen. Dtsch. Zahnaerztl. Z., *13*:1355, 1958.
24. Hruska, A.: Die frühzeitige Zahnlockerung in ihrer geographischen Verbreitung als Rassenfaktor und Pathoheredität trachtet. Zahnaerztl. Welt. *6*:95, 1951.
25. Dabbert, A.: Beobachtungen über Parodontose in Abessinien. Zahnaerztl. Rdsch. *44*:1443, 1935.
26. Leguay, J., and Mantelin, E.: Étude statistique sur les gingivopathies et les parodontolyses de la race berbère. Paradentologie *6*:52, 1952.

ADDITIONAL READING LIST

Greene, J. C., and Vermillion, J. R.: The simplified oral hygiene index. J. Am. Dent. Assoc. *68*:7, 1964.
Hruska, A.: Zahnanthropologisch-geographische Studien in Lappland. Zahnaerztl. Rdsch., *43*:2163, 1934.
Hruska, A.: Die Paradentose als Vererbungsfaktor. Osterr. Z. Stomatol., *37*:1348, 1939.
Kapellusch, W.: Anthropogeographische Paradentoseforschung. Paradentologie (Zurich), *7*:90, 1953.
Lovdal, A., Arno, A., and Waerhaug, J.: Incidence of clinical manifestations of periodontal disease in light of oral hygiene and calculus formation. J. Am. Dent. Assoc. *56*:21, 1958.
O'Leary, T. J., et al.: A screening examination for detection of gingival and periodontal breakdown and local irritants. Periodontics *1*:167, 1963.
Ramfjord, S. P.: Indices for prevalence and incidence of periodontal disease. J. Peridontol. *30*:51, 1959.
Russell, A. L.: International nutrition surveys: A summary of preliminary dental findings. J. Dent. Res. *42*:233, 1963.
Russell, A. L.: A system of classification and scoring for prevalence surveys of periodontal disease. J. Dent. Res. *35*:350, 1956.
Volpe, A. R., Manhold, J. H., and Hazen, S. P.: In vivo calculus assessment. I. A method and its examiner reproducibility. J. Periodontol. *36*:292, 1965.
Williams, N. B., Parfitt, G. J., and Richards, M. D.: A preliminary study of microbial smears as an aid in diagnosis of gingival health. J. Periodontol. *35*:197, 1964.
Zimmerman, E. R., and Baker, W. A.: Effect of geographic location and race on gingival disease in children. J. Am. Dent. Assoc. *61*:542, 1960.

CHAPTER SIX

Etiology of Periodontal Disease

Leonard Shapiro, D.M.D., M.S.
Richard E. Stallard, D.D.S., Ph.D.

The etiology of the inflammatory periodontal lesion is complex and, to a certain degree, obscure. It represents the interaction of extrinsic and intrinsic factors that result in the production of a group of symptoms collectively termed periodontal disease. While the lesion is the result of an interaction of various agents and circumstances, the nature and extent of the disease will vary from patient to patient and even from site to site in the same patient.

ANATOMICAL CONSIDERATIONS

The anatomy of the periodontium and the dentition must be considered as significant contributing factors in the development

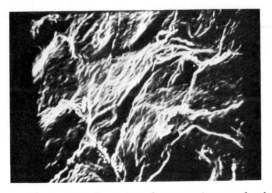

Figure 6–1 Scanning electron micrograph of the epithelium lining the gingival sulcus. Note the integrity of the epithelium and very little intercellular spaces. It is this epithelium that acts as a primary barrier in the etiology of periodontal disease.

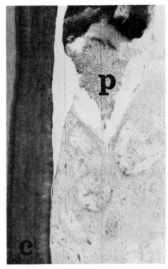

Figure 6–2 With the accumulation of dental plaque and calculus, downgrowth of the epithelium occurs, with destruction of underlying connective tissue. Note the v-shaped defect in the epithelium corresponding to the morphology of dental plaque, indicating the importance of dental plaque as the primary etiologic factor of periodontal disease (C = cementum, P = plaque).

of the inflammatory lesion. While the external surface of the gingiva has a relatively keratinized surface that acts as a barrier to extrinsic irritants, the lining of the sulcus (Fig. 6–1) and the col area are relatively unkeratinized and are therefore not afforded the protection of a keratin shield.[21] The col area has been described as the weakest link in the periodontal chain of defense.[14] While a sufficient zone of attached gingiva that can withstand functional forces can be subjected to a plethora of noxious stimuli and still maintain its structural integrity, the unkeratinized areas of the attachment apparatus react by undergoing successive inflammatory and degenerative changes, eventually leading to their destruction. An insufficient zone of attached gingiva resulting in detachment of the marginal tissue, on the other hand, reacts in a manner similar to that of the unkeratinized tissues, that is, marked inflammatory changes and apical migration of the epithelial adherence (Fig. 6–2).

The anatomy and integrity of the dental arch are also important factors in the defense mechanism of the periodontium, and conversely, an absence of this integrity contributes to the breakdown associated with the inflammatory lesion. Constricted arches and malposed teeth (Fig. 6–3) are associated with the relative absence of supporting bone. Rather than the osseous structures being relatively thick with an endosteal and periosteal blood supply, the endosteal supply is compromised, and nourishment is almost completely periosteal. Inflammatory reactions in the periodontium will affect the periosteal blood supply and lead to an early loss of osseous support. Missing and malaligned teeth also play an important role, owing to the lack of contiguous integrity of the dental arch (Fig. 6–4). With the resultant absence or malalignment of proximal contact, these areas become affected by the inordinate pressures of such extrinsic factors as food, leading to a breakdown of support.[7]

Dental anatomy also plays a role in the etiology of the inflammatory lesion. While the adherence of the periodontal fibers to cementum is relatively firm, there is an absence of adherence between periodontal fibers and enamel. A groove on the lingual surface of an upper incisor (Fig. 6–5) or an enamel projection into the furcation area provides a means of ingress[13] for noxious agents directly into the periodontal structures. These areas are not afforded a fiber barrier system as are the areas of the attachment apparatus that abut cementum.[21]

The fiber system of the periodontium has been well documented and is composed of fibers running between the soft and hard tissues consisting of relatively strong collagen fibers.[4] A thick network of these fibers in both the gingiva and the periodontal ligament affords a mechanism that protects the underlying structures from external irritants. Once the integrity of the fiber barrier system has been compromised, an avenue of ingress is afforded to extrinsic factors and also allows for an apical progression of the inflammatory process (Fig. 6–6).

It is apparent, therefore, that the anatomy of the periodontium and the dentition plays a role in the protective mechanism of the host against external stimuli, and conversely, a lack of anatomic integrity will affect the host response to noxious agents

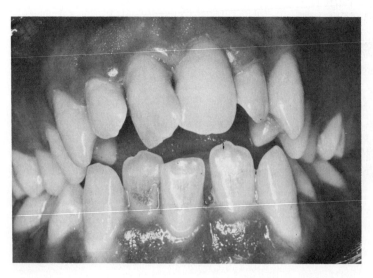

Figure 6–3 Constricted dental arches with accompanying malpositioning of the teeth often results in a deficiency of alveolar bone with the appearance of fenestrations or dehiscences. Any periodontal breakdown in this situation will result in rapid loss of periodontal supporting tissue.

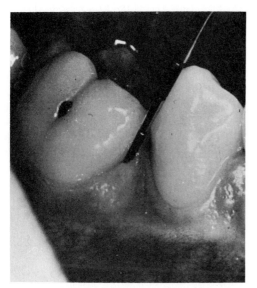 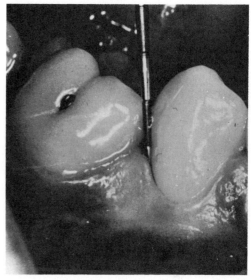

Figure 6–4 Loss of the second premolar and the resultant mesial migration and tipping of the first molar creates initially an apparent increase in sulcular depth on the mesial side of the first molar. Difficulty in maintaining oral hygiene in this area subsequently results in true pocket formation.

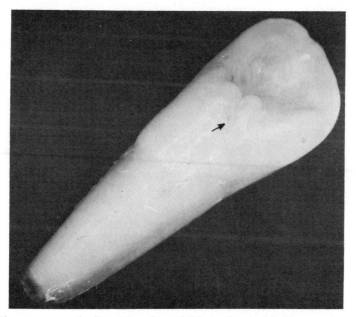

Figure 6–5 The groove on the lingual surface of this tooth provided ingress for toxic materials from dental plaque, contributing to the premature loss of this tooth from periodontal disease.

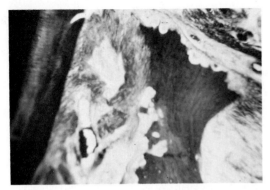

Figure 6-6 In this photomicrograph of human periodontal disease, disruption of the connective tissue elements of the periodontal ligament and gingiva affords ready access of extrinsic factors into the remaining supporting structures, with the resultant rapid continued periodontal breakdown.

and hence play an indirect role in the etiology of the lesion.

BACTERIAL AND IMMUNE FACTORS

A logical progression from anatomic factors is a consideration of bacterial factors that affect the integrity of the periodontium. Bacterial plaque appears to be the single most important extrinsic etiologic agent in the development of the inflammatory periodontal lesion. Bacterial plaque has been implicated more by its presence than by a fulfillment of Koch's postulates for infectious diseases. Conversely, the absence of bacterial plaque has led to a reversal of the inflammatory process, and as a logical consequence of this reasoning, it has been argued that the bacterial plaque is the etiologic factor in the disease process.

Bacterial plaque begins as a pellicle deposition on tooth structure. The primary source of the acquired pellicle is saliva, and it forms by a selective absorption of selected glycoproteins on the tooth. The acquired pellicle is covered by a bacteria-free matrix that subsequently is colonized by bacteria.[2]

The initial colonization of the bacterial plaque is predominately a gram-positive flora. Recent evidence indicates that *Actinomyces viscosus* plays a key role during the initiation of the inflammatory response. As the plaque flora becomes more heterogeneous with a relative increase in gram-negative species, the clinical inflammatory signs become more apparent.

It is of interest to note that, in the normal establishment of the plaque flora, coccoid cells initially colonize the tooth surface, followed by filamentous and fusiform cells, and lastly by spirochetes. In an experimentally induced plaque re-establishment, a similar sequence occurs with some slight modifications between the motile cells and coccoid cells. It is apparent, however, that the spirochetes take the longest to re-establish themselves.[18, 24] The time sequence of bacterial colonization is important, since it points out the unique nutritional interdependence between bacterial species. In addition, an experimentally induced plaque formation preceded by scaling may introduce bacterial antigens into the tissues, resulting in the exacerbation of the host immune response and a subsequent alteration in plaque re-establishment.

As the bacterial cells undergo metabolic changes and replicate, selected products are secreted into the surrounding sulcular exudate and are in direct contact with the

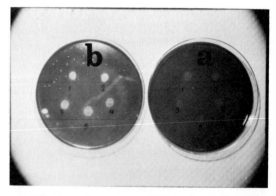

Figure 6-7 The activity of proteolytic enzymes present in dental plaque is demonstrated in this illustration. The medium consists of reconstituted collagen onto which a measured quantity of sonicated human dental plaque was placed. All five patients demonstrated the presence of the enzymes by digestion of the material as seen in Petri dish b. At this time a complete dental prophylaxis was performed. One week later similar samples were taken. Note the diminished enzymatic activity of the immature dental plaque (a).

gingival sulcular lining. The metabolic products of the bacteria rather than the bacteria themselves are responsible for the inflammatory changes occurring in the periodontium. Bacterial enzymes such as collagenase and hyaluronidase are present, are capable of degrading natural collagen (Fig. 6–7), and may play a significant role in the initiation of the inflammatory lesion. As a secondary stage, gram-negative bacteria produce endotoxin that may be responsible for the inflammatory reactions in the gingival tissue (Table 6–1).

Although the bacterial products play a role in the initiation of the inflammatory lesion, they also may play a secondary role in an immunologic reaction in the gingival tissues. The immunologic reaction can be considered to be biphasic to a certain degree. While its primary role is protection of the host, there is concurrent destruction of native tissue. While it may seem contradictory, the initial immune response in the gingival tissues is a cell-mediated type with a preponderance of lymphocytes on a histologic basis. As the lesion progresses, however, the cell-mediated response wanes, and a humoral reaction with an attendant increase in plasma cells predominates.

It was previously felt that the factors associated with destruction of the periodontal tissues were lymphocyte products, but it is now apparent that the plasma cell line of immune cells is capable of elaborating factors that can cause the connective tissue destruction associated with the advancing lesion. The cell-mediated response is now considered to have a helper function rather than a prime role in tissue destruction. It cannot be denied, however, that both reactions are occurring concurrently and work in concert with each other rather than as sole protective or destructive factors.

In addition to the role of bacterial plaque products in the humoral and cell-mediated immune responses, bacteria play an isolated role in the development of the inflammatory response. Bacterial products isolated from an immune response are chemotactic for inflammatory cells. The initial polymorphonuclear leucocyte response is a bacterial chemotactic response rather than an immune response as a function of the complement reaction. This reaction persists throughout the entire course of the disease process. It can occur even in immunosuppressed patients, indicating that the reaction is bacterial rather than immunologic.

DENTAL CALCULUS

While bacterial plaque may be the culprit in the initiation of the lesion, other secondary factors are present that contribute significantly to the etiology of the lesion. Calculus formation is the mineralized end product of plaque accumulation on the tooth surface.[28] With plaque acting as a nidus, there is a selective deposition of calcium and phosphate ions, with resultant calculus formation. The calculus that forms acts as both a mechanical irritant and a porous surface for additional plaque deposition with the consequent continuation of the inflammatory reaction.

Subgingival calculus, on the other hand, differs from supragingival calculus in its formation and composition.[27, 30] Rather than being a direct etiologic agent of the inflammatory reaction, it is a product of the reaction (Fig. 6–8). Selective deposition of miner-

TABLE 6-1 SUMMARY OF MEDIAN VALUES

SEVERITY OF INFLAMMATION	SALIVA *mcg/ml.*	TISSUE *mcg/ml.*	SULCULAR FLUID *mcg/ml.*	PLAQUE *mcg/ml.*
1	.130	.006	.002	1.6
2	.380	.0009	.768	2.4
3	.464	.003	.656	2.4
NUG	.544	.02	1.024	3.0
	$p < .01$	$p < .001$	$p < .001$	$p < .01$

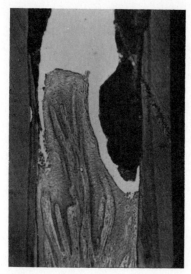

Figure 6–8 In this human biopsy specimen, subgingival calculus can be observed. The calculus represents mineralized dental plaque, and in the case of subgingival calculus, gingival crevicular fluid represents a major component of the matrix.

al ions from the sulcular exudate precipitates the formation of subgingival calculus and then acts as an irritant to further the inflammatory reaction.

OTHER FACTORS

The bacterial plaque and its resultant inflammatory reaction affect the supporting mechanisms of the tooth. If the fiber system of the attachment apparatus remains intact, an adequate barrier to the apical progression of the inflammatory exudate is present. If the bacterial products, however, react with the collagenous substances making up the fiber barrier system, breakdown occurs and the lesion progresses from a self-contained marginal lesion to one that attacks the support of the tooth. As the integrity of the fiber system is compromised, there is a progressive apical migration of the epithelial adherence, with subsequent destruction of the hard structures of the attachment apparatus.[25] Recent investigations have demonstrated that products of the gram-negative population of the dental plaque are capable of inducing osseous destruction[6] or preventing new bone

formation (Fig. 6–9). Prostaglandins, also abundant in the inflammatory exudate, may play a significant role in the destructive process when they are combined with bacterial products.[5]

Other factors must also be given consideration in the secondary etiology and progression of the lesion. Much stress has been placed on the role of the occlusion in the pathogenesis and progression of the lesion.[11] Traumatic occlusal forces may alter the arrangement of the fiber barrier system and allow the inflammatory exudate to progress directly into the osseous structures with the consequent development of intraosseous lesions (Fig. 6–10).[3] Abnormal occlusal forces alone cannot initiate the lesion, but they are probably capable of altering the progression of the inflammatory exudate into the attachment apparatus.

Also concerned with the occlusion is the iatrogenic consequence of faulty restorative dentistry. Like the occlusion, improper restorative dentistry cannot initiate a lesion. Improperly contoured restorations, however, act as a reservoir for plaque accumulation and are therefore capable of playing a significant role in the development of the lesion (Fig. 6–11).[26] Improper tooth contacts also allow food impaction, which causes pressure degenerative changes in the periodontium.

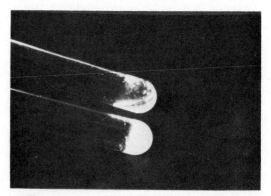

Figure 6–9 The presence of endotoxins produced by gram-negative organisms in human dental plaque can be visualized in these test tubes. Gel formation of the Limulus lysate occurred in the lower tube as a result of the presence of endotoxins. In the upper tube the lysate remains liquid, demonstrating the absence of endotoxins.

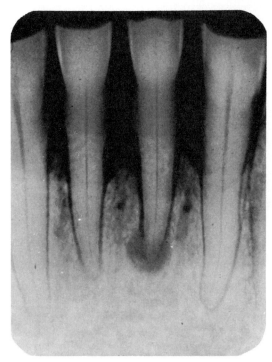

Figure 6–10 This radiograph demonstrates both horizontal and vertical bone loss accompanying trauma from occlusion combined with gingival inflammation resulting from accumulation of dental plaque and calculus. Note the significant incisal wear and the periapical lesion that has developed on the right central incisor.

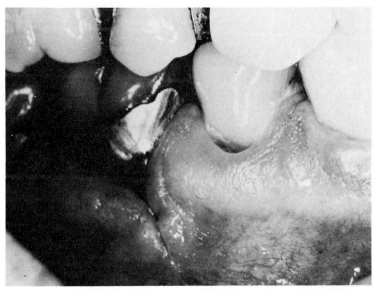

Figure 6–11 Placement of an improperly contoured buccal amalgam restoration has allowed further accumulation of dental plaque with alterations in the gingival morphology and cleft formation, together with bone loss.

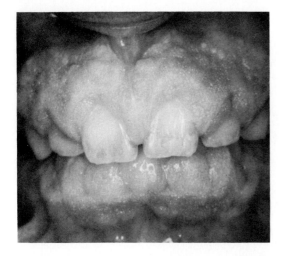

Figure 6–12 Dilantin hyperplasia in eighteen-year-old male. Courtesy of Dr. Sumner M. Sapiro.

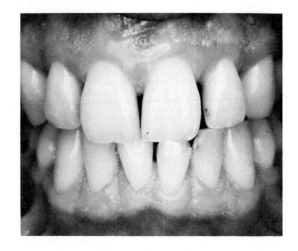

Figure 6–13 Dilantin hyperplasia six weeks post surgery. Courtesy of Dr. Sumner M. Sapiro.

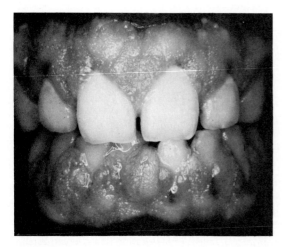

Figure 6–14 Dilantin hyperplasia eighteen months post surgery. Note recurrence of hyperplastic tissue. Courtesy of Dr. Sumner M. Sapiro.

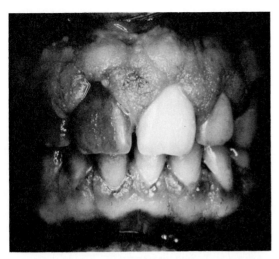

Figure 6–15 Dilantin hyperplasia, periodontal surgery performed on lower arch. Plaque control instituted on upper arch. Courtesy of Dr. Sumner M. Sapiro.

Tooth contacts that are too broad compromise the interdental papilla, making it more susceptible to inflammatory insults.

Although the etiology of the inflammatory periodontal lesion is basically extrinsic, certain intrinsic humoral factors may be present that are capable of altering the host response to external factors. Any systemic factors, such as diabetes,[15] pregnancy,[9] blood dyscrasias, and drugs such as Dilantin (Figs.

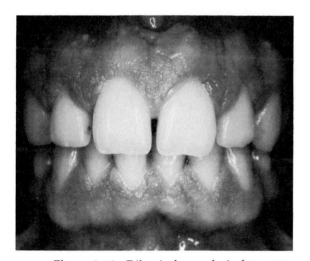

Figure 6–16 Dilantin hyperplasia four years after second surgical procedure. Note only plaque control without surgery done on upper arch. Courtesy of Dr. Sumner M. Sapiro.

6–12 to 6–16), that alter host resistance are capable of altering host responses to external irritants. The response of periodontal tissues to a generalized disease state can be expressed as being part of the overall tissue response to stress. Generalized disease states must be considered as modifying rather than initiating factors. It is reasonable to assume that patients with generalized disease states will react in an accentuated manner to local factors. This may be caused by an altered resistance or an interference with repair in the local tissues. The initiating insult, however, must be extrinsic in origin.

All the available data indicate that the periodontal lesion is extrinsic in nature, most likely of bacterial origin, and can be modified by intrinsic factors that alter the host resistance.

REFERENCES

1. Cohen, B.: Morphological factors in the pathogenesis of periodontal disease. Br. Dent. J. *107*:31–39, 1959.
2. Costeron, J. W., Gessey, G. G., and Cheng, K.-J.: How bacteria stick. Sci. Am. January, 1978, p. 86.
3. Glickman, I., and Weiss, L. A.: Role of trauma from occlusion in initiation of periodontal pocket formation in experimental animals. J. Periodontol. 26:14, 1955.
4. Goldman, H. M.: The behavior of transseptal fibers in periodontal disease. J. Periodontol. 30:249, 1957.
5. Goodson, J. M.: Prostaglandins: Potential mediators of periodontal disease. I.A.D.R. Abstracts. Abst. 375, 1972.
6. Hausman, E., Raisz, L. G., and Miller, W. A.: Endotoxin: Stimulation of bone resorption in tissue culture. Science 168:862, 1969.
7. Hirschfield, I.: Food impaction. J. Am. Dent. Assoc. *17*:1504, 1930.
8. Hodge, H. C., and Lueng, S. W.: Calculus formation. J. Periodontol. *31*:211, 1960.
9. Loe, H., and Silness, J.: Periodontal disease in pregnancy. I. Prevalance and severity. Acta Odontol. Scand. 21:533, 1963.
10. Loe, H., Tgeukade, E., and Jensen, S. B.: Experimental gingivitis in man. J. Periodontol. 36:177, 1965.
11. MacApanpan, I. C., and Weinmann, J. P.: The influence of injury to the periodontal membrane on the spread of gingival inflammation. J. Dent. Res., 33:263, 1957.
12. McDonald, J. B., Gibbons, R. J., and Socransky, S.: Bacterial mechanism in periodontal disease. Ann. N.Y. Acad. Sci. 85:467, 1960.
13. Masters, D. H., and Hoskins, S. W.: Projection of cervical enamel into molar furca bone. J. Periodontol. 35:49, 1964.

14. McHugh, W. D.: Some aspects of the development of gingival epithelium. Periodontics 1:239, 1963.

15. McMullen, J., Gottsegen, R., Legg, M., and Camerini-Davalos, R.: Microangiopathy in the gingival tissues in prediabetes. I.A.D.R. Abstracts. Abst. 56, 1965.

16. Meckel, A. H.: The formation and properties of organic films on teeth. Arch. Oral Biol. 10:585, 1965.

17. Mergenhagen, S.: Complement as a mediator of inflammation. Formation of a biologically active product after interaction of serum complement with endotoxins and antigen-antibody complexes. J. Periodontol. 41:202, 1970.

18. Mousgues, T., Listgarten, M., and Phillips, R.: Effect of scaling and root planing on the composition of the human subgingival microbial flora. J. Periodont. Res. 15:144, 1980.

19. Norton, L. A., Proffit, W. R., and Moore, R. R.: Inhibition of bone growth in vitro by endotoxin: Histamine effect. Nature 221:469, 1969.

20. Ritz, H. L.: Microbial population shifts in developing dental plaque. Arch. Oral Biol. 12:1561, 1967.

21. Schultz-Haudt, S. D., and Aas, E.: Dynamics of the periodontal tissues. II. The connective tissue. Odontol. Tidskr. 70:397, 1962.

22. Schultz-Haudt, S. D., and From, S.: Dynamics of the periodontal tissues. I. The epithelium. Odontol. Tidskr. 69:431, 1961.

23. Shapiro, L., Lodato, F. M., Courant, P. R., and Stallard, R. E.: Endotoxin determinations in gingival inflammation. J. Periodontol. 43:591, 1972.

24. Slots, J.: Microflora in the healthy gingival sulcus in man. Scand. J. Dent. Res. 85:247, 1977.

25. Stallard, R. E., Orban, J. E., and Hove, K. A.: Clinical significance of the inflammatory process. J. Periodontol., 41:20–24, 1970.

26. Waerhaug, J.: Effect of rough surfaces upon gingival tissues. J. Dent. Res. 35:323, 1956.

27. Waerhaug, J.: The source of mineral salts in subgingival calculus. J. Dent. Res. 34:563, 1955.

28. Wasserman, B. H., Mandel, I. D., and Levy, B. M.: In vitro calcification of dental calculus. J. Periodontol. 29:144, 1958.

29. Weinstein, E., and Mandel, I. D.: The fluid of the gingival sulcus. Periodontics 2:147, 1964.

30. Zander, H. A.: The attachment of calculus to root surfaces. J. Periodontol. 24:16, 1953.

ADDITIONAL REFERENCES

Lindhe, J., and Socransky, S. S.: Chemotaxis and vascular permeability induced by human periodontopathic bacteria. J. Periodont. Res. 14:138, 1979.

Patters, M. R., Sedransk, N., and Genco, R.: The lymphoproliferative response during human experimental gingivitis. J. Periodont. Res. 14:269, 1979.

Seymour, G. J., and Greenspan, J. S.: The phenotypic characterization of lymphocyte subpopulations in established human periodontal disease. J. Periodont. Res. 14:39, 1979.

CHAPTER SEVEN

Epidemiology of and Factors Related to Oral Cancer

Theodore E. Bolden, D.D.S., Ph.D.

EPIDEMIOLOGY

INCIDENCE AND PREVALENCE

The incidence of oral cancer varies in different populations. For males between 35 and 64 years of age, the six highest rates per 100,000 population are:

Bombay, India	61.3
Puerto Rico	26.6
Oceania (Caucasian)	16.8
Connecticut	11.5
Durban, South Africa	10.9
Cali, Colombia	9.0

The lowest rate, 1.3, occurs in Finland.[21] It is the commonest cancer in India, Ceylon, and other countries of South East Asia.[41]

Cancers of the mouth constitute three to five per cent of all human cancers.[70] They are most commonly seen on the tongue, on the lateral margin of the anterior two thirds. The disease may occur at any age in either sex but is seen more frequently between the fifth and sixth decade and in males approximately three to nine times more frequently than in females.

Oral cancer is a disease that strikes children as well as adults, but it occurs with increasing frequency with advancing age. Also, it is a disease that occurs more frequently in men than in women.

Of the estimated 6,950 deaths that resulted from oral cancer in 1967, approximately 5,200 deaths occurred in men and 1750 in women.[72] Presenting symptoms are usually an ulcer or a swelling that is painful. The symptoms of more advanced stages include dysphagia, dysphonia, a lump in the neck, or a pain in the ear.[70]

The prediction for new cases of oral cancer and deaths from oral cancer has steadily increased during the past decade.[16-18, 25] Table 7–1 shows the estimated new cases and deaths for the years 1971, 1976, 1978, and 1980. Twenty-five thousand five hundred new cases were predicted for 1980 as well as 9000 deaths. This estimated number of new cases for 1980 was nearly twice the estimate for 1971, and the estimated deaths totaled 2000 more than for 1971.

Twenty-five hundred new cases of oral cancer were estimated for New York as compared to 1,000 for New Jersey and 15 for Alaska for 1980.[17] In Britain more than 1850 cases of oral cancer are reported per annum (1963 to 1964). Approximately 900 deaths per year occur from oral cancer.

In Mississippi, the most common sites for oral cancers, in descending order, are the

TABLE 7–1 ESTIMATED NEW CASES OF CANCER AND ESTIMATED DEATHS — BUCCAL CAVITY AND PHARYNX (ORAL)*

YEAR	ESTIMATED NEW CASES	ESTIMATED DEATHS
1971	14,200	7,000
1976	23,800	8,300
1978	24,000	8,000
1980	25,500	9,000

*Compiled from Cancer Facts and Figures, American Cancer Society.

TABLE 7-2 DISTRIBUTION OF 347 CASES OF ORAL CANCER*

PRIMARY SITE	NUMBER OF CASES	PER CENT
Tongue	108	31
Lip	93	27
Alveolar mucosa	54	16
Floor of mouth	41	12
Buccal mucosa	28	8
Palate	23	6
Total	347	100

*From Weir, J. C. and Horton, C. A.: Oral squamous cell carcinoma in Mississippi. Miss. Dent. Assoc. J. *34:*27–29, 1978.

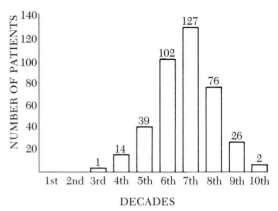

Figure 7–1 Age distribution of 388 cases of oral carcinoma. (From Weir, J. C., and Horton, C. A.: Oral squamous cell carcinoma in Mississippi. Miss. Dent. Assoc. J. *34:*27, 1978.)

tongue, lip, alveolar mucosa, floor of the mouth, buccal mucosa, and palate (Table 7–2).[87] The subject with oral cancer overwhelmingly tends to be white (70 per cent), male (63 per cent) and about 62 years of age with metastasis at the time of diagnosis (Table 7–3 and Fig. 7–1).[87]

The five-year survival rate in a series of 328 patients with oral carcinoma was only 42 per cent (Table 7–4). Carcinoma of the tongue had the worst five-year survival, that is, 18 per cent.[87]

Death from oral cancer is a worldwide problem. Those countries with the highest death rates from oral cancer per 100,000 people are shown in Table 7–5. The United States male ranks eighth in death rate from oral cancer, while the United States female

ranks twelfth. The highest death rate for both male and female is seen in Hong Kong.

Sex and Site Differences

The probability of a woman developing cancer of the lip is between 40 and 70 per cent above that for a man. The incidence of salivary gland tumors is equal in the two sexes. Malignant melanoma is more common in women than in men.[3]

The frequency at which oral cancer may occur at any intra-oral site has been tabulated by the Cancer Control Branch (CCB) of the

TABLE 7–3 CLINICAL DATA FOR 390 CASES OF ORAL SQUAMOUS CELL CARCINOMA*

SITE	Number of Patients	AGE Youngest	AGE Oldest	AGE Average	SEX Female	SEX Male	RACE White	RACE Black	STAGE Localized	STAGE Regional Involvement	STAGE Remote Metastasis	STAGE Not Stated	FIVE YEAR SURVIVAL Survived	FIVE YEAR SURVIVAL Not Survived	FIVE YEAR SURVIVAL Lost to Followup
All sites	390	28	93	62	143	247	248	106	164	179	14	33	138	190	1
Tongue	108	33	92	62	38	70	74	34	28	61	8	11	16	75	1
Lip	93	28	91	59	19	74	83	10	66	20	2	5	56	25	0
Gingiva/alveolar ridge	54	32	89	65	29	25	39	15	15	35	1	3	23	27	0
Floor of mouth	41	42	82	62	15	26	30	11	22	16	0	3	15	19	0
Buccal mucosa	28	43	93	64	17	11	16	12	18	7	0	3	9	13	0
Palate	23	39	79	62	10	13	14	9	7	14	0	2	7	14	0
†Misc.	43	45	87	62	15	28	28	15	8	26	3	6	12	17	0

*From Weir, J. C., and Horton, C. A.: Oral squamous cell carcinoma in Mississippi. Miss. Dent. Assoc. J. *34:*27–29, 1978.
†Includes cases in which a specific location was not stated and those that covered more than one anatomic site (i.e. tongue and floor of the mouth).

TABLE 7–4   SURVIVAL OF 328 CASES OF ORAL CANCER*

PRIMARY SITE	FIVE YEAR SURVIVAL RATE (%)	AVERAGE LENGTH OF SURVIVAL (MONTHS)
Tongue	18	31
Palate	33	69
Buccal mucosa	41	50
Floor of mouth	44	62
Alveolar mucosa	46	64
Lip	69	97
Overall	42	64

*From, Weir, J. C., and Horton, C. A.: Oral squamous cell carcinoma in Mississippi. Miss. Dent. Assoc. J. *34*:27–29, 1978.

United States Public Health Service as follows:

27 per cent	Lip
22 per cent	Tongue
16 per cent	Other oral mucosa
14 per cent	Salivary glands
11 per cent	Floor of mouth
10 per cent	Oral mesopharynx, including tonsil

The CCB has stated that the risk of oral cancer is highest at ages 45 to 54 for males and 65 to 74 for females. The incidence is 10 in 100,000 or greater. The rate is highest among those who use alcohol and tobacco products. The older the population and the greater the proportion of males, the greater the chances are that a significant number of oral cancers will be found.[81]

When the incidence of mouth cancer is compared to the world population between the ages of 35 and 64 years of age, it can be shown that in the populations of Bombay, Puerto Rico, and Hawaii, Caucasians have the highest incidence of mouth cancer, while Caucasian citizens of Manitoba and Connecticut and Hawaiian citizens of Hawaii have the highest incidence of leukemia (Table 7–6).

Oral Cancer Behavioral Characteristics

Oral cancer is essentially of two types — carcinoma and sarcoma. The carcinoma originates in the epithelium; the sarcoma originates in muscle, nerve, blood, or connective tissue.

The initial oral carcinoma has specific growth characteristics: (1) remarkable surface differentiation of epithelial growth with ortho- and parakeratosis, (2) neoplastic growth along minor salivary ducts, (3) lateral cancerization (Slaughter), (4) multicentric intraoral origin (Slaughter), and (5) multiple extraoral malignancies.[11] The squamous cell carcinoma may be indurated with a central depression or ulceration late in the disease. Pain is a late sign.[69] Salivary gland tumors are slow-growing, often asymptomatic swellings that seldom ulcerate.[69]

Sarcomas tend to grow fast, appear most often in the mandible, and either destroy bone or produce bone sclerosis (chondrosarcoma, osteosarcoma).[69] Patients are uniformly young, not aged (Fig. 7–2). When patients first present with tumors more than 2 cm in diameter, many are advanced and already involve lymph nodes. Oral sepsis, malnutrition and gross loss of weight, anemia, protein deficiency, avitaminosis and bronchopneumonia, emphysema, chronic bronchitis, atherosclerosis, and congestive heart

TABLE 7–5   DEATH RATES FROM ORAL CANCER BY COUNTRY HIGHEST INCIDENCE BY SEX

	MALE	FEMALE	FEMALE	
Hong Kong	17.95 (1)	6.29 (1)	6.29 (1)	Hong Kong
France	9.17 (2)	0.78 (28)	3.20 (2)	Taiwan
Puerto Rico	8.73 (3)	2.05 (7)	3.05 (3)	Venezuela
Switzerland	6.95 (4)	0.78 (29)	2.82 (4)	Philippines
Taiwan	6.60 (5)	3.20 (2)	2.36 (5)	Northern Ireland
South Africa	5.92 (6)	1.23 (13)	2.07 (6)	Ireland
Italy	5.44 (7)	0.88 (24)	2.05 (7)	Puerto Rico
United States	4.58 (8)	1.25 (12)	1.77 (8)	Panama
Portugal	4.57 (9)	1.07 (20)	1.47 (9)	England — Wales
Ireland	4.33 (10)	2.07 (6)	1.47 (10)	Sweden

TABLE 7–6 INCIDENCE OF DIFFERENT TYPES OF CANCER IN DIFFERENT POPULATIONS: ANNUAL RATES PER 100,000 PERSONS AGED 35–64 YEARS, STANDARDIZED FOR AGE

POPULATION	INCIDENCE OF CANCER Oral (141, 143–4)	Leukemia (204)	POPULATION	INCIDENCE OF CANCER Oral (141,143–4)	Leukemia (204)
AFRICA			EUROPE		
Mozambique,			°Austria	—	9.4
Lourenco Marques	8.5	4.2	°Belgium	—	9.8
Nigeria, Ibadan	2.3	9.1	°†Bulgaria	—	8.7
S. Africa			°Czechoslovakia	—	8.8
°(coloured)	—	3.0	Denmark	2.2	9.0
°(white)	—	8.0	England and Wales		
Durban			Birmingham region	4.4	6.2
(African)	10.9	4.8	Liverpool region	3.7	6.6
(Indian)	3.3	7.5	S. Metropolitan region	3.1	6.8
Johannesburg (African)	7.9	2.6	S. Western region	2.5	6.4
Uganda, Kyadondo	1.9	3.7	Finland	2.4	8.1
			°France	—	9.4
AMERICA			°‡Germany F.R.	—	9.2
Canada,			°Greece	—	9.0
Alberta	4.5	6.7	°Hungary	—	11.2
Manitoba	2.9	12.3	Iceland	1.3	10.7
New Brunswick	5.4	4.7	°Ireland	—	9.7
Newfoundland	3.8	4.2	°Italy	—	9.0
Saskatchewan	3.2	11.0	Netherlands (3 provinces)	3.1	5.4
Chile	2.3	4.4	°N. Ireland	—	7.9
Colombia, Cali	9.0	4.5	Norway	3.1	7.5
Jamaica, Kingston	7.9	5.7	°Poland	—	11.4
Puerto Rico	26.6	5.9	°Portugal	—	6.7
°Uruguay	—	9.4	°Rumania	—	6.5
°Venezuela	—	4.1	°Scotland	—	7.2
			Sweden	2.6	11.3
U.S.A.			°Switzerland	—	8.8
°(non-white)	—	8.3	°Yugoslavia	—	6.6
°(white)	—	10.6	Yugoslavia, Slovenia	5.0	6.5
Connecticut	11.5	11.6			
New York State	7.7	8.9	OCEANIA		
			°Australia	—	8.3
ASIA			New Zealand	3.9	7.8
°Hong Kong	—	3.1	U.S.A., Hawaii		
India, Bombay	61.3	3.7	(Caucasian)	16.8	5.9
Israel	3.0	10.6	(Hawaiian)	5.9	15.6
Japan, Miyagi	1.9	3.2	(Japanese)	1.9	6.7
Singapore (Chinese)	4.6	1.3			
°Taiwan	—	—			

°Estimated from mortality data.
†Estimated from data for ages 30–59 years.
‡Figures in parentheses refer to Hamburg only.

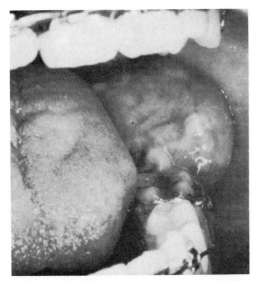

Figure 7–2 This rapidly growing lesion immediately distal to the mandibular left second molar in a 12-year-old girl under orthodontic treatment was clinically diagnosed as pyogenic granuloma, but was later identified by biopsy to be, in reality, a fibrosarcoma. (From Rowe, N. H., and Kwapis, B. W.: Oral and perioral cancer detection. Dent. Clin. N. Amer. 12:189–201, March 1968.)

failure are diseases that may accompany oral malignancy,[27] especially cancer of the floor of the mouth in males over 60 years old and females over 70 years old.

Less than one per cent of oral cancers metastasize to the oral cavity from a silent, primary site. Swelling and pain and loosening of one or more teeth in the area of the mandible or maxilla are common.[69] The spread is frequently hematogenous.

Geographic Considerations

THE NETHERLANDS

In the Netherlands, nearly 50 per cent of cancers of the buccal mucosa occur after the age of 70, and the majority occur in males of about 51 years of age. Some 85 patients with a squamous cell carcinoma of the buccal mucosa were seen in the Netherlands Cancer Institute and Free University Hospital, Amsterdam, from 1956 to 1972. The tumors tend to extend to the mandible from their site of origin along or inferior to the plane of occlusion. The condition was associated with

chewing tobacco, cigarette or cigar smoking, poor oral hygiene, dental caries, and perhaps dentures. A second primary tumor developed in the contralateral side. The majority were T_3 and were well differentiated. An overall five-year determinate cure rate of 58 per cent was achieved. Forty-five per cent survived five years with no evidence of disease.[80]

SWITZERLAND

The incidence of oral cancer was determined in two cities of Switzerland — Neuchatel and Geneva.[61] The highest incidence was seen in males for cancer of the lip, tongue, and buccal cavity. The incidence of cancer of the salivary glands was practically the same in both sexes. Cancer of the tongue and of the buccal cavity in Geneva was the highest in Europe. The majority of cases of cancer of the buccal cavity and pharynx in males occurred in the age range of 50 to 69 years. Less than 2.6 per cent of males with the disease were less than 40 years of age at the time of diagnosis. Some 2 to 20 per cent of the tumors were localized. However, at diagnosis, tumors of the tongue, especially, were well advanced. In Switzerland, the level of mortality from cancer of the tongue and pharynx is one of the highest in the world.

WESTERN CANADA

Oral cancer susceptibility in western Canada increases with age, and those who are 45 years old or over are in the high risk range. Men seem to be more susceptible, but this is decreasing. In Ontario, for males over 45 years old, the most susceptible oral sites (in decreasing order) are the lower lip (in rural residents), the lateral margins of the tongue, the anterior floor of the mouth, the remainder of the tongue, the buccal mucosa, and the lower gingiva.

In this province, a 1965 cancer incidence survey by site and status revealed 26,542 cases of cancer. There were 616 new cases of cancer involving the lip (268), tongue (100), and mouth (248), and 137 new cases of cancer of the pharynx. There were 9,282 deaths from cancer. Males had a higher incidence of cancer than females under 25 years old and at 65-years-old and over. There were 16 males to every one female with lip cancer, four to one for cancer of the pharynx, and about three to one for tongue and bladder cancer.[50]

Manitoba and Saskatchewan have a much higher incidence of lip cancer than Quebec and Ontario, with the reverse being true for intraoral cancer.

Age and sex are very significant factors in oral cancer incidence; older men have the higher rate of occurrence. Urban-rural resident distribution also appears to influence the incidence. Cancer of the floor of the mouth and gingival cancers appear more often in urban residents, and lip cancer is more frequent in rural residents.

Cancer of the hard palate has decreased in both sexes, but soft palate and floor of the mouth cancers have increased mainly in the 45 to 65 age group. The five-year survival rate in a Toronto group (1929 to 1958) was 44.7 per cent for floor and palate cancer and 44 per cent for buccal mucosa and gingival cancer.[1]

CANADIAN ESKIMOS

Carcinoma of the salivary glands in Eskimos is estimated to be approximately 30 times that of a white population of the same size over the same time span. The majority of malignant tumors observed are carcinomas.[84] Salivary tumors are unusually prevalent in Eskimos.

Fourteen tumors occurred in a population of about 11,500 Canadian Eskimos over a nine-year period. Eleven of the 14 tumors were diagnosed as malignant, and malignant tumors constituted about 28 per cent of all the cancers seen. One of the 14 tumors was a poorly differentiated carcinoma that tended to invade local tissue and regional nodes.

The evidence is strong that there is an increased susceptibility for salivary gland tumors in Eskimos. The incidence is calculated to be approximately 30 times that of the white population of the same size and over the same period of time in Saskatchewan.

This increased incidence of salivary gland tumors in Canadian Eskimos may be caused by either genetic or environmental factors. Support for a genetic factor comes from the fact that these Eskimos are such a small, close-knit group. Consideration of the environment of the patients gives no indication of the etiology of these tumors.

SOUTHWESTERN ALASKA: YUPEK ESKIMOS

During the ten and one-half year period from July, 1957 through December, 1967, there were 45 deaths from cancer among Eskimos of southwestern Alaska, with a male to female ratio of 1.37 to 1.0. In the same period, 82 malignant tumors were found in 82 patients. Forty-six per cent of the 82 malignant tumors originated in the alimentary tract. The most common site was the esophagus.[28] Four cases involved the buccal cavity, pharynx, and salivary glands. One squamous cell carcinoma was thought to have arisen in the submaxillary gland. There was complete absence of parotid malignancy, a finding that is in sharp distinction to that of other investigators who found 14 cases of parotid malignancies.[84]

AUSTRALIA

A total of 30,837 new cases of cancer were registered in Melbourne, Australia (1959 to 1964). The lip was the most common site of oral cancer in Australia (62.1 per cent) and represented 3.2 per cent of all malignancies reported.[74] The disease was predominant in males as compared to females (3,090 to 484), with a ratio of 64 to 1, and there was a predilection for the lower lip (99 to 1). In males the lower lip was involved about 15 times more often than the upper lip, in females, about one and a half times more often.

Histologic types included squamous cell carcinoma, basal cell carcinoma, malignant pleomorphic adenoma, mucoepidermoid carcinoma, adenocarcinoma, and mixed salivary gland tumors. The predominant tumors were the squamous cell carcinoma (88.1 per cent) and basal cell carcinoma (9.3 per cent).

Cancer of the lip was observed at every decade. However, most cases were found between 50 and 70 years old in males and between 55 and 75 years old in females. Surgery alone and radiotherapy alone gave comparable five-year survival rates: 87.3 versus 86.4, respectively.[74]

A review of 39 consecutive cases of local recurrence of squamous cell carcinoma of the lip revealed that those patients have more than a 50 per cent chance of survival for five years.[20] All lesions had originated on the vermillion border; radiotherapy was the initial therapy in 31 cases and excision in eight. The average age of the patients was 66 (22 to 88).

PUERTO RICO

One hundred fifty-seven cases of carcinoma of the floor of the mouth were seen in Puerto Rico between the years 1950 and 1965. Carcinoma of the floor of the mouth was the second most frequent form of cancer of the oral cavity seen at the I. Gonzales Martinez Oncologic Hospital. The incidence was approximately 1.8 per 100,000 population for

males and 0.7 for females. The most frequently occurring oral cancer involved the tongue, with an incidence of 4.97 per 100,000 population for males and 1.45 for females.[14]

These data had not changed significantly up to 1972.[26] In 1950, 10.8 new cases of oral cancer were seen; in 1972, the figure had risen to 13 new cases per 100,000 population. The tongue was still the most frequent site. With the exception of lip cancer, tongue cancer had the highest rate of occurrence in all countries studied. Metastases were more frequent in males than females at the time of diagnosis.

X-ray therapy and surgery were the treatments utilized in Puerto Rico, and survival rates were slightly less in Puerto Rico than in the U.S.A. Those factors most frequently associated with cancer of the floor of the mouth were tobacco, alcohol, poor oral hygiene, leukoplakia, and lues.

Radical surgery was considered best for the treatment of lymph node metastasis and for the management of recurrent and residual primary lesions of carcinoma of the floor of the mouth.

FACTORS RELATED TO ORAL CANCER

The use of tobacco, oral habits such as reverse smoking and betel chewing, poor oral hygiene, syphilis, inadequate diet, and chronic irritation from rough or broken teeth and ill-fitting dentures are several factors that have been considered responsible for causing oral cancer. Other important etiolog-

ic factors that have been associated with oral cancer are the consumption of alcohol, viruses, air pollution, sunlight, heredity, anemia, and certain occupations.

Most studies in the United States show a higher frequency of oral cancer in males (Tables 7–7 and 7–8). There seems' to be a

TABLE 7–7 AGE-ADJUSTING MORTALITY RATES FOR CANCER OF THE BUCCAL CAVITY AND PHARYNX AMONG THE WHITE POPULATION OF THE U.S. AS A WHOLE AND IN SELECTED REGIONS OF THE U.S. IN 1950*

POPULATION	U.S.	FIVE SOUTHERN STATES	NEW ENGLAND
White Male	5.66	5.54	7.28
White Female	1.41	2.36	1.19
Ratio M:F	4.0	2.3	6.1

*Death rate per 100,000 population. (From Vogler et al.: A retrospective study of etiological factor in cancer of the mouth, pharynx and larynx. Cancer 15:247–253, 1962.)

TABLE 7–8 INCIDENCE RATES FOR CANCER OF THE BUCCAL CAVITY AND PHARYNX IN 10 URBAN AREAS OF THE UNITED STATES IN 1947*

POPULATION	TOTAL *Ten Cities*	SOUTH *Four Cities*	NORTH *Four Cities*	WEST *Two Cities*
White Male	21.1	26.5	18.9	27.4
White Female	6.3	9.4	5.1	8.5
Ratio M:F	3.3	2.8	3.7	3.2

*Incidence per 100,000 population. (From Dorn, H. F., and Cutler, S. J.: Morbidity from Cancer in the United States [Public Health Monograph 56]. Washington, U.S. Government Printing Office, 1959.)

higher incidence of cancer of the upper gingiva, palate, buccal cavity, and pharynx among southern white females than in white males or females from other parts of the United States. Cancer of the lip and pharynx accounted for only nine per cent of oral cancers in females, while cancer in the same two sites accounted for nearly forty per cent of the oral cancers in males (Table 7–9).

The factor that apparently accounts for the excessive frequency of mouth cancers in southern (American) females is that many are habitual users of "snuff."

Location studies have shown three major concentration areas for oral cancer: the posterior alveolar-lingual sulcus on either side and the floor of the mouth.[56] The explanation is offered that materials suspended in saliva would have the greatest chance for concentration and pooling in these areas.

SYPHILIS

Clinical experience strongly supports a positive correlation between the incidence of syphilis and the onset of oral cancer. Late stages of syphilis involving the tongue are often complicated by cancer of the tongue.[55] Martin found syphilis in 24 per cent of patients with oral cancer.[51] Vitamin B deficiency and use of tobacco were also related to many of those cases. A positive Wassermann was reported in 18 per cent of Negro patients with oral cancer.[45]

The relationship between syphilis and oral cancer is variable, depending upon the population sample and the site of involvement. A high incidence of cancer and syphilis of the tongue has been reported.[30, 49] The figures reported are 11 per cent (in Indians),[83] 13.2 per cent,[31] 18 per cent,[30] and 33 per cent.[89] Syphilis is least associated with carcinoma of the buccal mucosa.[83]

AIR POLLUTION

Some investigators have suggested that oral cancer may be associated with high degrees of industrialization, atmospheric pollution by coal smoke, and exhaust fumes

TABLE 7–9 CANCERS OF THE ORAL CAVITY, PHARYNX AND LARYNX: DISTRIBUTION OF PRIMARY SITES BY SEX OF PATIENTS*

SITE	ALL PATIENTS *No.*	*Per Cent*	MALE PATIENTS *No.*	*Per Cent*	FEMALE PATIENTS *No.*	*Per Cent*
Lip	49	14.7	46	19.6	3	3.1
Min. saliv. glands	10	3.0	4	2.1	5	5.1
Tongue	55	16.5	39	16.6	16	16.3
Lower gingiva & floor of mouth	32	9.6	18	7.7	14	14.3

Upper gingiva,
  palate, &
  buccal mucosa
	82	24.6	40	17.0	42	42.9

Oropharynx	16	4.8	14	6.0	2	2.0
Other parts pharynx	36	10.8	26	11.1	10	10.2
Larynx	53	15.9	47	20.0	6	6.1
Total	333	99.9	235	100.1	98	100.0

*From Vogler, W. R., Lloyd, J. W., and Milmore, B. K.: A retrospective study of etiological factors in cancer of the mouth, pharynx, and larynx. Cancer 15:247–253, 1962.

TABLE 7–10 CASES OF LIP CANCERS AND THEIR MATCHED CONTROLS BY RACE*

| | CASES OF LIP CANCERS | | GENERAL CONTROLS† | |
	No.	Per Cent	No.	Per Cent
Whites	301	99.0	265	87.2
Negroes	3	1.0+	39	12.8‡
Totals	304	100.0	304	100.0

*From Keller, A. Z.: Cellular types, survival, race, nativity, occupations, habits and associated diseases in the pathogenesis of lip cancers. Am. J. Epidemiol. *91*(5):486–499, 1970.

†Males from all diagnostic categories of medical and surgical patients.

‡p < 0.00001.

containing benzopyrene and other polycyclic hydrocarbons.[57] A paradox is posed by the low incidence of oral cancers in rural areas.[33]

SUNLIGHT

The actinic rays of the sun may serve as a causative agent for cancer of the lip.[89] Most labial cancers in the United States are found on the lower lip as squamous cell carcinomas in white males who are farmers or sailors or who work out of doors, reside in the South, or emigrate from the South (Tables 7–10 and 7–11).

An increasing number of basal cell tumors appear on the skin and many of them begin in childhood. They appear to be directly related to the carcinogenic effects of actinic radiation on exposed skin. Usually, the basal cell carcinoma of the face is a solitary, slowly growing tumor that becomes apparent in middle age and beyond in fair-skinned individuals with deficient capacity to produce melanin.

RADIATION

The high rate of leukemia among dentists and physicians is thought to be caused

TABLE 7–11 OCCUPATIONAL CATEGORIES OF CASES OF LIP CANCERS AND THEIR CONTROLS — WHITE MALES ONLY[a]

| | CASES OF LIP CANCER | | CONTROLS | | | |
| | | | CANCER[b] | | GENERAL[c] | |
	No.	Per Cent	No.	Per Cent	No.	Per Cent
Professionals	16	5.3	14	4.7	13	4.9
Managerials	9	3.0[d]	13	4.3	20	7.5[d]
Clerical	8	2.7[d, e]	24	7.9[e]	16	6.0[d]
Salesworkers	8	2.7[d]	14	4.7	18	6.8[d]
Craftsmen	68	22.6	90	29.9	69	26.0
Operatives	51	16.9	33	11.0	34	12.8
Service workers	25	8.3[e]	44	14.6[e]	33	12.5
Laborers	28	9.3	40	13.3	27	10.2
Farmers	80	26.6[g]	25	8.3[g]	11	4.2[g]
Unknown	8	2.6[e]	4	1.3[f]	24	9.1[e,f]
Total	301	100.0	301	100.0	265	100.0

[a]From Keller, A. Z.: Cellular types, survival, race; nativity, occupations, habits and associated diseases in the pathogenesis of lip cancers. Am. J. Epidemiol. *91*(5):486–499, 1970.

[b]Males with squamous cell carcinoma of intra-oral cavity and pharynx.

[c]Males from all diagnostic categories of medical and surgical patients.

[d]p <0.05.

[e]p <0.01.

[f]p <0.0001.

[g]p <0.00001.

by overexposure to irradiation.[13] Ionizing radiations (alpha, beta, gamma) are recognized human environmental carcinogens acting on susceptible cells in the body.[35] Ionizing radiations are among the demonstrated causes of all lymphomas[5, 15, 34] and have been demonstrated to be antigenic for the malignant cells of Burkitt's lymphoma.

Normal mucous glands of the oral cavity frequently undergo squamous metaplasia with marked hyperplasia. This can occur as a result of incident radiation produced when squamous cell carcinoma is treated with 6000 to 6500 R delivered over a period of 23 to 28 days. Of 64 patients studied, 23 developed this change.[29] A relatively high percentage of patients with cancers of the major salivary glands subsequently developed breast cancer. This suggests the possibility of etiologic factors that are common to both diseases.[6]

ALCOHOL

The accumulated clinical evidence strongly suggests a positive correlation between alcohol consumption and the incidence of oral cancer. Approximately 94 per cent of the 189 patients with oral carcinoma examined by Gardner and associates consumed alcoholic beverages.[31] Thirty-three per cent of the patients with oral cancer examined by Wynder and coworkers (1957) consumed more than five ounces of alcohol per day.[89]

A positive correlation (r-6.82, t-0.26) appears when mouth cancer death rates are compared with national statistics of per capita alcohol consumption.[23] Per capita consumption of alcohol adjusted for males over 15 years of age is lowest in Israel and the Netherlands and highest in Switzerland and France. Oral cancer death rates are similar.

ALCOHOL PLUS

Alcohol consumption may not function as a single factor but may, in fact, be related to other habits and other carcinogenic agents. Heavy drinking and heavy smoking are frequently associated. Some studies suggest that the role of alcohol appears only when exposure to tobacco is also present.[77, 78, 88] Nearly six per cent of 1,916 patients in India with oral and oropharyngeal carcinoma were addicted to tobacco, had poor oral hygiene, and gave a history of taking alcohol over a number of years.[82]

One hundred fifty-three cases of epidermoid carcinoma of the mouth (115 in males and 38 in females) were studied in Puerto Rico. Cancer patients tended to use more alcohol, tobacco, hot beverages, and spices than did their sex-matched controls. Heavy drinkers were usually heavy smokers. Cigarette smoking was the principal type of tobacco use.[52]

There is further evidence to suggest the co-carcinogenesis of tobacco and alcohol. Data from 145 white females with intra-oral cancer and 1,973 controls seen at Roswell Park Memorial Institute between 1957 and 1966 revealed that exposure to both alcohol and tobacco can lead to the onset of oral cancer 15 or more years earlier than would occur if either alcohol or tobacco were used alone.[7] Exposure to alcohol only does not produce any clear shift in age of onset, while exposure to smoking only produces a smaller age shift.[7]

These data are supported by an analysis of the charts of 351 patients treated for oral tongue cancer between January 1, 1948 and December 31, 1967 at M.D. Anderson Hospital, Houston, Texas.[39] Of the 351 patients, 52 (13 male, 39 female) claimed no use of tobacco, 105 (49 male, 56 female) claimed no use of alcohol, and only 43 claimed no use of either tobacco or alcohol. Ninety-four per cent of males and 61 per cent of females with tongue cancer used tobacco. Seventy-six per cent of males and 41 per cent of females were chronic users of alcohol.

Of the 308 patients who used either tobacco or alcohol or both, 96 (31.2 per cent) died because of a tumor within five years. Only 6 of the 43 non-users (13.9 per cent) died because of tumors within five years.

Two hundred six (58.7 per cent) of the patients lived two years with no evidence of tumor. Of these 206, 106 patients were chronic users of both tobacco and alcohol, and 29 of these 106 (27.4 per cent) developed a second primary cancer. Twenty-seven of

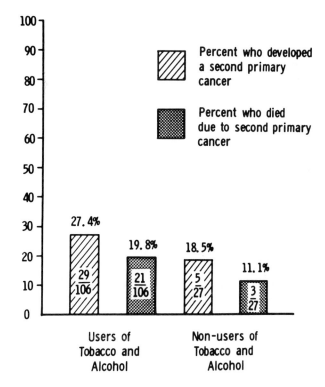

Figure 7–3 Incidence of second primary cancer in five to twenty year follow-up after treatment of primary cancer. There was a greater incidence of second primary cancer and deaths due to second primary cancer in users of tobacco and alcohol than in non-users. (From Johnston, W. D., and Ballantyne, A. J.: Prognostic effect of tobacco and alcohol use in patients with oral tongue cancer. Am. J. Surg. *134*:444–447, 1977.)

the 206 who were free of tumor at two years were non-users of tobacco and alcohol. Only five (18.5 per cent) of these developed a second primary cancer (Fig. 7–3). The data also demonstrated (Figs. 7–4 and 7–5) that non-users of tobacco and alcohol are older when they develop oral tongue cancer than users of tobacco and alcohol.

It seems clear that the greater the alcohol consumption at each level of smoking, the

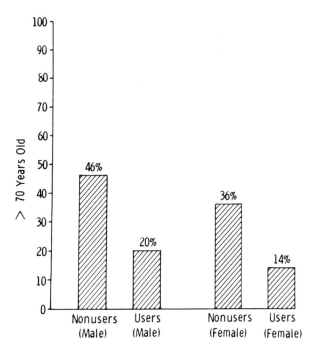

Figure 7–4 Percentage of users and nonusers of tobacco who develop oral tongue cancer at age seventy years or older. (From Johnston, W. D., and Ballantyne, A. J.: Prognostic effect of tobacco and alcohol use in patients with oral tongue cancer. Am. J. Surg. *134*:444–447, 1977.)

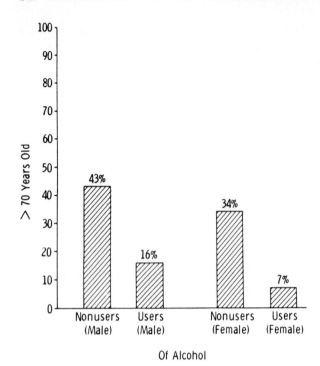

Figure 7–5 Percentage of users and nonusers of alcohol who develop oral tongue cancer at age seventy years or older. (From Johnston, W. D., and Ballantyne, A. J.: Prognostic effect of tobacco and alcohol use in patients with oral tongue cancer. Am. J. Surg. *134*:444–447, 1977.)

greater the risk of intraoral cancer.[67] This risk is greatest for cancer of the floor of the mouth.

SMOKING

Smoking has been estimated to increase the likelihood of developing a mouth cancer by two to four times.[89] As early as 1859, the observation was made that out of 68 patients with cancer of the buccal cavity, 66 smoked pipes, one chewed tobacco, and one apparently used tobacco in some form.[32] Prior to World War I, tobacco consumption was primarily in the form of snuff, chewing tobacco, pipe tobacco, and cigars.[64] Cigarette consumption drastically increased after World War I.[57]

Nearly 36 per cent of the oral cancer patients reported by Mills and Porter gave a history of smoking cigarettes only, while approximately 55 per cent smoked pipes, cigars, or some combination of these.[53] There seems to be a link between tobacco use and cancer of the lower lip and oral cavity.[9] Heavy smoking (40 or more cigarettes daily) has been found to be significant for cases of

tongue cancer and cancer of the floor of the mouth. The death rate for heavy smokers (25 grams of pipe or cigar tobacco or more per day) from oral-pharyngeal cancer has been demonstrated to be more than five times that of the light smoker rate.[86]

Recent evidence suggests that acrolein and cyanide, substances present in the gas-vapor phase of tobacco smoke, might contribute to malignant transformation by causing a reduction in cellular respiration.[24] Acrolein has also been shown to produce inhibition of RNA synthesis, loss of RNA, pyknosis, and cell destruction within 24 hours after exposure of mouse kidney and slime mold cell cultures to cigarette smoke gas phase.[2, 48]

Ash was able to list nine possible predisposing or etiologic factors for oral cancer observed over a 25-year period (Table 7–12). It is interesting to note that in his series trauma (dental, mechanical) and tobacco lead the list at 14 per cent each.[2]

Analysis made of puffs of commercial cigarettes with and without sodium nitrate ($NaNO_3$) by gas chromatography[76] showed that the addition of $NaNO_3$ reduces the components and properties of cigarette smoke

TABLE 7–12 ORAL CARCINOMA, 1929–1958: RECORDED ETIOLOGIC FACTORS*

ETIOLOGY	PER CENT	
Trauma (dental, mechanical)	13.8	
Tobacco	13.7	
Leukoplakia	8.7	
Syphilis alone	2.5	
		68.2
Syphilis with other factor	2.1	
Alcohol	1.8	
Anemia	0.8	
Chronic inflammation	1.0	
Other, or combination	23.8	
Not stated	19.1	
		31.8
None	12.7	

*From Ash, C. L.: Oral cancer: A twenty-five year study. Am. J. Roentgenol. Radium Ther. Nucl. Med. 87(3):417–430, March 1962.

that are associated with tumorigenicity. Cigarettes with $NaNO_3$ added produce smoke that is less tumorigenic and toxic (in mice).[75] The effect is due to thermal decomposition of the nitrate into oxygen and nitrogen oxides; the fumes enhance combustion of tobacco and later inhibit free radical reactions leading to formation of benzo [α] pyrene.

Other investigators have shown that in the absence of smoking the occurrence of cancer of the oral cavity is quite rare.[90] Duration and quantity of tobacco exposure are significantly correlated with the risk of oral cancer.[60]

Cigar and pipe smoking have been implicated in the etiology of oral cavity and esophagus cancer, but to a lesser extent than cigarette smoking. Cessation of tobacco usage causes a decrease in the risk of developing cancers of the lung, larynx, pharynx, oral cavity, and esophagus.[90]

REVERSE SMOKING

Reverse smoking has been reported as part of the cultural habits of Andhrans (India), Pygmy Negritos (Bantu Peninsula), Sardinians, Jamaicans, Venezuelans, Colombians, Panamanians, and South Caribbean islanders. Leukoplakias and cancers of the palate are frequent among the females of

Maracaibo and appear to be related to the frequent habit of smoking with the burning end of the cigarette inside the mouth.[47] Women of Visakhapatnam smoke cigars with the burning end inside the mouth and have a high incidence of palatal cancer. The cancer usually appears in the center of the palate where the burning end of the cigar is held. An ulcerated plaque in the center of a wide leukoplakic area is the earliest lesion observed.[66] Chutta cancer is a palatal cancer that is seen in smokers of Chutta (India) and is related directly to the habit of smoking a homemade cigar with the lighted end in the mouth.[42]

SNUFF DIPPERS

"Snuff dippers" squamous cell carcinoma of the oral cavity has been reported as a disease of males in a ratio 2:1 and as high as 10:1. The sex ratio was reversed in patients with the carcinoma site in the gingivobuccal sulcus. This is where most females place their quid. There is evidence that prolonged use of snuff is conducive to the development of squamous cell carcinoma at or near the site of application. These carcinomas are often multicentric with recurrence.

Onset of the lesion that precedes the oral cancer in a chronic snuff dipper may well be extensive leukoplakia and the breakdown of periodontal tissues, as reported in a 36-year-old male.[10] The patient had dipped snuff for 13 years. Routine intraoral inspection showed a quid of snuff in the region of the

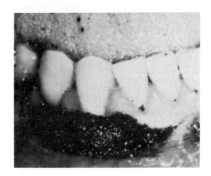

Figure 7–6 Snuff in place in right mandibular mucobuccal region. (From Christen, A. G., et al.: Intraoral leukoplakia, abrasion, periodontal breakdown, and tooth loss in a snuff dipper. J.A.D.A. *98*:584, 1979.)

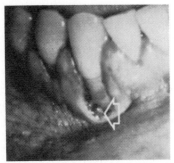

Figure 7–7 After tobacco was rinsed away, extensive area of clinical leukoplakia was seen. Biopsy was done of area at gingiva of mandibular canine (arrow). There was extensive gingival recession, abrasion, and periodontal involvement of entire segment. Fissured, white appearance of alveolar mucosa is characteristic of "snuff-dippers' keratosis." (From Christen, A. G., et al.: Intraoral leukoplakia, abrasion, periodontal breakdown, and tooth loss in a snuff dipper. J.A.D.A. *98*:584–586, 1979.)

right mucobuccal fold directly over the gingiva of the right mandibular lateral incisor, canine, and first and second premolars (Fig. 7–6); an area of extensive leukoplakia; and periodontal breakdown (Figs. 7–7 and 7–8).[10] Healing after biopsy was uneventful (Fig. 7–9).

The five-year survival of 84 cases of snuff users (all females) with buccal and gingival squamous cell carcinoma was 44 per cent. Treatment consists of wide local excision.[57] Carcinomas of the maxillary antrum among rural Africans who insert homemade snuff into their nostrils may be directly related to the presence of high concentrations of nickel, chromium, and zinc.[4]

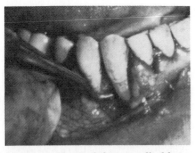

Figure 7–8 Vertical three-walled bony defect on distal proximal surfaces of mandibular right canine root is shown after biopsy was completed. (From Christen, A. G., et al.: Intraoral leukoplakia, abrasion, periodontal breakdown, and tooth loss in a snuff dipper. J.A.D.A. *98*:584–586, 1979.)

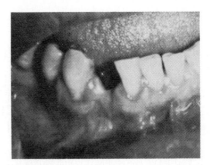

Figure 7–9 Healing of surgical area six weeks later. Clinical leukoplakia is not present. (From Christen, A. G., et al.: Intraoral leukoplakia, abrasion, periodontal breakdown, and tooth loss in a snuff dipper. J.A.D.A. *98*:584–586, 1979.)

TOBACCO CHEWING

The initial lesions presenting on the oral mucosa of South Lancashire coal miners who chewed tobacco were described histologically as leukoplakia and pre-leukoplakia. Twenty-two individuals were observed to have lesions. Approximately five years later, one lesion had progressed to form an exophytic squamous cell carcinoma (Figs. 7–10 and 7–11).[79] One lesion arose at a site where the subject, a 57-year-old male, had held tobacco for some 30 years.

In another study smoking or chewing tobacco or both were found to be associated with a 70 per cent chance for cancer of the oral cavity, an 84 per cent chance for cancer of the oropharynx, and about a 75 per cent chance for cancer of the hypopharynx and larynx.[38] Data were analyzed from 2,005 patients with oral, pharyngeal, and esophageal cancers and from an equal number of controls comparable in sex, age, and religion. Chewers were shown to have a higher risk of cancer of the oral cavity and hypopharynx with risk factors of 5.98 per 100,000 population and 6.21 per 100,000 population, respectively. Smokers had a higher risk of cancer of the oropharynx and larynx, that is, risk factors of 11.82 and 7.74, respectively.[38]

NUTRITION

Avitaminosis may play a role in the etiology of oral cancer.[44] A protracted defi-

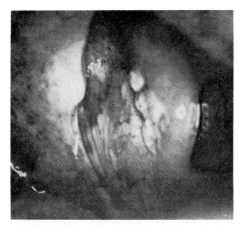

Figure 7–10 Leukoplakia of buccal mucosa, April 1970. (From Tyldesley, W. R.: Tobacco chewing in English coalminers (2). Malignant transformation in a tobacco-induced leukoplakia. Brit. J. Oral Surg., *14*:93–94, 1976.)

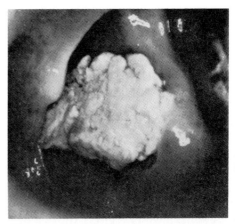

Figure 7–11 Exophytic carcinoma arising in site of leukoplakia, July 1974. (From Tyldesley, W. R.: Tobacco chewing in English coalminers (2). Malignant transformation in a tobacco-induced leukoplakia. Br. J. Oral Surg. *14*:93, 1976.)

ciency of vitamin B yielded a higher level of susceptibility of the cutaneous tissues of the mouse to the irritating effects of tobacco smoke.[43] However, no significant changes were noted in hamsters under the same experimental regime.[89] A lower vitamin B excretion level has been found in many patients with oral cancer.[85]

In one series, low serum vitamin A was found in 76.2 per cent of patients with oral carcinomas and was considered an adjuvant in the carcinogenic process.[83] A diet of rice and tapioca, extremely deficient in protein and vitamin A, might predispose to oral cancer. This diet was found among the Indian coolie class in Travancore, where oral cancer rates are extremely high.[63, 68]

OCCUPATION

A high incidence of oral cancer has been noted in male textile workers.[62] Excess deaths (77 per cent) from oral and pharyngeal cancers in male textile workers of England and Wales (1959 to 1963) involved the tongue, mouth, and pharynx. The excess was concentrated predominately in fiber preparers (wool).

A more recent study included male and female patients from two main textile regions in England: Northwest region (cotton) and West Yorkshire (wool). Fifty-seven women with squamous cell carcinoma in oral and pharyngeal sites were interviewed during 1973 and 1974 along with age-matched controls. An association was found between oral and pharyngeal cancers and industrial exposure to textiles that could not be accounted for by wearing of dentures, by smoking or drinking habits, or by tobacco chewing.[58]

Male leather workers, persons employed in the leather industry, were recently shown to have a higher or elevated risk for cancer of the buccal cavity and pharynx and cancer of the larynx.[22] The risk is increased by long-term employment and is confined to workers over 60 years of age. The risk of buccal cavity and pharynx cancer was also increased among men employed as shoemakers or shoe repairers.[22]

VIRUSES

Cancer viruses are nucleoprotein macromolecules. They consist mainly of DNA with a covering of protein.[15] The evidence to support the postulate that viruses may play a significant role in the etiology of human oral cancers is non-substantive. Recent studies have related herpes simplex virus to cancer in humans. An association between squamous cell carcinoma of the lip and recurrent infection of the lip by type 1 herpes virus has been postulated. To date, research has not succeeded in demonstrating unequivocally that there is a tumor virus in man.[36]

Human Disorders and Cancers

Chédiak-Higashi Syndrome. The Chédiak-Higashi syndrome is a rare familial disorder characterized by partial albinism, photophobia, nystagmus, and anomalous granulations in leukocytes and other cells.[8, 37] Patients suffer recurrent severe infection and death because of malignant lymphoma. The circulating leukocytes of children with the Chédiak-Higashi syndrome have been shown to contain virus-like particles. They are oval with a dense inner nucleoid and a surrounding membrane-like capsule and are approximately 70 mm in diameter.[83]

Leukemias. Structures resembling virus particles (type C murine leukemia particles) and mycoplasma have been found in specimens of blood plasma from acute lymphocytic leukemia patients and also from cases of monocytic leukemia. They were not found in chronic lymphocytic or granulocytic leukemias. Bone marrow specimens failed to reveal virus particles (except in one case of reticulum-cell sarcoma). Structures resembling virus particles (type C) have been found in material obtained from tissue culture. Many more patients with different types of leukemia and lymphoma will have to be examined before, during, and after treatment before a meaningful correlation between the various parameters can be attempted.[54]

Burkitt's Lymphoma. A reovirus,[5] a herpes-type virus, a vaccine virus, a leukovirus, and an echovirus[59] are among the several viruses isolated from Burkitt's lymphoma tissue. Epstein-Barr virus has been isolated from cases of infectious mononucleosis and Burkitt's lymphoma.[34] It is interesting to note that the female mosquito (*Aedes aegypti*) is capable of transmitting viable reticulum cell sarcoma cells. However, no responsible insect virus vector has been reported.

SOCIOECONOMIC STATUS AND HEREDITY

The majority of patients with oral cancers seem to belong to a low socioeconomic group.[82] A general hereditary disposition to cancer as a whole, however, has not been demonstrated.[12] One evidence for heredity as a cancer factor is seen in Gardner's syndrome. Gardner's syndrome is a group of inherited traits with a Mendelian autosomal-dominant inheritance. The onset of symptoms secondary to diffuse polyposis usually does not occur until late childhood or early adult life. The osseous tumors are benign osteomas or exostoses ranging from simple cortical thickening to protuberant bony masses. Although there may be involvement of almost any part of the skeletal system, the mandible is the most common site. Other sites frequently involved are the maxilla, sphenoid, frontal, ethmoid, and temporal bones. These tumors usually attain full size in a few years early in life and remain dormant with slight or no increase in size thereafter.

Another characteristic of Gardner's syndrome is that most patients have poor teeth with numerous caries. The mandible or maxilla may show loss of the normal bony trabecular pattern and replacement by irregular dense bone formation throughout. It is also common to have both unerupted and supernumerary teeth. A characteristic symptom of the syndrome is multiple colonic polyposis. The incidence of carcinoma in the retained rectal or colonic segment after subtotal colectomy has been reported to be 5.2 per cent.[40]

MULTIPLE CANCER

The available evidence suggests that "the risk of a secondary primary tumor in a person once affected with cancer does not exceed that of other persons not previously affected."[12] Plummer-Vinson's syndrome, however, carries the associated tendency to develop multiple oral cancers.[65] A glandular carcinoma, adenocarcinoma, of the accessory salivary gland of the upper lip was reported in the sections of the upper lip of a 70-year-old Caucasian male.[19] The patient presented with multiple submucosal, cystic, movable nodules on the upper lip. The nodules were deep in the stroma and in direct relationship with the accessory glands of the lip. The accessory salivary gland lobules adjacent to the clinical nodules — the mucosal surface on the left side near the midline and on the right side, approximately one-half cm in diameter, and clearly separated from each other — were lined by similar cancer cells. Invasion into the connective tissue by the cancer cells was absent.

RELIGIOUS BELIEFS

Seventh Day Adventists, whose religious beliefs prohibit the use of alcohol and tobacco, experience 90 per cent less chance of death from mouth cancer compared to a similarly constituted non–Seventh Day Adventist population.[46] Moslem males and·females have a greater incidence of carcinoma of the buccal mucosa than do Hindus.[83] In Lebanon, Moslem males and females have a lower incidence of cancer of the buccal cavity, mouth, and pharynx than do Christians. Moslem females have a lower incidence of cancer of the salivary glands.

MENTAL STRESS

Mental stress may be a factor in the pathogenesis of cancer.[71] The results of one study suggest that the five-year cure rates obtained in 306 determinate cases of squamous cell carcinoma of the lip and 74 of the tongue were not related to the pretherapeutic duration of the lesion as expressed by the patient.[73]

REFERENCES

1. Anderson, D. L.: Oral cancer incidence in central and western Canada. J. Can. Dent. Assoc. *34*:180–189, 1968.
2. Ash, C. L.: Oral cancer: A twenty-five year study. Am. J. Roentgenol. Radium Ther. Nucl. Med. *87*:417–430, 1962.
3. Ashley, D. L.: Sex differences in the incidence of tumors at various sites. Brit. J. Cancer *23*:26–30, 1969.
4. Baumslag, N., Keen, P., and Petering, H. G.: Carcinoma of maxillary antrum and its relationship to trace metal content of snuff. Arch. Environ. Health *23*:1–5, 1971.
5. Bell, T. M., Massie, A., Ross, M. G. R., and Williams, M. C.: Isolation of a reovirus from a case of Burkitt's lymphoma. Brit. Med. J. *1*:1212, 1964.
6. Berg, J. W., Hatter, R. V. P., and Foot, F. W., Jr.: Unique association between salivary gland cancer and breast cancer. J.A.M.A. *204*:771–774, 1968.
7. Bross, I. D. J., and Coombs, J.: Early onset of oral cancer among women who drink and smoke. Oncology *33*:136–139, 1976.
8. Chédiak, M.: Nouvelle anomalie leucocytaire de caractère constitutionnel et familial. Rev. Hemat. *7*:362–367, 1952.
9. Christen, A. G.: The clinical effects of tobacco on oral tissue. J. Am. Dent. Assoc. *81*:1378–1382, 1970.
10. Christen, A. G., Armstrong, W. R., and McDaniel, R. I.: Intraoral leukoplakia, abrasion, periodontal breakdown, and tooth loss in a snuff dipper. J.A.D.A. *98*:584–586, 1979.
11. Chomet, B.: Some features of oral carcinoma. Proc. Inst. Med. Chicago *27*:347, 1969.
12. Clemmesen, J.: Statistical studies in the aetiology of malignant neoplasms. I. Review and results. Acta Pathol. Microbiol. Scand. Suppl. *174*, Part 1, 1965.
13. Committee on Genetic Effects of Átomic Radiation: National Academy of Sciences. Science *123*:1157, 1956.
14. Correa, J. N., Bosch, A., and Marcial, V. A.: Carcinoma of the floor of the mouth: Review of clinical factors and results of treatment. Am. J. Roentgenol. Radium Ther. Nucl. Med. *99*:302, 1967.
15. Cowdry, E. V.: Etiology and Prevention of Cancer in Man. New York, Appleton-Century-Crofts, 1968.
16. '80 Cancer Facts and Figures, American Cancer Society.
17. '78 Cancer Facts and Figures, American Cancer Society.
18. '71 Cancer Facts and Figures, American Cancer Society.
19. De La Pava, S., Karjoo, R., Mukhtar, F., and Pickreu, J. W.: Multiple carcinoma of accessory salivary gland. A case report. Cancer *19*:1308–1310, 1966.
20. Dickie, W. R., Colville, J., and Graham, W. J. H.: Recurrent carcinoma of the lip. Oral Surg. *24*:449–454, 1967.
21. Doll, R.: The geographical distribution of cancer. Brit. J. Cancer *23*:1–8, 1969.
22. Decoufle, Pierre: Cancer risks associated with employment in the leather and leather products industry. Arch. Environmental Health *4*:33–37, 1979.
23. Efron, V., and Keller, M.: Selected Statistical Tables on the Consumption of Alcohol and on Alcoholism. New Brunswick, N.J., Rutgers Center for Alcohol Studies, 1963.
24. Eichel, B., and Shahrik, H. A.: Tobacco smoke toxicity: Loss of human oral leukocyte function and fluid-cell metabolism. Science *166*:1424–1427, 1969.
25. Epstein, M. A., and Barr, Y. M.: Cultivation *in vitro* of human lymphoblasts from Burkitt's malignant lymphoma. Lancet *1*:252–253, 1964.
26. Fishman, S. L., and Martinea, Isidro: Oral cancer in Puerto Rico. J. Surg. Oncol. *9*:163–169, 1977.
27. Fleming, W. B.: Cancer of the floor of the mouth: A survey of the problem in Victoria. Med. J. Aust. *2*:434–436, 1968.

28. Fortiune, R.: Characteristics of cancer on the Eskimos of southwestern Alaska. Cancer 23:468–474, 1969.

29. Friedman, M., and Hall, J. W.: Radiation induced squamous cell metaplasia and hyperplasia of normal mucous glands of the oral cavity. Radiology 55:848–851, 1950.

30. Frieger, N., Ship, I. I., Taylor, G. W., and Weisberger, D.: Cirrhosis and other predisposing factors in carcinoma of the tongue. Cancer J. N.Y. 11:357–361, 1958.

31. Gardner, A. F., Hamburger, S., and Love, S.: Oral carcinoma: Analysis of one hundred and eighty-nine cases. J. Am. Dent. Assoc. 66:456–465, 1963.

32. Hammond, E. C.: Effects of smoking. Sci. Am. 207:39, 1962.

33. Hammond, E. C., and Horn, D.: The relationship between human smoking and death rates. J.A.M.A. 155:1316–1328, 1955.

34. Heule, G., Heule, W., and Dilhl, V.: Relation of Burkitt's tumor-associated herpes type virus to infectious mononucleosis. Proc. Nat. Acad. Sci. 59:94, 1968.

35. Heuper, W. C.: Carcinogens in the human environment. Arch. Pathol. 71:237, 267, 355, 1961.

36. Holland, J. J.: Biochemistry of Cell and Virus Multiplications. Sixth National Cancer Conference Proceedings. Philadelphia, J. B. Lippincott Co., 1968, pp. 265–277.

37. Itigashi, O.: Congenital gigantism of peroxidase granules — First case ever reported of qualitative abnormality of peroxidase. Tohoku J. Exp. Med. 59:315–332, 1954.

38. Jayant, K., Balakrishman, V., Sanghvi, L. D., and Jussawalla, D. J.: Quantification of the role of smoking and chewing tobacco in oral, pharyngeal and oesophageal cancers. Br. J. Cancer 35:232–234, 1977.

39. Johnston, William D., and Ballantyne, A. J.: Prognostic effect of tobacco and alcohol use in patients with oral tongue cancer. Am. J. Surg. 134:444–447, 1977.

40. Jones, E. L., and Cornell, W. P.: Gardner's syndrome. Arch. Surg. 92:287–299, 1966.

41. Khanna, N. N., Pant, G. C., Tripathi, F. M., Sanyal, B., and Gupta, S.: Some observations on the etiology of oral cancer. Indian J. Cancer 12:77, 1975.

42. Khanolkar, V. R., and Suryabai, B.: Cancer in relation to usages. Three new types in India. Arch. Pathol. 40:351–361, 1945.

43. Kreshover, S.: Observations on the effect of tobacco on epithelial tissues of vitamin deficient mice. J. Dent. Res. 34:789, 1955.

44. Kreshover, S., and Salley, J.: Predisposing factors in oral cancer. J. Am. Dent. Assoc. 54:509, 1957.

45. Leffall, L. D., and White, J. E.: Cancer of the oral cavity in Negroes. Surg. Gynec. Obstet. 120:70–72, 1965.

46. Lemmon, F. R., Walden, R. T., and Woods, R. W.: Cancer of the lungs and mouth in Seventh Day Adventists. Cancer 17:486–497, 1964.

47. Lepp, H., and Wenger, F.: Leucoplasias y cancer buccal por el habito de fumar coy el cigarrillo invertido. Boletin de la Sociedad de Cirugia 19:471–481, 1955.

48. Leuchtenberger, C., Schumacher, M., and Haldiman, T.: Z Praeventinied 13:130, 1968 (cited by Eichel et al., 1969).

49. Lund, C. C.: Epidermoid carcinoma of the buccal mucosa. Surg. Gynec. Obstet. 66:810–813, 1938.

50. Mackey, E. N., and Sellers, A. H.: The Ontario cancer incidence survey, 1968. A progress report. Can. Med. Assoc. 103:51–52, 1970.

51. Martin, H.: Mouth cancer and the dentist. J. Am. Dent. Assoc. 33:845–861, 1946.

52. Martinez, I.: Factors associated with cancer of the esophagus, mouth, and pharynx in Puerto Rico. J. Natl. Cancer Inst. 42:1069–1094, 1969.

53. Mills, C. A., and Porter, M. M.: Tobacco smoking habits and cancer of the mouth and respiratory system. Cancer Res. 10:539–542, 1950.

54. Mochowski, L., Yumoto, T., and Greg, C. E.: Electron microscopic studies of human leukemia and lymphoma. Cancer 20:760–777, 1967.

55. Moertal, C., and Foss, E.: Multicentric carcinomas of the oral cavity. Surg. Gynec. Obstet. 106:652–654, 1958.

56. Moore, C., and Catlin, D.: Anatomic origins and locations of oral cancer. Am. J. Surg. 114:510–513, 1967.

57. Moore, G., and Bock, F.: A summary of research technics for investigating the cigarette smoking–lung cancer problem. Surgery 39:120–130, 1956.

58. Moss, E.: Oral and pharyngeal cancer in textile workers. Ann. N.Y. Acad. Sci. 271:301–307, 1976.

59. Munube, G. M. R., and Bettl, T. M.: Isolation of echovirus type II from two cases of Burkitt's tumor and three cases of other tumors. Int. J. Cancer 2:613, 1967.

60. Mushinski, M. H., and Stellman, S. D.: Impact of new smoking trends on women's occupational health. Preventive Medicine 7:349–365, 1978.

61. Obradovic, M., Roch, R., and Pellaux, S.: Incidence of cancer of the mouth and pharynx in the cantons of Geneva and Neuchatel, especially in males. Rev. med. Suisse rom. 99:62–66, 1979.

62. Binnie, W. H., Cawson, R. A., Hill, C. B., and Soaper, A. E. (eds.): Office of Population Censuses and Surveys. 1972, Studies on Medical and Population Subjects No. 23 — Oral Cancer in England and Wales. H.M.S.O. London, England (Cited by Moss, E., 1976).

63. Orr, I.: Oral cancer in betel nut chewers in Travancore. Lancet II:575–580, 1933.

64. Peacock, E. E., and Brawley, B. W.: An evaluation of snuff and tobacco in the production of mouth cancer. Dent. Abstr. 5:269, 1960.

65. Pindborg, J. J.: Oral cancer from an international point of view. J. Can. Dent. Assoc. 31:219–226, 1965.

66. Reddy, D. G., and Rao, V. K.: Cancer of the palate in Costal Andhra due to smoking cigars with the burning end inside the mouth. Indian J. Med. Sci. 11:791–797, 1957.

67. Rothman, Kenneth J.: The effect of alcohol consumption on risk of cancer of the head and neck. The Laryngoscope LXXXVIII (Suppl. 8):1–5, 1978.

68. Rowe, N. H.: Epidemiological concepts relative to cancer of the oral cavity. Missouri Med. J. 65:660–664, 1968.

69. Rowe, N. H., and Kwapis, B. W.: Oral and perioral cancer detection. Dent. Clin. N. Am. 12:189–201, 1968.

70. Sisson, G. A., and Goldstein, J. C.: Intraoral carci-

noma. Arch. Otolaryngol. *89*:646(108)–651(113), 1960.

71. Solomon, G. F., and Moss, R. H.: Emotions, immunity and disease. Arch. Gen. Psychiat. *11*:657–674, 1964.

72. Statistics on Cancer. New York, American Cancer Society, 1967, p. 5.

73. Sutton, P. R. N.: Prognosis of carcinoma of the lip or tongue in relation to mental stress: Speculation of an anomalous finding. Med. J. Australia *2*:312–313, 1968.

74. Tan, K. N.: Cancer of the lip in Australia. Aust. Dent. J. *15*:179–184, 1970.

75. Tennekoon, G. E., and Bartlett, G. C.: Effect of betel chewing on the oral mucosa. Br. J. Cancer *23*:39–43, 1969.

76. Terrell, J. H., and Schweltz, I.: Cigarettes: Chemical effect of sodium nitrate content. Science *160*(3835):1456, 1968.

77. Tuyns, A. J.: Association tabac et alcool dans le cancer. Bull. Schweiz. Akad. Med. Wiss. *35*:151–158, 1979.

78. Tuyns, A. J.: Epidemiology of alcohol and cancer. Cancer Research *39*:2840–2843, 1979.

79. Tyldesley, W. R.: Tobacco chewing in English coal miners (2). Malignant transformation in tobacco-induced leukoplakia. Brit. J. Oral Surg. *14*:93–94, 1976.

80. Vegers, J. W. M., Snow, G. B., and van der Waal, I.: Squamous cell carcinoma of the buccal mucosa. A review of 85 cases. Arch. Otolaryngol. *105*:192–195, 1979.

81. Vital Statistics for the United States. 1965. Mortality, Part B. Mortality Figures for Malignant Neoplasms Given by Age. U.S. Department of Health, Education and Welfare, Public Health Service (National Center for Health Statistics), Washington, Government Printing Office, 1967.

82. Vogler, W. R., Lloyd, J. W., and Milmore, B. K.: A retrospective study of etiological factor in cancer of the mouth, pharynx, and larynx. Cancer *15*:247–253, 1962.

83. Wahi, P. N., Kebar, U., and Lahiri, B.: Factors influencing oral and oropharyngeal cancers in India. Brit. J. Cancer *19*:642–660, 1965.

84. Wallace, A. C., MacDougal, J. J., Hildes, J. A., and Lederman, J. M.: Salivary gland tumors in Canadian Eskimos. Cancer *16*:1338–1353, 1963.

85. Waravdekar, V. S., Mangaonkar, V. G., and Khanolkar, V. R.: Vitamin B excretion in oral cancer patients. Acta Un. Internat. Ctr. Cancer *6*:1017–1022, 1950.

86. Weir, J. M., Dunn, J. E., Jr., and Buell, P. E.: Smoking and oral cancer: Epidemiological data, educational responses. Am. J. Public Health *59*:959–966, 1969.

87. Weir, J. C., and Horton, C. A.: Oral squamous cell carcinoma in Mississippi. Miss. Dent. Assoc. J. *34*:27–29, 1978.

88. Wynder, E. L.: The epidemiology of cancers of the upper alimentary and upper respiratory tracts. Laryngoscope *88*(Suppl.8):50–51, 1978.

89. Wynder, E., Bross, I., and Friedman, R. A.: Study of the etiological factors in cancer of the mouth. Cancer *10*:1300–1323, 1957.

90. Wynder, E. L., Mushinski, M. H., and Spivak, J. C.: Tobacco and alcohol consumption in relation to the development of multiple primary cancers. Cancer *40*:1872–1878, 1977.

CHAPTER EIGHT
Nutrition in Oral Health and Disease

Juan M. Navia, Ph.D.

Oral tissues, like all other tissues in the human body, are dependent on their trophic environment to supply the nutrients essential for growth, development, and maintenance of health. From the moment of conception, the availability of nutrients necessary for full expression of the genetic potential of the cell determines the intensity and direction of growth and development in tissues and organs. These nutritional needs are not limited only to developmental periods but also exist at later stages when tissues have reached maturity and require nutrients to maintain the integrity of the body and to compensate for catabolic losses. Nutrients are also involved in health-related problems associated with intake of excess amounts or imbalanced proportions of nutrients that may contribute to disease processes. These nutrient effects are quite different from those induced by a deficiency, which specifically affects the normal metabolic activity of the tissue and thus contributes to the breakdown of specific cellular events that are essential to growth or maintenance of tissues. Nutrients, therefore, are essential to growth, development, and maintenance of tissues, and under certain circumstances they can contribute to disease processes, particularly infectious ones, in a synergistic or antagonistic manner. Such interactions between nutrition and infection are recognized as being of extreme importance and are being carefully studied and evaluated to obtain a clear understanding of the magnitude of their contribution to general oral health.

One other aspect of nutrition that has received a great deal of attention is the concept of critical periods of human development, periods when specific nutrients are especially required by organs developing with different chronologies and rates.[129] A vitamin deficiency or a lack of good quality protein during one of these critical stages of development can result in severe, irreversible changes affecting the growth of the tissue or organ. The changes that lead to these drastic effects may result in clearly detectable morphologic and morphometric alterations of organs and also in less noticeable changes in the fine structure and biochemical characteristics of their cells and tissues, possibly decreasing their resistance to a disease challenge imposed later.

Heredity, nutrition, and infection affect the development of oral tissues, just as they influence other organs and tissues. The teeth, particularly enamel and dentin, begin forming *in utero* and the developmental process for different teeth spans a period of 12 to 15 years. Thus, critical periods occur for specific tooth surfaces at different times. For tooth enamel, deleterious effects of malnutrition and infection become important not only because of the irreversible nature of effects imposed during critical periods of development but also because tooth enamel has no cellular mechanisms to repair tissue damage after tooth eruption. The ability of teeth to withstand a caries attack becomes impaired and susceptibility to such a disease may be markedly increased. Other organs such as salivary glands and the immune

90

system can also be affected by the synergistic action of nutrition and infection imposed early in development. In spite of the ability to reorganize and to repair tissue damage, once these organs have reached maturity, developmental insults may contribute to a decreased ability to protect the tooth against dental caries.

The interaction between nutrition and infection affects oral tissues early during their formative stages, but dietary patterns affect teeth after eruption through dental plaque bacteria. The quality, quantity, and intake frequency of foods included in a diet contribute to the implantation, colonization, and metabolic activity of specific bacteria in dental plaque, thus contributing to the caries virulence of these plaque bacteria. While posteruptive dietary influences on the oral environment are generally accepted, the systemic, nutritional effect on growth and development of oral tissues and the relative magnitude of these effects in humans remains unresolved and requires further investigation.

In general, investigations conducted using experimental animals and some epidemiologic studies suggest that nutrients in the diet can influence oral disease in the following ways: (1) by modifying the biochemical environment of cells responsible for formation of tissues, such as enamel, thus changing tooth structure and its composition and physicochemical properties preeruptively; (2) by altering biosynthetic reactions (proteins, proteoglycans, and lipids) and thereby modifying the nature of the calcifying organic matrix of mineralized tissues; (3) by influencing either directly, or indirectly through calcemic hormones, the cellular activity involved in mineralization processes; (4) by altering the quantity and flow of saliva and its physical, chemical, or immunologic properties; (5) by enhancing or inhibiting the remineralization process taking place normally on the enamel surface of erupted teeth; and (6) by influencing implantation, colonization, and metabolic activity of plaque flora on the tooth surface or in the gingival crevice.

Failure to recognize the importance of the different systemic effects of nutrients has led to serious misunderstanding of the total influence of diet on the etiology and development of oral diseases. In plaque-dependent diseases such as caries and periodontal disease, the outcome is usually determined by the interaction of host, microbial, and nutritional factors. Host factors include, among others, the integrity and perfection of enamel and dentin, the morphology of the teeth, the size ratio of the teeth to the mandible, the degree of salivation, and the chemical and immunologic compositions of saliva and gingival fluids. The microbial factor is represented by the bacterial masses in contact with oral tissues. These microorganisms secrete metabolic end products that affect the oral tissues with which they come in close contact. Under the influence of the nutrient composition of the diet and other associated factors, plaque bacteria may develop such a degree of virulence that disease (caries or periodontal disease) can become rampant if left untreated.

It is of interest to point out that frequently dietary habits and specific foods are made responsible for the type of oral health exhibited by specific groups of people. Oddly enough, when solutions to problems in oral health are studied and formulated, the nutritional or dietary aspects are not fully considered or recognized.

Efforts to prevent disease by only controlling the etiologic microbial agent may be frustrating. However, a broad approach to the prevention of disease through modification of all three etiologic factors would be both practical and rewarding. In human populations, the nutritional factors may be of greater importance than can be surmised from experimental studies. Laboratory studies are usually carried out using highly susceptible animals infected with a virulent organism that readily implants in the oral cavity. Under these experimental circumstances, studies on the influence of malnutrition usually yield little information, for the virulence of the microorganisms overwhelms and obscures whatever effect malnutrition may have contributed. The conditions prevailing among human populations are, however, quite different and are described in Figure 8–1. If host conditions are such that

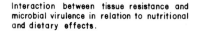

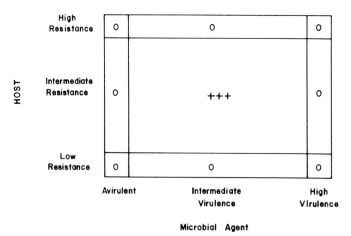

O: Area in which nutrition is ineffective in Influencing disease process.

+++: Area where nutrition will influence the prognosis of disease.

Figure 8–1 Nutritional effects on disease processes will not be seen in extreme cases in which the virulence of the microbial agent is high or the resistance of the host is extremely low. However, because of the heterogeneous genetic and metabolic background of humans and microorganisms, nutrition will be able to influence the outcome of human disease in a large number of cases.

they confer a high degree of resistance to the tooth relative to the virulence of the microbial agent, then the disease process resulting from infection will not develop, regardless of the nutritional state during tooth formation. The same would be true if the conditions were reversed, so that if natural or constitutional resistance is very low in relation to the virulence of the microbial agent, then the disease process will develop regardless of the beneficial effects provided by adequate nutrition during growth and development. Since people and microorganisms have heterogeneous genetic and metabolic backgrounds, nutritional and dietary factors have various effects on the course of human oral disease, and these effects usually fall between the extremes just described. These multifactorial properties of the etiology of oral disease have made it difficult to evaluate the true extent of the contribution of nutritional factors.

One final point should be discussed, and this relates to the concept of nutrition. The word has many different connotations, depending on the scientific background and approaches used to study nutritional problems. Nutrition is an applied science that is essentially concerned with the main effects and interactions of nutrients and other substances in foods available from the trophic environment on growth, health, and disease of living organisms. Human nutrition can be considered and studied at various levels of complexity: (1) the *cellular or tissue level,* which involves biochemical reactions of the tissues and cellular metabolism of nutrients; (2) the *organismal level,* which is mainly concerned with diets, food intake patterns, and nutrient composition, and metabolism of food nutrients including digestion, absorption, transport, utilization, and excretion; and (3) the *community level,* in which cultural, religious, and socioeconomic factors as well as agricultural, industrial, and commercial factors are considered in determining the nutritional status of the community or group. Obviously, the disciplines and scientific expertise required to contend with each of these three approaches will vary. The cellular level is the domain of biochemists and cell biologists; the organismal level requires input from physicians, dentists, human and animal nutritionists, physiologists, dietitians, dental hygienists, nurses, and other health professionals; finally, the third level of complexity involves economists, sociologists, anthropologists, psychologists, educators, technologists, and engineers, among others.

From this description, it is obvious that the perception of what nutrition is depends on the particular interest and emphasis of the individual working in this field, and yet all of them can contribute to the overall result of nutrition, which is to allow normal development as well as maintenance of oral and general health. It is through the concerted effort of many different professionals that we will be able to identify lifestyles compatible with health for individuals, resulting in an awareness of the importance of the factors involved and a willingness to incorporate them into daily behavior.

NUTRITION AND ORAL HEALTH

Nutritional Aspects of Oral Tissue Growth and Development

Cell processes are profoundly influenced by nutritional factors, but two have special importance for oral tissues: protein synthesis and calcification. Protein synthesis is constantly being carried out by all cells during both growth and maintenance states. Cell life is therefore dependent on the ability to synthesize a large number of proteins. Protein synthesis requires the presence within cells of different nutrients such as amino acids, vitamins in the form of cofactors, and minerals that are essential to the process and have to be supplied by the diet. The basic mechanism by which these different amino acids are organized into proteins is well understood. The assembly of a protein in a cell depends on transcription from DNA of a characteristic messenger RNA, which has a code indicating the sequence in which amino acids are to be organized into the specific protein being formed. Another group of RNA molecules helps to transport amino acids to the messenger strands, which are associated with the ribosomes in the cell. Each messenger RNA strand is associated in an aggregate with ribosomes, referred to as a polyribosome. The number of ribosomes on a messenger strand is reflective of the protein-synthetic capacity of this organelle. It has been shown that amino acids play an important role in maintaining the integrity of this organelle and therefore regulate to

some extent the protein-synthetic activity of the cell. In mammalian cells some polysomes are attached to a system of intracellular membranes, the endoplasmic reticulum, which is usually associated with production of exportable proteins. Free within the cytoplasm are other polysomes that are thought to make proteins intended to remain within the cell.

The regulation of protein synthesis is one of the fundamental aspects of this phenomenon, and in mammalian cells it is carried out partly through regulation of RNA synthesis in the nucleus. The amount of RNA made increases after observable increases in the enzyme RNA polymerase and also by a change in the availability of its nucleotide substrate or by varying the amount of DNA template exposed to the enzyme. Nutrition can influence the amount of protein in the cell cytoplasm by controlling the amounts of amino acids available to the tissue and thus, in a way, regulating the translation by the messenger. In addition, other nutrients can influence the stability of the protein that is formed and therefore influence protein synthesis by changing the rate of degradation. The iron-containing protein, ferritin for example, seems to be stabilized by iron; therefore, the concentration of this mineral nutrient determines the rate of breakdown of ferritin protein in the cell and hence the absolute amount present at any one time.

The biosynthesis of collagen protein, because of its important role in bone, dentin, and the supporting structures of teeth, deserves a closer look. The synthesis of this protein is influenced by nutrition to an even greater extent than other proteins. Collagen contains amino acids such as hydroxyproline and hydroxylysine, which are incorporated initially into the polypeptide chain as proline and lysine and subsequently hydroxylated. One of the nutrients involved in the hydroxylation reaction is ascorbic acid, a vitamin whose role in tissue repair and growth is well documented.

Copper is a nutritionally essential element that also participates in the biosynthesis of collagen and of another structural protein, elastin. There are several types (I to IV) of collagen molecules with a triple-helical, fibrous structure composed of three chains of about 1000 amino acid residues.[24, 102] Crosslinking of collagen (as well as elastin) is carried out by a copper-dependent oxidase. Much of the evidence for this comes from studies in which β-amino propionitrile, a lathyrogen, is fed to animals. The lathyritic α chains of collagen appear to be normal; however, the ϵNH_2 groups of the lysyl residues, which are involved in crosslinkage, are not oxidatively deaminated and crosslinking does not occur. Thus, normal maturation of collagen does not proceed in the absence of adequate amounts of copper. Other minerals, such as manganese, are necessary for the glycosilation reactions. These reactions are essential to the formation of the proteoglycans that are needed for proper bone formation.

Calcification Processes and Nutrition

Collagen formed by certain cells such as osteoblasts and odontoblasts undergoes a process of mineralization in which a number of vitamins and mineral elements must take part to fulfill either a structural or a catalytic role.

For many years it has been observed that dietary systems in which there is a low calcium-high phosphate content or a deficiency of vitamin D are usually associated with bone deformities referred to as rickets. While identification and synthesis of antirachitic substances were achieved in the late 1930's, it was not until 30 years later that the metabolism and function of vitamin D were established, and recently, active metabolites have been identified and described by DeLuca and coworkers.[35]

As it is understood today, vitamin D undergoes several transformations in the body before forming the final active metabolite. Cholecalciferol (D_3) from the diet or from irradiation of 7-dehydrocholesterol in the skin is transported in the blood to the liver, where cholecalciferol is transformed to 25-hydroxycholecalciferol (25-OH-D_3). This compound is then transported by the blood to the kidneys, where it is hydroxylated again to form the 1,25-dihydroxycholecalciferol (1,25-OH)$_2 D_3$ (Fig. 8–2). This metabolite and others such as 24,25(OH)$_2 D_3$ cause a more rapid enhancement of calcium absorption than either vitamin D_3 or 25-OH-D_3 in rachitic chicks. Current evidence suggests that 24,25(OH$_2$)D_3 could be an inactivation form of the vitamin. It also was found to be more effective at lower concentrations than these two parent steroids. The presence of the various vitamin D_3 metabolites, under the regulation of the kidney and liver hydroxylase systems, allows for the maintenance of a homeostatic control of calcium in the extracellular fluids. Absorption of calcium from the intestine, mobilization from bones, and excretion of calcium in urine regulates serum calcium concentration with the help of the parathyroid gland and the vitamin D endocrine system (see Fig. 8–2).

Many other nutrients are involved in the process of calcification. Proteins, vitamins A, C, and K, and minerals such as Mg, Mn, Cu, Zn, and F are all involved in the process. Some of these nutrients, such as protein, vitamin C, and copper, are essential for collagen formation. Vitamin A[114] and Mn affect glycosaminoglycan metabolism. Still others, like vitamin K, are involved in the synthesis of specific components of bones such as γ carboxyglutamic acid-rich peptides. The presence of these factors seems to be necessary for the successful formation and maintenance of calcified tissues such as bones and teeth. Severe and even mild deficiencies of these essential elements during the mineralization of teeth may cause the deposition of defective enamel and dentin, which may in turn have a deleterious effect on dental health. It should be remembered that enamel, in contrast to bone, has only one opportunity to be formed normally. Defects during development cannot be cellularly repaired and constitute irreversible lesions.

Stages in Tooth Development: Concept of Critical Periods

To evaluate the possible impact of nutrition and infectious stresses upon tooth development, it is necessary to describe the stages of dental development. Deciduous teeth are known to begin forming at about 6 weeks *in utero* in the ectoderm-lined, primitive oral cavity or stomadeum. From this

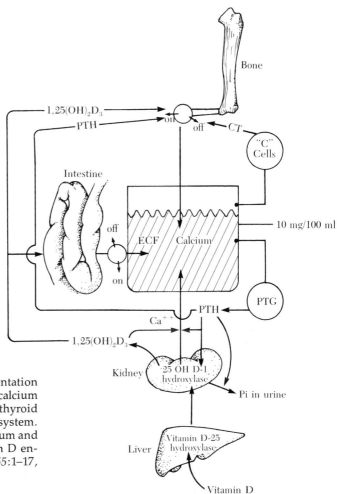

Figure 8–2 Diagrammatic representation of the mechanisms whereby serum calcium concentration is regulated by the parathyroid gland and the vitamin D endocrine system. (From Deluca, H. F.: The control of calcium and phosphorus metabolism by the vitamin D endocrine system. Ann. N.Y. Acad. Sci. 355:1–17, 1980.)

moment, differential growth, characterized by rapid mitosis, leads to formation of the dental lamina. The process continues through evolution into the cap stage and formation of the dental sac until it reaches the bell stage when cells differentiate into ameloblasts and odontoblasts. At this time, appositional growth of enamel and dentin begins by a regular, layer-like deposition of an extracellular matrix. This *Stage I* (which includes initiation, proliferation, morphodifferentiation, histodifferentiation, and finally, appositional cellular activities) requires the availability of nutrients, which in the case of deciduous dentition, are provided through the placenta and, in the permanent dentition, from circulating fluids.

Stage II is characterized by active mineralization of enamel and dentin. Enamel mineralization, which has been studied by several investigators,[6, 7, 19, 57, 122, 137, 161]

differs from that of other hard tissues such as bone. In amelogenesis, the ameloblasts begin to secrete the organic matrix in a thin layer along the dentin shortly after dentin formation has started. Mineralization starts in the matrix and the interprismatic areas soon after secretory activity has begun. It is characterized by the appearance of numerous long, thin crystals of apatite-like material.[48] The initial mineralization[122] is followed by a second phase in which crystals increase in thickness, water is lost from enamel, and the matrix protein concentration is reduced. This process spreads from the dentino-enamel junction toward the surface of the enamel, and from the height of the crown it progresses cervically toward the cemento-enamel junction and also into the fundus of the fissures. The incisal and occlusal regions of the tooth are more fully mineralized than the cervical areas which lag behind during development. *Stage II* ends when enamel matrix has completed its primary mineralization, and amelolasts cease functioning as mineralizing cells. At this time, a cell layer forms a stratified epithelial covering over the enamel to protect it until time of eruption, which varies from a few months to years depending on the tooth.

Stage III involves the peri-eruptive period when the mineral in enamel continues to acquire calcium, phosphorus, and trace elements and undergoes phase changes toward more stable crystals of hydroxyapatite and also fluoroapatite, which occurs through fluoride substitution of hydroxyl ion in surface positions of crystal lattices. This process takes place before, during, and just after eruption, and can be considered a maturation process for hypomineralized areas of enamel (HAE) that were not fully mineralized during the previous developmental stage. These HAE can be remineralized quickly at this time under the action of minerals and proteins in saliva, which contribute actively to the process of remineralization. *Stage III* is definitely a critical stage that could determine the susceptibility of the tooth to carious attack.

Stage IV represents the final period when the tooth is functionally present in the oral cavity, and enamel is subjected sequentially to the mineralization and demineralization action of the oral environment.

From a nutritional and dietary viewpoint, these four stages represent four different periods that are characterized by different tooth developmental activities and different environmental conditions, which may influence final tooth susceptibility to caries. Failure to obtain the necessary nutrients during the first three stages may therefore affect the internal structure and chemical composition of enamel and dentin, as well as possibly affecting the morphology and time of eruption of the tooth. Dietary imbalances and excesses during *Stage IV* affect mainly pellicle and plaque bacteria, thus modifying the mineralization-demineralization processes in the tooth environment.

Within the last 15 years, an important concept has been developed that emphasizes the importance of critical periods in development when nutritional insults may have detrimental and irreversible effects. While working with whole rat brain, Winick and Noble[162] observed that there is a definite pattern and sequence in the changes of DNA and total protein. These studies and others[129] suggest that for most organs there are three major periods of cell growth (Fig. 8–3): (1) a period characterized by hyperplastic activity or an increase in the number of cells; (2) a subsequent phase during which cells continue to increase in numbers but also start to increase in size; and (3) a final stage in which hypertrophic growth of the tissue is the main characteristic. The major nutritional importance of these distinct phases of growth is that nutritional or systemic disturbances imposed early in the process, during the hyperplastic initial phase, tend to be irreversible, and the tissue alterations produced cannot be compensated for. Nutritional insults to developing tissues of the tooth early in the formation of the organic matrix can lead to clinically detectable hypoplasia of enamel characterized by pitting, furrowing, or in the extreme case, absence of enamel. If the stress is imposed later when the hydroxyapatite crystals are in the process of obtaining their maximum size and degree of perfection, the result may be a hypocalcification, manifested by opaque or chalky areas surrounded by normal-looking enamel. This latter phase is also the time when, depending on atomic size and chemical properties, various inorganic ions including fluoride are incorporated into the crystal lattice or into the hydration layer surrounding the apatite crystals, thus contributing to the chemical composition of enamel. Both hypoplasia and hypocalcification can also be induced by environmental stresses[105] such as febrile episodes, chemical intoxications, and genetic defects.

Enamel represents for the tooth what the skin is to the body. Both tissues are ectodermal in origin, and each serves as a protective barrier between the systemically controlled internal environment and the variable and potentially pathologic external environment. Like skin, enamel has a bacterial load and may harbor pathogens capable of disrupting the integrity of this tissue, thus penetrating to the underlying tissues. For these reasons,

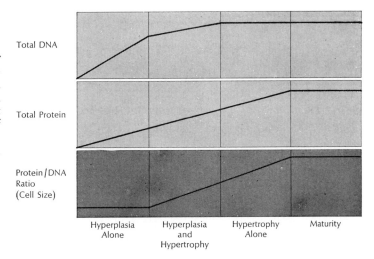

Total DNA

Total Protein

Protein/DNA Ratio (Cell Size)

| Hyperplasia Alone | Hyperplasia and Hypertrophy | Hypertrophy Alone | Maturity |

Figure 8–3 Periods of cellular growth. Plotted are the relationships between DNA and protein during the three phases of organ growth. It will be observed that DNA content crests and levels off well before organ size, as determined by protein accretion and weight gain, reaches its maximum. (From Winick, M.: Fetal malnutrition and growth processes. Hosp. Pract. 5:33, 1970.)

a sound enamel surface is critical, since it determines to some extent whether the tooth is healthy or carious. Adequate nutrition can allow enamel formation to take place, while malnutrition and infection can interfere with normal amelogenesis. Malnutrition is undesirable for all tissues, but it is even worse for enamel. This tissue, once the tooth erupts into the oral cavity, has no cellular mechanisms to repair whatever developmental damage has taken place. Therefore, the lesion is to a large extent irreversible. It is true that the enamel surface is constantly exposed to the reparative effect of saliva and its components, but this can be interfered with and completely neutralized by the destructive activity of bacterial plaque.

It is important to notice that there is an extended period of time between completion of enamel formation and time of eruption *(Stage III)* when human enamel can undergo extensive changes in mineralization of the surface layer and acquire elements such as fluoride that contribute to formation of large, stable crystals of hydroxyapatite containing fluoride in selected sites on the crystal surface.[23] Some of these trace elements tend to enhance maturation of enamel and thus reduce caries susceptibility of the tooth after eruption. Further research is necessary to understand the mechanisms of preeruptive maturation of enamel in humans as well as in experimental animals such as the rat, which have, in contrast to the long human amelogenesis, a 20-day period between beginning

of amelogenesis and eruption of the tooth into the oral cavity.

NUTRITIONAL REQUIREMENTS AND ASSESSMENT SCREENING

Recommended Dietary Allowances

The evidence presented in the previous section clearly indicates that cells have specific nutritional requirements at different stages in their growth and development. These nutritional requirements also exist for tissues undergoing certain processes, such as calcification, and they have to be met if their different functions are to be completed successfully.

Humans can be considered as a conglomerate of cells, tissues, and organs, each with their specific chronology of development. Individual nutritional requirements of these tissues, when considered at a whole, organismal level, become the nutritional requirements of an individual. Furthermore, these requirements of individuals constitute, collectively, the requirements of a group or community of people with a similar genetic background, living under approximately similar environmental and social conditions. Figure 8–4 depicts the various factors that influence the nutritional requirements of a community. Such estimated values are the recommended dietary allowances (RDA) suggested by the Food and Nutrition Board

FACTORS DETERMINING NUTRITIONAL STATUS

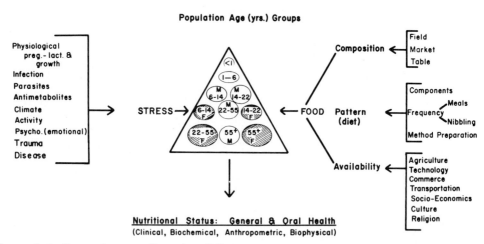

Figure 8–4 Stress factors affect the different population groups to increase the nutritional requirements that must be supplied by the foods consumed by individuals. From the interactions of these different factors emerges a specific nutritional status that determines to a large extent general health. (From Navia, J. M.: Nutrition and Wound Healing. *In* Menaker, L. (ed.): *Biologic Basis of Wound Healing.* Hagerstown, Md., Harper & Row Publishers, 1975.)

of the U.S. National Research Council.[107] The RDA are defined as "the levels of intake of essential nutrients considered, in the judgment of the Committee on Dietary Allowances of the Food and Nutrition Board on the basis of available scientific knowledge, to be adequate to meet the known nutritional needs of practically all healthy persons."[107]

The RDA can be used (1) as a guide in planning nutritionally adequate diets for population groups in the United States, (2) for interpreting food consumption records, (3) for facilitating implementation of public health and welfare programs, (4) for devising nutrition education programs, (5) for helping in the development of new manufactured foods and labeling procedures, and (6) as a standard reference to interpret the adequacy of nutrient intake of individuals in dietary surveys of population groups in the United States.

It is important to point out that, although these RDA figures provide a margin of safety to allow for individual variations, they cannot be used to determine the nutritional adequacy of the diet of one individual. This would also require knowledge of the

current and past nutrient intake of the individual together with an evaluation of clinical signs and symptoms and biochemical data on tissue and excretory levels of nutrients. Individuals whose diets meet the RDA are not necessarily free of malnutrition, nor should individuals consuming diets that fail to meet the RDA standards be judged necessarily as undernourished. The evaluation of the nutritional adequacy of an individual diet must take more into consideration. The RDA figures are given for groups of people, while nutritional requirements of an individual are determined by the needs of the cells and tissues to grow and function.

The recommended dietary allowances include nutritional recommendations for 17 categories of men, women, children, and infants arranged according to age. Recommendations for 17 nutrients are tabulated (Table 8–1): protein; vitamins A, D, E, ascorbic acid, folacin, thiamine, riboflavin, niacin, and vitamins B_6 and B_{12}; and the minerals calcium, phosphorus, magnesium, iron, and zinc. Estimation of the RDA is considered to meet the nutritional needs of the population because in its formulation the

TABLE 8-1 FOOD AND NUTRITION BOARD, NATIONAL ACADEMY OF SCIENCES-NATIONAL RESEARCH COUNCIL RECOMMENDED DAILY DIETARY ALLOWANCES,[a] (REVISED 1980) – DESIGNED FOR THE MAINTENANCE OF GOOD NUTRITION OF PRACTICALLY ALL HEALTHY PEOPLE IN THE UNITED STATES*

	Age (years)	Weight (kg)	Weight (lb)	Height (cm)	Height (in)	Protein (gm)	Vitamin A (µg RE)[b]	Vitamin D (µg)[c]	Vitamin E (mg α-TE)[d]	Vitamin C (mg)	Thiamin (mg)	Riboflavin (mg)	Niacin (mg NE)[e]	Vitamin B_6 (mg)	Folacin[f] (µg)	Vitamin B_{12} (µg)	Calcium (mg)	Phosphorous (mg)	Magnesium (mg)	Iron (mg)	Zinc (mg)	Iodine (µg)
Infants	0.0–0.5	6	13	60	24	kg × 2.2	420	10	3	35	0.3	0.4	6	0.3	30	0.5[g]	360	240	50	10	3	40
	0.5–1.0	9	20	71	28	kg × 2.0	400	10	4	35	0.5	0.6	8	0.6	45	1.5	540	360	70	15	5	50
Children	1–3	13	29	90	35	23	400	10	5	45	0.7	0.8	9	0.9	100	2.0	800	800	150	15	10	70
	4–6	20	44	112	44	30	500	10	6	45	0.9	1.0	11	1.3	200	2.5	800	800	200	10	10	90
	7–10	28	62	132	52	34	700	10	7	45	1.2	1.4	16	1.6	300	3.0	800	800	250	10	10	120
Males	11–14	45	99	157	62	45	1000	10	8	50	1.4	1.6	18	1.8	400	3.0	1200	1200	350	18	15	150
	15–18	66	145	176	69	56	1000	10	10	60	1.4	1.7	18	2.0	400	3.0	1200	1200	400	18	15	150
	19–22	70	154	177	70	56	1000	7.5	10	60	1.5	1.7	19	2.2	400	3.0	800	800	350	10	15	150
	23–50	70	154	178	70	56	1000	5	10	60	1.4	1.6	18	2.2	400	3.0	800	800	350	10	15	150
	51+	70	154	178	70	56	1000	5	10	60	1.2	1.4	16	2.2	400	3.0	800	800	350	10	15	150
Females	11–14	46	101	157	62	46	800	10	8	50	1.1	1.3	15	1.8	400	3.0	1200	1200	300	18	15	150
	15–18	55	120	163	64	46	800	10	8	60	1.1	1.3	14	2.0	400	3.0	1200	1200	300	18	15	150
	19–22	55	120	163	64	44	800	7.5	8	60	1.1	1.3	14	2.0	400	3.0	800	800	300	18	15	150
	23–50	55	120	163	64	44	800	5	8	60	1.0	1.2	13	2.0	400	3.0	800	800	300	18	15	150
	51+	55	120	163	64	44	800	5	8	60	1.0	1.2	13	2.0	400	3.0	800	800	300	10	15	150
Pregnant						+30	+200	+5	+2	+20	+0.4	+0.3	+2	+0.6	+400	+1.0	+400	+400	+150	h	+5	+25
Lactating						+20	+400	+5	+3	+40	+0.5	+0.5	+5	+0.5	+100	+1.0	+400	+400	+150	h	+10	+50

[a] The allowances are intended to provide for individual variations among most normal persons as they live in the United States under usual environmental stresses. Diets should be based on a variety of common foods in order to provide other nutrients for which human requirements have been less well defined.

[b] Retinol equivalents: 1 retinol equivalent = 1 µg retinol or 6 µg β-carotene.

[c] As cholecalciferol. 10 µg cholecalciferol = 400 IU vitamin D.

[d] α-Tocopherol equivalents. 1 mg d-α-tocopherol = 1 α-TE.

[e] 1 NE (niacin equivalent) is equal to 1 mg of niacin or 60 mg of dietary tryptophan.

[f] The folacin allowances refer to dietary sources as determined by *Lactobacillus casei* assay after treatment with enzymes ("conjugases") to make polyglutamyl forms of the vitamin available to the test organism.

[g] The recommended dietary allowance for vitamin B_{12} in infants is based on average concentration of the vitamin in human milk. The allowances after weaning are based on energy intake (as recommended by the American Academy of Pediatrics) and consideration of other factors such as intestinal absorption.

[h] The increased requirement during pregnancy cannot be met by the iron content of habitual American diets nor by the existing iron stores of many women; therefore the use of 30 to 60 mg of supplemental iron is recommended. Iron needs during lactation are not substantially different from those of nonpregnant women, but continued supplementation of the mother for 2 to 3 months after parturition is advisable in order to replenish stores depleted by pregnancy.

* Reproduced from Recommended Dietary Allowances, 9th ed., 1980, by permission of the National Academy of Sciences, Washington, D.C.

following procedure has been used: (1) estimation of the average requirement for a given nutrient and the variability of the requirement; (2) addition to the average of an amount to ensure that needs of nearly all members of the population are covered; and (3) increasing the allowance further to account for inefficient utilization. Thus, the estimate of the RDA should represent a safe recommendation for most people in the United States.

Obviously, adjustments have to be made whenever there is a departure from standard conditions. The RDA table has taken such adjustments into consideration and tabulates requirements for different age groups and for certain physiologic states, such as lactation and pregnancy, when nutritional demands are higher. These dietary allowances do not take into consideration nutritional requirements under extreme stress or disease conditions in humans when nutritional demands are even higher.

Assessment of Nutritional Status

Dental clinicians recognize that even though their main concern involves tissues in the oral cavity to which they direct their observation and treatment, they still should have enough peripheral vision to evaluate the patient *in toto*. In many cases nutritional deficiencies are manifested in such a way that they are readily available for diagnosis by the dentist rather than by other health professionals. Sandsted[132] reports the following:

This happened last summer, when a well-known American adventurer and his wife, bound across the North Atlantic in their 40-foot yacht, sailed into port on the northern coast of Iceland, and the woman went to see a local doctor. She complained of tiredness and lassitude. Her shoes seemed too tight, and her teeth ached. The physician apparently did not think women should be making such ocean passages and quickly concluded there was nothing really wrong that couldn't be cured if she would only go home where housewives belong. While this advice might have

TABLE 8–2 24-HOUR RECALL FORM AND FOOD GROUP EVALUATION*

The following question pattern may be used for conducting the 24-hour recall. The information should then be recorded in the chart at the end.

"In order to get a more complete picture of your family's health, I need to know more about your eating habits. Would you please tell me everything you ate or drank, all day yesterday. Let's begin with:"

1. What time did you go to bed the night before last? _____ (typical versus atypical day)
   Was this the usual time? _____
2. What time did you get up yesterday? _____
   Was this the usual time? _____
3. When was the first time you had anything to eat or drink? _____ What did you have and how much?

_____

4. When did you eat again? _____ Where? _____ What and how much?_____

_____

5. When did you eat next? _____ What did you eat and how much? _____

_____

6. Did you eat or drink anything else? _____
   a. Anything from 1st to 2nd "meal?" _____
   b. Anything from 2nd to 3rd "meal?" _____
   c. Anything from 3rd "meal" to bedtime? _____
7. Was this day's food intake different from usual? _____ If so, how? _____
8. Is weekend eating different? _____ If so, how?_____

*From Krause, M. V., and Mahan, L. K.: Food, Nutrition, and Diet Therapy, 6th ed. Philadelphia, W. B. Saunders Co., 1979.

Table continued on opposite page

TABLE 8–2 24-HOUR RECALL FORM AND FOOD GROUP EVALUATION (*Continued*)

FOOD AND FLUID INTAKE FROM TIME OF AWAKENING UNTIL
THE NEXT MORNING—24-HOUR RECALL

TIME	FOOD AND DRINK CONSUMED		NUMBER OF SERVINGS IN THE FOOD GROUPS							
	Name and Type	*Amount*	*Milk Grp.*	*Meat Grp.*	*Vit A Grp.*	*Vit C Grp.*	*Other F & V*	*Bread & Cereal*	*Butter, Fat, Oil*	*Miscellaneous (Candy, etc.)*
TOTALS										
	Amount	*Milk Grp.*	*Meat Grp.*	*Vit A Grp.*	*Vit C Grp.*	*Other F & V*	*Bread & Cereal*	*Butter Fat, Oil*	*Miscellaneous (Candy, etc.)*	
Recommended No. of Servings Daily										
Children 6 or under		2–3 c.	2	3/wk	1	2	4	2 TBSP.*	†	
Adolescent		4 c.	2	3/wk	1	2	4	2TBSP.		
Adult		2 c.	2	3/wk	1	2	4	2 TBSP.		
Pregnant or Lactating		4 c.	2	3/wk	1	2	4	2 TBSP.		
		Milk Grp.	Meat Grp.	Vit A Grp.	Vit C Grp.	Other F&V	Bread & Cereal	Butter, Fat, Oil	Miscellaneous (Candy, etc.)	
Evaluation L = Low A = Adequate E = Excessive										

*2 Tbsp./day recommended to meet calorie and essential fatty acid needs. Excessive amounts in this group usually mean excessive caloric intake.

†Servings of high calorie, low nutrient items such as sugar, candy, soda pop. Excessive amounts in this group usually mean excessive caloric intake and are contributory to dental caries.

seemed sensible, it was not very helpful. However, the sportswoman accepted the conclusion that she was not really sick and sailed on around the island to the capital, Reykjavik. By the time they got there, she was obviously quite ill. In fact, what alarmed her most was that her gums were bleeding. She immediately sought a dentist instead of a physician. The dentist took one look at her mouth and exclaimed, "Scurvy." Two weeks ashore with plenty of fresh foods and fruit juices and she was cured.

In the United States, nutritional deficiencies are not as common as in technically underdeveloped countries, but the HANES[58] and Ten State[155] surveys indicate that certain economically deprived sectors of our society may show nutritional deficiency syndromes, and another sector suffers from overnutritional syndromes (for example, obesity). Between these two extremes there are groups of people that frequently show borderline and, in some cases, clear malnutrition. There are teenagers with bizarre diets, alcoholics, and elderly persons who, living alone, have neither the motivation nor the facilities to feed themselves properly. In many cases these problems are compounded and made more severe by loss of teeth, inadequate prosthetic appliances, or mucosal lesions that make it difficult for them to masticate and swallow. Children in households where both parents and other members of the family work long and unconventional hours, thus disrupting the management and orderly preparation of foods, are also prime targets for malnutrition.

Dentists are unusual in the sense that in many cases they are the only clinicians that have an opportunity to examine such individuals for complaints other than nutritional problems. Their understanding of the expression of nutrition deficiencies in the oral cavity can be valuable in the diagnosis of incipient problems before they bloom into overt chronic deficiencies. Some of the le-

---

TABLE 8–3 A GENERAL FOOD FREQUENCY QUESTIONNAIRE*

For the frequency of food use, the following pattern of questions may be useful. However, you may have to modify questions after learning some information from the 24-hour recall. For instance, if the patient has said he had a glass of milk yesterday, you wouldn't ask "Do you drink milk?", but rather "How much milk do you drink?" Record answers as 1/day, 1/wk., 3/mo., for example, or as accurately as possible. It may just have to be noted as "occasionally" or "rarely."

1. Do you drink milk? If so, how much? _____ What kind? Whole _____ Skim _____
2. Do you use fat? If so, what kind? _____ How much? _____
3. How many times do you eat meat? _____ eggs _____ cheese _____ beans _____
4. Do you eat snack foods? If so, which ones? _____ How often? _____ How much? _____
5. What vegetables do you eat? (in each group) How often?
   a. Broccoli _____ greenpeppers _____ cooked greens _____ carrots _____
      sweet potato _____
   b. Tomatoes _____ raw cabbage _____
   c. Asparagus _____ beets _____ cauliflower _____ corn _____
      cooked cabbage _____ celery _____ peas _____ lettuce _____
6. What fruits and how often?
   a. Apples or applesauce _____ apricots _____ banana _____ berries _____
      cherries _____ grapes or grape juice _____ peaches _____ pears _____
      pineapple _____ plums _____ prunes _____ raisins _____
   b. Oranges _____ orange juice _____ grapefruit _____ grapefruit juice _____
7. Bread and cereal products
   a. How much bread do you usually eat with each meal? _____ between meals _____
   b. Do you eat cereal (daily, weekly) cooked _____ dry _____
   c. How often do you eat foods such as macaroni, spaghetti, noodles, etc. _____
8. Do you use salt? _____ Do you salt your food before tasting it? _____
   Do you cook with salt? _____ Do you "crave" salt or salty foods? _____
9. How many tsp. of sugar do you use/day (1 packet = 1 tsp.)? _____
   (Be sure and ask patient about sugar on cereal, fruit, toast and in coffee, tea, etc.)
10. Do you drink water? _____ How often during the day? _____
    How much each time? _____ How much would you say you drink each day? _____
11. Do you drink alcohol? _____ How often? _____ How much? _____
    Beer, wine, liquor? _____

*From Krause, M. V., and Mahan, L. K.: Food, Nutrition, and Diet Therapy, 6th ed. Philadelphia, W. B. Saunders Co., 1979.

sions are not completely diagnostic of malnutrition but generally indicate a malnourished situation that makes the tissue susceptible to disease. The information obtained by the dentist about nutritional status of the patient can be used to decide the best treatment plan to control oral disease. In general, if severe deficiency states are present, patients should be prescribed appropriate nutritional supplementation and encouraged to see their physician for further evaluation and treatment if systemic complications are suspected.

The assessment of the nutrition status of an individual is essentially derived from the following information:

1. Anthropometric data.
2. Dietary history and food intake record.
3. Biochemical data.
4. Clinical examination and medical history.
5. Cultural and psychosocial information.

Generally, dentists in their practice do not need to do the in-depth type of nutritional assessment that should be reserved for the nutritionist and physician prior to treatment of a severe nutritional disorder. However, anthropometric evaluation, dietary intake assessment, and clinical evaluation of orofacial nutritional signs should be part of the data-gathering process performed prior to formulation of a treatment plan. Tables 8–2 and 8–3 describe the type of information to be obtained in a 24-hour recall for which the patient records the food consumed the previous day.[87] More complete food records are obtained from a 3-day recall evaluation in which 2 days of the week and 1 holiday are included in the evaluation to obtain a more complete and representative picture of the dietary habits of the patient. It should be pointed out that such dietary evaluation is intended to provide information on the nutritional status of the individual being assessed. Further interpretation of the data (as indicated later) is necessary in order to use the dietary data in the management and control of specific oral diseases such as dental caries.

The anthropometric information in general should be simple and designed to provide some data on overall physical development of the subject and normally could include height, weight, and mid-arm circumference. Table 8–4 tabulates some anthropometric measurements used in nutritional assessment, and texts such as that of Krause and Mahan[87] describe some of the major approaches used in obtaining such measurements with the necessary degree of accuracy and precision.

The dentist could extend the evaluation to a more detailed procedure that calls for biochemical assessment and complete physical examination. However, generally this is unnecessary and should really be done by nutritionists and physicians specialized in this area who can report their various findings to the dentist. The health team, not the individual professional, are the ones who are most competent to deliver the best overall care for the patient.

Oral Manifestations Associated with Malnutrition

Clinical evaluation of a patient may show specific pathologic changes in oral tissues caused by malnutrition. Some of the oral tissue lesions associated with malnutrition are discussed in the following paragraphs.[78]

LIPS

Changes in lips are usually observed on exposed mucosa and angles of the mouth. Riboflavin, niacin, and iron deficiencies are associated with these lesions. Other factors such as environment, exposure to extreme cold, or dry conditions may also produce similar lesions. In certain cases, poorly fitting prosthetic appliances, diseases such as herpes and syphilis, or allergic reactions to drugs or cosmetics may also produce similar lesions. The most common lesions are:

Cheilosis. This is characterized by edematous, swollen lips. In some cases, desquamation and chapping are present with increase in the vertical markings. In *atrophic cheilosis*, the exposed mucosa has a parch-

TABLE 8–4 SOME ANTHROPOMETRIC MEASUREMENTS APPLIED IN
NUTRITIONAL ASSESSMENT*

MEASUREMENTS	AGE GROUPS	NUTRITIONAL INDICATION	ADVANTAGES	DISADVANTAGES
1. Weight	All groups	Present nutr. status; under and over	Common in use	Difficult in field; can't tell body composition; need accurate age; need proper scales
2. Height	All groups	Chronic nutr. status (under) Chronic under nutr. in early childhood	Common in use Simple to do in field	Differs by time of day Other factors play a role
3. Head circumference	0–4 yr.	Intrauterine & childhood nutr. (chronic undernutrition; mental abilities)	Simple	Other factors play a role
4. Mid-arm circumference	All groups	Present under- and overnutrition	Simple, age independent; child need not be denuded; suitable for rapid survey	No limits for over-nutrition; no standard for adult
5. Skin-fold thickness	All groups	Present under- and over nutrition	Measure body composition; detect obesity in adults	Need expensive callipers Difficult with child and in the field
6. Weight/height ratio	All ages	Present under- and over nutrition	Index of body build; age independent; 1–4 yr. and adults	Need proper scales; need trained personnel
7. Mid-arm/head ratio	3 mo. to 48 mo.	Present undernutrition	Simple; age independent; sex independent; any person can do it for field	No standard for adults
8. Chest/head circs. ratio	1–5 yr.	Present undernutrition	Simple; age independent	For limited age; no classification method
9. Mid-arm/ height ratio	0–10 yr.	Present over and undernutrition	Simple; age and sex independent; only tape measure needed	

°Adapted from Bengoa, J. M.: Nutrition, National Development and Planning. Massachusetts, MIT Press, 1972, p. 110 as published in Krause, M. V., and Mahan, L. K.: Food, Nutrition, and Diet Therapy, 6th ed. Philadelphia, W. B. Saunders Co., 1979. For information on the interpretation of these measurements, see text of Krause and Mahan.

ment-like appearance and vertical fissures disappear.

Angular Lesions. Pallor and erythema are sometimes associated with monilial infections at the corner of the mouth. The broken or macerated integument in this area can usually be observed bilaterally when the mouth is held half open. Angular scars can sometimes be observed at the angle of lips, sometimes spreading up and down and with a pink or bleached color, depending on how recently the lesion was formed.

TEETH

Dental Caries. Caries involves microbial breakdown of teeth caused by the presence of cariogenic bacteria in dental plaque. The implantation and metabolism of these bacteria are stimulated by poor dietary habits, such as consumption of large amounts of carbohydrates and frequent intake of sugar-containing snacks.

Mottled Enamel. Stained teeth sometimes associated with aplastic pitted enamel should not be confused with developmental anomalies and tetracycline stains. This lesion is usually seen in areas where fluoride concentration in drinking water and foods is excessively high (in the U.S., more than 2 ppm F in water supply).

Linear Hypoplasia. The lesions can be seen in deciduous maxillary incisors. The hypoplastic line stains brown and corresponds in position to the neonatal line. It has been associated with infectious disease attacks, changes in serum calcium levels,[119] and malnutrition at an early age.

Melanodontia. Extensive yellowish-brown staining of teeth and high caries susceptibility are characteristics of this condition. Epidemiologic data suggest overall undernutrition at critical stages during tooth development as part of its etiology.

Malposition. Crowding and malposition of teeth may have a nutritional origin either because of lack of protein at an early age that has interfered with jaw development or because of early loss of deciduous teeth. Genetic factors may be solely responsible and should be considered in evaluating the etiology of this condition.

GUMS

Inflammatory changes in gingival tissues are seen commonly and should be differentiated to ascertain their origin.

Scorbutic Type. This is the classical symptom associated with vitamin C deficiency. Gums are red and spongy, with swollen interdental papillae and spontaneous bleeding. This syndrome is associated with other signs and does not develop when teeth are absent.

Gingivitis. This condition has a number of stages from a mild inflammation at the marginal gum tissue to a severe periodontal condition in which there is detachment of the gingiva with apical migration of the epithelial attachment, bone loss, and formation of deep periodontal pockets. Although vitamin and protein deficiencies may influence this tissue response, this syndrome commonly results from local bacterial action alone and is aggravated by other local factors such as malocclusion, poor restorations, prostheses, or calculus, or systemic diseases such as diabetes.

Hypertrophic Gingivitis. The gingiva enlarges to such an extent that it may cover the teeth in certain non-nutritional manipulations, such as occurs with the administration of drugs, for example, phenytoin. This condition, too, probably requires an associated local bacterial action.

TONGUE

The tongue has been found to be a sensitive indicator of many pathologic conditions characterized by changes in texture and color. Chronic glossitis has been associated with deficiency of most of the B complex vitamins, particularly niacin, riboflavin, folic acid, and B_{12}. Chronic iron deficiency is also known to induce glossitis. Certain syndromes, such as "geographic tongue" or "furrow tongue," are known to exist in otherwise healthy individuals in whom no nutritional deficiency is suspected. Infections such as candidiasis, as well as drug reactions, late syphilis, malignancy, and some of the aphthous lesions may cause glossitis.

Filiform and Fungiform Papillary Atrophy. This is the earliest lesion of chronic glossitis and produces a completely smooth tongue when both types of papillae atrophy. It can change to a red and fissured appearance, depending on whether or not some of the papillae become hypertrophied and fused.

Papillary Hypertrophy or Hyperemia. This may usually be observed by running a tongue depressor over the anterior two thirds of the tongue. Red dots indicate the presence of hyperemia.

Magenta Tongue. The tongue seems cyanotic, and the syndrome is usually related specifically to riboflavin deficiency. It is generally found in association with angular stomatitis and dermatitis.

Scarlet-Red Glossitis. This condition is characteristic of acute niacin deficiency (pellagra) and sprue. In advanced stages, oral mucous membranes also become bright red.

Beefy-Red Glossitis. This condition differs from the previous one in that the tongue is darker in color, resembling raw beef. It is usually associated with a niacin deficiency, although other B-complex vitamins may contribute to this syndrome.

OTHER POSSIBLE ORAL MANIFESTATIONS OF NUTRITIONAL DEFICIENCIES

Besides the classical signs and symptoms previously described that are associated with nutritional deficiencies, there are other oral manifestations of malnutrition that can be detected by the dentist better than by any one else. These include ulcerations and keratotic lesions on the mucosa, oral pain and burning sensations, xerostomia or sialorrhea, diminished or absent taste perception (hypogeusia and sometimes also anosmia associated with zinc deficiency), and pallor of the oral or lingual mucosa.

Anemias, subclinical B-complex deficiencies (such as folic acid deficiency), and vitamin A and zinc deficiencies have been found to have a part in the causation of these symptoms either directly or indirectly by diminishing the resistance or the function of the tissue. Under the influence of different stresses (for example, infection, functional stimulation, or local irritants), a breakdown takes place and a diseased state is established.

NUTRITION AND ORAL DISEASE

Nutrition and Dental Caries

In most oral disease processes the prognosis is usually determined by the interaction of host, microbial, and nutritional factors. When they interact, disease will result, and when these factors are unbalanced, the pathosis may be retarded or even prevented. Host factors involve genetic determinants that affect the quality of enamel, the morphology of teeth, the size ratio of the teeth to the mandible, the degree of salivation, and the composition of saliva (lysozyme, IgA, and so on), tissue biochemistry, and other factors. The microbial factor is represented by specific bacteria in dental plaque, which accumulate on the tooth surfaces in close contact with oral tissues. Dental plaque represents a highly dense layer of microorganisms, which secrete metabolic products that are in constant contact and interaction with oral tissues. These organisms, under the influence of the nutrient composition of the diet and other undefined factors, may develop such a degree of virulence that disease (caries or periodontal disease) will become rampant if the condition is not treated.

Caries is a chronic disease with a complex etiology characterized by the interaction of three previously mentioned factors (bacteria, diet, and host) acting over a period of time.[116] The direct etiologic factor in dental caries is specific, acid-producing bacteria present in dental plaque covering the tooth surface. A carious lesion is characterized by a progressive demineralization of enamel and subsequently dentin, which advances intermittently along predetermined anatomical pathways in those tissues. If this process is uncontrolled, it usually ends in total decay or destruction of the tooth. The virulence of plaque bacteria is enhanced by the availability of substrate provided by: (1) food residues retained on soft oral tissues and in interproximal dental sites, (2) foods coming into direct contact during mastication, and (3) salivary and gingival fluid components. Other factors influencing the oral environment of the host include saliva composition, tooth morphology and composition, immune competency of the host, positioning of the dentition, degree of occlusal erosion and abrasion, and other factors that can modify the clinical expression of the disease.[111] The health status of the teeth and the periodontium in an individual is therefore largely determined by the interaction of these factors.

The early work by Keyes[80] and Fitzgerald and Keyes,[47] who worked with hamsters, demonstrated the bacterial specificity of the disease and its infectious nature. *Streptococcus mutans* is now considered one of the most important cariogenic microorganisms associated with smooth surface enamel lesions and fissure lesions.[30, 56] Other bacteria found in pits and fissures include *Strep. sanguis, Strep. mitis,* enterococci, *Actinomyces,* lactobacilli, and others.[50] Frequently, close associations between *Strep. mutans* and filamentous microorganisms such as *Actinomyces viscosus* (both cariogenic strains of bacteria) can be commonly seen in dental plaque.[125]

Plaque varies widely in its bacterial components, and this heterogenicity is clearly reflected in its fermentative potential.[113] Therefore, biochemical utilization of available substrate in the oral cavity depends on the types of bacteria present, the metabolic interactions among them, the specific ecological site in the mouth, and previous exposures to a particular substrate.

These bacterial and ecological reactions leading to caries activity are clearly understood and are predictable under experimental conditions. However, the appearance and severity of clinical human caries is more difficult to predict from a given number of circumstances, because caries development in humans is determined principally by a combination of the following factors:

1. Tooth morphology and space relationships of the dentition.
2. Structure and compositon of enamel.
3. Structure and composition of dentin.

4. Fluoride status (available concentration in oral fluids, plaque, and in external layers of enamel).
5. Presence of a virulent cariogenic strain of bacteria in dental plaque.
6. Oral hygiene status.
7. Type, amount, and frequency of exposure to fermentable dietary carbohydrates.
8. Salivary (flow rate and composition, including minerals, proteins, and immunoglobulin) and gingival fluids.

Each of these factors can influence the caries susceptibility of individuals to make them either highly resistant or highly susceptible. Therefore, when the epidemiologic literature is searched, there will be unexpected examples of people consuming low levels of sugars and yet having caries[133] and examples of communities where people consume moderate to high amounts of sugar but have low levels of caries.[59, 128]

EPIDEMIOLOGIC DATA ON NUTRITION AND DENTAL CARIES

Some epidemiologic studies relating the incidence of dental caries to nutrition illustrate difficulties encountered in interpreting results. Russell[131] reported on his extensive field work to determine oral disease prevalence in people from different parts of the world. These findings show that prevalence of caries is not the same around the world, but rather that groups of people living in different areas have a characteristic level of caries activity, thus forming regional patterns (Fig. 8–5). This has enabled Russell to group populations and regions into areas of high, intermediate, and low prevalence of caries (Table 8–5).

Evaluation of the degree to which nutrition contributes to the disease patterns of these people is difficult because of the multiplicity of previously mentioned factors that enter into the etiology of the disease. Caries prevalence in some of these different populations is found to be closely related to excessive consumption of foods rich in carbohydrates. People from areas in which fluoride is present in the drinking water (sometimes in

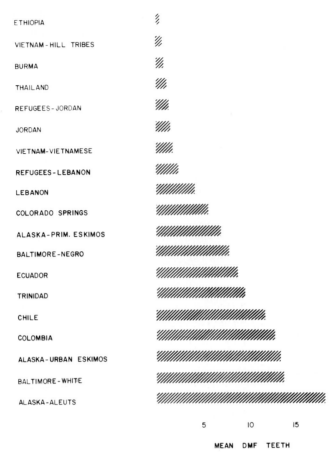

Figure 8–5 Caries prevalence of inhabitants of various parts of the world (Russell, A. L.: J. Dent. Res. *42*:233–244, 1963.)

TABLE 8–5 POPULATIONS AND REGIONS WITH RELATIVELY HIGH, INTERMEDIATE, AND RELATIVELY LOW PREVALENCES OF DENTAL CARIES°

RELATIVELY HIGH	INTERMEDIATE	RELATIVELY LOW
Most populations in:	Fluoride areas in:	Ethiopia
North America	United States	
South America	Ecuador	
Europe	Bolivia	Burma, Thailand, Viet Nam
New Zealand	Greece	India, China, Taiwan
Australia	Israel	
Tahiti	Lebanon	
Hawaii	Egypt	
		Remote areas of Alaska
Urban Alaska	Malaya	
	Indonesia	Jordan
Trinidad		
		New Guinea

°From Russell, A. L.: International Nutrition Surveys. A summary of preliminary dental findings. J. Dent. Res. *42*:233–244, 1963.

excess quantities) have been found to have low caries prevalence. Comparisons between the nutritional status of a population at the time when the survey was conducted and its accumulated lifetime total of decayed, missing, or filled permanent teeth have not yielded evidence that optimum nutrition inhibits caries. Despite the widespread consumption of diets low in vitamin A in Alaska and Ethiopia or diets low in thiamine and riboflavin in Vietnam and Thailand, the people in these countries exhibit surprisingly low levels of caries prevalence.[131] This same pattern has been observed by other investigators, and Russell has summarized this concept by stating that "freedom from dental caries commonly observed in primitive peoples cannot be ascribed to any superiority of nutrition."[131]

Such interpretation of this data should be made cautiously, as many qualifying factors in the area of nutrition determine the outcome of disease. Two have been mentioned previously: carbohydrate consumption and fluoride level in the diet. The increased consumption of refined carbohydrates at the expense of proteins is a factor that, when present, will forcibly incline the balance toward disease. Experiments done in our laboratories[108] indicate that if rats are undernourished during the time that molars are being formed, and then they are fed at weaning time a mild caries-promoting diet containing 5 per cent sucrose and 62 per cent cornstarch, they exhibit 50 per cent higher caries scores than control animals receiving a normal diet during tooth mineralization. If a high sucrose (67 per cent) caries-promoting diet is offered at weaning, then all the rats exhibit the same high degree of caries activity regardless of their pre-eruptive nutritional status. The intensity of the cariogenic potential of sugar overwhelms the protective effect of the diet during tooth formation.

Fluoride availability is another factor that has been clearly shown to interfere with the course of the disease. Water-drinking patterns and proportions of fluids such as tea, milk, water, or fruit juices consumed by people around the world vary enormously. Whereas in some areas young children are weaned early and start to consume water, fruit juices, or even beverages such as tea, which has high fluoride content, in other parts of the world the consumption of milk is continued for long periods of time to the practical exclusion of water. It is well known that while the nutritional value of milk is outstanding, a child raised on water containing fluoride or tea will obtain the benefit of a higher fluoride intake, while a child who is relatively better nourished by milk will have a lower fluoride intake. A child raised on milk may be better nourished overall, but the protective value of fluoride on caries incidence will be absent. Therefore, total fluoride intake of diets in different areas should be determined to evaluate the contribution of this parameter to the disease pattern.

Differences in the water intake pattern of children may have a profound influence on caries experience, especially if water contains trace elements that may not be present in other beverages such as milk. Curzon and coworkers[33, 34] have carried out an epidemiologic study comparing 251 children living in an Ohio town that uses water containing a high level of boron and strontium against a control group of 338 children drinking water with low levels of these elements. These authors suggest that the significantly lower caries prevalence in the former group is related to the boron and strontium content of the water. In this case changes in the amount of water consumed and the drinking pattern may be reflected in a difference in the caries experience of the child. Minerals are extremely important to the development of teeth and their susceptibility to disease.[109]

Two other factors must be considered in order to understand the role of nutrition in a disease such as dental caries. One important point is the particular distribution of food within the family depending on sex, economic status, and lifestyle (rural, urban, and so on). Food has strong social and cultural connotations and its distribution within the family unit may vary, depending on the factors listed above. Thus, its influence on the development of teeth and the outcome of the disease may differ and therefore obscure the interpretation of the contribution of nutritional status to oral diseases.

Another important consideration is that the frequency of consumption of snack foods containing high sugar levels has been clearly shown to increase the severity of caries. Malnourished populations not only consume foods with low nutritional quality, but they also eat less frequently. A man working in the field in Latin America may have only one or two meals a day interspaced with consumption of some beverage such as black coffee, while a white collar worker in an urban economy will have two or three meals together with several snacks during the day. Again, the overall nutritional requirements are better fulfilled in the latter situation, but the incidence of oral disease in these individuals is higher than in their counterparts in the rural Latin American community.

Notwithstanding these considerations, several vitamin deficiencies, especially vitamin A and D deficiencies, and protein-energy malnutrition have been associated with dental abnormalities in malnourished populations. For a long time it has been observed that children in underprivileged groups have a high prevalence of dental dysplasias that have been ascribed to inadequate nutrition during tooth development. Baume and Meyer[13] studied the dental condition and dietary habits of several thousand school children in French Polynesia and described two types of dental dysplasias possibly related to malnutrition: an odontoclasia in the deciduous dentition and a "yellow teeth" condition seen in permanent teeth. Both of these defects were highly susceptible to rampant decay. These authors described a third dysplastic condition referred to as "infantile melanodontia," which was occasionally seen as mottled enamel in children living on distant islands; these children seemed to be caries resistant. Baume[11, 12] made an extensive study of these epidemiologic findings and suggested that probably these enamel alterations were related to malnutrition experienced early in life, when the teeth were undergoing active mineralization. The enamel of these carious "yellow teeth" contained half the fluoride concentrations of the slightly mottled teeth from caries-resistant counterparts.[14] Microradiograph studies[15] using teeth from malnourished individuals showed extensive areas of hypomineralized enamel, which they referred to as "developmental hypomineralization."

Hypoplasia of enamel has been described in remains of prehistoric populations,[31] and recently in many parts of the world these hypoplastic defects have been observed and described. Sweeney and coworkers[152] described a linear hypoplasia of deciduous incisor teeth in Guatemalan children, and Moller[104] described a similar condition in Icelandic children. The timing of occurrence for these dysplasias seemed to correspond to birth or to the postnatal period. This defect is similar to those described by Nicholls and coworkers[118] in Asiatic, underprivileged children (referred to as "bar decay") and by Enwonwu[43] in Nigerian children. Jelliffee and Jelliffee[76] have called attention to the fact that in rural Jamaica[73] and also in Haiti[74] a characteristic "carved out" erosion of deciduous incisors is frequently found in 3- to 6-year-olds, which affects adjacent tooth sides particularly in the maxillary teeth. The same defect with an even higher prevalence (31 per cent) was reported in 1- to 4-year-old Cuna Indians in the San Blas Islands off the Caribbean coast of Panama.[75]

From these epidemiologic studies, it is apparent that a linear hypoplasia resulting in increased susceptibility to dental decay (provided the cariogenic challenge is present) is a common occurrence in young children in areas where malnutrition and infection are rampant. The exact etiologic factor for these lesions is difficult to ascertain. However, epidemiologic data suggest that malnutrition or hypovitaminosis A synergistically combined with infection[150, 151] has a profound influence on the development of these enamel lesions.

In 1979, Nikiforuk and Fraser[119] described the strong association existing between hypophosphatemia in children and the presence of extensive interglobular dentin in both primary and permanent teeth. Hypocalcemia, however, was strongly correlated with enamel hypoplasia. In this long-term investigation, children with X-linked hypophosphatemia who had low plasma P_i but were normocalcemic did not have hypoplastic enamel, yet all had severe interglobular dentin. Children with recessive vitamin D-dependent rickets, which results in hypocalcemia and secondary hypophosphatemia, had enamel hypoplasia and a mild interglobular dentin. Children with a hypoparathyroid condition, which determined a hypocalcemia and hyperphosphatemia, had clear signs of enamel hypoplasia but no interglobular dentin. These authors proposed an interesting unifying hypothesis that enamel hypoplasia, in situations where there are disturbances of calcium and phosphate homeostasis, is caused by hypocalcemia and interglobular dentin by hypophosphatemia. In view of the number of metabolic and nutritional circumstances that lead to chronic alterations of calcium and phosphorus plasma levels, it is perhaps possible to extrapolate these findings to include in the etiology of such lesions the effect of gastrointestinal infections, mineral and trace element deficiencies and imbalances, and vitamin-mineral interactions that frequently occur during tooth formation, affecting Ca and P balance, thus possibly interfering with the normal development of enamel or dentin.

The overall impact that such disturbances of enamel and dentin may have on caries experience is not fully documented. However, Infante and Gillespie[69, 70] reported a high incidence in Guatemalan children of maxillary anterior linear enamel hypoplasia, which often became carious. In this study, caries scores for posterior teeth alone were found to be greater than those reported for total decayed, extracted, and filled teeth in U.S. children. In another study, Infante and Gillespie[71] found that Guatemalan children with anterior linear enamel hypoplasia (LEH) had significantly greater caries experience in posterior dentition than their peers who did not have anterior LEH. Their findings are highly significant, because they suggest that synergistic mechanisms of undernutrition and infection are not only etiologic factors for the development of LEH but may contribute also to the caries experience of seemingly clinically normal molar teeth.

Clinical evidence is not yet available to support directly the concept that malnutrition and infectious diseases influence dental caries. It has been difficult to discern these nutritional effects in epidemiologic studies. High caries incidence has been reported in people living in areas of affluence, whereas in less technologically advanced countries, where individuals frequently have poor nutritional status, low caries has been consistently reported. Some of the main reasons for these apparent discrepancies may be summarized as follows:

1. Caries is an infectious chronic disease produced by one or more types of cariogenic bacteria with varying degrees of virulence, which may account, in part, for differences in the incidence and severity of the disease.

2. Diet is highly influential in caries development and can act preeruptively, as described for mineral, protein, and vitamin A malnutrition, or posteruptively by enhancing the implantation and metabolic activity of cariogenic microorganisms. This posteruptive influence of diet can be overwhelming and capable of determining rampant caries despite the beneficial effects that may have been contributed preeruptively. Additionally, some malnourished populations consume foods with high caries potential infrequently and in small quantities, in contrast to the nibbling eating pattern that is customary in some affluent countries. These underfed populations may lack adequate nutrition during tooth formation, but they also lack the cariogenic challenge that is necessary for the disease to develop. Therefore, their dental caries prevalence is low. It is only upon exposure to cariogenic conditions that their teeth seem to "melt" under such undue stress.

3. Fluoride is well known to be an excellent cariostatic agent and its varying availability in different geographic areas frequently confounds the interpretation of epidemiologic studies. Water drinking patterns and the amount of other fluids consumed, such as tea (high in F), milk (low in F), and juices, vary, depending on the region of the world and the predominating dietary habits. Nutritional effects can be masked by availability of fluoride; therefore, interpretation of epidemiologic data is difficult if all

these factors are not taken into consideration.

Epidemiologic studies are useful in evaluating associations and broad patterns of oral disease and dietary habits, but they can also be highly misleading if they are not properly carried out. Oral disease is a multifactorial problem, which can be influenced in a number of ways at different anatomic and physiologic ages of the tissues involved. Nutritional factors are essential to the expression of the genetic information and continue to be important from conception to death. The provision of the right nutrient at the right developmental stage and in the proper amount and chemical combination is essential to the growth, development, and function of the tissue. These conditions are characteristic for each tissue; therefore, optimum formation and functioning of oral tissues demands that their special nutritional requirements, in the form of proteins, vitamins, minerals, and other compounds, be satisfied at the proper time during development. Unfortunately, we have limited knowledge about the individual requirements of teeth and other oral tissues, but more is being understood of processes that are common to many tissues, such as cell reproduction, protein synthesis, and calcification mechanisms.

EXPERIMENTAL STUDIES: PROTEIN-ENERGY MALNUTRITION, VITAMIN A DEFICIENCY, AND DENTAL CARIES

It has been our hypothesis that infectious diseases and nutritional stresses such as protein malnutrition and other nutrient deficiencies or excesses imposed during tooth development will increase the susceptibility of teeth to disease. The nutritional status of an individual during tooth development may contribute to some extent to the susceptibility or resistance of teeth to dental caries. This hypothesis has been supported mainly by evidence from animal experiments,[145] although some previously mentioned epidemiologic investigations also support this concept.

The experimental studies have involved manipulation of diets and interchange of rat pups between underfed and normally fed rat dams, to distinguish and characterize the developmental effect of undernutrition during pregnancy and lactation on body growth, on incisor and molar weight, and on dental caries susceptibility.[108] A low-protein diet fed to pregnant or to lactating dams provided the nutritional stress. In lactating dams, consumption of low-protein diets reduced the amount, but not the quality of their milk and therefore, pups suckled by these dams were underfed. When these undernourished pups were fed a moderate caries-promoting diet for 15 days after weaning, they were found to be retarded in growth and had higher caries scores than well-nourished, control rats.[115] The suckling period in the rat pup is particularly important, because active tooth mineralization takes place during this period until day 17 when first molars start to erupt. These effects on caries were not observed when a nutritional stress was imposed during gestation.

Another study[39] has been conducted to differentiate the effects of protein malnutrition from those of overall protein-energy deprivation. Rat dams were fed a low-protein diet during lactation to induce a protein-energy deficiency. Rat pups from these dams were intubated with isocaloric supplements that contained either protein or carbohydrates and fats in a formula that simulated rat milk in composition. A specific protein deficiency was thus imposed on suckling pups that received calories and no protein during the critical period for molar development. This deficiency limited the growth of incisors and molars of rat pups and delayed eruption by one day compared to well-nourished, control rats.

These experiments were repeated with the modification that pups from control and experimental groups were fed, after tooth eruption, a caries-promoting diet (that was nutritionally adequate) to determine the response of these rat pups to a standardized caries challenge provided after weaning.[98] In this and the previous study, feeding the protein supplement to the undernourished rats during development allowed rat pups to compensate for the loss in body weight.

Significantly, it was noted that protein-malnourished pups had higher caries scores than did well-nourished controls. In undernourished rats that received isocaloric supplements without protein, caries levels were similar to those of control, undernourished rats that were intubated with distilled water. Thus, these controlled animal experiments suggest that marginal protein malnutrition during tooth development contributes to caries susceptibility.

The experimental studies showing that protein-energy malnutrition (PEM) imposed during tooth formation had an effect on caries susceptibility were followed by a series of investigations to determine some of the factors explaining these effects.[112] These studies indicated that protein deficiency affected the salivary flow and composition[99] and the immune system.[101] Investigations have shown that PEM imposed on rat dams during lactation also increased the acid solubility of the enamel surface of molars from rat pups suckling from these dams.[8] The increase in acid solubility of surface enamel seems to be caused by differences in chemical composition of the outer enamel layers, and this may contribute to the increased caries susceptibility associated with PEM.

Protein-energy malnutrition is not the only nutritional deficiency contributing to the caries experience. In studies[60] in which rat pups were made vitamin A-deficient specifically during critical periods of tooth development, it was concluded that there was an increased caries susceptibility of rat molars from experimental rats compared to that of control rats, without altering the morphology and function of salivary glands or the solubility of the enamel surface. These rat pups seemed to be mainly affected in the dentinal caries scores, thus indicating that the effect was more related to the integrity of the dentin rather than to that of the enamel.

These experimental studies, therefore, seem to suggest that marginal nutritional disturbances may affect either enamel or dentin, increasing the susceptibility to a standardized caries challenge. Studies are in progress to determine the possible synergistic effects of other factors associated with malnutrition, such as infectious episodes that frequently occur concomitantly in human populations.

FOOD AND DIETARY FACTORS IN CARIES DEVELOPMENT

Once the tooth has erupted into the oral cavity, nutritional effects are mostly directed to salivary gland function or the periodontium, and not to enamel and dentin, which have by then completed their development and are fully functional. Effects of foods and their intake pattern become mainly dietary effects on the bacterial flora associated with the enamel surface and other niches in the oral cavity rather than nutritional, systemic effects.

Most food components have an effect on implantation, colonization, and metabolism of dental plaque bacteria. Food carbohydrates are the most important dietary factors affecting the type and number of plaque bacteria and their metabolic activity. The type, amount, texture, and intake frequency of carbohydrates determine to a large extent the chemical composition of plaque, and the nature and quantity of bacteria, the extracellular and intracellular polysaccharides that are formed in plaque. Other food components such as protein and fats can also modify plaque metabolism by: (1) providing basic amino acids, which could neutralize the glycolytic effect of sugars; (2) stimulating the flow rate of saliva, which could buffer acids produced by plaque; or (3) modifying the residence times of food, which could limit the availability of fermentable substrate to the plaque. These dietary effects and food interactions are complex and are being investigated.[49, 68, 130]

Dietary carbohydrates are major sources of energy for plaque bacteria and also contribute the essential substrate to form intracellular and extracellular polysaccharides used as storage material and also as adhesive molecules in the colonization process. The major carbohydrate components of foods are the polymeric carbohydrates such as starches, dextrins, and gums; disaccharides; monosaccharides; and sugar alcohols. Recently, some modified sugars that have been proposed as sugar substitutes and some synthetic sweeteners have been added to foods. The latter are not readily metabolized by plaque bacteria and to a very limited extent by the human body. Synthetic sweeteners, although sweet, cannot be classified chemically as carbohydrates, and they have a variety of molecular structures that determine the sweet chemoreception.[140] It is important to review briefly the effects of some of these different carbohydrates and sweeteners on plaque metabolism and caries activity.

Food starches are not easily digested by plaque bacteria, but it should be noted that dietary carbohydrates could influence plaque metabolism as they come in contact with the tooth surface during mastication and also later when they remain in the oral cavity as food debris. Starches are then hydrolyzed by salivary amylases to readily fermentable units of maltose and glucose. Food snacks that combine starch and sugars may be far more detrimental to oral health than commonly considered. The residence time of foods in the oral cavity, as suggested by Caldwell,[32] is important because it not only extends the availability of sugars in foods to plaque bacteria but also generates new fermentable substrates from substances previously considered inert. Starch fermentation is not only aided by salivary action, but also by metabolic activity of several microorganisms that are present in the oral cavity of humans and that have powerful hydrolyzing enzymes to degrade starch residues.

Sucrose is a disaccharide commonly found in manufactured foods and beverages (and also in some fruits), which provides a source of energy, a desirable sweet taste, and specific technologic properties to the food.[136] The sucrose generally used for these different purposes is obtained from sugar cane or beets. It is highly refined to yield a purified food ingredient that consequently keeps well in storage and whose only nutritional contribution is energy. Therefore, foods that are made up essentially of sugar as a major ingredient provide mainly calories. Examples of these types of foods are confectionary products that contain 60 to 100 per cent sugar.

Other major disaccharides besides sucrose are lactose and maltose, which, upon hydrolysis, can yield monosaccharides such as glucose, fructose, and galactose. These sugars are readily fermented by plaque bacteria as a source of energy to produce ATP and a variety of acids. Disaccharides such as sucrose can be hydrolyzed by a β-D-fructofuranoside fructohydrolase (invertase: EC 3.2.1.26) to glucose and fructose. This enzyme has been identified[96] as an intracellular enzyme that can be induced by sucrose in *Strep. sanguis* but was found to be constitutive in *Strep. mutans*. An amylomaltase that can hydrolyze maltose also has been found in *Strep. mutans*. The latter is important as it could be a metabolic step in the utilization of starch breakdown products such as maltose and maltodextrins. Metabolism of sucrose by dental plaque has been extensively evaluated,[22, 103] and the total sucrolytic capacity of plaque[3, 4] points to a key role of this sugar for plaque growth and caries-associated metabolic activity, which includes not only acid production but also formation of extracellular and intracellular polysaccharides contributing to the caries virulence of plaque. The contributory role of sucrose in concentrations ranging from 1 to 65 per cent to the colonization of enamel surfaces by *Strep. mutans* has been clearly described as being caused by: (1) preformed glucans associated with cells or teeth, and (2) new glucan polymers synthesized by cells that are weakly attached initially to the tooth surface.[157] These microbial polysaccharides serve not only for colonization purposes but also as substrates for streptococci and other plaque bacteria; therefore, they play an important role in the development and maintenance of dental plaque.[124]

Fermentation of dietary carbohydrates by plaque yields lactic acid in concentrations of about 50 per cent of the total acid concentration. However, it is not uncommon in many plaque samples to find that acetic and formic acids represent the major acids present. Whether lactic or formic acid is produced could make a vast difference, considering the fact that formic acid is a stronger acid. Larger amounts of formic acid could be expected to be produced in the deeper layers of plaque next to enamel, where a carbon-limited environment may be predominant.

The acid produced by the fermentation of monosaccharides brings about an increase in plaque acidity. Following exposure to a 0.1 per cent glucose solution, the pH of human plaque may decrease by one unit within 5 minutes and will not return to the original value for 20 to 30 minutes.[82] Higher sugar concentrations (10 per cent) will lower the pH further to values below 5.0 and proportionally increase the time necessary to return to original pH values. Stephan[149] first described this behavior of plaque and also reported that plaques on the labial surfaces of maxillary and mandibular teeth differed in pH minima obtained by these procedures. Relating this phenomena to caries activity on these tooth surfaces and taking into consideration the physicochemical characteristics of enamel, he postulated the existence of a critical pH (4.5 to 5.5) below which enamel would demineralize and loose its integrity. Other investigators[83] have extended these studies and made significant contributions to the understanding of the acid-base reactions of plaque and their significance to demineralization and remineralization processes on the tooth surface.

The literature pertaining to the relation between caries and sucrose, glucose, and fructose is voluminous and when evaluated as a whole, indicates that there are specific roles for sucrose relative to plaque metabolism that make it more contributory to plaque formation than glucose and fructose. However, there is no experimental evidence[28] to support the contention that if these monosaccharides were substituted for sucrose in the diet of people, a reduction in caries would follow. The health aspects of sucrose, glucose, fructose, and invert sugar have been reviewed,[90-92] and no evidence was found that their consumption is a health hazard, except for their contribution to dental caries.

Three sugar alcohols, mannitol, sorbitol, and xylitol, have been evaluated as possible substitutes for sucrose to reduce the caries-promoting properties of sugar-containing foods. Evaluation of clinical and experimental data show that there is a potential usefulness in such substitutions.[135] The health aspects of xylitol[93] and sorbitol[94] used as sugar substitutes have been reviewed recently. No major hazard has been identified, in spite of the fact that the results of studies at the Huntingdon Research Centre in England showed bladder tumors and stones in male mice fed diets containing 20 per cent xylitol. These studies are now being re-evaluated to determine whether the nutritional composition of the diet used was adequate or not. Other problems associated with sorbitol and xylitol ingestion were diarrhea and flatulence caused by delayed intestinal absorption of these two sugar alcohols, which is limited and occurs through passive transport mechanisms. The Turku sugar studies[134] suggest that there are no major laxative effects if the xylitol dose is kept under 30 g and is provided at intervals of not less than 4 hours between doses. The critical dose for sorbitol to avoid osmotic diarrhea and flatulence is lower and of the order of 20 to 25 g. Adaptation to large doses of these sugar alcohols can take place when the doses are progressively increased.

Energy metabolism by plaque bacteria of these sugar alcohols seems to differ. Glucose and fructose enter the glycolytic metabolic pathway directly through formation of glucose-6-phosphate and fructose-6-phosphate by hexokinases. Polyol sugars, such as sorbitol and mannitol, can be fermented through this glycolytic pathway too. Studies[22] in which *Strep. mutans* cells adapted to grow on mannitol or sorbitol showed the presence of induced mannitol-1-phosphate dehydrogenase and sorbitol-6-phosphate dehydrogenase. This allows the conversion of these polyols to fructose-6-phosphate, which then can enter the glycolytic pathway. *Strep. mutans* has, as a specific biochemical characteristic, the ability to ferment mannitol and sorbitol, and when grown in the presence of these substrates, the concentrations of these dehydrogenases are increased. It is possible that fermentation of sorbitol (which, in the case of *Strep. mutans* adapted cells, is marked by production of high levels of alcohol dehydrogenase[20, 21] and a shift away from the homolactic fermentation) might not represent an important contribution to acid plaque production. However, ability to utilize and ferment polyols such as sorbitol, which are widely used in some types of confectionary products, might contribute to the metabolism of *Strep. mutans* and other bacteria, thus providing a nutritional advantage in the colonization process and subsequent metabolic activities within plaque.

Xylitol differs from sorbitol and mannitol in that it is not metabolized by streptococci, especially *Strep. mutans*;[84] therefore, from the standpoint of plaque biochemistry, it cannot contribute to lowering of the pH. Human studies suggest that this polyol could be administered without danger of accommodation or adaptation of plaque streptococci. Some questions that arise relative to this polyol and other sugars proposed as substitutes for dietary sugars include: (1) whether the other numerous bacteria in dental plaque and the oral cavity at large are capable of metabolizing the polyol; (2) what, if any, will be the bacterial interactions (synergisms or antagonisms) stimulated by continuous presence of this new substrate in the oral cavity; (3) what will be the net oral health effect obtained by partial substitution, in view of the ubiquitousness of other sugars; and (4) what will be the cost, safety, and organoleptic acceptability of snack foods manufactured with such sugar substitutes?

In vitro studies[17, 41] to determine the potential of other different sugar alcohols such as maltitol and Lycasin (a hydrogenated partial hydrolysate of starch, which contains free sorbitol, disaccharides, and oligosaccharides) indicated that they were fermented by plaque at a slower rate than glucose, sucrose, and invert sugar. In these studies, acid production from sorbitol was observed among more than 80 per cent of the strains of streptococci and most of the lactobacilli strains tested, while no acid production was produced by xylitol added to plaque. Only two strains of bacteria, which are not normal components of human plaque (*Strep. avium* [ATCC 14025] and *L. salvarius* subsp. *salivarius* [ATCC 11741]), fermented xylitol.

Other sugar substitutes that have been recently proposed include: (1) L sorbose,[106] which is not fermented by *Strep. mutans* or *A. viscosus*; (2) lactitol (β-D-galactopyranosido-1, 4-sorbitol) and isomaltitol (α-D-glucopyranosido-1, 6-sorbitol), for which there is limited information about their metabolism by intestinal bacteria and dental plaque; (3) Palatinit, an equimolar mixture of isomaltitol and α-D-glucopyranosido-1, 6-mannitol,[79] which was tested in programmed feeding experiments with rats and found to be less cariogenic than sucrose and lactose and roughly comparable to L-sorbose; (4) coupling sugars free of sugar (CSSF), which are prepared from starch as a white powder containing a large number of components including glucose, fructose, and maltose in various combinations[67] and which reduced caries scores in rats in comparison to sucrose; and (5) 2-deoxy-D-glucose, which has been suggested as a sugar substitute, although another report of a caries study in rats[153] found no caries inhibitory properties.

Several conferences[45, 61, 142] as well as some recent reviews[97, 117, 135] have discussed the many complicated scientific, legal, industrial, regulatory, and technologic aspects of the use of sugar substitutes. At this time there are a variety of substances that have been proposed and as indicated previously, that have different degrees of caries activity, sweetening power, undesirable side effects, cost, and availability. To this list, we can also add a variety of synthetic, non-calorie sweeteners such as cyclamates, aspartame, monellin, chlorosucrose derivatives,[81] dehydrochalcones, and many others that have been proposed. These synthetic sweeteners are used in extremely small concentrations in a food because of their intense sweetness, and they are not readily metabolized by plaque to produce acids and other metabolic end products. Therefore, they are not caries promoting. They are also potential candidates as sugar substitutes, but it will take a long time before their effectiveness and safety are demonstrated to such an extent that regulatory agencies will approve their use in snack foods intended for humans.

Nutrition and Periodontal Disease

The relation between nutrition and periodontal disease has been evaluated in epidemiologic, animal, and metabolic studies.[1, 2, 36, 44] Barros and Witkop[10] surveyed the prevalence of periodontal disease in a Chilean population and related nutritional status in nearly 2,000 individuals of various age groups. Significant in their findings was the increase in prevalence and severity of the disease with age increase. Periodontal disease, assessed by pocket depth, was found to be generally severe and widespread in older persons, even though 50 per cent of all persons between 15 and 19 years of age suffered from the disease in a milder form. Periodontal disease was even detected in children nine years old and younger. This same pattern was found in a nutritional survey done by INCAP (Instituto de Nutricion de Centro America y Panama) in Honduras in 1969,[77] in which periodontal index (PI) scores were even higher. The disease was present in young people, although the most severe levels were found among the older persons. In both of these groups of people, oral hygiene status was assessed by presence or absence of soft debris and dental calculus. A marked, statistically significant correlation was found in each age group between the presence of debris, calculus, or both and the severity of the periodontal disease.

The assumption that nutritional deficiencies may play a major role in the etiology of periodontal disease was tested in the Chilean study by determining serum and urinary vitamin levels and relating these values to the periodontal status of the individual. Persons with acceptable or high vitamin levels showed no less severe disease than persons with deficient or low levels.

Studies done by Russell[131] in different parts of the world to evaluate the relation between biochemical findings and periodontal disease in humans have yielded no significant correlations. The highest correlation was always found to be with a high oral debris index. To conclude from this epidemiologic data that nutritional factors do not enter at all into the etiology of the disease is incorrect because:

1. The etiology of the disease is multifactorial, and no single factor is solely responsible for its pathologic expression in humans.

2. Recognition should be given to the fact that the disease has a variety of clinical expressions that may involve a different etiologic group of factors that respond differently to systemic, nutritional manipulations.

3. The data have usually been gathered from individuals with a high disease severity. At these late stages nutritional factors have only a minor role. Nutritional effects on periodontal disease, if they are present, should be detected at the initial stages of the disease when the delicate balance between a healthy or a diseased tissue is being established.

4. The evaluation of nutritional status in most surveys is really limited to biochemical determinations carried out on a certain day, and this does not provide adequate understanding about the previous nutritional history of the individual.

5. Periodontal disease demonstrates several stages of progression, which extend from a mild gingivitis to extensive bone resorption, deep pocket formation, bleeding, and finally, complete disruption of the periodontium with loss of teeth. It is important to understand the relation of nutrition to the various stages of the disease process.

6. Further understanding of the influence of malnutrition on the humoral and cell immunity system is necessary.

Epidemiologic evidence does not support the assumption that broad or specific nutritional deficiencies induce formation of deep periodontal pockets in the absence of local irritants such as subgingival plaque and calculus. However, this type of information does not indicate whether transient or chronic deficiencies are a factor at the initial stages of the disease (which are poorly diagnosed in most surveys) or whether undernutrition or malnutrition modifies the course and prognosis of the disease.

In general, two major effects of foods and nutrients in foods have been postulated to affect periodontal disease: a local effect and a systemic effect. The proposed local effects of diet include the following: (1) provision by food residues of substrate material for specific bacteria in dental plaque; (2) removal of large accumulations of plaque in close apposition to the gingival tissues; (3) stimulation of saliva flow and functional stimulation of the periodontium and the alveolar bone by masticatory action; and (4) immunologic stimulation of periodontal tissues brought about by food antigens. Of these, the first two have been shown to be untrue, but the last two have been supported by results of several investigators.[126, 147, 148]

The systemic effects of nutrition are most important and are mainly related to the repair and defense mechanisms of the host. These involve: (1) oral fluids such as saliva and the gingival fluids, (2) maintenance of the epithelial barrier, (3) specific and nonspecific immunity, and (4) repair and maintenance processes of the periodontium and alveolar bone.

Marginal nutritional deficiency in protein, ascorbic acid, folic acid,[40] vitamin A, or minerals such as iron or calcium may contribute to: (1) alterations in the mucosal barrier, which affect the permeability of these tissues to a number of toxic compounds; (2) induction of "end organ deficiencies,"[1] which interfere with repair processes normally contributing to maintenance of the integrity of the tissue; and (3) impairment and disorganization of the immune defense system, which contributes to the host resistance mechanism.

Studies that have addressed the behavior of gingival tissue response to local irritations in particular indicate that malnutrition directly influences the metabolic behavior of the tissue and, indirectly, the course of the disease. Because of the rapid turnover of the connective tissue of the periodontium, nutrients such as protein and ascorbic acid, which, as previously seen, intervene in collagen synthesis, have been studied in detail.

Vitamin C deficiency has been reported to be associated with edema, hemorrhage, osteoporosis of alveolar bone, tooth mobility, and changes in periodontal fibers. Although inflammation of the gingiva is frequently seen in humans deficient in ascorbic acid, gingivitis in animals is only observed in association with some form of local irritation.

Attempts to show clear relations between ascorbic acid nutriture, as determined by blood ascorbic acid levels, and severity of periodontitis have not been clear. The same

is true for protein malnutrition. Some investigators have found protein supplementation to have a beneficial effect on the health of the periodontium, while others have not observed a clear effect.

The study of the etiologic factors involved in periodontal disease has been severely handicapped and, to a certain point, confused by the following experimental limitations:

1. Lack of an appropriate experimental animal model to study periodontal disease.

2. Difficulties in evaluation and objective quantitation of initial stages of gingivitis.

3. Technical limitations in the administration and standardization of the local stress factor in experimental models.

In spite of the limitations outlined above, a definite understanding of the role of nutrition in periodontal disease is emerging today. While nutritional deficiencies do not independently initiate the pathologic breakdown of the periodontal tissues, they may set the stage and definitely modify the severity and extent of lesions by influencing the response and repair properties of the tissues. This effect, together with other biochemical changes, such as the ones brought about by aging, determines the outcome of the interaction between pathologic stresses and resistance mechanisms. Even aging processes are known to be influenced by nutritional factors, as shown by the general appearance and increased oral disease (for example, noma) susceptibility of children and young adults in nutritionally deprived areas compared to same age but well-fed individuals in other communities.[43] Other factors such as hormones, immunologic response, and enzymatic activities play a definite role in periodontal diseases, but their mode of action and the degree of contribution to the pathologic process varies in different individuals in such a way that their effect is difficult to evaluate clinically. Standardized and well-defined animal models would be helpful in the study of these interactions.

The influence of nutrition on periodontal disease, therefore, appears to be exerted mainly at three different levels: (1) on the metabolism of the gingival crevice-plaque flora,[146] (2) on the repair process in the connective tissue at the local site, and (3) on the immunologic response to microbial antigens.

The role of nutrition in the etiology and management of periodontal disease can be considered to be secondary, in the sense that it can only help by facilitating the repair process necessary to re-establish healthy tissue, provided that therapeutic procedures are used to remove specific components of the bacterial flora, as well as local irritants and debris interfering with tissue healing. However, once oral hygiene has been established, the role of nutrition becomes primary and vitamins such as ascorbic acid, folic acid, and vitamin A, some minerals such as calcium, copper, and manganese, and the essential amino acids become necessary for protein synthesis, calcification, and final re-establishment and maintenance of the integrity of the periodontium.

Nutrition and Oral Cancer

Cancer is the second leading cause of death in the U.S. and is exceeded only by cardiovascular disease. In 1980, approximately 405,000 persons died of cancer. Incidence of lung cancer has increased; colon-rectum and breast cancer have maintained the same incidence; and oral cancer has shown a definite increase. Approximately 5 per cent of all tumors are found in the oral cavity with a male to female ratio of 5 to 3. However, in certain regions in the U.S. this ratio has been reduced to 1 to 1.

Reasons for these changes are unknown, since the etiology and pathogenesis of oral tumors are poorly understood. Several factors have been suggested as potentiating cancer development. These include ionizing radiations; exposure over long periods of time to solar radiations, which seems to be related to cancer of the lower lip; tobacco in its various forms: cigarette and pipe smoking, chewing tobacco, and snuff; alcohol consumption over long periods of time and in excessive quantities; and finally

chronic infectious lesions such as tertiary syphilis. All these factors represent either a chronic stress factor to the oral tissues or a debilitating habit, which may interfere with normal nutrition and development of systemic defenses.

The relationship between nutrition and cancer can be viewed at three levels:

1. Diet as a factor in cancer causation (etiology).
2. The effect of cancer and its treatment on nutritional status.
3. Nutritional management of the cancer patient.

Epidemiologic studies of cancer indicate that its incidence varies worldwide and seems to change with migration of individuals from one region to another. This has led to the concept that environmental factors play an important role in carcinogenesis, and that diet and nutrition are related to approximately 50 per cent of all cancers in men and women. Examples of these studies are the Japanese data[65] on the relationship between food consumption and cancer of the stomach and colon and also the correlations between mortality from breast cancer and per capita consumption of dietary fat.[26, 51]

Some of the major aspects of the relationship between food components and the etiology of cancer are:[25]

1. Presence of carcinogens or pro-carcinogens in foods (saccharin, nitrites, aflatoxin, cycasin, bracken fern toxins, and so on).
2. Oxidative damage to cells and tissues (lack of antioxidants such as tocopherols, ascorbic acid, and so on).
3. Excessive intake of certain nutrients (particularly animal fat and its consequence on bile metabolism).
4. Altered metabolism of carcinogens by diet components (particularly by fiber in foods).
5. Altered fecal bacterial populations caused by dietary factors (*Clostridium* vs. *Lactobacillus*).
6. Chromosome damage (nutritional deficiency of vitamins such as folic acid).
7. Abnormal repair of chromosome damage.

8. Altered metabolism of hormones (for example, resulting in obesity).

9. Impaired immunity to tumor cells and viruses.

10. Special interactions between genetic susceptibility and dietary factors.

The other major relationship between nutrition and cancer relates to the nutritional impact of cancer and its treatment.[62] Table 8–6 describes the major effects of cancer cachexia and anorexia on nutritional status. Oral cancer, because of the physical impediment it produces on food mastication and ingestion, is especially detrimental to the nutritional status of the patient. Table 8–7 describes some of the consequences of cancer treatment predisposing to nutrition problems. In these patients, assessment of nutritional status is important in order to monitor their progress and to decide on the best

TABLE 8–6 SOME EFFECTS OF NEOPLASTIC DISEASES ON NUTRITIONAL STATUS

1. Malnutrition secondary to persistent anorexia.
2. Malnutrition associated with impaired food intake secondary to obstruction.
3. Malabsorption associated with:
   A. Deficiency of pancreatic enzymes or bile salts.
   B. Infiltration of small bowel by neoplasms, such as lymphoma or carcinoma.
   C. Fistulous bypass of small bowel.
   D. Gastric hypersecretion inhibiting pancreatic enzymes (in Zollinger-Ellison syndrome).
   E. Blind loop secondary to partial upper small bowel obstruction.
   F. Malnutrition−induced villous hypoplasia.
4. Protein-losing enteropathy (e.g. in gastric carcinoma, lymphoma, or with lymphatic obstruction).
5. Electrolyte and fluid balance disturbances associated with:
   A. Persistent vomiting in obstruction.
   B. Vomiting secondary to increased intracranial pressure from tumors.
   C. Small-bowel fluid losses from fistula.
   D. Diarrhea associated with hormone-secreting tumors (e.g. carcinoid syndrome, Zollinger-Ellison syndrome, Verner-Morrison syndrome) and villous adenoma of the colon.
   E. Inappropriate antidiuretic hormone secretion associated with certain tumors.
   F. Hyperadrenalism secondary to excessive corticotropin or corticosteroid production by tumors.

(From Goodhart, R. S., and Shils, M. E.: Modern Nutrition in Health and Disease. Philadelphia, Lea and Febiger, 1980.)

TABLE 8–7 CONSEQUENCES OF CANCER TREATMENT PREDISPOSING TO NUTRITION PROBLEMS

1. Radiation treatment.
   A. Radiation of oropharyngeal area.
      (1) Destruction of sense of taste; xerostomia and odynophagia; loss of teeth.
   B. Radiation to lower neck and mediastinum.
      (1) Esophagitis with dysphagia.
      (2) Fibrosis with esophageal stricture.
   C. Radiation of abdomen and pelvis.
      (1) Bowel damage, acute and chronic, with diarrhea, malabsorption, stenosis and obstruction, fistulization.
2. Surgical treatment.
   A. Radical resection of oropharyngeal area.
      (1) Chewing and swallowing difficulties.
      (2) Tube feeding possibly required.
   B. Esophagectomy and esophageal reconstruction.
      (1) Gastric stasis and hypochlorhydria secondary to vagotomy.
      (2) Steatorrhea.
      (3) Diarrhea.
   C. Gastrectomy (high subtotal or total).
      (1) Dumping syndrome.
      (2) Malabsorption.
      (3) Achlorhydria and lack of intrinsic factor.
      (4) Hypoglycemia.
   D. Intestinal resection.
      (1) Jejunum.
         (a) Decreased efficiency of absorption of many nutrients.
      (2) Ileum.
         (a) Vitamin B_{12} deficiency.
         (b) Bile salt losses with diarrhea.
         (c) Hyperoxaluria.
      (3) Massive bowel resection.
         (a) Life-threatening malabsorption.
         (b) Malnutrition.
         (c) Metabolic acidosis.
      (4) Ileostomy and colostomy.
         (a) Complications of salt and water balance.
   E. Blind-loop syndrome.
   F. Pancreatectomy.
      (1) Malabsorption.
      (2) Diabetes mellitus.
3. Chemotherapy treatment.
   A. Corticosteroids.
      (1) Fluid and electrolyte problems.
      (2) Nitrogen and calcium losses.
      (3) Hyperglycemia.
   B. Antimetabolites, alkylating agents and other drugs.

(From Goodhart, R. S., and Shils, M. E.: Modern Nutrition in Health and Disease. Philadelphia, Lea and Febiger, 1980.)

nutritional therapy, which can be supportive, adjunctive, or definitive, depending on the condition of the patient and the antitumor treatment being used.

Nutrition and Infection

In considering the interactions between nutritional status and infection in the individual, two aspects should be recognized:

1. An infection usually precipitates or aggravates the malnourished state of an individual by a combination of mechanisms to be discussed later.

2. Nutritional status influences host susceptibility to infections. Scrimshaw and coworkers[138] have discussed this relationship thoroughly, pointing out that some of these influences are synergistic in nature. Infections involving bacteria, rickettsiae, and various parasites have been enhanced by nutritional deficiencies as well as nutritional excess, for example, obesity. Antagonistic interactions have been described in which malnutrition reduces the severity of infection. This type of interaction has been observed in animal experiments involving certain viral, protozoan, or helminthic infections. These interactions are of special interest to oral pathologic conditions such as periodontal disease and extraction or surgical wounds.

The effect of stress factors such as infections, including severe oral infections, is primarily on protein metabolism, especially protein catabolism. This effect will in turn affect the maintenance of normal tissue barriers, the production of enzymes essential to repair processes, production of antibody proteins, and the activity of phagocytic cells.

The interference with protein synthesis alters the ability of specific cells to initiate, maintain, or increase the rate of production of proteins essential for maintaining tissue integrity. Clinically, these events, if important enough, determine wasting of the body. If localized to a certain tissue area, as in the oral cavity, it leads to pathologic changes in the tissue that may eventually affect the whole organism. Biochemically, these effects of infectious stress can be detected as an altered metabolic balance of nutrients. Nutrients are on a positive or negative balance depending on whether there is a net gain or a net loss of the nutrient from the body. Infection, trauma, emotional disturbances, and other stresses precipitate a loss of nitrogen from the body, thus producing a negative nitrogen balance. This is produced by interference with protein synthesis, increased catabolism, and other body reactions, which have been collectively referred to by Selye[139] as the alarm reaction. This reaction is probably triggered by hormones, such as the glucocorticoids and others. The effect of these reactions is not only to increase nitrogen loss but also to induce losses of electrolytes such as sodium and potassium in the urine. This is further compounded by losses of these electrolytes in febrile sweats, vomiting, diarrhea, and blood loss. Other mineral elements are also affected in these stress situations. In association with fever, surgery, trauma, or bed immobilization, urinary losses of calcium, phosphate, zinc, and iron are commonly seen in patients.

At the beginning of the chapter the nutrient requirements of a healthy human were discussed and the importance of fulfilling these needs for growth, development, and maintenance of body functions was indicated. Most of these allowances, however, do not take into consideration the stressed or the diseased state. If the stress is mild or transiently applied, the nutritional insult will not have lasting consequences, for individuals will be able to compensate for it from their own stores or from their diet. Supplementation of the losses will not really be necessary, for the reaction to the stress is mild. If, however, the stress is one that is chronically present and of enough severity, then patients will continue to debilitate, with undue prolongation of their diseased state and discomfort. It is especially important under these circumstances to evaluate the nutrient losses and supplement the patient's diet with the nutrients that are essential for the defense mechanisms and general well-being of the patient.

Nutrition and Surgical Stress

The relation between nutrition and surgical stress, although generally recognized,[156] has not received proper attention. Oral surgery is especially stressful to the patient, because together with the usual lack of appetite characteristic of disease and depressed emotional status seen in surgery patients, there can be physical disability, pain, or discomfort in the oral tissues with which food must come in contact. The inability to masticate, the increased physiologic need for certain nutrients, and the metabolic losses previously discussed tend to induce rapid nutritional degradation in surgery patients. It is the surgeon's responsibility to determine when and how to start adequate feeding of seriously ill patients. If surgery is drastic, it is usually not realistic to offer complete nourishment during the first 24 to 72 hours, but soon after this initial period the patient should be offered the full recommended dietary allowance plus any supplements that might be deemed necessary. In cases in which the surgical stress is not as severe, soft or liquid diets can be given by tube or conventional means, depending on the condition of the patient.

The nutritional requirements of a surgical patient can be determined by evaluating the following:

1. The previous nutritional state of the individual.

2. The nature and severity of the surgery performed.

3. The amount and type of nutrients that are being lost from the body.

4. The anticipated duration of the injury or disease.

One aspect of special consideration in many of these cases is the question of calorie density of the diet fed to patients. It is important to note that while the rate of energy expenditure of a person sleeping and reclining is approximately 1 kcal per minute, this rate is three times larger when walking and may increase four- or five-fold during active exercise. The patient confined to bed will have a low energy requirement because of immobilization, but it should be noted that restlessness in a bed patient may increase energy requirements by 10 or 20 per cent, and fever increases caloric needs by approximately 13 per cent for each degree C rise in body temperature (7.2 per cent for each degree F). If large protein losses are known to have taken place, then a 50 to 100 per cent increase in the caloric density of the diet is in order. In severe disease or trauma, therefore, an energy requirement of 2500 to 4000 calories per day is not unusual, and if such a level cannot be achieved through the diet, parenteral administration should then be considered.

The other nutritional aspect in which control is of extreme importance is the nitrogen balance. If a person sustains a fracture of the jaw in an accident or undergoes extensive surgery, the first response is an increased urinary nitrogen excretion, reflecting protein degradation. As indicated previously, this is characteristic of the alarm reaction. It reaches a peak in four to seven days and may continue for three to seven weeks, depending on severity or duration of the stress. If immobilized in bed, nitrogen losses from immobilization may vary between one and two g per day. Fracture of a long bone, for example, may lead to a loss of 9 per cent of body protein in one to two weeks. It is desirable, therefore, to bring the patient as soon as possible into positive nitrogen balance as this will enhance the therapeutic measures and shorten the recovery period.

Among the vitamins, ascorbic acid has a special role in stress conditions such as surgery or trauma. Numerous vitamin C studies have pointed out that besides the role in hydroxylation of proline in the newly formed collagen to be used in repair of tissues, this vitamin is involved in the function of the adrenal cortex. During the alarm reaction, the body loses large amounts of vitamin C from the adrenal cortex and probably its rate of utilization is increased two or three times. Administration of vitamin C is recommended in those cases in which the demand of the organism for this nutrient is increased.

It is not possible to give definite recommendations for the administration of vitamins to surgical patients, but the following guidelines can be used in establishing the best levels for each case:

1. A previously healthy patient with a minor illness expected to last less than ten days, who is ambulatory and eating well and who has no history of previous inadequate nutrition, needs to be given no special consideration concerning his vitamin requirements.

2. When the foregoing qualifications are not met, the patient is given a maintenance level that is approximately twice the minimum requirement.

3. When the patient receives his nutrition by the intravenous route, he should be given a maintenance level supplemented with vitamin C.

4. When a serious illness or severe trauma exists, the requirement for the first few days should be supplied at the therapeutic level. Thereafter, the patient should receive the maintenance level until recovery is complete.

A discussion of nutritional rehabilitation is not really complete without consideration of water, electrolytes, and trace-element requirements. Water accounts for 50 to 75 per cent of body weight, depending on age and body fat. Numerous factors determining water loss preclude the setting of a general value for a minimal requirement. However, under ordinary circumstances, a reasonable allowance is 1.0 ml/kcal for adults and 1.5 ml/kcal for infants. Special attention to water intake should be paid in situations involving (1) infants being offered high protein diets, (2) comatose patients, and (3) patients with fever, polyuria, diarrhea, or excessive sweating.

Electrolytes such as sodium and potassium should be carefully controlled. Sodium (Na), since it is an extracellular cation, enters into the maintenance of osmotic equilibrium and body fluid volume, and potassium (K) acts intracellularly to control cellular enzyme function. The normal adult intake of sodium is approximately 100 to 300 mEq per day and that of K ranges between 50 and 150 mEq per day. Because sweat contains 20 to 50 mEq of Na per liter, the losses from this source during high fever can be up to 350 mEq per day. Monitoring Na and K is important, therefore, during prolonged intravenous feeding.

Other elements, such as magnesium, iron, zinc, and manganese, present in low concentrations in body tissues and fluids, are severely depleted during stress conditions of different types. While little is known about the specific amounts of zinc and manganese required under stress conditions,

they are still important, and current research suggests that they may play an important role in healing of hard and soft tissues.

NUTRITIONAL AND DIETARY MEASURES IN THE PREVENTION AND MANAGEMENT OF ORAL DISEASE

Dietary Patterns in the U.S.

Discussion of nutritional and dietary factors affecting oral health requires a brief overview of the present dietary habits of people living in the U.S. in order to understand the nature of the problem and to evaluate how reasonable and realistic the proposed solutions to these problems seem to be.

The food supply, the dietary patterns, and indeed, the lifestyle in general in the U.S. has changed markedly during the last 50 years. The U.S.D.A. Economic Research Service has compiled average per capita food consumption estimates based on food disappearance statistics that indicate that certain food commodity groups such as cereal products, potatoes, and sweet potatoes have shown a steady decline; other foods such as meat, poultry, and fish have shown an increase; and still other foods such as eggs showed an increase in consumption during the fifties, but their use (and also that of butter) has decreased in the last 30 years.[52] Although there have been changes in dietary patterns and food supply, total sugar and sweetener consumption and total caloric intake estimates during these years have remained essentially unchanged at approximately 119 lbs/capita/year and 3,300 calories intake per day per person.[123] Today, as 50 years ago, approximately 12 per cent of these calories are supplied by protein in foods. However, 42 per cent of total calories are now supplied by fats (representing a 10 per cent increase) and the rest, or approximately 46 per cent, are supplied by carbohydrates and alcoholic beverages. Since total caloric intake has not changed appreciably and fat consumption has increased, carbohydrate consumption has decreased, mostly through a decline in the use of flour, starches, and cereal foods. This decrease, which mainly took place in the fifties, is being essentially maintained today.[123] While the per capita consumption of sucrose has remained essentially constant over the last fifty years (except for the war years), the disappearance data on total sweeteners, high fructose syrups, and glucose syrups indicate a steady increase in consumption. Interestingly, the use of refined sugar has also changed.[29, 123] While household use has diminished, sugar utilization in total processed foods and soft drink beverages has increased. Today, approximately two thirds of the sucrose used in the U.S. is for industrial purposes, particularly soft drinks and bakery industries, rather than for household use.[66]

One more recent change in the dietary trend in the U.S. should be pointed out in relation to carbohydrate consumption. There is a generalized increase in snacking between meals with foods that contain high concentrations of sugar. Snack foods include some products that are new foods, but there are also many items that are not new to supermarket shelves. Most of the latter (cookies, crackers, ice cream, soft drinks, and candy) have been traditionally considered as desserts, but increasingly they are being consumed throughout the day as snacks. This dietary change could have been brought about by new consumer attitudes associated with better income, informal lifestyle, and increased leisure time when snacking is frequent. These behavioral preferences have been reinforced by manufacturer's marketing and advertising strategies, which are directed to fit these new, consumer attitudes.[66]

This brief description of our present dietary habits, the changes that have taken place over the last fifty years, and the new dietary trends of people in the U.S. can be summarized as follows:

1. Total sucrose consumption has not increased substantially, and therefore the total amount consumed cannot be made wholly responsible for the fluctuations seen in caries prevalence.

2. There has been an increase in the consumption of glucose and fructose, which have replaced sucrose in various products.

3. Sugar use in the manufacture of numerous snack foods that are consumed frequently throughout the day, particularly between meals, has increased. This remains a finding that needs further study and attention. It is possibly the most important factor in the relationship between sugar-containing foods and dental caries.

4. The rate of obesity among American adults (50 per cent) and children (as high as 35 per cent) is a clear indication of excessive consumption of calories, lack of energy expenditure, or both. The estimated per capita consumption of calories per day is 3,300. Given the age distribution of the U.S. population and considering the recommended levels of intake for the different age groups (that is, preschoolers — 1,300 to 1,800 calories, elementary school children — 1,800 to 2,400, adult females — 2,000, and males — 2,700),[107] it can be concluded that per capita calorie intake should be reduced. Sugar and fats, because they are virtually devoid of nutrients except calories, are likely candidates for reduction of use. However, care should be exercised in the implementation of such broad dietary recommendations, since decisions on reduction of calorie sources have to be made at an individual level, taking into consideration the type of diet consumed, as well as other factors such as physical activity, sex, age, and climate that are relevant to the determination of the energy requirement of an individual.

These characteristics of sugar consumption are especially detrimental to oral health when they are combined with the increase in the nibbling habit that also has taken place over the last twenty years. Frequent nibbling of sugar-containing foods stimulates implantation, colonization, and metabolic activity of cariogenic microorganisms, thus enhancing the formation of dental plaque and the development of plaque-dependent diseases such as caries. The evidence for this comes from human studies such as the Vipeholm, where a small amount of candy distributed over several feedings during the day was associated with a significant increase in caries.[55] The most convincing evidence, however, is provided by animal experiments in which the severity of caries is seen to be proportional to the number of feedings. The maximum caries scores occurred when the animals were allowed to feed *ad libitum*, in the nibbling fashion commonly observed in rats that eat throughout the night.[86, 88, 141]

Each time foods containing fermentable carbohydrates are brought in contact with dental plaque, bacteria metabolize them and produce acid and other metabolic end products in proportion to the amount and time of exposure to the sugars in foods.[68, 83] Therefore, the combined experience of clinical, animal, and *in vitro* studies indicates the undesirability of exposing teeth frequently to sugars. No data are yet available to indicate what concentration of sugar or what number of exposures is considered to be safe for human teeth.

Dietary Patterns Compatible with Oral Health: Behavioral Modifications and Management

Dentists can and should use nutrition in the prevention and cure of oral disease.[38, 42, 63, 64, 100, 121, 143, 144] Furthermore, they can provide a valuable service to the community by guidance of the dietary habits of their patients even after treatment is completed. Some oral diseases such as dental caries can be prevented or controlled if appropriate diets are used consistently and early enough after tooth eruption. In other diseases, as well as in surgical stress and trauma, nutrition can alleviate and shorten the recovery and convalescence period.

Several approaches have been devised to carry out dietary counseling, such as the ones designed at Tufts University by Dr. A. E. Nizel,[120, 121] at the University of Texas Dental Branch by Dr. K. O. Madsen,[95] and at Ohio State University by Dr. L. P. DiOrio.[37, 38] Most of these programs involve a personalized approach in which, through a series of organized interviews, patients are able to define their own dental-diet problem. Motivation is elicited by understanding that the problem and the preventive measures applied involve dietary and oral hygiene measures. In most recommended approaches there is extensive involvement of patients in defining their problem and thus facilitating implementation of preventive procedures.

Regardless of the approach used, there are some considerations that constitute the basis for successful modification of dietary behavior:

1. A rapport or confidence has to be established between the patient and the dentist to achieve proper communication.

2. Proper clinical and dietary evaluation has to be made of the nutritional status of the patient. This can be done by evaluation of signs and symptoms of malnutrition and by identification of foods consumed and a description of the eating pattern of the patient. In this area we strongly recommend that use be made of a professional dietitian, nutritionist, or dental hygienist trained in this field. This person is an invaluable link between the dentist and the patient. Being technically competent in nutrition, this auxiliary professional is best equipped to evaluate the dietary pattern of the individual.

3. Finally, under the guidance of the dentist, the dietitian will help the patient in identifying the diet that will fulfill his or her nutritional, emotional, economic, and cultural needs, as well as the therapeutic requirements established by the dentist.

In general, the process of changing behavior involves a series of steps that provide an orderly approach to the problem.[160] These include:

1. *Identification and definition of the problem.* The health professional and the patient exchange information about nutrition and the impact it may have on oral problems and establish the need for skills and attitudes necessary to carry out the program.

2. *Collection of baseline data.* Patients will record their own dietary habits and intake patterns and the situations that lead to specific uses of foods and snacks.

3. *Determination of achievable, specific goals and objectives.* Once the patient is informed and the baseline data is established, the person is usually motivated to go on with the help of the dentist or nutritionist to establish concrete goals such as "eliminating consumption of in-between sugar-containing snacks from Monday to Friday" or "including green leafy vegetables at dinner 3 times a week." The establishment of such a contract is most important to the success of the program.

4. *Plannification: intervention.* This represents devising a strategy to help change the pinpointed behavior and includes developing a reward schedule and eliminating obstruction by using response substitution (diet soft drinks for regular carbonated drinks) and avoidance of cues that trigger undesirable behavior (avoid watching television at certain times when it is associated with consumption of snacks).

5. *Monitoring activities.* Normally it is difficult to obtain initial total compliance with the contract terms; therefore, it is necessary to record failures and successes in order to modify the plan accordingly, if necessary.

6. *Plannification of behavior that has internalized the new modifications.* Once new habits have become self-perpetuating skills, plans should be made to disengage the health professional from the process and to allow the patient to self-maintain the new habits without fear of backsliding into old behavior.

The technique of behavioral modification has been studied extensively[27, 127, 159, 160] and applied to various disciplines and circumstances and should be carefully researched to ensure success in instituting dietary modifications beneficial to oral health.

General Principles for Dietary Counseling

If a discussion of nutrition and oral disease were to stop at a description of problems, hypotheses, and conditions without suggesting solutions, it would not be complete. Even though there are many areas that have not been sufficiently investigated, enough is understood today to enable the dentist to use dietary manipulations in the preventive or therapeutic procedures used in the office or the hospital. Nutritional and dietary information will not only be useful to the patient, but will be carried to the patient's home where it may influence the eating patterns of the whole family. The effectiveness of preventive dentistry relies heavily on patient self-care, a fundamental aspect of disease prevention.

There are three areas in the professional activity of the dentist in which nutritional and dietary knowledge are required:

1. Clinical diagnosis, where the total health status of the patient is evaluated.

2. Therapeutic procedures, which can be supplemented and made more effective by dietary counseling directed to the clinical problem under consideration.

3. Health education offered to the patient and through the patient to the family unit as a whole. This preventive aspect becomes especially important in the practice of pedodontics, where young patients can be influenced to incorporate into their living pattern those dietary practices that will enable them to maintain not only oral, but also general health.

Regardless of whether the diet is intended for healthy or for diseased people,[62, 87] it is usually based on the same foods used by a healthy person, with the exception that, in the diseased state, nutrient intake or texture is changed and the food composition of the diet has to be altered to accommodate such requirements. Knowledge about normal diet is thus essential.

In designing a normal diet the following should be kept in mind:

1. For growth and maintenance certain nutrients (approximately 50) are required that cannot be synthesized by the cells and therefore have to be provided in the foods consumed daily. Thus nutrients are the essential factors, not the foods consumed in the diet, which may vary from region to region.

2. These nutrients are especially required for certain body functions, and they interact with other nutrients and food substances in such a way that an excess of one may interfere with the activity of others, so the balance between these nutrients is also essential to health.

3. The requirements of these nutrients vary with age, sex, activity, climate, physiologic conditions, and health status.[107] The RDA's represent an estimate of the nutritional needs for people living in the U.S.

4. Nutrients are present in more than one food in different proportions and degrees of availability. It is important to understand that calcium can be provided by milk

in the U.S., but it can also be derived from sesame seed or tortilla in other countries. This concept emphasizes the importance of consuming a *variety of foods,* since no single food has all the nutrients required for full growth and health. A well-balanced daily diet can only be obtained if many types and combinations of foods are used.

THE FOOD GROUP METHOD

The formulation of a diet that fulfills the nutritional requirements of an individual, is palatable and attractive, and does not pose a threat to oral health is not really a difficult task. Several approaches have been devised to guide in the selection of foods to be consumed daily. In one of these approaches foods have been divided into groups depending on the major nutritional components that they contribute, and suggestions as to the number of servings of these groups of foods are given (Fig. 8–6). This food classification for diet formulation has been found useful by some nutritionists, while others stress the limitations it has. For example, there are a large number of manufactured foods that are widely consumed that do not easily fit this classification. The important consideration is that the food group classification represents a daily dietary pattern that can provide the foundation for a nutritious diet. The recommended servings (Table 8–8) from the food groups are intended to provide adults with approximately 1,200 calories per day, and adjustment has to be made for energy expenditures of the individual. It is essential that people become familiar with the basic concepts of nutrition and that with this information they make the habit of reading the nutritional information on food labels to guide themselves in making the appropriate dietary choices.

It should be recognized that there are four types of dietary counseling that can be performed in the dental office:

1. Behavioral modification procedures to eradicate deleterious dietary habits for oral health.

2. Nutritional counseling related to special diets (liquid, soft, supplements, and so on) used in the management of oral treatments and surgery.

3. Nutritional counseling related to reduction of carbohydrates for diabetic patients or those afflicted with rampant caries.

4. Dietary counseling for maintenance of oral and general health.

It is important to emphasize again that the dentist should make use of the professional nutritionist or dietitian in implementing these various programs in order to extend his dental and nutrition expertise. The dentist should be knowledgeable in nutritional matters so that he can supervise the counseling done by specially trained professionals in nutrition and dietary manipulations.

THE EXCHANGE LIST APPROACH

The Food Group approach is a useful approach to maintain an adequate nutritious diet in most patients whose behavior has been modified to eliminate excessive use of sugar-containing foods between meals and who do not have an in-depth knowledge of nutrition.

In certain cases, for instance, in the treatment of rampant dental caries, strict control of the amount of a nutrient such as carbohydrate might be necessary. The dentist can then make use of the food exchange method prepared by committees of the American Dietetic Association and the American Diabetes Association in cooperation with the Chronic Disease Program of the Public Health Service of the Department of Health, Education, and Welfare. This approach requires more knowledge and dedication to master the procedure, but once it is learned, it becomes a simple matter to follow.

In this procedure the foods are divided into six major groups of food portions (exchanges), which contribute different amounts of carbohydrate, protein, or fat (Tables 8–9 and 8–10) and which can be exchanged in the preparation of a diet.

Eight different diets (Table 8–11) are offered, of which two diets (numbers 5 and 6) are especially intended for children because they contain a higher proportion of milk exchanges. Diet suggestions for children and teenagers have to take into account

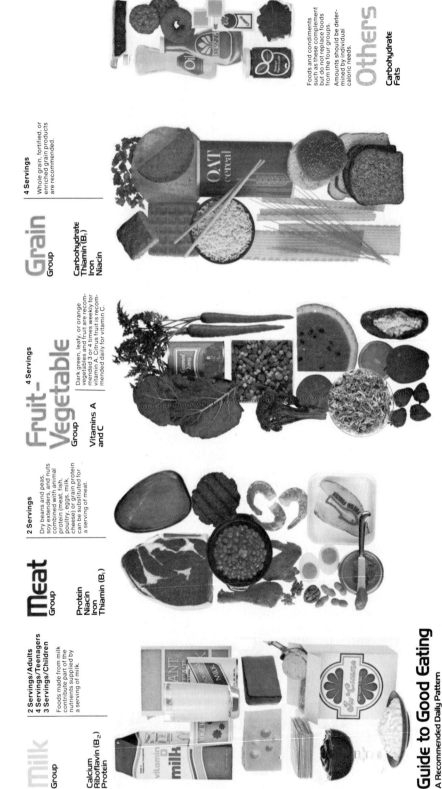

Figure 8-6 A guide to good eating. Courtesy, National Dairy Council.

their energy requirement, so Diet Plan 5 provides 1,800 calories and should be used for children about 4 to 6 years of age. Diet Plan 6 provides 2,600 calories and is usually appropriate for children 7 to 10 years of age. Table 8–12 illustrates the method to be used in planning a diet that has 1,500 calories and provides 184 g of carbohydrate, 60 g of protein, and 58 g of fat using the food exchanges. Adult diets and diets for special situations can be easily developed with this approach by consulting the table of recommended dietary allowances, depending, as indicated previously, on age, sex, activity, height, weight, and other special considerations. A number of food ingredients and beverages can be used freely, depending on taste preferences and dietary needs:

Seasonings (examples)

Chopped Parsley	Mint
Garlic	Onion
Celery	Nutmeg
Mustard	Cinnamon
Pepper and other spices	Saccharin
Lemon	Vinegar

Various foods and beverages

Coffee	Gelatin, unsweetened
Tea	Pickles, sour
Clear broth	Pickles, unswee-
Bouillon (without fat)	tened dill

This valuable therapeutic approach to diet counseling, when used with understanding of the nutrition principles and awareness of the patient's preferences, can be an effective way for the dentist to help the patient in the control of severe disease as well as in the maintenance of overall health.

If the patient requires other dietary modifications involving the consistency of diets, reference should be made to handbooks on diet therapy[62, 87] that describe the formulation and preparation of a variety of soft and liquid diets.

DIETARY CONSIDERATIONS PERTINENT TO ORAL HEALTH

Because foods not only provide nutrients for the host but also for the bacterial flora in the different parts of the oral cavity, the dentist has to pay attention to three other dietary factors with which nutritionists are not normally concerned: (1) frequency with which foods are consumed, (2) sugar content of foods, and (3) texture of foods.

Dentists interested in caries control understand that high frequency of food intake, especially foods containing large amounts of carbohydrates, is probably the most likely means of inducing the accumulation of virulent plaque associated with either dental decay or periodontal disease. Several investigations have clearly shown that increased frequency of snack consumption is definitely associated with caries increase. Diet planning, therefore, should take into account this important factor by advising not only on the nutrient composition of the diet, but also on the manner and frequency with which it is consumed.

The second important aspect relates to the sugar content of foods and its role in promoting dental plaque and caries. The relationship of sugar to health[18, 154] has been extensively discussed and its effect on oral health identified. However, it should be understood that sugar is not the only etiologic agent in dental caries, and that factors such as (1) the pattern and form of sugar consumption; (2) food consumption and texture; (3) type and virulence of specific bacteria colonizing tooth surfaces; and (4) other host factors related to saliva composition, enamel structure, tooth morphology, and fluoride status are important contributors to the expression and severity of the disease.

The effect of diet after the tooth has erupted is mostly related to plaque bacteria.[113] Under the influence of abundant and frequently available carbohydrates, bacteria colonize the enamel surface[158] and produce a number of metabolic end products that destroy the integrity of enamel. Each time a sugar-containing food is consumed, it stimulates bacterial cariogenicity and thus challenges enamel, which, unlike other tissues, has no cells to repair the damage. Therefore, the more frequent and prolonged is the exposure to such foods, the more likely that caries will develop, although there are reported differences in these effects.[89]

By evaluating the research data obtained over the last 25 years, it can be said that the

Text continued on page 139

TABLE 8–8   THE FOOD GROUP METHOD FOR FORMULATION OF A DIET*

Guide to Good Eating...

A Recommended Daily Pattern

The recommended daily pattern provides the foundation for a nutritious, healthful diet.

The recommended servings from the Four Food Groups for adults supply about 1200 Calories. The chart below gives recommendations for the number and size of servings for several categories of people.

Food Group	Recommended Number of Servings				
	Child	Teenager	Adult	Pregnant Woman	Lactating Woman
Milk 1 cup milk, yogurt, OR **Calcium Equivalent:** 1½ slices (1½ oz) cheddar cheese* 1 cup pudding 1¾ cups ice cream 2 cups cottage cheese*	3	4	2	4	4
Meat 2 ounces cooked, lean meat, fish, poultry, OR **Protein Equivalent:** 2 eggs 2 slices (2 oz) cheddar cheese* ½ cup cottage cheese* 1 cup dried beans, peas 4 tbsp peanut butter	2	2	2	3	2
Fruit-Vegetable ½ cup cooked or juice 1 cup raw Portion commonly served such as a medium-size apple or banana	4	4	4	4	4
Grain, whole grain, fortified, enriched 1 slice bread 1 cup ready-to-eat cereal ½ cup cooked cereal, pasta, grits	4	4	4	4	4

*Count cheese as serving of milk OR meat, not both simultaneously.

"Others" complement but do not replace foods from the Four Food Groups. Amounts should be determined by individual caloric needs.

B164 5 1980. Copyright © 1977, 4th Edition, National Dairy Council, Rosemont, IL 60018 All rights reserved.

---

*Courtesy, National Dairy Council.

Nutrients for Health

Nutrient	Important Sources of Nutrient
Protein	Meat, Poultry, Fish Dried Beans and Peas Egg Cheese Milk
Carbohydrate	Cereal Potatoes Dried Beans Corn Bread Sugar
Fat	Shortening, Oil Butter, Margarine Salad Dressing Sausages
Vitamin A (Retinol)	Liver Carrots Sweet Potatoes Greens Butter, Margarine
Vitamin C (Ascorbic Acid)	Broccoli Orange Grapefruit Papaya Mango Strawberries
Thiamin (B_1)	Lean Pork Nuts Fortified Cereal Products
Riboflavin (B_2)	Liver Milk Yogurt Cottage Cheese
Niacin	Liver Meat, Poultry, Fish Peanuts Fortified Cereal Products
Calcium	Milk, Yogurt Cheese Sardines and Salmon with Bones Collard, Kale, Mustard, and Turnip Greens
Iron	Enriched Farina Prune Juice Liver Dried Beans and Peas Red Meat

Table continued on opposite page

TABLE 8–8   THE FOOD GROUP METHOD FOR FORMULATION OF A DIET (*Continued*)

Nutrients are chemical substances obtained from foods during digestion. They are needed to build and maintain body cells, regulate body processes, and supply energy.

About 50 nutrients, including water, are needed daily for optimum health. If one obtains the proper amount of the 10 "leader" nutrients in the daily diet, the other 40 or so nutrients will likely be consumed in amounts sufficient to meet body needs.

One's diet should include a variety of foods because no *single* food supplies all the 50 nutrients, and because many nutrients work together.

When a nutrient is added or a nutritional claim is made, nutrition labeling regulations require listing the 10 leader nutrients on food packages. These nutrients appear in the chart below with food sources and some major physiological functions.

Some major physiological functions		
Provide energy	Build and maintain body cells	Regulate body processes
Supplies 4 Calories per gram.	Constitutes part of the structure of every cell, such as muscle, blood, and bone; supports growth and maintains healthy body cells.	Constitutes part of enzymes, some hormones and body fluids, and antibodies that increase resistance to infection.
Supplies 4 Calories per gram. Major source of energy for central nervous system.	Supplies energy so protein can be used for growth and maintenance of body cells.	Unrefined products supply fiber — complex carbohydrates in fruits, vegetables, and whole grains — for regular elimination. Assists in fat utilization.
Supplies 9 Calories per gram.	Constitutes part of the structure of every cell. Supplies essential fatty acids.	Provides and carries fat-soluble vitamins (A, D, E, and K).
	Assists formation and maintenance of skin and mucous membranes that line body cavities and tracts, such as nasal passages and intestinal tract, thus increasing resistance to infection.	Functions in visual processes and forms visual purple, thus promoting healthy eye tissues and eye adaptation in dim light.
	Forms cementing substances, such as collagen, that hold body cells together, thus strengthening blood vessels, hastening healing of wounds and bones, and increasing resistance to infection.	Aids utilization of iron.
Aids in utilization of energy.		Functions as part of a coenzyme to promote the utilization of carbohydrate. Promotes normal appetite. Contributes to normal functioning of nervous system.
Aids in utilization of energy.		Functions as part of a coenzyme in the production of energy within body cells. Promotes healthy skin, eyes, and clear vision.
Aids in utilization of energy.		Functions as part of a coenzyme in fat synthesis, tissue respiration, and utilization of carbohydrate. Promotes healthy skin, nerves, and digestive tract. Aids digestion and fosters normal appetite.
	Combines with other minerals within a protein framework to give structure and strength to bones and teeth.	Assists in blood clotting. Functions in normal muscle contraction and relaxation, and normal nerve transmission.
Aids in utilization of energy.	Combines with protein to form hemoglobin, the red substance in blood that carries oxygen to and carbon dioxide from the cells. Prevents nutritional anemia and its accompanying fatigue. Increases resistance to infection.	Functions as part of enzymes involved in tissue respiration.

TABLE 8-9 NUTRIENT COMPOSITION OF FOOD EXCHANGES*

LIST	EXCHANGE GROUP	AMOUNT	C	P	F
1	Milk, whole	1 cup	12 g	8 g	10 g
1	Milk, skim	1 cup	12 g	8 g	—
2	Vegetable	~½ cup	5 g	2 g	—
3	Fruit	Varies	10 g	—	—
4	Bread	Varies	15 g	2 g	—
5a	Meat, lean	1 oz	—	7 g	3 g
5b	Meat, medium fat	1 oz	—	7 g	5 g
5c	Meat, high fat	1 oz	—	7 g	8 g
6	Fat	1 tsp	—	—	5 g

*Data from American Dietetics Association: Handbook of Clinical Dietetics. New Haven, Conn., Yale University Press, 1981.

TABLE 8-10 SIMPLIFIED LIST OF EXCHANGE FOODS

An 1,800 Kcal Diet: 90 g protein, 60 g fat, 225 g carbohydrate
Translation into Food Exchanges

Food	Total for day	Carbohydrate (g)	Protein (g)	Fat (g)
Milk, skim	2	24	16	0
Vegetables	2	10	4	0
Fruit	7	70	0	0
Bread	8	120	16	0
Meat, lean	6	0	42	18
Meat, medium fat	2	0	14	11
Fat	6	0	0	30
Total distribution		224	92	59

Example of Caloric Distribution by Meals/Snacks

	A.M.	Noon	P.M.	Between meals
Milk, skim	½ cup	½ cup	½ cup	½ cup
Vegetables	0	1	1	0
Fruit	3	3	1	0
Bread	2	2	3	1
Meat, lean	0	3	3	0
Meat, medium fat	1	0	0	1
Fat	3	2	1	0
Total carbohydrate	66	71	66	21
Total kilocalories	513	580	520	218
Fractional Distribution	$\frac{3}{10}$	$\frac{3}{10}$	$\frac{3}{10}$	$\frac{1}{10}$

Note: There are many possible variations, depending on the individual's needs and preferences and the dosage and type of insulin administered.

Exchange Lists

List 1—Nonfat Milk Exchanges   One Exchange of nonfat milk contains 12 grams of carbohydrate, 8 grams of protein, a trace of fat and 80 kilocalories.

Milk is the leading source of calcium. It is a good source of phosphorus, protein, some of the B complex vitamins, including folacin and vitamin B_{12}, and vitamins A and D. Magnesium is also found in milk.

Whole milk contains 12 grams of carbohydrate, 8 grams of protein, 9 grams of fat and 160 kilocalories.

Table continued on opposite page

TABLE 8–10 SIMPLIFIED LIST OF EXCHANGE FOODS (*Continued*)

List 1 — Nonfat Milk Exchanges (*Continued*)	The milk shown on your meal plan can be used to drink, to add to cereal, in coffee or tea, or with other foods.

This list shows the kinds and amounts of milk or milk products to use for one nonfat exchange:

Nonfat fortified milks	*Amount to use*
Skim or nonfat milk	1 cup
Powdered (nonfat dry)	⅓ cup
Canned, evaporated—skim	½ cup
Buttermilk made from skim milk	1 cup
Yogurt made from skim milk (plain, unflavored)	1 cup
1% skim	1 cup
2% fortified skim (omit 1 Fat Exchange)	1 cup

Whole milks: (omit 2 Fat Exchanges)

Whole milk	1 cup
Canned, evaporated	½ cup
Buttermilk made from whole milk	1 cup
Yogurt made from whole milk (plain, unflavored)	1 cup

List 2— Vegetable Exchanges	One Exchange of most vegetables on this list is ½ cup and contains about 5 grams of carbohydrate, 2 grams of protein, and 25 kilocalories.

Dark green and deep yellow vegetables are leading sources of vitamin A. Some vegetables such as asparagus, broccoli, brussels sprouts, cauliflower, cabbage, green peppers, greens, and tomatoes contain vitamin C. Green leafy vegetables contain folacin; and broccoli, cabbage, carrots, spinach, and tomatoes are good sources of vitamin B_6. Brussels sprouts, greens, tomatoes, and broccoli contain potassium. Spinach is a source of zinc, and magnesium is found in green beans, broccoli, and tomatoes. Vegetables are good sources of fiber.

Serve vegetables cooked or raw. If fat is added in preparation, omit the equivalent number of fat exchanges.

Asparagus	Greens:
Bean sprouts	Mustard
Beets	Spinach
Broccoli	Turnip
Brussels sprouts	Mushrooms
Cabbage	Okra
Carrots	Onions
Cauliflower	Radishes
Celery	Rhubarb
Cucumbers	Rutabaga
Eggplant	Sauerkraut
Green pepper	String beans, green or yellow
Greens:	Summer squash
Beet	Tomatoes
Chards	Tomato juice
Collards	Turnips
Dandelion	Vegetable juice cocktail
Kale	Zucchini

Raw celery, chicory, chinese cabbage, cucumbers, endive, escarole, lettuce, and watercress can be used, as desired.

Starch vegetables are found in the **Bread Exchanges**

Table continued on following page

TABLE 8–10 SIMPLIFIED LIST OF EXCHANGE FOODS (*Continued*)

List 3— Fruit Exchanges	One Exchange of fruit contains 10 grams of carbohydrate and 40 kilocalories.

Fruits are valuable for vitamins and minerals and fiber. Oranges, tangerines, grapefruit, strawberries, cantaloupe, and honeydew melon are good sources of vitamin C. Apricots and peaches contain vitamin A. Mangoes and papaya contain both vitamin A and vitamin C. Bananas, nectarines, oranges, plums, and dried fruits are sources of potassium. Canteloupe, oranges, and strawberries contain folacin. Magnesium and vitamin B_6 are found in bananas.

Fruit may be used fresh, dried, canned or frozen, cooked or raw, as long as no sugar is added. Read the label on the can or package to be certain no sugar or sorbitol has been added.

This list shows the kinds and amounts of fruits to use for one fruit exchange:

	Amount to use		*Amount to use*
Apple	1 small	Mango	½ small
Apple juice	⅓ cup	Melon	
Applesauce		Cantaloupe	¼ small
(unsweetened)	½ cup	Honeydew	⅛ medium
Apricots, fresh	2 medium	Watermelon	1 cup
Apricots, dried	4 halves	Nectarine	1 small
Banana	½ small	Orange	1 small
Berries		Orange juice	½ cup
Blackberries	½ cup	Papaya	¾ cup
Blueberries	½ cup	Peach	1 medium
Raspberries	⅔ cup	Pear	1 small
Strawberries	¾ cup	Persimmon, native	1 medium
Cherries	10 large	Pineapple	½ cup
Cider	⅓ cup	Pineapple juice	⅓ cup
Dates	2	Plums	2 medium
Figs, dried	1	Prunes	2 medium
Figs, fresh	1	Prune juice	¼ cup
Grapefruit	½	Raisins	2 tbsp
Grapefruit juice	½ cup	Tangerine	1 medium
Grapes	12		
Grape juice	¼ cup		

For variety serve fruit as a salad or in combination with other foods for dessert.

Cranberries may be used as desired if no sugar is added.

List 4—Bread, Cereal, and Starchy Vegetables Exchange	One Exchange contains 15 grams of carbohydrate, 2 grams of protein and 70 kilocalories

Whole grain or enriched breads and cereals are good sources of iron and some of the B vitamins, as are dried beans and peas and the vegetables on this list. Magnesium is found in dried cooked beans and whole grain cereals. Dried beans, peas, and lentils are sources of zinc. Dried peas and beans, and whole grain breads and cereals are excellent sources of fiber.

Table continued on opposite page

TABLE 8–10 SIMPLIFIED LIST OF EXCHANGE FOODS (*Continued*)

| List 4—Bread, Cereal, and Starchy Vegetables Exchange (*Continued*) | This list shows the many kinds and amounts of breads, cereals, and starchy vegetables to use for one Bread Exchange: |

	Amount to use		*Amount to use*
BREAD		*CEREAL*	
White (including French and Italian)	1 slice	Bran flakes	½ cup
Whole wheat	1 slice	Other ready to eat unsweetened cereal	¾ cup
Rye or pumpernickel	1 slice	Puff cereal, unfrosted	1 cup
Raisin	1 slice	Cereal, cooked	½ cup
Bagel, small	½	Grits, cooked	½ cup
English muffin, small	½	Rice or barley, cooked	½ cup
Plain roll, bread	1	Pastas, cooked	
Frankfurt roll	½	spaghetti, noodles	½ cup
Hamburger bun	½	macaroni	½ cup
Dry bread crumbs	3 tbsp	Cornmeal, dry	2 tbsp
		Flour	2½ tbsp
Pancake, 5″	1	Wheat germ	¼ cup
Waffle, 5″	1		
Tortilla, 6″	1		
CRACKERS		*MISCELLANEOUS*	
Arrowroot	3	Biscuit, 2″ dia.	1
Graham 2½″	2	(Omit 1 Fat Exchange)	
Matzoth 4″ × 6″	½	Corn muffin 2″ dia.	1
Oyster	20	(Omit 1 Fat Exchange)	
Pretzels 3⅛″ long ⅛″ dia.	25	Crackers, round butter type	5
		(Omit 1 Fat Exchange)	
DRIED BEANS, PEAS, AND LENTILS		Muffin, plain small	1
Beans, peas, lentils, dried and cooked	½ cup	(Omit 1 Fat Exchange)	
		Popcorn, popped	3 cups
Baked beans, no pork	¼ cup	Potatoes, French fried, length 2 to 3½″ (Omit 1 Fat Exchange)	8
STARCHY VEGETABLES			
Corn	⅓ cup	Potato or corn chips (Omit 2 Fat Exchanges)	15
Corn on cob	1 small		
Lima beans	½ cup		
Parsnips	⅔ cup		
Peas, green—canned or frozen	½ cup		
Potato, white	1 small		
Potato, mashed	½ cup		
Pumpkin	¾ cup	*CRACKERS*	
Winter squash, acorn or butternut	½ cup	Rye wafers 2″ × 3½″	3
		Saltines	6
Yam, or sweet potato	¼ cup	Soda 2½″ sq.	4

Table continued on following page

TABLE 8–10 SIMPLIFIED LIST OF EXCHANGE FOODS (*Continued*)

List 5—Lean Meat, Protein Rich Exchanges	One Exchange of meat (1 oz) contains 7 grams of protein, 3 grams of fat, and 55 kilocalories

Meat, poultry, fish, cheese and eggs are important sources of protein, iron, vitamin B_{12}, and other B-complex vitamins. Liver and eggs also contain Vitamin A. Oysters and peanut butter contain magnesium. Liver is a good source of iron and both liver and peanut butter contain folacin. Zinc is found in lean beef, cheddar type cheese, crab, liver, peanut butter, oysters, and the dark meat of turkey.

Cholesterol is of animal origin; therefore, peanut butter and dried peas and beans contain no cholesterol.

To plan a diet low in saturated fat and cholesterol, choose only those exchanges in **bold type.**

You may use the meat, fish, etc. that is prepared for the family when no fat or flour have been added. If meat is fried, use the fat included in the meal plan. Meat juices with the fat removed may be used with your meat or vegetables for added flavor. Be certain to trim off *all* visible fat and measure meat after it has been cooked. A 3-oz serving of cooked meat is about equal to 4 oz of raw meat.

This list shows the kinds and amounts of meat and protein rich foods to use for one Low Fat Meat Exchange:

Beef:	**Baby beef; chipped beef; chuck; flank steak; tenderloin; plate ribs: plate skirt steak: round (bottom, top); all cuts rump; spare ribs; tripe**	**1 oz**
Lamb:	**Leg; rib; sirloin; loin (roast and chops); shank; shoulder**	**1 oz**
Pork:	**Leg (whole rump, center shank); ham, smoked (center slices)**	**1 oz**
Veal:	**Leg; loin; rib; shank; shoulder; cutlets**	**1 oz**
Poultry:	**Meat without skin of chicken, turkey, cornish hen, guinea hen, pheasant**	**1 oz**
Fish:	**Any fresh or frozen;**	**1 oz**
	canned salmon, tuna, mackerel, crab, and lobster;	**¼ cup**
	clams, oysters, scallops, shrimp;	**5 or 1 oz**
	sardines, drained	**3**
Cheeses containing less than 5% butterfat		**1 oz**
Cottage cheese, dry and 2% butterfat		**¼ cup**
Dried peas and beans (Omit 1 Bread Exchange)		**½ cup**

Medium Fat Meat and Protein Rich Exchanges contain 7 grams of protein, 5 grams of fat, and 75 kilocalories (1 oz)

Table continued on opposite page

TABLE 8-10 SIMPLIFIED LIST OF EXCHANGE FOODS (*Continued*)

List 5—Lean Meat, Protein Rich Exchanges (*Continued*)	This list shows the kinds and amounts of meat and protein rich foods to use for one Medium Fat Meat Exchange:	
	Beef:	Ground, 15% fat; corned beef, canned; rib eye; round, ground (commercial)	1 oz

Beef:	Ground, 15% fat; corned beef, canned; rib eye; round, ground (commercial)	1 oz
Pork:	Loin (all cuts); tenderloin; shoulder arm, picnic; shoulder blade (Boston butt); Canadian bacon, boiled ham; loin, shoulder, picnic ham	1 oz
Liver, heart, kidney and sweetbreads (these are high in cholesterol).		1 oz
Cottage cheese, creamed		¼ cup
Cheese, mozzarella, ricotta, farmer's cheese, Neufchâtel		1 oz
Cheese, Parmesan		3 tbsp
Egg (high in cholesterol).		1
Peanut butter (Omit 2 Fat Exchanges)		2 tbsp

High Fat Meat and Protein Rich Exchanges contain 7 grams of protein, 8 grams of Fat, and 100 kilocalories (1 oz)

This list shows the kinds and amounts of meat and protein rich foods to use for one High Fat Meat Exchange:

Beef:	Brisket; corned beef (brisket); ground beef, more than 20% fat; hamburger (commercial); chuck, ground (commercial); roasts, rib; steaks, club and rib	1 oz
Lamb:	Breast	1 oz
Pork:	Spare ribs; loin (back ribs); pork, ground; country style ham; deviled ham; spare ribs	1 oz
Veal:	Breast	1 oz
Poultry:	Capon, duck (domestic); goose	1 oz
Cheese, cheddar type		1 oz
Cold cuts		4½" × ⅛" slice
Frankfurter		1

Table continued on following page

TABLE 8–10   SIMPLIFIED LIST OF EXCHANGE FOODS (*Continued*)

List 6—Fat Exchanges	One Exchange of fat contains 5 grams of fat and 45 kilocalories.

Since all fats are high in kilocalories, foods on this list should be measured carefully to control weight. Margarine, butter, cream and cream cheese contain vitamin A. Use the fats on this list in the amounts on the meal plan.

To plan a diet low in saturated fat select only those exchanges which appear in **bold type** and are polyunsaturated.

This list shows the kinds and amounts of fat containing foods to use for one Fat Exchange:

	Amount to use
Margarine, Soft, tub or stick*	1 tsp
Avocado (4″ in diameter)†	⅛
Oil, corn, cottonseed, safflower, soy, sunflower	1 tsp
Oil, olive†	1 tsp
Oil, peanut†	1 tsp
Walnuts	6 small
Nuts, other†	6 small
Olives†	5 small
Margarine, regular stick	1 tsp
Butter	1 tsp
Bacon fat	1 tsp
Bacon, crisp	1 strip
Cream, light	2 tbsp
Cream, sour	2 tbsp
Cream, heavy	1 tbsp
Cream cheese	1 tbsp
French dressing‡	1 tbsp
Italian dressing‡	1 tbsp
Lard	1 tsp
Mayonnaise†	1 tsp
Salad dressing, mayonnaise type‡	2 tsp
Salt pork	¾″ cube

* Made with corn, cottonseed, safflower, soy or sunflower oil only.
† Fat content is primarily monounsaturated.
‡ If made with corn, cottonseed, safflower, or soy oil, can be used on fat modified diet.

TABLE 8-11 SAMPLE DIET PLANS

| DIET | CARBO-HYDRATE (G) | PROTEIN (G) | FAT (G) | CALORIES | CARBOHYDRATE DISTRIBUTION* | | | |
					Breakfast	*Lunch*	*Dinner*	*Other*
1	135	60	45	1200	27	40	38	30
2	150	70	70	1500	25	52	47	26
3	190	80	80	1800	40	56	52	42
4	265	80	80	2100	53	80	76	56
5†	180	90	80	1800	37	52	61	30
6†	335	90	100	2600	67	100	98	70
7	335	90	100	2600	70	95	90	80
8	435	90	100	3000	90	100	150	95

Total Day's Food in Sample Meal Plans

DIET	WHOLE MILK	VEGETABLES	FRUITS	BREAD EX.	MEAT (A)	MEAT (B)	FAT EX.
1	2 pt.	3	2	5	2	2	2
2	2 pt.	3	2	6	3	2	6
3	2 pt.	3	3	8	3	3	7
4	2 pt.	5	5	11	2	3	7
5†	4 qt.	6	3	5	3	2	4
6†	4 qt.	7	7	12	2	1	10
7	2 pt.	7	8	13	3	2	12
8	2 pt.	7	10	18	2	2	12

*In these meal plans, the total carbohydrate content has been divided approximately into fifths. About one fifth is alloted for breakfast, and the other four fifths are distributed between lunch, dinner, and other meals. The division of the carbohydrate is flexible and can be varied to meet the patient's needs. For example, it may be desirable for some patients to take a part of the food at some time other than during regular meals.

†These diets contain more milk and are especially suitable for children.

Modified from American Dietetics Association: Handbook of Clinical Dietetics. New Haven, Conn., Yale University Press, 1981.

abuse and misuse of sugar-containing foods has contributed to dental decay. Administration of sugar-containing foods at frequent intervals stimulates implantation of cariogenic microorganisms, production of acids, and consequently, lowers plaque pH to a level that is incompatible with the stability of enamel. Therefore, efforts should be made to exercise moderation in consumption of those sugar-containing foods that stimulate caries. As is true with other issues related to the role of certain food ingredients in the etiology of specific diseases, it is difficult to identify the level of sugar intake that leads to caries development or, conversely, the level that does not produce adverse caries effects. Nevertheless, since sugar is a caries promoting substance, efforts should be made to avoid its excessive intake and, furthermore, to reduce its consumption to sensible levels. This means that there should be a concerted effort to lower the level of sugar in manufactured foods and to limit the addition of sugar to foods prepared at home. It also means re-stricting the consumption of such sugar-containing foods to dessert time, rather than snacking on them throughout the day. For a few, even this controlled dietary behavior would not deter the development of caries, for there are individual differences in caries susceptibility. However, for the majority, reduction in the amount and frequency of sugar intake should prove beneficial in terms of oral health. Use of sugar substitutes or foods containing additives with cariostatic agents such as trimetaphosphate[46] are viable alternatives in the future but are not widely available to the public at the present time.

Dietary manipulations characterized by restriction or elimination of carbohydrates[16, 72] have been known to control dental caries and plaque formation. However, it has been difficult to identify a dietary carbohydrate intake that would be associated with absence of virulent, cariogenic streptococci from human plaque. At this time, the consequence for oral health of extreme dietary behaviors are clearly understood. Those who

TABLE 8–12 EXAMPLE OF A METHOD FOR PLANNING A DIET USING FOOD EXCHANGES

Diet Prescription: Calories = 1,500   C = 184g (49%), P = 60g (16%), F = 58g (35%)

Total Day's Food

Exchange Group	List	Amount	C	P	F
Milk, skim	1	2 cups	24	16	
Vegetables	2	3 cups	15	6	
Fruit	3	7 cups	70		

C from sources other than bread exchange			109	
Total C in prescription			184	
Less C from non-bread sources			− 109	
			75 ÷ 15 = 5 bread exchanges	

Bread	4	5	75	10	

P from sources other than meat exchange		32
Total P in prescription		60
Less P from non-meat exchange		−32
		28 ÷ 7 = 4 meat exchanges

Meat, lean	5a	2		14	6
Meat, med. fat	5b	2		14	11

F from sources other than fat exchange	17
Total F in prescription	58
Less F from non-fat sources	−17
	41 ÷ 5 = 8 fat exchanges

Fat	6	8			40

			C	P	F
Totals			184	60	58
			× 4	× 4	× 9
Calories			736	240	522
TOTAL = 1,498 calories					

Procedure for Calculations.

1. Estimate amounts of milk, vegetables, and fruits to be included:

Minima	Milk	2 exchanges — adults
		3–4 exchanges — children and pregnant and lactating women
	Vegetables	2 exchanges
	Fruit	2 exchanges

2. Fill in C, P, and F values for tentative amounts of milk, vegetables, and fruits, using composition per exchange from Table 8–10.
3. To determine number of bread exchanges, subtract total C from Step 2 for total C prescribed. Divide by 15 (C from 1 bread exchange). Use nearest whole number. Total the C and P values.
4. Recalculate if C deviates from prescribed amount by more than 3–4 grams.
5. To determine number of meat exchanges, subtract total P of milk, vegetables, and bread exchanges from total P prescribed. Divide by 7 (P from 1 meat exchange). Use nearest whole number. Total P and F values.
6. To determine number of fat exchanges, subtract total F values for milk and meat from total F prescribed. Divide by 5 (F from 1 fat exchange). Use nearest whole number. Total F values.
7. Check computations. Use 4 kcal/g for C and P and 9 kcal/g F to calculate total kcal.

   C = carbohydrate; P = protein; F = fat.

meticulously avoid all types of sugar-containing foods, such as individuals afflicted with heredity fructose intolerance, have low caries experience, while those who frequently are exposed to sugars, such as infants fed sugared drinks in nursing bottles or workers in sweets industries[5] who consume sucrose frequently, have poor oral health. Identification of in-between dietary behavior that might be safe for teeth is difficult. Therefore, considering the bacterial composition of dental plaque and the mechanisms of action of the many metabolic reactions that take place within plaque, it is sensible to avoid the frequent consumption of snacks containing sugar between meals and restrict the intake of sweet desserts to mealtime. Professionals involved in nutritional counseling to control plaque and prevent oral disease can offer more specific advice by using the previously described approaches that involve obtaining nutritional histories and dietary evaluations and correlating them with plaque indexes, the presence of cariogenic bacteria, and the overall clinical impression. Gradual limitation of carbohydrate consumption and frequency of intake will indicate which dietary regimen will yield acceptable oral health conditions for a specific patient.

The third important point has been fully discussed by Caldwell[32] and involves the question of the physical properties of foods and their caries-promoting potential. A few clinical studies[53, 54, 85] have been conducted to explore the relation between such physical properties of food as adhesiveness, solubility, viscosity, hardness, and so on and their caries-promoting potential. There are indications that these properties do influence the amount of residues left on and around teeth. It is important to understand the role of food texture in caries in order to select appropriate foods for diet counseling. Eventually, this understanding will be used in formulation and manufacture of foods with low caries-promoting potential. Studies are going on in several laboratories around the world using animal models, plaque pH measurements in humans, and *in vitro* tests that will allow the estimation of caries-promoting properties of foods and thus help the health professional

to carry out dietary counseling based on use of foods that are safe for oral health.

CONCLUSION

Advances in the understanding of the nutritional and dietary factors involved in the etiology and control of caries will help in the design of preventive disease programs for the benefit of individuals who are willing to incorporate this knowledge into a comprehensive oral health program. These same approaches can be implemented at a community or public health level to combat caries around the world.[9]

Oral health cannot be exclusively maintained through one approach, that is, through nutritional guidance, dietary manipulations, chemotherapeutic agents, or restorative procedures. The chances for preserving oral health, however, are improved by lifelong disciplined dedication of the individual who understands the benefits to be derived from the combined effects of oral hygiene, fluorides, and adequate nutrition and diet and who incorporates this knowledge into his or her daily habits.[110]

Research has given us a better understanding of our nutritional needs and of how the fulfillment of such requirements contributes to the prevention of disease. Through the combined efforts of individuals together with health professionals and food scientists we can begin, today, to provide and to ensure better oral health for all people.

REFERENCES

1. Alfano, M. C.: Controversies, perspectives and clinical implications of nutrition in periodontal disease. Dent. Clin. North Am. *20*:519–548, 1976.
2. Alfano, M. C.: Nutrition in periodontal diseases. J. Cont. Dent. Ed. (U.S.C.) *1*:160–173, 1980.
3. Aksnes, A.: Relative effects of sucrolytic enzymes in human dental plaque. Scand. J. Dent. Res. *84*:372–376, 1976.
4. Aksnes, A.: Sucrolytic enzymes from human dental plaque in saliva. Scand. J. Dent. Res. *85*:101–105, 1977.
5. Anaise, J. Z.: Prevalence of dental caries among workers in the sweet industry in Israel. Comm. Dent. Oral Epid. *6*:286–289, 1978.
6. Angmar-Mänsson, B.: A quantitative microradiographic study of the organic matrix of develop-

ing human enamel in relation to the mineral content. Arch. Oral Biol. *16*:135–145, 1971.

7. Angmar-Mänsson, B.: A polarization microscopic and micro x-ray diffraction study on the organic matrix of developing human enamel. Arch. Oral Biol. *16*:147–156, 1971.

8. Aponte-Merced, L., and Navia, J. M.: Preeruptive protein malnutrition and acid solubility of rat molar enamel surfaces. Arch. Oral Biol. *25*:701–705, 1980.

9. Barmes, D. E.: Global problems of oral disease. J. Dent. Res. *56*:C9–C13, 1977.

10. Barros, L., and Witkop, C. J., Jr.: Oral and genetic study of Chileans. III. Periodontal disease and nutritional factors. Arch. Oral Biol. *8*:195–206, 1963.

11. Baume, L. J.: Report on a dental survey among the school population of French Polynesia. Arch. Oral Biol. *13*:787, 1968.

12. Baume, L. J.: Caries prevalence and caries intensity among 12,344 school children of French Polynesia. Arch. Oral Biol. *14*:181, 1969.

13. Baume, L. J., and Meyer, J.: Dental dysplasia related to malnutrition with special reference to melanodontia and odontoclasia. J. Dent. Res. *45*:726, 1966.

14. Baume, L. J., and Vulliemoz, J. P.: Dietary fluoride intake into the enamel of caries susceptible "yellow" permanent teeth and of caries-resistant permanent and primary teeth of Polynesians. Arch. Oral Biol. *15*:431, 1970.

15. Baume, L. J., and Vulliemoz, J. P.: Variations in the mineral content of the enamel of Polynesian teeth. Int. Dent. J. *22*:193, 1972.

16. Becks, H.: Carbohydrate restriction in the prevention of dental caries using the L. A. count as an index. J. Calif. St. Dent. Assoc. *26*:1–6, 1950.

17. Birkhed, D.: Automatic titration method for determination of acid production from sugars and sugar alcohol in small samples of dental plaque material. Caries Res. *12*:128–136, 1978.

18. Bowen, W. H.: Role of Carbohydrates in Dental Caries. *In* Shaw, J. H., et al. (eds.): Sweeteners and Dental Caries. Sp. Suppl. Feeding, Weight and Obesity Abstract, Washington, D.C., Information Retrieval Inc., 1978, pp. 147–155.

19. Boyde, A., and Jones, S. J.: Scanning Electron Microscopic Studies of the Formation of Mineralized Tissues. *In* Slavkin, H. C., and Bavetta, L. O.: Developmental Aspects of Oral Biology. New York, Academic Press, 1972.

20. Brown, A. T., and Patterson, C. E.: Ethanol production and alcohol dehydrogenase activity in *Streptococcus mutans*. Arch. Oral Biol. *18*:127–131, 1973.

21. Brown, A. T., and Christian, C. P.: Characterization of a novel nicotinamide adenine dinucleotide-depending alcohol dehydrogenase from a strain of *Streptococcus mutans*. Arch. Oral Biol. *19*:397–406, 1974.

22. Brown, A. T.: The Role of Dietary Carbohydrates in Plaque Formation and Oral Disease. *In* Present Knowledge in Nutrition, 4th ed. New York, Nutrition Foundation, 1976.

23. Brown, W. E., and König, K. G. (eds.): Cariostatic mechanisms of fluoride. Proceedings of ADA-NIDR Conference. Caries Res. *11*:1–327, 1977.

24. Butler, W. T., and Richarson, W. S., III: Biochemistry of Tooth Proteins. *In* Menaker, L. (ed.):

Biologic Basis of Dental Caries, New York, Harper & Row, 1980, pp. 168–190.

25. Butterworth, C. E., Jr.: New concepts in nutrition and cancer: Implications for folic acid. Contemp. Nutr. *5*:1–2, 1980.

26. Carroll, K. K., and Khor, H. T. (eds.): Dietary Fat in Relation to Tumorigenesis. *In* Paoletti, R. (ed.): Progress in Biochemical Pharmacology, Vol. 10. White Plains, New York, Albert J. Phiebig Inc., 1975.

27. Chambers, D. W.: Behavior Modification. *In* Randolph, P. M., and Dennison, C. I. (eds.): Diet, Nutrition and Dentistry. St. Louis, The C. V. Mosby Co., 1981.

28. Colman, G., Bowen, W. H., and Cole, M. F.: The effects of sucrose, fructose and a mixture of glucose and fructose on the incidence of dental caries in monkeys *(M. fascicularis)*. Br. Dent. J. *142*:217–221, 1977.

29. Cantor, S. K.: Patterns of use in sweeteners: Issues and uncertainties. Washington, D.C., NAS Fourth Academy Forum, 1975.

30. Carlsson, J.: Presence of various types of non-hemolytic streptococci in dental plaque and other sites of the oral cavity in man. Odontol. Rev. *18*:55–74, 1967.

31. Cook, D. C., and Buikstra, J. E.: Health and differential survival in prehistoric populations: Prenatal dental defects. Am. J. Phys. Anthrop. *51*:649–664, 1979.

32. Caldwell, R. C.: Physical properties of foods and their caries-producing potential. J. Dent. Res. *49*:1293–1298, 1970.

33. Curzon, M. E. J., Adkins, B. L., Bibby, B. G., and Losee, F. L.: Combined effect of trace elements and fluorine on caries. J. Dent. Res. *49*:526–528, 1970.

34. Curzon, M. E. J., and Crocker, D. C.: Relationship of trace elements in human tooth enamel to dental caries. Arch. Oral Biol. *23*:647–653, 1978.

35. DeLuca, H. F.: The control of calcium and phosphorus metabolism by the vitamin D endocrine system. Ann. N. Y. Acad. Sci. *355*:1–17, 1980.

36. DePaola, D. P., and Alfano, M. C.: Diet and oral health. Nutr. Today *12*:6–32, 1977.

37. DiOrio, L. P., and Madsen, K. O.: Patient education — A health service for the prevention of dental disease. Dent. Clin. North Am. *15*:905–917, 1971.

38. DiOrio, L. P., and Madsen, K. O.: A personalized program: Educating the patient in the prevention of dental disease. Chicago, Ill., March Publishing Co., Inc., 1972.

39. DiOrio, L. P., Miller, S. A., and Navia, J. M.: The separate effects of protein and calorie malnutrition on the development and growth of rat bones and teeth. J. Nutr. *103*:856–865, 1973.

40. Dreizen, S., Levy, B. M., and Bernick, S.: Studies on the biology of the periodontium of marmosets. VII. The effect of folic acid deficiency on the marmoset oral mucosa. J. Dent. Res. *49*:616–620, 1970.

41. Edwardsson, S., Birkhed, D., and Mejare, B.: Acid production from Lycasin, maltitol, sorbitol and xylitol by oral streptococci and lactobacilli. Acta. Odont. Scand. *35*:257–263, 1977.

42. Enwonwu, C. O.: Elements of dietetics for the

general practitioner. Int. Dent. J. 23:317–327, 1973.

43. Enwonwu, C. O.: Influence of socio-economic conditions on dental development in Nigerian children. Arch. Oral Biol. 18:95–107, 1973.

44. Enwonwu, C. O.: Role of biochemistry and nutrition in preventive dentistry. J. Am. Soc. Prev. Dent. 4:6–17, 1974.

45. FAO/WHO: Symposium on carbohydrates in human nutrition. September 17–26, Geneva, 1979.

46. Finn, S. B., Frew, R. A., Leibowitz, R., Morse, W., Manson-Hing, L., and Brunelle, J.: The effect of sodium trimetasphosphate (TMP) as a chewing gum additive on caries increments in children. J. Am. Dent. Assoc. 96:651–655, 1978.

47. Fitzgerald, R. J., and Keyes, P. H.: Demonstration of the etiologic role of streptococci in experimental caries in the hamster. J. Am. Dent. Assoc. 61:9–19, 1960.

48. Frazier, P. D.: Adult human enamel: An electron microscopic study of crystallite size morphology. J. Ultrastruc. Res. 22:1–11, 1968.

49. Geddes, D. A. M., Edgar, W. M., Jenkins, G. N., and Rugg-Gunn, A. J.: Apples, salted peanuts and plaque pH. Br. Dent. J. 142:317–319, 1977.

50. Gibbons, R. J., and Van Houte, J.: Dental caries. Ann. Rev. Med. 26:121–136, 1975.

51. Gori, B. G.: Diet and cancer. J. Am. Dent. Assoc. 71:375–379, 1977.

52. Gortner, W. A.: Nutrition in the United States 1900–1974. Cancer Res. 35:32–46, 1975.

53. Grenby, T. H.: The stickiness of cereal products and the composition of cereal diets as factors in their cariogenicity in the rat. Arch. Oral Biol. 14:1253–1258, 1969.

54. Grenby, T. H.: The influence of sticky foods of high sugar content on dental caries in the rat. Arch. Oral Biol. 14:1259–1265, 1969.

55. Gustafsson, B., Quensel, C., Lanke, L., et al.: The Vipeholm dental caries study: The effect of different levels of carbohydrates intake on caries activity in 436 individuals observed for five years. Acta Odontol. Scand. 11:232–252, 1954.

56. Guggenheim, B.: Streptococci of dental plaque. Caries Res. 2:147–163, 1968.

57. Gwinett, A. J.: The ultrastructure of the "prismless" enamel of permanent teeth. Arch. Oral Biol. 12:381–387, 1967.

58. HANES: Health and Nutrition Examination Survey United States 1971–72: Dietary intake and biochemical findings. Rockville, Md., U.S. Dept. H.E.W. (D.H.E.W. Publication No. [HRA] 74-1219-1), Jan., 1974.

59. Harris, S., and Cleaton-Jones, P.: Oral health in a group of sugar-cane chewers. J. Dent. Assoc. S. Afr. 33:255–258, 1978.

60. Harris, S. S., and Navia, J. M.: Vitamin A deficiency and caries susceptibility of rat molar. Arch. Oral Biol. 25:415–421, 1980.

61. Hefferren, J. J. (ed.): Conference on Foods, Nutrition and Dental Health: Role of sugar and other foods in dental caries. Am. Dent. Assoc., Chicago, Ill., 1978.

62. Goodhart, R. S., and Shils, M. E.: Modern Nutrition in Health and Disease, 6th ed. Philadelphia, Lea & Febiger, 1980.

63. Hartles, R. L., and Leach, S. A.: Effect of diet on dental caries. Br. Med. Bull. 31:137–141, 1975.

64. Hazen, S. P.: The role of nutrition in periodontal disease. J. Ala. Med. Sci. 5:328–335, 1968.

65. Hirayama, T.: Epidemiology of cancer of the stomach with special reference to its recent decrease in Japan. Cancer Res. 35:3460–3463, 1975.

66. Hoskins, W. A.: Industrial potential of sweeteners other than sucrose and simple carbohydrates. In Shaw, J. H., et al. (eds.): Sweeteners and Dental Caries. Sp. Suppl. Feeding, Weight and Obesity Abstr., Washington, D.C., Information Retrieval Inc., 1978.

67. Ikeda, T., Shiota, T., McGhee, J. R., et al.: Virulence of Streptococcus mutans: Comparison of the effects of coupling sugar and sucrose on certain metabolic activities and cariogenicity. Infect. Immun. 19:477–480, 1978.

68. Imfeld, T., Hirsch, R. S., and Muhlemann, H. R.: Telemetric recordings of interdental plaque pH during different meal patterns. Br. Dent. J. 144:40–45, 1978.

69. Infante, P. F., and Guillespie, G. M.: An epidemiologic study of linear enamel hypoplasia of deciduous anterior teeth in Guatemalan children. Arch. Oral Biol. 19:1055–1061, 1974.

70. Infante, P. F., and Guillespie, G. M.: Dental caries experience in the deciduous dentition of rural Guatemalan children ages 6 months to 7 years. J. Dent. Res. 55:951–957, 1976.

71. Infante, P. F., and Guillespie, G. M.: Enamel hypoplasia in relation to caries in Guatemalan children. J. Dent. Res. 56:493–501, 1977.

72. Jay, P.: The reduction of oral Lactobacillus acidophilus counts by the periodic restriction of carbohydrate. Am. J. Orth. Oral Surg. 33:162–184, 1947.

73. Jelliffee, D. B., Williams, L. L., and Jelliffee, E. F. P.: A nutrition survey in rural Jamaica. J. Trop. Med. Hyg. 57:27, 1954.

74. Jelliffee, D. B., and Jelliffee, E. F. P.: The nutritional status of Haitian children. Acta. Trop. 18:1, 1961.

75. Jelliffee, D. B., Jelliffee, E. F. P., Garcia, I., and DeBarrir, G.: The children of the San Blas Indians of Panamá. J. Ped. 59:271, 1961.

76. Jelliffee, D. B., and Jelliffee, E. F. P.: Linear hypoplasia of deciduous incisor teeth in malnourished children. Am. J. Clin. Nutr. 24:893, 1971.

77. INCAP: Evelucion Nutricional de la Poblacion de Centro America y Panama: INCAP, Guatemala City, Guatemala, Pub. V-29, pp. 6, 1969.

78. Jolliffee, N.: The physical signs of malnutrition. In The Control of Malnutrition in Man. New York, American Public Health Association, pp. 8, 1960.

79. Karle, E. J., and Gehring, F.: Palatinit: A new sugar substitute and its caries prophylactic evaluation. Dtsch. Zahnaerztle Z. 33:189–191, 1978.

80. Keyes, P. H.: The infectious and transmissible nature of experimental dental caries. Findings and implication. Arch. Oral Biol. 1:304–320, 1960.

81. Khan, R.: Advances in sucrose chemistry. In Birch, G. G., and Parker, K. J. (eds.): Sugar: Science and Technology. London, Applied Science Publishers, LTD, 1978.

82. Kleinberg, I.: Studies on dental plaque. I. The effect of different concentrations of glucose on

the pH of dental plaque *in vivo*. J. Dent. Res. *40*:1087–1111, 1961.

83. Kleinberg, I.: Formation and accumulation of acid on the tooth surface. J. Dent. Res. *49*:1300–1315, 1970.

84. Knuuttila, M. L. E., and Makinen, K.: Effect of xylitol on the growth and metabolism of *Streptoccocus mutans*. Caries Res. *9*:177–189, 1975.

85. König, K. G.: Caries induced in laboratory rats. Posteruptive effect of sucrose and of bread of different degrees of refinement. Br. Dent. J. *123*:585–589, 1967.

86. König, K. G., Schmid, P., and Schmid, R.: An apparatus for frequency controlled feeding of small rodents and its use in dental caries experiments. Arch. Oral Biol. *13*:13–26, 1968.

87. Krause, M. V., and Mahan, L. K.: Food, Nutrition and Diet Therapy, 6th ed. Philadelphia, W. B. Saunders, Co., 1979.

88. Larson, R. H., Rubin, M., and Zipkin, I.: Frequency of eating as a factor in experimental dental caries. Arch. Oral Biol. *9*:705–712, 1962.

89. Littleton, N. W., Kakehashi, S., and Fitzgerald, R.: Study of differences in the occurrence of dental caries in Caucasian and Negro children. J. Dent. Res. *49*:742–751, 1970.

90. LSRO-FASEB: Dietary sugars in health and disease. I. Fructose. Bethesda, Md. Life Science Research Office, Fed. Am. Soc. Exptl. Biol., 1976.

91. LSRO-FASEB: Evaluation of the health aspects of corn sugar (dextrose), corn syrup and invert sugar as food ingredients. Bethesda, Md. Life Science Research Office, Fed. Am. Soc. Exptl. Biol., 1976.

92. LSRO-FASEB: Evaluation of the health aspects of sucrose as a food ingredient. Bethesda, Md., Life Science Research Office, Fed. Am. Soc. Exptl. Biol., 1976.

93. LSRO-FASEB: Dietary sugars in health and disease. II. Xylitol. Bethesda, Md., Life Science Research Office, Fed. Am. Soc. Exptl. Biol., 1978.

94. LSRO-FASEB: Dietary sugars in health and disease. III. Sorbitol. Bethesda, Md., Life Science Research Office, Fed. Am. Soc. Exptl. Biol., 1979.

95. Madsen, K. O.: Nutritional Basis of Oral Health. *In* Dental Biochemistry, 2nd ed. Philadelphia, Lea & Febiger, pp. 289–347, 1976.

96. McCabe, M. M., Smith, E. E., and Cowman, R. A.: Invertase activity in *Streptococcus mutans* and *Streptococcus sanguis*. Arch. Oral Biol. *18*:525–531, 1973.

97. MacKay, D. A.: Sucrose and sucrose substitutes: Industrial considerations. Pharmacol. Ther. Dent. *3*:69–74, 1978.

98. Menaker, L., and Navia, J. M.: Effect of undernutrition during the perinatal period on caries development in the rat. II. Caries susceptibility in underfed rats supplemented with protein or caloric additions during the suckling period. J. Dent. Res. *52*:680–687, 1973.

99. Menaker, L., and Navia, J. M.: Effect of undernutrition during the perinatal period on caries development in the rat. III. Effect of undernutrition on biochemical parameters in the developing submandibular salivary glands. J. Dent. Res. *52*:688–691, 1973.

100. Menaker, L., Morehart, R., and Navia, J. M. (eds.): The Biologic Basis of Dental Caries. Harper & Row, New York, 1980.

101. Michalek, S. M., McGhee, J. R., Navia, J. M., and Narkates, A. J.: Effective immunity to dental caries: Protection of malnourished rats by local injection of *Streptococcus mutans*. Infect. Immun. *13*:782–789, 1976.

102. Miller, E. J.: The Collagen of Joints. Chapter 5 *in* The Joints and Synovial Fluid. Vol. 10, pp. 205–242. New York, Academic Press, 1978.

103. Minah, G. E., and Loesche, W. J.: Sucrose metabolism in resting-cell suspensions of caries-associated and non-caries–associated dental plaque. Infect. Immun. *17*:43–54, 1977.

104. Moller, P.: Dental caries and non-fluoride enamel hypoplasia in Icelandic children aged 6–14 years. Birmingham, Alabama, Univ. Ala. School Dent., 1981.

105. Molnar, S., and Ward, S. C.: Mineral metabolism and microstructural defects in primate teeth. Am. J. Phys. Anthrop. *43*:3–11, 1974.

106. Muhlemann, H. R., Iselin, W., and Marthaler, T. M.: Anti-plaque effects of sorbose. Helv. Odont. Acta. *87*:1273–1279, 1977.

107. NAS/NRS: Recommended Dietary Allowances, Washington, D.C., National Academy of Sciences, National Research Council, 1980.

108. Navia, J. M.: Evaluation of nutritional and dietary factors that modify animal caries. J. Dent. Res. *49*:1213–1227, 1970.

109. Navia, J. M.: Effects of Minerals on Dental Caries. *In* Dietary Chemicals vs. Dental Caries. Adv. Chem. Series *94*:123–160, 1970.

110. Navia, J. M.: Prevention of dental caries: Agents which increase tooth resistance to dental caries. Int. Dent. J. *22*:427–440, 1972.

111. Navia, J. M.: Nutritional and Dietary Aspects of Dental Caries. J. Cont. Dent. Ed. *1*(2):136–159, 1980.

112. Navia, J. M.: Nutrition in dental development and disease. *In* Winick, M. (ed.): Human Nutrition — A Comprehensive Treatise. Vol. I: Nutrition — Pre- and Postnatal Development. New York, Plenum Press, 1979.

113. Navia, J. M.: Plaque Biochemistry. *In* Menaker, L., Morehart, R., and Navia, J. M. (eds.): Biologic Basis of Dental Caries, New York, Harper & Row, 1980.

114. Navia, J. M., and Harris, S. S.: Vitamin A influence on calcium metabolism and calcification. Ann. N. Y. Acad. Sci. *355*:45–57, 1980.

115. Navia, J. M., DiOrio, L. P., Menaker, L., and Miller, S.: Effect of undernutrition during the perinatal period on caries development in the rat. J. Dent. Res. *49*:1091–1098, 1970.

116. Newbrun, E.: Cariology. Baltimore, Md., Williams and Wilkins Co., 1978.

117. Newbrun, E., and Frostell, G.: Sugar restriction and substitution for caries prevention. Caries Res. *12*(Suppl. 1):65–73, 1978.

118. Nicholls, L., Sinclair, H. M., and Jelliffee, D. B.: Tropical Nutrition and Dietetics, 4th Ed. London, Balliere, Tindall and Cox, 1961.

119. Nikiforuk, G., and Fraser, D.: Etiology of enamel hypoplasia and interglobular dentin: The roles of hypocalcemia and hypophosphatemia. Metab. Bone Dis. Rel. Res. *2*:17–23, 1979.

120. Nizel, A.: The Science of Nutrition and Its Applica-

tion to Clinical Dentistry. Philadelphia, W. B. Saunders Co., 1966.

121. Nizel, A. E.: Nutrition in Preventive Dentistry: Science and Practice, 2nd ed. Philadelphia, W. B. Saunders Co., 1981.

122. Nylen, M. U.: Recent electron microscopic and allied investigations into the normal structure of human enamel. Int. Dent. J. 17:719–733, 1967.

123. Page, L., and Friend, B.: The changing United States diet. Bio-Science 28:192, 1978.

124. Parker, R. B., and Creamer, H. R.: Contribution of plaque polysaccharides to growth of cariogenic microorganisms. Arch. Oral Biol. 16:855–862, 1971.

125. Poole, D. F. G., and Newman, H. N.: Dental plaque and oral health. Nature 234:329–331, 1971.

126. Radentz, W. H., Baker, J., Altman, L. C., and Oppenheim, P.: Human lymphoproliferative reaction to food products. Possible role in periodontal inflammation. J. Periodontol. 46:562–566, 1975.

127. Redd, W. H., and Sleator, W.: Take Charge: A Personal Guide to Behavior Modification. New York, Random House Inc., 1976.

128. Retief, D. H., Cleaton-Jones, P. E., and Walker, A. R. P.: Dental caries and sugar intake in South African pupils of 16 to 17 years in four ethnic groups. Br. Dent. J. 138:463–469, 1975.

129. Rozovski, S. J., and Winick, M.: Nutrition and cellular growth. In Winick, M. (ed.): Human Nutrition — A Comprehensive Treatise, Vol. I: Nutrition: Pre- and Postnatal Development. New York, Plenum Publishing Co., 1979.

130. Rugg-Gunn, A. J., Edgar, W. M., Geddes, D. A. M., and Jenkins, G. N.: The effect of different meal patterns upon plaque pH in human subjects. Br. Dent. J. 139:361–366, 1975.

131. Russell, A. L.: International Nutrition Surveys: A summary of preliminary dental findings. J. Dent. Res. 42:233–244, 1963.

132. Sandstead, H. D., Carter, J. P., and Darby, W. J.: How to diagnose nutritional disorders in daily practice. Nutr. Today 4:20–26, 1969.

133. Schamschula, R. G., Adkins, B. L., Barmes, D. E., et al.: WHO Study of Dental Caries Etiology in Papua and New Guinea. WHO Offset Publication No. 4. Geneva, WHO, 1978.

134. Scheinin, A., and Mäkinen, K. K. (eds.): Turku sugar studies I–XXI. Acta. Odontol. Scand. 33(Suppl. 70), 1975.

135. Scheinin, D.: Sugar substitutes in relation to the incidence of clinical and experimental caries. Pharm. Ther. Dent. 3:95–100, 1978.

136. Schultz, H. W., Canin, R. R., and Wrolstad, R. W.: Symposium on Foods: Carbohydrates and Their Roles. The Avi Publishing Co., Inc., Westport, Connecticut, 1969.

137. Scott, D. B., Simmelink, J. W., Swancar, J. R., and Smith, T. J.: Apatite crystal growth in biological systems. In Brown, U., and Young, R. A. (eds.): Structural Properties of Hydroxyapatite and Related Components. Gordon and Breach, Science Publishing, Inc., New York, 1972.

138. Scrimshaw, N. W., Taylor, C. F., and Gordon, J. E.: Interactions of nutrition and infection. Am. J. Med. Sci. 237:367–403, 1959.

139. Selye, H.: The story of the adaptation syndrome. Montreal, Acta Medica Publishers, 1952.

140. Shallenberger, R. S.: Predicting sweeteners from chemical structure and knowledge of chemoreception. Food Tech. 34:65–66, 1980.

141. Shaw, J. H.: An evaluation in rats of the relationship between the frequency of providing food and the caries-producing ability of diets. Arch. Oral Biol. 13:1003–1013, 1968.

142. Shaw, J. H., and Roussos, G. G.: Sweeteners and Dental Caries. Sp. Supp. Feeding, Weight and Obesity, Abstr. 403. Washington, D.C., Information Retrieval Inc., 1978.

143. Shaw, J. H.: Nutrition. Chapter 11 in Shaw, J. H., et al.: Textbook of Oral Biology. Philadelphia, W. B. Saunders Co., 1978.

144. Shaw, J. H.: Nutritional guidance in the prevention of oral disease. Dent. Clin. North Am. 16:733–746, 1972.

145. Shaw, J. H., and Griffith, D.: Dental abnormalities in rats attributable to protein and deficiency during reproduction. J. Dent. Res. 80:123–141, 1963.

146. Socransky, S. S.: Relationship of bacteria to the etiology of periodontal disease. J. Dent. Res. 49:203–222, 1970.

147. Sreebny, L. M.: Effect of physical consistency of food on the "crevicular complex" and the salivary glands. Int. Dent. J. 22:394–401, 1972.

148. Sreebny, L. M.: Food consistency and periodontal disease. In Hazen, S. P. (ed.): Diet Nutrition and Periodontal Disease. Chicago, Ill., Am. Soc. Prev. Dent., pp. 78–93, 1975.

149. Stephan, R. M.: Changes in hydrogen-ion concentration on tooth surfaces and in carious lesions. J. Am. Dent. Assoc. 27:718–723, 1940.

150. Sweeney, E. A., and Guzman, M.: Oral conditions in children from three highland villages in Guatemala. Arch. Oral Biol. 11:687, 1966.

151. Sweeney, E. A., Cabrera, J., Urrutia, J., and Mata, L.: Factors associated with linear hypoplasia of human deciduous incisors. J. Dent. Res. 48:1275–1279, 1969.

152. Sweeney, E. A., Saffir, A. J., and DeLeon, R.: Linear hypoplasia of deciduous incisor teeth in malnourished children. Am. J. Clin. Nutr. 24:29, 1971.

153. Tanzer, J. M., and Fitzgerald, R. J.: Lack of caries inhibitory property of 2-deoxy-D-glucose in rats. J. Dent. Res. 57:440, 1978.

154. Sipple, H. L., and McNutt, K. W.: Sugars in Nutrition. Nutrition Foundation Series, New York, Academic Press, 1974.

155. Ten-State Nutrition Survey in the United States 1968–1970. Washington, D.C., U. S. Dept. H. E. W. Health Services and Mental Health Administration (D.H.E.W. Publ. No. [HSM] 72-8134), 1972.

156. Therapeutic Nutrition. National Academy of Sciences, National Research Council, Publication No. 234, 1951.

157. Van Houte, J., and Upeslacis, V. N.: Studies of the mechanism of sucrose-associated colonization of Streptococcus mutans on teeth of conventional rats. J. Dent. Res. 55:216–222, 1976.

158. Van Houte, J., Upeslacis, V. N., Jordan, H. V., et al.: Role of sucrose in colonization of Streptococcus mutans on teeth of conventional

Sprague-Dawley rats. J. Dent. Res. *55*:202–215, 1976.

159. Watson, D. L., and Tharp, R. G.: Self-directed Behavior. Monterey, California, Brooks-Cole Publishing Co., 1977.

160. Weinstein, P., and Getz, T.: Changing Human Behavior: Strategies for Preventive Dentistry. Chicago, Ill., Scientific Research Associates, Inc., 1978.

161. Weinstock, A.: Matrix development in mineraliz-ing tissues as shown by radioautography: Formation of enamel and dentine. *In* Slavkin, H. C., and Bavetta, L. A. (eds.): Developmental Aspects of Oral Biology. New York, Academic Press, 1972.

162. Winick, M., and Noble, A.: Quantitative changes in DNA, RNA and protein during prenatal and postnatal growth in the rat. Dev. Biol. *12*:451–456, 1965.

CHAPTER NINE
Water Fluoridation and Other Methods for Delivering Systemic Fluorides

Herschel S. Horowitz, D.D.S., M.P.H.

Dental caries is the most nearly preventable of all diseases of the mouth. Three conditions must be present for dental caries to occur. (1) There must be a susceptible host. Inasmuch as any tooth will develop caries if challenged sufficiently, all persons with teeth must be considered susceptible. (2) Bacteria that produce acids that attack the teeth must be present in plaque. (3) There must be a diet suitable for bacterial fermentation.[1, 2]

In correspondence with these conditions, our efforts to prevent dental caries have focused upon attempts to (1) increase the resistance of teeth with various fluorides and adhesive pit and fissure sealants,[3-8] (2) lower the number of bacteria in contact with the teeth by mechanical means or reduce their cariogenic activity with chemical agents,[9-12] and (3) modify dietary practices by urging people to eat cariogenic foods less frequently.[13-15]

In the United States, mechanical removal is now the only way to control accumulations of dental plaque. It is unrealistic to believe and data do not support the conclusion that dental caries can be controlled simply by urging people to remove dental plaque fastidiously each day. Because persuading people to change their diet in order to improve oral health is difficult, the prospects for reducing dental decay by altering

dietary habits are equally unpromising. Today, the most feasible way to prevent dental caries is to increase the resistance of teeth to decay, and the most practical way to accomplish that goal is by the proper use of fluorides. Fluorides have been and continue to be the best weapon to defend our teeth against dental decay.

MECHANISMS OF ACTION OF FLUORIDE

An agent used to prevent or treat a disease may be given systemically or topically. Systemic agents are taken into the body and circulate through the blood stream to reach the sites where they produce benefits. In contrast, topical agents are applied directly to the body tissues selected for treatment. The precise mechanisms by which fluorides protect teeth from dental caries are not completely understood, but clearly, more than one mechanism is involved, and both topical and systemic exposures are important.

Until about ten years ago, most dental experts believed that fluorides worked principally by increasing the resistance of enamel to acids produced in dental plaque by bacteria.[16] More recent research clearly shows that other actions of fluoride, such as remineralization of initial or pre-carious lesions and a host of antimicrobial effects, are also important.[17-19]

Figure 9–1 shows schematically what happens to fluoride when it is ingested. Fluoride is readily absorbed into the body, although the presence of ions that complex with fluoride, such as calcium and aluminum, may interfere with its absorption from the gastrointestinal tract. Usually, little fluoride is eliminated in the feces. There is a temporary rise in the fluoride concentration of the blood shortly after its ingestion. The elevated fluoride level quickly subsides because fluoride is rapidly taken up by mineralizing tissue (bones and teeth) or excreted by the kidneys.[20, 21] Fluoride concentrations in blood reach peak levels about 30 minutes after ingestion and, within a few hours, return to fasting levels.[21] Fasting levels of fluoride in blood are low — about 0.02 to 0.03 parts per million (ppm). These levels rise somewhat with increasing age, probably because reservoirs of fluoride in mature skeletal tissues are continually released into the blood stream. Fluoride does not accumulate in non-calcified soft tissues.

While teeth are forming, small amounts of fluoride are incorporated into the enamel as hydroxyfluorapatite, which is more resistant to dissolution by acids than hydroxyapatite, the principal inorganic mineral of enamel. In the presence of high concentrations of plasma fluoride, the enamel surface continues to incorporate fluoride during the period of pre-eruptive maturation when the developing tooth is contained in its bony crypt within the jaws.

Because the enamel of newly erupted teeth is incompletely mineralized, appreciable diffusion of fluoride into enamel probably continues for an indefinite period of time following eruption. Of course, this type of uptake occurs only if fluorides are available at the enamel surface. Many researchers believe that the increasing concentration of fluoride in the enamel surface is crucial to establishing resistance to carious attack.

Bacterial plaque on teeth tends to concentrate fluoride from the oral environment.[22] The drop in pH that occurs in plaque when acid-producing foods are consumed facilitates the uptake of fluoride and other minerals by the underlying enamel. In simple terms, the preceding sentences describe the process of remineralization.

As Figure 9–1 indicates, systemic fluoride is excreted in small amounts into the oral fluids through the salivary glands and crevicular fluid around the teeth. Some researchers believe that these continuous secretions of low concentrations of fluoride are responsible for a large part of the anticariogenic effects of fluoride. Although this may be so, fluoride must be ingested, circulated in the blood, and excreted into the mouth for this protective topical effect to be produced.

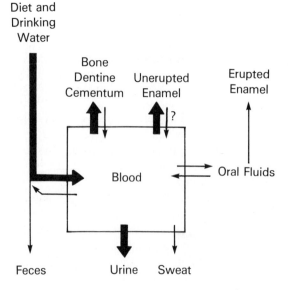

Figure 9–1 The kinetics of ingested fluoride.

An understanding of this process re-emphasizes the importance of systemic fluorides.

The mechanisms by which fluorides prevent decay vary, depending upon the agent used, its route of administration, the age at which it is administered, its concentration, its frequency of use, and the vehicle used to deliver it.[23] Several mechanisms may operate simultaneously, with one or another pre-eminent at different times because of local conditions at the tooth surface.

COMMUNITY WATER FLUORIDATION

Fluoride compounds are among the most common components of the earth's crust. Because all of these compounds are soluble to some degree in water, nearly all natural water sources contain a measurable quantity, which varies according to the amount and solubility of the fluoride in adjacent mineral deposits. Only distilled water and uncontaminated rain and snow are completely free of fluoride.

Many common foods also contain appreciable amounts of fluoride. Fish and tea are particularly rich sources. Fluoride is also found in fowl and other meats and in such cereals as rye, wheat, and rice. In fact, fluoride is present in so many foods that some is probably ingested at every meal.

Because naturally occurring water-borne fluoride is not always present in a concentration sufficient to produce dental benefits, it is recommended that the natural level be adjusted. The process of adjusting the amount of fluoride in a community's water to an optimal concentration for the prevention of dental caries is known as community water fluoridation. Because the original water is likely to contain some fluoride already, a key word in this definition is adjustment.

History of Fluoridation

The history of water fluoridation is colorful and consists of many studies in which classic epidemiologic methods were used. In the 1800's, scientists knew that fluoride was contained in calcified tissues of animals and humans. By the middle of the 19th Century, they had established that fluoride occurred in varying amounts in water and food. Drinking water was even suspected as the source of the fluoride present in animal tissue.

In 1902, an American dentist working for the U.S. Immigration Service in Naples, Italy reported a condition of discolored teeth known locally as "denti di chiaie," among Italians from certain towns who were immigrating to the United States, but he made no association between the condition and fluoride.[24] The same condition was also observed in the early 1900's by McKay in several Colorado towns, where it was called "Colorado brown stain." McKay sought the advice and help of G. V. Black, Dean of Northwestern University Dental School in Chicago, who visited Colorado in 1909 and was amazed to find that a dental condition that affected so many people was unmentioned in the literature.[25] After conducting several large-scale surveys of children in Colorado and other states, McKay realized that persons who had spent their entire lives in these particular towns had the discolored teeth, whereas those who had spent their childhood in other communities before moving to the endemic areas had unaffected teeth. He concluded that a mysterious element in the water supply was responsible.[26] McKay also noted that mottled teeth, as the condition came to be called, were no more susceptible to dental caries than were unaffected teeth.[27] Not all of his early investigations, however, were on target; in one survey, he attempted to correlate mottled enamel with freckles.

McKay's enthusiasm in studying dental fluorosis came from a desire to discover its cause so that a way could be found to prevent the unsightly pitted and stained teeth. Because he was convinced that something in the water supply was responsible, he persuaded the town of Oakley, Idaho, where native children were affected by fluorosis, to change its water supply.[28] The community decided to bring its water from another town, which happened to have a low concentration of fluoride in its water supply. Several years later, children born in Oakley subsequent to the change in water supply showed no evidence of mottled permanent teeth.[29] Another town, Bauxite, Arkansas, had inadvertently changed its drinking water in 1909 from a source with a low fluoride concentration to another with a high concentration. A survey done by Kempf and McKay[30] showed that people who grew up in Bauxite before the change had no fluorosis, whereas those reared in Bauxite after 1909 had severely mottled teeth.

The final proof that excessive fluoride in water causes dental fluorosis occurred in 1931. The chief chemist for the Aluminum Company of America (ALCOA), C. V. Churchill, analyzed water from Bauxite for some rare elements that were not usually assessed. He found that the water contained 13.7 parts per million (ppm) of fluoride. He contacted McKay and obtained samples of water from other communities with endemic fluorosis; all had 2 ppm fluoride or more.[31] Working independently, H. V. Smith and M. C. Smith had fed water from a community with endemic fluorosis to rats, which produced dull white and pitted teeth. Unaware of Churchill's work, the two investigators reported their findings just a few weeks after Churchill's initial report was published.[32] Thus, it was nearly 30 years after McKay's first observations that the cause of mottled teeth was identified.

Beginning in 1931, a U.S. Public Health Service dentist, H. Trendly Dean, continued McKay's work. He was assigned the task of determining the extent and geographic distribution of dental fluorosis in the United States. During the next ten years or so, he and his associates (including McKay) conducted hundreds of surveys throughout the country and identified 375 communities in 26 states with various degrees of dental fluoro-

sis.[33] In order to rate the severity of fluorosis, Dean developed an index for classifying the condition.[34] These surveys showed conclusively that the prevalence and severity of fluorosis increased as concentrations of fluoride in drinking water increased above 1 ppm. Scientists during this period focused on identifying endemic areas of fluorosis and gave little attention to the possible caries-preventive effects of fluoride.[35, 36]

Dean was aware of McKay's observation that teeth with fluorosis were not more susceptible to dental caries than teeth without fluorosis.[27] Others had also made this observation, including Ainsworth, a British dentist.[37] During his own surveys, Dean also noted that children who were mildly affected by fluorosis seemed to have teeth that were remarkably free from dental caries. To test the hypothesis of an inverse relationship between dental caries and dental fluorosis, Dean, in 1939, conducted a survey in four Illinois towns, two with negligible concentrations of fluoride in their water (Macomb and Quincy) and two with fluoride concentrations of about 1.7 ppm (Galesburg and Monmouth). As shown in Table 9–1, the survey indicated that caries prevalence was twice as great in Macomb and three times as great in Quincy as in Galesburg and Monmouth.[38] In the early 1940's, a larger study of 7,257 children 12 to 14 years old living in 21 cities in four states confirmed the inverse relationship between dental caries and fluoride concentration of drinking water up to a level of 1.0 ppm of fluoride.[39, 40] As the fluoride concentration increased beyond that level, the prevalence and severity of dental fluorosis increased without a concomitant, appreciable decrease in the prevalence of dental caries. It seemed paradoxical that the

TABLE 9–1 AVERAGE NUMBER OF DMF TEETH IN 12 TO 14-YEAR-OLD CHILDREN IN 4 ILLINOIS COMMUNITIES

COMMUNITY	WATER FLUORIDE CONCENTRATION (ppm)	NUMBER OF EXAMINED CHILDREN	MEAN NUMBER DMF TEETH
Galesburg	1.8	319	2.01
Monmouth	1.7	148	2.05
Macomb	0.2	112	4.01
Quincy	0.2	306	6.33

same element could benefit teeth at one concentration but harm them at another concentration, but it was true.

These findings led to the hypothesis that dental caries could be prevented by adjusting the existing fluoride concentration of community water supplies to optimal levels. In 1945, the U.S. Public Health Service began to fluoridate the drinking water of Grand Rapids, Michigan, at 1.0 ppm.[41] Muskegon, Michigan, was to serve as a control community, so that findings in Grand Rapids could be assessed. After six and a half years, the caries-preventive effects of fluoridation in Grand Rapids were already so pronounced[42] that the people of Muskegon decided to fluoridate their own water supply. From that point on, findings in Grand Rapids had to be compared retrospectively with conditions that existed in the community before fluoridation began.

In the mid 1940's, three other independent clinical trials of fluoridation at 1.0 ppm were initiated in North America: Newburgh, New York;[43] Evanston, Illinois;[44] and Brantford, Ontario.[45] In each of these communities, as in Grand Rapids, after 15 or more years the prevalence of dental caries in children was reduced overall by 50 to 70 per cent compared with the prevalence in control communities with similar demographic characteristics or in the same community before fluoridation was initiated.[44, 46-48] Table 9–2 shows the change in dental caries prevalence among children 12 through 16 years old after 15 years of community water fluoridation in Grand Rapids. Interim results from these studies were so impressive that in the 1950's many additional fluoridation programs or evaluations were begun in the United States and in other countries.[49-51]

Advantages of Community Water Fluoridation

Fluoridation of community water supplies is the least expensive and most effective way to provide fluoride to large groups of people.[52-56] Optimal adjustment of the fluoride concentration of community water supplies should be the foundation for all programs of dental health because this public health method is nearly ideal. First and foremost, community fluoridation is highly effective.[57, 58] Hundreds of studies done throughout the world have shown that children who consume optimally fluoridated water from birth have from 50 to 70 per cent less dental decay than they would have experienced without fluoridation. Consumption of fluoridated water is eminently safe.[57, 58] No other health measure has been more critically analyzed than fluoridation of city water supplies. The procedure is also inexpensive and greatly reduces the per capita costs of dental treatment.[59-61] On the average, community fluoridation currently costs about 20 cents per person per year to operate in the United States.[56, 57] In addition, the entire community benefits from the procedure, regardless of socioeconomic level, educational achievement, individual motivation, or the availability of dentists. No cooperative effort or direct action need be taken by those who will benefit. Moreover, the improvement in dental health continues for life if consumption of fluoridated water continues.[62, 63] A recent report shows that

TABLE 9–2   AVERAGE NUMBER OF DMF TEETH IN 12 TO 16-YEAR-OLD CHILDREN IN GRAND RAPIDS BEFORE AND AFTER 15 YEARS OF COMMUNITY WATER FLUORIDATION

| | DMF TEETH | | |
AGE	1944–45 Before Fluoridation	1959 After 15 Years of Fluoridation	PERCENTAGE DIFFERENCE
12	8.07	3.47	57.0
13	9.73	3.58	63.2
14	10.94	5.38	50.8
15	12.48	6.22	50.2
16	13.50	7.03	47.9

life-long consumption of fluoridated water also significantly lowers the prevalence of root surface caries in older persons.[64]

Although the benefits of community fluoridation are truly impressive, the procedure is not a panacea for dental caries. Unfortunately, its implementation is limited to areas with central water supplies. Moreover, other methods of preventing decay are still necessary for particularly susceptible persons living in fluoridated communities, and obviously, the use of fluoridated water is not a license for unrestricted consumption of confections between meals or for abandoning oral hygiene procedures.

Current Status of Community Fluoridation

Published estimates show that 185 million persons living in 6,470 communities in 40 countries drink water with an optimally adjusted fluoride concentration.[65] Another 39 million persons living in 4,096 communities in 39 countries consume drinking water with naturally occurring amounts of fluoride at optimal or greater concentrations. Nineteen of these 39 countries also have communities with controlled fluoridation. Thus, there are at least 60 countries in the world with adjusted or natural fluoridation, serving more than 10,000 communities and 224 million persons.[65] The Republic of Ireland implemented legislation for national fluoridation in the early 1960's. The municipal water supplies in Hong Kong and Singapore are fluoridated. Thirty million persons in 85 communities in the Soviet Union consume fluoridated water.

Unfortunately, administrative and political developments have caused some major setbacks for fluoridation in Sweden[66] and the suspension of new fluoridation activities in the Netherlands.[67] For many years, Denmark has had a law that prohibits the addition of fluoride to food and cosmetics. This law has been interpreted to include the prohibition of fluoridation.[57] In other countries, governments or health authorities have been totally or relatively inactive with regard to community fluoridation. Less than five million persons in Britain currently receive the benefits of this important public health measure.[68] In

Europe's 30 countries, only 15.5 million of the continent's 750 million persons — about two per cent — are consuming fluoridated water.[69]

In the United States, by the end of 1975, which was the last time a nationwide census of community water fluoridation was taken, an estimated 105 million persons were consuming water with optimum or greater concentrations of fluoride.[70] Since then, the metropolitan Boston area has fluoridated its water, as have New Orleans and Memphis. Of the estimated U.S. population of 224 million persons, approximately 112 million persons live in communities served by fluoridated water supplies or by water that contains optimal or greater concentrations of fluoride as a natural constituent. About 11 million people live in communities in the latter category. Thus, 50 per cent of the U.S. population consumes water with sufficient amounts of fluoride. About 37 million persons cannot benefit from fluoridation because they live in largely rural areas that lack community water supplies. Thus, those who consume water with adequate amounts of fluoride in the U.S.A. compose 60 per cent of the population with access to community water supplies. However, about 75 million persons in the U.S. live in communities that could fluoridate but have not yet adopted the procedure for economic or political reasons, or because of lack of interest, perceived need, or motivation.

According to the U.S. Environmental Protection Agency, there are 61,500 community water supplies in the United States. Eighty-six per cent of these supplies serve fewer than 2500 people. Perhaps the difficulty of achieving universal fluoridation in the United States is best highlighted by the fact that the half of the U.S. population now consuming fluoridated water is served by only 13 per cent of the central water supplies in the country.[57] Consequently, 87 per cent of the supplies must still be fluoridated in order to achieve complete fluoridation in the United States. As might be surmised from these statistics, most of the large cities in the country are already fluoridated; in fact, about 70 per cent of U.S. cities with populations of 100,000 or more have fluoridated water, and many of these, for example, Baltimore, Pittsburgh, San Francisco, and Washington, have been fluoridated for about 30 years. There are still several large cities in the U.S., however, that have failed to implement the procedure, including Los Angeles, Phoenix, San Antonio, and Portland.

Eight of the 50 states in the U.S. have passed laws making fluoridation mandatory.[57] These are Connecticut, Minnesota, Illinois, Michigan, Ohio, South Dakota, Georgia, and Nebraska. Five states — Delaware, Maine, New Hampshire, Nevada, and Utah — require referenda before fluoridation may be implemented. It is interesting to note that 65 per cent of the population in the eight states with mandatory fluoridation laws consume fluoridated water, whereas only 19 per cent of the population in the five states that require referenda drink fluoridated water. Referenda are a deterrent to fluoridation. Not only are they costly, they frequently are merely advisory to decision-making bodies. Some communities have had repeated referenda that reversed decisions on fluoridation after fluoridating equipment had already been installed. Plebiscites frequently result in rejection of fluoridation because they are conducted in an atmosphere of near-hysteria. During the campaigns, the opponents have often resorted to scare tactics and the dissemination of false, irrelevant, and misleading information.[57] Some states, for example, Hawaii, New Hampshire, and New Jersey, have fewer than 25 per cent of their total population served by adjusted or natural fluoridated water. By contrast, more than 75 per cent of the total populations of Colorado, Connecticut, and Michigan consume fluoridated water.[70]

Effects of Fluoridation on the Dental Health of Children and Adults

Abundant data show that fluoridated water not only acts systemically during tooth formation to produce teeth with enamel more resistant to dental caries but also acts directly as a topically applied agent. Therefore, the procedure benefits both children and adults.

Studies of the effects of fluoridation in young children prove that the procedure effectively reduces the prevalence of dental caries in primary teeth by about 40 per cent.[71-75] For example, in 1944, five-year-old children in South Shields, England (F = 1.4 ppm) were found to have 41 per cent fewer decayed, missing, and filled (dmf) primary teeth than did children of the same age in North Shields (F = 0.4 ppm).[74] Marthaler has shown that consumption of fluoridated water should begin at birth to provide maximal protection to primary teeth.[75]

Many studies have confirmed the finding that fluoridation reduces the prevalence of dental caries in permanent teeth by an average of about 60 per cent.[57, 58] However, the benefits are not uniformly conferred to all tooth surfaces. Approximal and other smooth tooth surfaces are protected to a far greater extent than are pit and fissure surfaces.[75-77] For example, data from the Culemborg-Tiel study in the Netherlands showed a caries-inhibitory effect of 86 per cent in gingival areas of buccal-lingual surfaces. The reduced prevalence of dental caries in approximal surfaces was 73 per cent, but fluoridation produced only about 37 per cent fewer pit and fissure carious lesions in fluoridated Tiel compared with those in fluoride-deficient Culemborg.[78]

Using data from several studies, Marthaler has shown rather conclusively that maximal caries protection to permanent teeth occurs only when children begin to consume fluoridated water at birth.[75] The protection lessens gradually as the age of the children at the start of fluoridation increases (Figure 9–2). Although the cariostatic effects of fluoridation are greater in smooth surfaces than in pit and fissure surfaces, the systemic or pre-eruptive effects are more critical to the protection of pit and fissure tooth surfaces than to smooth surfaces.[75]

Arnold's 1943 forecast for dental benefits from controlled fluoridation based on observations in areas with naturally occurring fluoride have been substantiated by nearly 40 years of observations.[76] He specifically predicted that, after fluoridation, there would be (1) about six times as many children who are free from dental caries, (2) about a 60 per cent lower prevalence of dental caries, (3) almost a 75 per cent decrease in extracted first permanent molars,

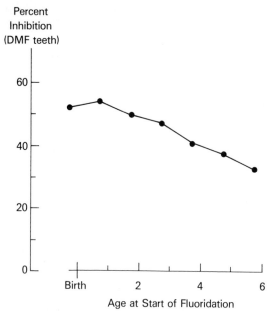

Figure 9–2 Percentage inhibition of dental caries in permanent teeth of children in Grand Rapids, Michigan, according to age when first exposed to fluoridated water. (From Marthaler, T. M.: Fluoride supplements for systemic effects in caries prevention. Reprinted by permission of Westview Press from *Continuing Evaluation of the Use of Fluorides* edited by Erling Johansen, Donald R. Taves, and Thor O. Olsen. Copyright 1979 by the American Association for the Advancement of Science.)

and (4) approximately 95 per cent fewer carious lesions in approximal surfaces of maxillary incisors.

Although the caries prevention derived from community fluoridation is substantial, other methods of preventing caries in fluoridated communities cannot be ignored. Several studies have shown that the regular use of a therapeutic, fluoride-containing dentifrice by children in a fluoridated community produces an additional moderate lowering of the incidence of dental caries.[79, 80] Therefore, their use in both fluoridated and low-fluoride communities should be recommended. At least two studies have shown that mouthrinsing in school with a dilute fluoride solution produces measurable protection from dental caries in children in a fluoridated community.[81, 82] The findings of studies in which professional topical applications of fluoride have been given to children in fluoridated communities are mixed.[83, 84] Therefore, public health programs in fluoridated cities in which all

school children of certain ages are scheduled to receive these treatments cannot be recommended. However, individual children in fluoridated communities who are especially susceptible to dental decay should definitely be given topical applications of fluoride.

Studies carried out among adults who lived continuously in fluoride and non-fluoride areas have demonstrated that the dental benefits from fluorides in water are not limited to children. For example, as shown in Figure 9–3, adults 20 to 44 years of age in Colorado Springs, who had consumed water that contained 2.5 ppm of fluoride all their lives, had lower DMF tooth scores than did adults of the same age in Boulder, Colorado, who had consumed water with only trace levels of fluoride.[63] For each five-year age grouping between 20 and 44, the average DMF score was approximately 60 per cent lower in Colorado Springs than in Boulder. Natives of Boulder had lost three to four times as many teeth because of dental caries as had natives of Colorado Springs.

Findings were similar in comparisons of adults in Aurora, Illinois (1.2 ppm F) and Rockford, Illinois (fluoride-free).[85] In another study of British adults between the ages of 15 and 65 in Hartlepool (natural fluoride) and York (low fluoride), the DMF values in Hart-

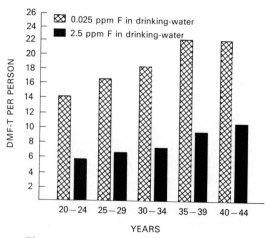

Figure 9–3 Mean numbers of DMF teeth per adult. Natives of Boulder (0.025 ppm F) and Colorado Springs (2.5 ppm F), excluding third molars. (From Russell, A. L., and Elvove, E.: Domestic water and dental caries. VII. A study of the fluoride dental caries relationship in an adult population. Public Health Rep. *66*:1389, 1951.)

lepool were lower than those observed in York for all ages up to and including the 60 to 65 age group. Hence, continuous residence in a fluoride-sufficient area has life-long beneficial effects.[86] Consuming drinking water with adequate amounts of fluoride, therefore, does not merely delay the development of dental caries, but gives substantial life-long protection.

Effects of Fluoridation on Need for Dental Care

Because fluoridation protects smooth tooth surfaces best, which include approximal surfaces of posterior teeth, proportionally fewer complex, multi-surface fillings are placed in optimally fluoridated communities than in areas with fluoride-deficient water. Pits and fissures of teeth also receive protection from consumption of fluoridated water, but to a lesser extent. Hence, caries in pits and fissures persist as the predominant type of decay in fluoridated communities. These cavities are easy to detect and, because they are generally easier to restore than approximal cavities, they require less of the dentist's time.

Analysis of cost and time factors required to provide regular, periodic dental care for children in fluoridated Newburgh, N.Y., and fluoride-deficient Kingston, N.Y., demonstrated that costs of treating the backlog of accumulated dental needs at the initiation of the care program were 60 per cent lower in Newburgh than in Kingston, and the costs for incremental care for six years were 50 per cent lower. The average chairtime required to provide both initial and incremental care was 1.6 times greater in Kingston than in Newburgh.[59, 87, 88] Similar findings have been reported from New Zealand[60] and, relative to the need for care of primary teeth, from Canada.[89]

Optimal Concentrations for Community Fluoridation

In the 1950's, Galagan and his coworkers studied environmental factors that affect the consumption of fluoridated water.[90, 91] They concluded that only the mean annual maximum daily temperature of an area determines how much drinking water is consumed (Table 9–3). The fluoride concentration of a water supply should be adjusted according to this climatic variable because persons in hotter climates consume more water than do those in colder climates.

As Table 9–3 shows, recommended fluoride concentrations for community fluoridation range from 0.7 to 1.2 ppm depending on temperature. A community located in a cold climate, for example, in Maine, should fluoridate its water at 1.2 ppm, whereas a community in a hot climate, for example, in southern Texas, should fluoridate at 0.7 ppm. These concentrations are currently recommended for the water supply in addition to the fluoride that occurs in various foods.

Engineering and Surveillance of Fluoridation

Adding fluoride to a community's water supply resembles the addition of other materials to treat water.[92] The compounds com-

TABLE 9–3 MEAN MAXIMUM DAILY TEMPERATURES AND CORRESPONDING OPTIMAL FLUORIDE CONCENTRATIONS FOR COMMUNITY WATER FLUORIDATION

RANGES OF MEAN MAXIMUM DAILY TEMPERATURES (°F)	RECOMMENDED OPTIMAL F CONCENTRATION FOR COMMUNITY FLUORIDATION (ppm)
50.0 to 53.7	1.2
53.8 to 58.3	1.1
58.4 to 63.8	1.0
63.9 to 70.6	0.9
70.7 to 79.2	0.8
79.3 to 90.5	0.7

monly used for fluoridation are sodium fluoride, hydrofluosilicic acid, and sodium silicofluoride. Important factors in selecting a specific process and chemical for fluoridation include size of the water system, number of sites of application, volume of water used, costs for equipment, water pressure at points of application, storage space, and convenience of maintenance and handling. The chemicals are automatically fed in either solution or dry form.

For most communities, the maintenance and surveillance of fluoridation equipment can be done by existing water works personnel, but for complex installations additional personnel are sometimes needed. The fluoride concentration must be monitored regularly, usually by colorimetric assay. Ion-specific electrodes for fluoride are now commercially available for this purpose and have greatly simplified the accurate determination of fluoride concentrations in water.

However, installing fluoridation equipment does not assure maximum protection against tooth decay. A survey conducted in 1972 of 104 fluoridated public water supply systems in nine states of the U.S. revealed that 44 per cent did not contain adequate concentrations of fluoride ion.[93] Continual surveillance of the installation is required for maintenance of the desired concentration of fluoride in the system. Improved training programs for water plant operators must be implemented in order to improve surveillance.

Opposition to and Support of Community Water Fluoridation

Efforts to implement fluoridation have frequently been unsuccessful.[94] The National Health Federation (NHF), a group ". . . dedicated to the protection of health freedoms," is a major center for the organized opposition to community fluoridation.[95] The NHF not only opposes water fluoridation, but also takes issue with such basic health practices as pasteurization of milk and immunization. It supports the use of Laetrile, megavitamins, chelation therapy and other health care practices of undemonstrated medical value. Despite these questionable positions, the NHF seeks to create an image of legitimate authority in the field of health and attracts support by appealing to popular issues, such as individual rights, freedom of choice, pollution, environmental carcinogens, and natural diets.

A report by the former Scientific Director of the NHF purported to demonstrate a relationship between increased cancer mortality and water fluoridation. Although the report has been severely criticized by many recognized health authorities and researchers for violating fundamental precepts for the design of epidemiologic surveys,[97, 98] the findings have been widely disseminated in this country and abroad.

The opponents of community fluoridation often employ surprise and intimidation in their campaigns against the procedure. They have organized referenda to prohibit the procedure in some communities. Moreover, they increasingly are apt to sue those who support the procedure or who allegedly impugn the reputations of their chosen experts.[95]

It is unfortunate that a public health measure as inexpensive, safe, easily implemented, and effective as fluoridation should create, on occasion, such public controversy. In many areas, proposals to fluoridate have become political issues, decided on by public referendum or by elected officials without expertise in health. Doubts raised in voters' minds have frequently led them to reject fluoridation.

Evans has outlined five steps that must be taken to overcome the obstacles to community water fluoridation: Supporters of fluoridation must recognize that the decision to fluoridate has become a political issue; the public must be made aware of its benefits; a national strategy and information exchange for fluoridation matters must be developed; federal agencies must provide incentives for communities to fluoridate; and schools of dentistry must stress the benefits of fluoridation in their curricula.[95]

The American Dental Association has endorsed fluoridation since 1950,[99] and, in 1958, the World Health Organization first recognized it as a practicable and effective public health measure.[100] In fact, community water fluoridation continues to have the unqualified approval of every major health organization in the United States and of many other countries as well.

Dental Fluorosis and Defluoridation

When drinking water contains too much fluoride, children who consume the water from birth are likely to develop teeth with dental fluorosis. The prevalence and severity of fluorosis is directly proportional to the extent that the concentration of fluoride in the water exceeds the recommended optimal level. Dean's modified system for classifying fluorosis contains six categories: normal, questionable, very mild, mild, moderate, and severe.[101] In its mildest forms, fluorosis is not in the least disfiguring; in fact, many prefer the lustrous, vitreous, translucent appearance of these teeth, occasionally highlighted with small paper-white flecks, to that of the dull, more yellowish enamel generally found in life-time residents of communities with negligible levels of fluoride in water.[102] Moreover, reports show that the prevalence of idiopathic or unexplained non-fluoride opacities in enamel is lower in areas with optimal fluoride levels than in fluoride-free areas.[103] Also, persons reared in fluoridated communities have fewer missing teeth and fewer carious lesions and, therefore, a lower risk of having unsightly dental restorations than those reared in areas without protective levels of fluoride in the water.

Moderate and severe fluorosis is unattractive and, in its worst forms, it can be disfiguring. According to Dean's classification,[101] when the amount of fluoride in water exceeds twice the optimal concentration for fluoridation, dental fluorosis may begin to be a public health problem that becomes increasingly severe as the fluoride concentra-

tion becomes greater.[104] Dean's work, however, was done many years ago. Since then, many changes have occurred in the types, origins, and distribution of foods and beverages that people consume. Studies are underway in various climatic zones to determine the current relationships between fluoride concentrations in drinking water, dental caries, and dental fluorosis.

Congress passed the Safe Drinking Water Act (Public Law 93-523) in 1974, which was intended to improve the quality and safety of drinking water supplies. The Environmental Protection Agency (EPA), which administers the Act, unfortunately included fluoride in excessive amounts (greater than two times the optimum level of fluoride for dental health [1.4 to 2.4 ppm F], depending on climatic zone) as a contaminant of drinking water.[105] The maximum contaminant levels were based on Dean's research, which indicated that beyond those levels cosmetically objectionable fluorosis might occur. The EPA's regulations required communities with contaminant levels of fluoride in their water to reduce the concentrations to tolerable levels. Communities can sometimes obtain an alternative source of drinking water with a lower fluoride concentration, and sometimes they can dilute the original to optimal levels by blending water supplies.[29] It is not always possible or practical, however, to find a new water supply. Community water supplies with excessive fluoride concentrations can be defluoridated to optimal levels. Bartlett, Texas[106] and Britton, South Dakota[107] have successfully done so with activated alumina and bone char, respectively. Fluorosis was reduced greatly in both communities by means of partial defluoridation. Table 9–4 shows a percentage distribu-

TABLE 9–4 PERCENTAGE DISTRIBUTION OF CHILDREN IN BARTLETT, TEXAS, BY FLUOROSIS CLASSIFICATION, 1954 AND 1969

YEAR	FLUOROSIS ABSENT			FLUOROSIS PRESENT				
	Normal	Questionable	Total	Very Mild	Mild	Moderate	Severe	Total
1954 (N = 132)	2.3	1.5	3.8	3.0	43.9	34.9	14.4	96.2
1969 (N = 157)	49.0	32.5	81.5	12.1	5.7	0.6	0.0	18.4

tion of children in Bartlett according to their classification of fluorosis before defluoridation (1954) and after 15 years of partial defluoridation (1969). Only four per cent of the children were free of fluorosis in 1954, but the number increased to 81 per cent by 1969.

However, defluoridation is expensive, and several states, such as Arizona, Texas, and South Dakota, that have many communities with excessive fluoride concentrations have sought exemptions from the EPA regulations concerning fluorides. Awareness of the technical problems and economic hardships of small communities in implementing defluoridation has recently led the EPA to relax and delay its enforcement priorities for excessive fluorides.[108]

SCHOOL WATER FLUORIDATION

Children who live in areas without public water supplies cannot benefit from optimally fluoridated drinking water. One effective way to bring them these benefits is to fluoridate their school water supplies. Rural schools usually have private wells, and the water from these wells can easily be fluoridated. Researchers in the late 1950's hypothesized that prevention of dental caries could be produced by part-time consumption of fluoridated water only on school days, even if consumption did not begin until age 5 or 6. Higher than optimal fluoride concentrations for community fluoridation were suggested for school fluoridation to compensate for the part-time and belated exposure. Studies of school fluoridation have been conducted in the U.S. Virgin Islands,[109] Kentucky,[110] Pennsylvania,[111] and North Carolina[112] in which fluorides were added to school water supplies at levels of 2.3, 3.0, 5.0 and 6.3 ppm, respectively.

After 12 years of school fluoridation at 5.0 ppm, or four and a half times the optimum level recommended for community fluoridation in the same geographic area, children at Elk Lake School in Pennsylvania demonstrated 40 per cent fewer DMF surfaces than their baseline counterparts.[111] The findings showed a differential effectiveness according to time of tooth eruption (Table 9–5); earlier erupting teeth (incisors and first molars) that were already in place when the children began to attend school showed a protective effect that resulted in 31 per cent fewer DMF surfaces, whereas surfaces of later erupting teeth (canines, premolars, and second molars) that could derive both topical and systemic exposure to the fluoridated water in school yielded 57 per cent fewer DMF surfaces. Both eruptive classes of teeth showed superior effects in proximal surfaces — as great as a 69 per cent lower prevalence of decay in proximal surfaces of later erupting teeth. The rate of extractions per 100 teeth decreased overall by 65 per cent during the 12-year period of the study. No objectionable dental fluorosis resulted from the procedure.

After eight years of school fluoridation at 6.3 ppm, that is, seven times the recommended optimum for community fluoridation in the geographic area, interim findings in Seagrove, North Carolina suggest that school water fluoridation at seven times the

TABLE 9–5   AVERAGE DMF SURFACE SCORES BY ERUPTIVE STATUS
AMONG SCHOOL CHILDREN IN ELK LAKE, PA. BEFORE (1958) AND
AFTER 12 YEARS (1970) OF SCHOOL FLUORIDATION

YEAR	DMFS		
	In All Teeth	*In Early Erupting Teeth*	*In Late Erupting Teeth*
1958 (N = 1,030)	13.51	9.03	4.47
1970 (N = 1,149)	8.13	6.23	1.91
% Difference from 1958	40	31	57

optimum may produce only marginally greater caries inhibition than at 4.5 times the optimum.[112] No objectionable fluorosis, however, is produced by consuming the higher concentration of fluoridated water at school.

More than 400 schools in 14 states of the U.S. are now fluoridating their water supplies at about 4.5 times the concentration appropriate for community fluoridation in the same geographic area.[57, 113] North Carolina and Kentucky have the largest programs.

One major disadvantage of school fluoridation is that its application is limited to geographic areas where both school and home water supplies of the students have uniformly low concentrations of fluoride. If some students drink nearly optimal concentrations of fluoride in water at home and others only trace levels, it is impossible to determine the proper concentration for the school's water supply.

The engineering aspects of fluoridating school water resemble those of community water fluoridation.[114, 115] In both instances, the maintenance of equipment and the surveillance of fluoride levels must be done regularly and conscientiously.

DIETARY FLUORIDE SUPPLEMENTS

In communities with insufficient fluoride in drinking water, dietary fluoride supplements in the form of tablets, lozenges, solutions, or drops are recommended for children for the prevention of dental caries. In order to protect primary and permanent teeth as well as consuming fluoridated water does, fluoride supplements must be taken daily in the correct dosage from birth until

about age 13 when all permanent teeth other than third molars have erupted.[116] A high degree of motivation, dedication, and perseverance from both parents and children is needed when such a long period of time is involved. For this reason, fluoride supplements lose some of their effectiveness for the community. In addition, they are more costly than water fluoridation. Therefore, dietary fluoride supplements should not be regarded as a substitute for community water fluoridation. Rather, they are best suited for low-fluoride areas without public water systems and as an interim measure in those communities with central water systems that have not yet implemented community fluoridation.

Dosages for Dietary Fluoride Supplementation

The Council on Dental Therapeutics of the American Dental Association recommends the dosage schedule for dietary fluoride supplements shown in Table 9–6.[117] The schedule is applicable in areas with negligible fluoride in water and in areas with significant but suboptimal levels. The dosages may be used for fluoride drops as well as 0.25, 0.5, and 1.0 mg. fluoride tablets. The Committee on Nutrition of the American Academy of Pediatrics has adopted a nearly identical dosage schedule.[118] Until 1979, the Academy had recommended 0.5 mg. of fluoride from birth until age three.

The dosage schedule in Table 9–6 applies in areas in moderate temperature zones where the optimal concentration of fluoride for community fluoridation is 1 ppm. Table 9–7 shows recommended dosages of dietary fluoride supplements according to the natu-

TABLE 9–6 SUPPLEMENTAL FLUORIDE DOSAGE SCHEDULE* (IN MG F/DAY)

AGE (YEARS)	CONCENTRATION OF FLUORIDE IN WATER (PPM)		
	Less Than 0.3	*0.3 to 0.7*	*Greater Than 0.7*
Birth to 2	0.25	0	0
2 to 3	0.50	0.25	0
3 to 13	1.00	0.50	0

*Approved by the Council on Dental Therapeutics of the American Dental Association.

ral fluoride content of an area's drinking water supply expressed as a percentage of the optimal fluoride concentration for that area. For example, in a community where the fluoride concentration of drinking water should be 1.2 ppm but which has 0.75 ppm (or 62.5% of the optimal), a supplement of 0.25 mg of fluoride should be prescribed for a two and a half year old child. According to Table 9–6, which does not take into account the range of recommended levels for fluoridation according to climate, no fluoride would be recommended for a child in the community just described. The dosage schedule in Table 9–7 requires knowing both the existing fluoride concentration in drinking water and the desirable concentration for that area based on the climate. The best dosage may be determined by using the schedule in Table 9–7.

No occurrences of esthetically unacceptable dental fluorosis have been reported following the use of the dosages recommended by the Council on Dental Therapeutics. The only study that has mentioned significant dental fluorosis is one in which 0.5 mg of fluoride was administered during the first two years of life,[119] rather than the 0.25 mg recommended by the ADA's Council on Dental Therapeutics. The investigators reported that 67 per cent of the participating children had fluorosis, most of which was very mild or mild and of no esthetic concern. However, a few of the children had unattractive, moderate fluorosis.[119] Five years after supplementation was discontinued the fluorosis scores were lower.[120] The investigators suggested that milder types of fluorosis may diminish with time because of enamel mineralization or abrasion.[120] The caries-protection in primary and permanent teeth at the end of their study was a striking 80 per cent.

One group of investigators recommended in 1977 that fluoride supplements should not be prescribed for children under six months of age except for breast-fed infants.[121] This recommendation emanated from a report that fluoride intake from commercial infant formulas and foods is higher than desirable.[122] Other investigators, however, have estimated smaller amounts of ingested fluoride from such foods.[123, 124] Moreover, in the last few years, the manufacturers of infant formula have taken steps to ensure that the amounts of fluoride in their products are acceptably low.

Because primary teeth undergo substantial mineralization during infancy, it is important to provide adequate fluoride during this period. Ingestion of fluorides from formulas and supplements has not been shown to be harmful to the dentition. Moderate and severe enamel fluorosis is exceedingly rare in primary teeth even when fluoride levels are high.[125] Moreover, mineralization of the permanent dentition during the first six months of age is limited essentially to incisal edges of anterior teeth and to the cusp tips of six-year molars. Thus, there is little opportunity for objectionable fluorosis to occur in permanent teeth even if there is over-ingestion of fluoride during the first six months of life. Because the risk of fluorosis is very small and the expected benefit to primary teeth is large, fluoride supplementation should begin at birth, as recommended by the Council on Dental Therapeutics.

TABLE 9–7   SUPPLEMENTAL FLUORIDE DOSAGE SCHEDULE (IN MG F/DAY) ACCORDING TO THE EXISTING FLUORIDE CONCENTRATION IN DRINKING WATER AS A PERCENTAGE OF THE RECOMMENDED OPTIMAL CONCENTRATION

NATURAL FLUORIDE CONTENT AS PERCENTAGE* OF OPTIMAL CONCENTRATION	FLUORIDE DOSAGE (MG F/DAY)		
	Age		
	0–2	2–3	3–13
70% or greater	None	None	None
40% to 60%	0.125	0.25	0.5
30% or less	0.25	0.5	1.0

*Rounded to nearest 10%

Fluoride Supplementation for Breast-fed Infants

Because the concentration of fluoride in breast milk is very low, some health practitioners have suggested giving fluoride supplements to breast-fed infants in fluoridated communities.[126] However, this suggestion should be viewed with caution because the period of breast feeding for infants is highly variable. Moreover, some mothers supplement breast feeding with bottle feedings that may be prepared with fluoridated water, or they may give drinking water to their infants between feedings. These factors make it difficult to determine whether a supplement should be given and to calculate the proper dosage, especially when close contact with mothers is not maintained. Consequently, in public health settings, it is advisable to dispense fluoride supplements to breast-fed infants residing in fluoridated communities only when a child's health practitioner has good rapport with a mother and can ascertain her exact breast-feeding practices. In private pediatric practices, the potential for ascertaining exact breast-feeding practices is greater than in public health settings. For children who are solely breast-fed, dietary fluoride supplements should be prescribed during that interval. The prescribed dosage should be the same as that recommended for use by infants in areas having negligible amounts of fluoride in the water supply.

Prenatal Fluoride Administration

In 1966, the U.S. Food and Drug Administration (FDA) banned manufacturers of fluoride supplements from claiming that dental caries would be prevented in the offspring of women who used their products during pregnancy because clinical evidence to substantiate such a claim was insufficient.[127] The FDA did not question the safety of the procedure because there was no indication that the recommended dosages of fluoride harmed either the pregnant woman or the fetus. Although the ban effectively stopped the pharmaceutical industry from promoting fluoride supplements for prenatal use, it did not prohibit physicians and dentists from prescribing them for pregnant women. Therefore, some practitioners who believe the procedure has value have continued to prescribe prenatal fluorides for their patients.

Of seven studies in which the caries-preventive effects of prenatal exposure to water-borne fluorides were evaluated, only two showed that such exposure benefits primary teeth.[128, 129] In these studies, children who received fluoride in water both prenatally and postnatally had less caries in deciduous teeth than children who had only postnatal exposure. The other five studies report no meaningful additional benefits from maternal ingestion of fluoridated water if the offspring also ingests fluoridated water from birth.[130-134]

Seven reports of dietary fluoride supplements address the question of the value of their prenatal use.[135-141] All these studies support the practice of prenatal fluoride administration but, without exception, they all have major shortcomings in design or execution that undermine their conclusions.[142]

From a theoretical standpoint, primary teeth could benefit from prenatal exposure to dietary fluoride supplements, but permanent teeth are unlikely to benefit from the procedure. Nevertheless, prenatal administration of dietary fluoride supplements cannot be recommended at this time because conclusive clinical evidence of their value is lacking.[142]

Types of Available Fluoride Supplements

Fluoride supplements are commercially available in the form of drops, solutions, lozenges, and tablets. The selection of a particular form of supplement should depend primarily on the personal preferences of the practitioner and patient, after consideration of the patient's age and the relative costs of various preparations. Fluoride drops are particularly convenient for use with infants because they can be dispensed directly into a child's mouth from a medicine dropper or drip bottle, or they can be added to foods or liquids. Tablets or lozenges for infants must be crushed or dissolved in liquids, which makes the procedure more difficult for the parent. Fluoride tablets are most commonly prescribed for children whose primary teeth have all erupted (about two years of age). Erupted teeth can derive a significant topical benefit from fluoride supplements if the supplement remains in contact with the teeth for a period of time before it is swallowed.[143-146] Therefore, tablets and lozenges should be chewed and the resulting salivary fluoride solution forcefully swished around the teeth before swallowing. They can also be slowly dissolved in the mouth. Similarly, if a solution is used by children with erupted teeth, they should swish it thoroughly in the mouth before swallowing.

Neutral sodium fluoride and acidulated phosphate-fluoride preparations are both available as dietary supplements and produce similar reductions in the incidence of dental decay.[144] Therefore, the choice between these preparations should depend upon their relative costs and the taste preferences of patients. Sodium fluoride tablets are absorbed entirely when ingested on an empty stomach However, bioavailability is reduced to about 70 per cent when fluoride is given with milk or with a calcium-rich meal.[147] The reduced absorption is probably produced by a complex interaction between the calcium, the tablet components, and the pH in the gastrointestinal tract.[148] Therefore, concomitant use of supplements with high calcium foods should be avoided.

Prescriptions for Dietary Fluoride Supplements

Prescriptions for fluoride supplements should state the precise dosage and indicate clearly the manner in which the supplements should be used. The following example illustrates a prescription for a child who is three years of age or older and resides in a community having less than 0.3 ppm fluoride in its drinking water supply:

Name___Johnny Jones___

Address___128 Peaks Street___ Age _5_

___Buchanan, Virginia___

Rx Sodium Fluoride Tablets, 2.2 mg
   (1.0 mg F)
   Dispense 120 tablets
Sig. One tablet each day: chew and swish for one minute before swallowing or allow to dissolve in mouth.

Signed ___Robert L. Smith, D.D.S.___

A prescription for fluoride drops should specify the number of drops required to deliver one mg of fluoride. For example, it should state that 4 drops of liquid contain 1.0 mg fluoride (2.2 mg NaF). One drop of this preparation provides the desired dosage (0.25 mg F) for a child younger than two years of age who lives in a fluoride-deficient community, and two drops provide the desired dosage (0.5 mg F) for a child between two and three years of age.

Although acute overdoses of fluoride supplements have not been reported, the recommendation of the Council on Dental Therapeutics that no more than 264 mg of sodium fluoride (120 mg of fluoride) be dispensed at any one time for home use should be strictly followed. This amount of fluoride, even if ingested in its entirety, would not be fatal to a small child, although symptoms of stomach discomfort probably would occur. Parents should oversee the administration of supplements, and the supply of supplements should be stored in a safe place out of the reach of small children. Because a prescription for each child requires refilling at most only once every four months, a limitation to 120 mg of fluoride does not greatly inconvenience parents.

Fluoride-Vitamin Preparations

Dietary fluoride supplements may be obtained as fluoride-vitamin combinations. Several clinical studies have shown that fluoride-vitamin combinations reduce dental caries effectively,[119, 120, 126, 149-151] and in one study, as effectively as fluoride supplements without vitamins.[151] There is no evidence that vitamins enhance the effect of fluoride. The determining factor in choosing a fluoride-vitamin combination should be a clear indication that a vitamin supplement is needed. If a need does not exist, then a fluoride supplement without vitamins should be prescribed; vitamins should not be used merely as a vehicle for delivering fluoride. However, if vitamins as well as fluorides are indicated, it is sometimes convenient to prescribe a combined fluoride-vitamin supplement. When a combined supplement is prescribed, parents should know the importance of the fluoride itself aside from the value of the vitamin component because the need for fluoride supplementation usually continues beyond the age at which vitamins are usually discontinued.

An important disadvantage of fluoride-vitamin combinations in capsule form is that, because they are swallowed directly, they cannot provide a topical effect to erupted teeth. This effect may be sizable.

School-based Fluoride Tablet Programs

The success of dietary fluoride supplementation depends upon the interest of prescribers and the cooperation of parents and children in following the consistent and continuous regimen required from birth to age 13. Strong motivation and a clear realization of the need for daily intake are essential. These demands limit the effectiveness of home consumption of dietary fluoride supplements as a broadly applicable procedure for preventing dental caries.

The problems of compliance associated with home use can be largely overcome by using fluoride supplements in a school-based program. With this approach, dentists or physicians have the responsibility of prescribing the supplements and of directing the program, whereas the actual administration of the supplements is carried out in classrooms under the supervision of classroom teachers, teachers' aides, or volunteers.

The effectiveness and feasibility of these programs have been demonstrated in several studies in which fluoride supplementation began at school age and was given only on days of school attendance.[143-146, 152-155] Per-centage reductions in caries have ranged from about 20 to 35 per cent after two or more years of fluoride ingestion. Although these benefits are lower than those derived from daily use of supplements from birth, the practical advantages of a school-based program are noteworthy. Table 9-8 shows the results of a study in which children initially in grades 1 and 2 ingested 1 mg fluoride tablets in school on school days for six years.[145] The findings show greater benefits in late erupting teeth than in early erupting teeth, although both types of teeth clearly showed benefits.

In order to derive maximum benefits from tablet administration in school, the procedure should begin in the lowest school grade. If the procedure can be initiated in kindergarten, most incisors and six-year molars will receive some pre-eruptive exposure to fluoride, followed by topical exposure after they erupt. Cuspids, bicuspids, and second molars will receive extensive pre-eruptive exposure, as well as topical exposure after they erupt at ages 11 to 13. Primary teeth may also derive some benefit from topical exposure to the supplement when use begins in kindergarten. In order to provide maximal benefit, school-based programs should continue at least through junior high or middle school and, if administratively feasible, through high school.

The research results of these school-based studies should indicate to health practitioners that a child of early school age is not too old to begin a program of daily dietary fluoride supplementation at home if the necessary motivation is present. Benefits derived from daily home use may be better than those derived from using supplements only on school days.

TABLE 9-8 MEAN INCREMENTAL DMF SURFACES ACCORDING TO ERUPTION STATUS AFTER SIX YEARS OF FLUORIDE TABLET USE IN WAYNE COUNTY, N.C.

| | | MEAN DMFS INCREMENT | | |
STUDY GROUP	NO. OF CHILDREN	All Teeth	Early Erupting Teeth	Late Erupting Teeth
Control	153	7.25	5.30	1.95
Test	150	5.22	4.13	1.09
% Difference		28	22	44

SALT FLUORIDATION

The successful use of salt enriched with iodine to prevent goiter has facilitated the use in some countries of salt as a vehicle for administering fluoride to prevent dental caries. Salt was first used for this purpose in 1946 in Switzerland.[156] By 1961, fluoridated salt was available in 16 of the 25 cantons of Switzerland. Several studies in Switzerland, Hungary, and Colombia have established the value of fluoridated salt.[156-159] In the early programs and studies, 90 mg of fluoride per kg of salt produced a limited caries-preventive benefit, which led to recommendations that the concentration of fluoride in salt be raised to between 200 and 300 mg per kg.[156, 160, 161] It is thought that when the concentration of fluoride in salt is such that excretion levels of urinary fluoride are similar to those found in communities with optimally fluoridated water, the caries-preventive effects are similar.[162]

Sources of ingested salt vary. It may be purchased directly by consumers and used to season food during its preparation or at the table. It may occur as pre-seasoning in some items or in processed foods, which are being increasingly consumed in many countries. Apparently, much of the salt purchased for households is not actually ingested.[162] For example, only a small part of the salt added to water for cooking pasta and vegetables is actually ingested. Therefore, determinations of the most effective concentrations of fluoride for enrichment of kitchen salt are difficult to make. Reliance on urinary excretion levels of fluorides for groups of persons is probably the best way to determine target levels for enrichment.[162]

Some find it paradoxical that salt, which has been associated with hypertension, should be a vehicle for preventing another disease. Proponents of salt fluoridation point out that the concentration of fluoride in salt can be adjusted so that a small amount of salt will still provide an optimal amount of fluoride for caries prevention. However, the inconsistency of advising reduced consumption for one purpose while implicitly encouraging ingestion for another purpose jars the sensibilities of some public health officials. Nevertheless, fluoridation of salt may be an effective and practical method to prevent caries in some countries where water fluoridation is uncommon or unattainable, and where the production or importation of salt is state-controlled.

Additional information is needed to establish optimal dosages for different age groups, for various ethnic groups with different food preferences, and for different geographic areas. One inherent disadvantage of salt fluoridation is the difficulty of adjusting consumption and distribution to accommodate varying suboptimal levels of fluoride that occur naturally in water supplies.

MILK FLUORIDATION

There are only a few studies with human beings that have explored the use of milk as a vehicle for fluoride supplementation, and these have had few participants.[163, 164] Although the results have been encouraging, more clinical data are needed before the fluoridation of milk can be recommended as a caries-preventive measure. Interest in this research persists thanks to the support of the Borrow Dental Milk Foundation in Great Britain.

Theoretically, milk fluoridation has certain inherent disadvantages. The amount of milk consumed by children, particularly among those in different socioeconomic groups, varies considerably. Also, unlike consumption of water, the consumption of milk tends to decrease as a child grows older; whereas the need for fluoride to prevent dental decay increases with age. Therefore, the long-term benefits of milk fluoridation may be less than those afforded by continual exposure to fluoridated drinking water. Moreover, the absorption of fluoride from milk has been shown to be lower than from water,[165] and fluoride is incompletely ionized in milk.[148, 165, 166]

Milk fluoridation also has some technical disadvantages not shared by water fluoridation. For example, water fluoridation can usually be accomplished by installing fluoridating units at only one or, at most, a few main points in a water system. In contrast, milk often is processed in many different facilities within or surrounding a community. Thus, the problems of inspecting facilities and monitoring fluoride concentrations are likely to be more complex with milk fluoridation. Problems of distribution, particularly in areas with varying levels of natural fluoride in the drinking water, and of costs also are likely to restrict the widespread adoption of milk as a vehicle for fluoride administration.

Fluoridated milk could be useful in a school-based program in which an optimal daily dosage is provided at one time. However, the costs of fluoridating milk for distribution in schools are likely to be much greater than corresponding costs for a school-based fluoride tablet program.

REFERENCES

1. Carlos, J. P. (ed.): Prevention and Oral Health, Fogarty International Center Series, DHEW Publ. No. (NIH) 74–707, Washington, Government Printing Office, 1973.
2. Newbrun, E.: Cariology, 5th ed. Baltimore, Williams & Wilkins, 1978.
3. Brudevold, F., and Naujoks, R.: Caries-preventive fluoride treatment of the individual. Caries Res. 12(Suppl. 1):52, 1978.
4. Duckworth, R.: Fluoride dentifrices. A review of clinical trials in the United Kingdom. Br. Dent. J. 124:505, 1968.
5. Horowitz, H. S.: Increasing the resistance of teeth. In Advances in Caries Research. Chicago, American Dental Association, 2:v–xiii, 1974.
6. Murray, J. J.: Fluorides in Caries Prevention. Bristol, John Wright and Sons, 1976.
7. Silverstone, L. M.: Operative measures for caries prevention. Caries Res. 12(Suppl. 1):103, 1978.
8. Stookey, G. K., and Katz, S.: Chairside procedures for using fluorides for preventing caries. Dent. Clin. N. Am. 16:681, 1972.
9. Frostell, G., and Ericsson, Y.: Antiplaque therapeutics in caries prevention. Caries Res. 12(Suppl. 1):74, 1978.
10. Heløe, L. A., and König, K. G.: Oral hygiene and educational programs for caries prevention. Caries Res. 12(Suppl. 1):83, 1978.
11. Loesche, W. J.: Chemotherapy of dental plaque infections. Oral Sci. Rev. 9:65, 1976.
12. Theilade, E., and Theilade, J.: Role of plaque in the etiology of periodontal disease and caries. Oral Sci. Rev. 9:23, 1976.
13. Mäkinen, K. K.: The role of sucrose and other sugars in the development of dental caries: A review. Internat. Dent. J. 22:363, 1972.
14. Newbrun, E., and Frostell, G.: Sugar restriction and substitution for caries prevention. Caries Res. 12(Suppl. 1):65, 1978.
15. Winter, G. B.: Sucrose and cariogenesis. A review. Br. Dent. J. 124:407, 1968.
16. Jenkins, G. N.: The mechanism of action of fluoride in reducing caries incidence. Internat. Dent. J. 17:552, 1967.
17. Brown, W. E., and König, K. G. (eds.): Cariostatic mechanisms of fluorides. Caries Res. 11(Suppl. 1), 1977.
18. Ericsson, S. Y.: Cariostatic mechanisms of fluorides: Clinical observations. Caries Res. 11(Suppl. 1):2, 1977.
19. Kleinberg, I.: Prevention and dental caries. J. Prevent. Dent. 5:9, 1978.
20. Armstrong, W. D., and Singer, L.: Distribution of fluoride in body fluids and soft tissue. In Fluorides and Human Health. Geneva, World Health Organization, 1970, p. 94.
21. Weatherell, J. A., et al.: Assimilation of fluoride by enamel throughout the life of the tooth. Caries Res. 11(Suppl. 1):85, 1977.
22. Hardwick, J. L., and Leach, S. A.: The fluoride content of the dental plaque. Arch. Oral Biol. 8(Suppl.):151, 1963.
23. Mellberg, J. R.: Enamel fluoride and its anti-caries effects. J. Prevent. Dent. 4:8, 1977.
24. Caldwell, R. C., and Nornoo, D. C.: Water fluoridation and systemic fluoride therapy. In Caldwell, R. C., and Stallard, R. E. (eds.): A Textbook of Preventive Dentistry. Philadelphia, W. B. Saunders, 1977, p. 154.
25. Black, G. V.: Mottled teeth. Dent. Cosmos 58:129, 1916.
26. McKay, F. S.: Progress of the year in the investigation of mottled enamel with special reference to its association with artesian water. J. National Dent. Assoc. 5:721, 1918.
27. McKay, F. S.: An investigation of mottled teeth (I). Dent. Cosmos 58:477, 1916.
28. McKay, F. S.: The relation of mottled teeth to caries. J. Am. Dent. Assoc. 15:1429, 1928.
29. McKay, F. S.: Mottled teeth: The prevention of its further production through a change in the water supply at Oakley, Idaho. J. Am. Dent. Assoc. 20:1137, 1933.
30. Kempf, G. A., and McKay, F. S.: Mottled enamel in a segregated population. Public Health Rep. 45:2923, 1930.
31. Churchill, H. V.: Occurrence of fluorides in some waters of the United States. Indust. Engineer. Chem. 23:996, 1931.
32. Smith, H. V., and Smith, M. C.: Mottled Enamel in Arizona and its Correlation with the Concentration of Fluoride in Water Supplies. Bull. Ariz. Agric. Experiment Station, No. 32, 1931.
33. Dean, H. T.: Distribution of mottled enamel in the United States. Public Health Rep. 48:704, 1933.
34. Dean, H. T.: Classification of mottled enamel diagnoses. J. Am. Dent. Assoc. 21:1421, 1934.
35. Dean, H. T.: Chronic endemic dental fluorosis (mottled enamel). J.A.M.A. 107:1269, 1936.
36. Dean, H. T., and Elvove, E.: Some epidemiological aspects of chronic endemic dental fluorosis. Am. J. Public Health 26:567, 1936.
37. Ainsworth, N. J.: Mottled teeth. Br. Dent. J. 60:233, 1933.
38. Dean, H. T., et al.: Domestic water and dental

caries, including certain epidemiological aspects of oral *L. acidophilus*. Public Health Rep. *54*:862, 1939.

39. Dean, H. T., et al.: Domestic water and dental caries. II. A study of 2,832 white children aged 12–14 years of eight suburban Chicago communities, including *L. acidophilus* studies of 1,761 children. Public Health Rep. *56*:761, 1941.

40. Dean, H. T., Arnold, F. A., Jr., and Elvove, E.: Domestic water and dental caries. V. Additional studies of the relation of fluoride domestic water to dental caries experience in 4,425 white children, aged 12 to 14 years, of 13 cities in 4 states. Public Health Rep. *57*:1155, 1942.

41. Dean, H. T., et al.: Studies on mass control of dental caries through fluoridation of public water supplies. Public Health Rep. *65*:1403, 1950.

42. Arnold, F. A., Jr., Dean, H. T., and Knutson, J. W.: Effect of fluoridated public water supplies on dental caries prevalence. Results of the seventh year of study at Grand Rapids and Muskegon, Mich. Public Health Rep. *68*:141, 1953.

43. Ast, D. B., Finn, S. B., and McCafferty, I.: The Newburgh-Kingston caries fluoride study. I. Dental findings after three years of water fluoridation. Am. J. Public Health *40*:116, 1950.

44. Blayney, J. R., and Hill, I. N.: Fluorine and dental caries. J. Am. Dent. Assoc. *74*:233, 1967.

45. Hutton, W. L., Linscott, B. W., and Williams, D. B.: Brantford fluoride experiment. Canad. J. Public Health *42*:81, 1951.

46. Arnold, F. A., Jr., et al.: Fifteenth year of the Grand Rapids fluoridation study. J. Am. Dent. Assoc. *65*:780, 1962.

47. Hillboe, H. E., et al.: Newburgh-Kingston caries-fluorine study: Final report. J. Am. Dent. Assoc. *52*:290, 1956.

48. Brown, H. K., and Poplove M.: The Brantford-Sarnia-Stratford fluoridation caries study: Final survey, 1963. J. Canad. Dent. Assoc. *31*:505, 1965.

49. Backer Dirks, O., Houwink, B., and Kwant, G. W.: The results of 6½ years of artifical fluoridation of drinking water in the Netherlands. The Tiel-Culemberg experiment. Arch. Oral Biol. *5*:284, 1961.

50. Ludwig, T. G.: The Hastings fluoridation project V — dental effects between 1954 and 1964. N. Z. Dent. J. *61*:175, 1965.

51. World Health Organization: Report of Expert Committee on Water Fluoridation. Geneva, WHO Tech. Rep. Series No. 146, 1958.

52. Backer Dirks, O., Künzel, W., and Carlos, J. P.: Caries-preventive water fluoridation. Caries Res. *12*(Suppl. 1):7, 1978.

53. Davies, G. N.: Cost and benefits of fluoride in the prevention of dental caries. Geneva, World Health Organization, Offset Publ. No. 9, 1974.

54. Horowitz, H. S., and Heifetz, S. B.: Methods for assessing the cost-effectiveness of caries preventive agents and procedures. Internat. Dent. J. *29*:106, 1979.

55. Künzel, W.: The cost and economic consequences of water fluoridation. Caries Res. *8*(Suppl. 1):28, 1974.

56. Newbrun, E.: Systemic use of fluorides: Assessment of cost-benefit features and practicality. *In* Burt, B. A. (ed.): The Relative Efficiency of Methods of Caries Prevention in Dental Public Health. Ann Arbor, University of Michigan, 1978, p. 27.

57. Leukhart, C. S.: An update on water fluoridation: Triumphs and challenges. Pediatr. Dent. *1*:32, 1979.

58. Newbrun, E.: Systemic fluorides — an overview. J. Canad. Dent. Assoc. *46*:31, 1980.

59. Ast, D. B., et al.: Time and cost factors to provide regular, periodic dental care for children in a fluoridated and non-fluoridated area: Final report. J. Am. Dent. Assoc. *80*:770, 1970.

60. Denby, G. C., and Hollis, M. J.: The effect of fluoridation on a dental public health programme. N. Z. Dent. J. *62*:32, 1966.

61. Rugg-Gunn, A. J., et al.: Fluoridation in Newcastle and Northumberland. A clinical study of 5-year-old children. Br. Dent. J. *142*:395, 1977.

62. Murray, J.: Adult dental health in fluoride and non-fluoride areas. I. Mean DMF values by age. J. Dent. Res. *131*:391, 1971.

63. Russell, A. L., and Elvove, E.: Domestic water and dental caries. VII. A study of the fluoride dental caries relationship in an adult population. Public Health Rep. *66*:1389, 1951.

64. Stamm, J. W., and Banting, D. W.: Comparison of root caries in adults with lifelong residence in fluoridated and non-fluoridated communities. Abstract, J. Dent. Res. *59*(Spec. Issue A):405, 1980.

65. Federation Dentaire Internationale: Basic Fact Sheets. London, Federation Dentaire Internationale, 1975.

66. Petterson, E. O.: Abolition of the right of local Swedish authorities to fluoridate drinking water. J. Public Health Dent. *32*:243, 1972.

67. Division of Dental Health, Health Resources Administration, U.S. Dept. Health, Education and Welfare: Status of fluoridation in the Netherlands (news item). Oct., 1973.

68. Whittle, J. G., and Downer, M. C.: Dental health and treatment needs of Birmingham and Salford school children. Br. Dent. J. *147*:67, 1979.

69. Leatherman, G. H.: Water fluoridation — scientifically accepted but politically rejected. Presentation at 67th Annual World Dental Congress, Paris, Federation Dentaire Internationale, 1979.

70. U.S. Department of Health, Education, and Welfare, Public Health Service, Center for Disease Control: Fluoridation Census. Atlanta, DHEW, 1975.

71. Tank, G., and Storvick, C. A.: Caries experience of children one to six years old in two Oregon communities (Corvallis and Albany). I. Effect of fluroride on caries experience and eruption of teeth. J. Am. Dent. Assoc. *69*:749, 1964.

72. Murray, J. J.: Caries experience of five-year-old children from fluoride and non-fluoride communities. Br. Dent. J. *127*:128, 1969.

73. Winter, G. B., et al.: The prevalence of dental caries in pre-school children aged 1–4 years. Br. Dent. J. *130*:271, 1971.

74. Weaver, R.: Fluorosis and dental caries on Tyneside. Br. Dent. J. *76*:29, 1944.

75. Marthaler, T. M.: Fluoride supplements for systemic effects in caries prevention. *In* Johansen, E.,

Taves, D., and Olsen, J. (ed.): Continuing Education on the Use of Fluorides. Boulder, Colorado, Westview Press 1979, p. 33.

76. Arnold, F. A., Jr.: Role of fluorides in preventive dentistry. J. Am. Dent. Assoc. 30:499, 1943.

77. Russell, A. L., and Hamilton, P. M.: Dental caries in permanent first molars after eight years of fluoridation. Arch. Oral Biol. 6(Special Suppl.):50, 1961.

78. Backer Dirks, O.: The benefits of water fluoridation. Caries Res. 8(Suppl.):2, 1974.

79. Gish, C. W., and Muhler, J. C.: Effectiveness of a SnF₂-Ca₂P₂O₇ dentifrice on dental caries in children whose teeth calcified in a natural fluoride area. II. Results at the end of 24 months. J. Am. Dent. Assoc. 73:853, 1966.

80. Mergele, M.: An unsupervised brushing study on subjects residing in a community with fluoride in the water. Acad. Med. New Jersey Bull. 14:251, 1968.

81. Radike, A. W., et al.: Clinical evaluation of stannous fluoride as an anticaries mouthrinse. J. Am. Dent. Assoc. 86:404, 1973.

82. Driscoll, W. S., et al.: Caries-preventive effects of daily and weekly oral rinsing with sodium fluoride solutions in an optimally fluoridated community: Findings after 18 months. Pediat. Dent., in press.

83. Muhler, J. C.: The anticariogenic effectiveness of a single application of stannous fluoride in children residing in an optimal communal fluoride area. II. Results at the end of 30 months. J. Am. Dent. Assoc. 61:431, 1960.

84. Horowitz, H. S., and Heifetz, S. B.: Evaluation of topical applications of stannous fluoride to teeth of children born and reared in a fluoridated community: Final report. J. Dent. Child. 56:65, 1969.

85. Englander, H. R., and Wallace, D. A.: Effects of naturally fluoridated water on dental caries in adults. Public Health Rep. 77:887, 1962.

86. Jackson, D., Murray, J. J., and Fairpo, C. G.: Life-long benefits of fluoride in drinking water. Br. Dent. J. 134:419, 1973.

87. Ast, D. B., et al.: Time and cost factors to provide regular, periodic dental care for children in a fluoridated and non-fluoridated area. Am. J. Public Health 55:811, 1965.

88. Ast, D. B., et al.: Time and cost factors to provide regular, periodic dental care for children in a fluoridated and non-fluoridated area: Progress report II. Am. J. Public Health 57:1635, 1967.

89. Lewis, D. W., et al.: Initial dental care time, cost, and treatment requirements under changing exposure to fluoride during tooth development. J. Canad. Dent. Assoc. 38:497, 1953.

90. Galagan, D. J., and Lamson, G. G.: Climate and endemic fluorosis. Public Health Rep. 68:497, 1953.

91. Galagan, D. J., and Vermillion, J. R.: Determining optimum fluoride concentrations. Public Health Rep. 72:491, 1957.

92. Maier, F. J.: Manual of Water Fluoridation Practice. New York, McGraw-Hill Book Co., 1963.

93. Hushower, T. N.: Adequacy of community water supply fluoridation. Presented at annual meeting. Am. Dent. Assoc., San Francisco, Oct. 30, 1972.

94. Evans, C. A., Jr., and Pickles, T.: Statewide antifluoridation initiatives: A new challenge to health workers. Am. J. Public Health 68:59, 1978.

95. Evans, C. A., Jr.: Challenges to the adoption of community water fluoridation. Family Community Health 3:33, 1980.

96. Yaimonyiannis, J. A.: Fluoridation and cancer. Age dependence of cancer mortality related to artificial fluoridation. Fluoride 10:102, 1977.

97. Doll, R., and Kinlen, L.: Fluoridation of water and cancer mortality in the USA. Lancet 1(8025): 1300, 1977.

98. Hoover, R. N., McKay, F. W., and Fraumeni, J. F.: Fluoridated drinking waters and the occurrence of cancer. J. Natl. Cancer Inst. 57:757, 1975.

99. Council on Dental Health, American Dental Association: Policies on Community Dental Health. Chicago, American Dental Association, 1975.

100. World Health Organization: Expert Committee on Water Fluoridation: First Report. WHO Tech. Report Series No. 146. Geneva, World Health Organization, 1958.

101. Dean, H. T.: Chronic endemic dental fluorosis (mottled enamel). In Gordon, S. M. (ed.): Dental Science and Dental Art. Philadelphia, Lea & Febiger, 1938.

102. Diefenbach, V. L., Nevitt, G. A., and Frankel, J. M.: Fluoridation and the appearance of teeth. J. Am. Dent. Assoc. 71:1129, 1965.

103. Forrest, J. R.: Caries incidence and enamel defects in areas with different levels of fluoride in the drinking water. Br. Dent. J. 100:195, 1956.

104. Hodge, H. C., and Smith, F. A.: Fluorine Chemistry, Vol. IV. New York, Academic Press, 1965.

105. Environmental Protection Agency, Office of Water Supply: National Interim Primary Drinking Water Regulations, Washington, D.C., U.S. Government Printing Office, 1977, p. 66.

106. Horowitz, H. S., and Heifetz, S. B.: The effect of partial defluoridation of a water supply on dental fluorosis — final results in Bartlett, Texas, after 17 years. Am. J. Public Health 62:767, 1972.

107. Horowitz, H. S., Heifetz, S. B., and Driscoll, W. S.: Partial defluoridation of a community water supply and dental fluorosis. Health Services Rep. 87:451, 1972.

108. Environmental Protection Agency: Small system strategy for public water supply systems — Safe Drinking Water Act. Fed. Regist. 45: 40222, 1980.

109. Horowitz, H. S., Law, F. E., and Pritzker, T.: Effect of school water fluoridation on dental caries, St. Thomas, V.I. Public Health Rep. 80:381, 1965.

110. Horowitz, H. S., et al.: School fluoridation studies in Elk Lake, Pennsylvania and Pike County, Kentucky — results after eight years. Am. J. Public Health 58:2240, 1968.

111. Horowitz, H. S., Heifetz, S. B., and Law, F. E.: Effect of school water fluoridation on dental caries: Final results in Elk Lake, Pennsylvania, after 12 years. J. Am. Dent. Assoc. 97:193, 1972.

112. Heifetz, S. B., Horowitz, H. S., and Driscoll, W. S.:

Effect of school water fluoridation on dental caries: Results in Seagrove, N. C., after eight years. J. Am. Dent. Assoc. 97:193, 1978.

113. Horowitz, H. S.: School fluoridation for the prevention of dental caries. Internat. Dent. J. 23:346, 1973.

114. Bellack, E.: School Water Fluoridation. Environmental Protection Agency Public., Washington, D.C., U.S. Government Printing Office, 1972.

115. Murphy, R. F., and Bowden, B. S.: School water fluoridation in North Carolina. J. North Carolina Dent. Soc. 53:27, 1970.

116. Driscoll, W. S., and Horowitz, H. S.: A discussion of optimal dosage for dietary fluoride supplementation. J. Am. Dent. Assoc. 96:1050, 1978.

117. American Dental Association. Prescribing fluoride supplements. In Accepted Dental Therapeutics, 38th ed. Chicago, American Dental Association 1979, p. 319.

118. American Academy of Pediatrics, Committee on Nutrition: Fluoride supplementation: Revised dosage schedule. Pediatrics 63:150, 1979.

119. Aasenden, R., and Peebles, T. C.: Effects of fluoride supplementation from birth on human deciduous and permanent teeth. Arch. Oral Biol. 19:321, 1974.

120. Aasenden, R., and Peebles, T. C.: Effects of fluoride supplementation from birth on dental caries and fluorosis in teenaged children. Arch. Oral Biol. 23:111, 1978.

121. Wei, S. H. Y., Wefel, J. S., and Parkins, F. M.: Fluoride supplements for infants and preschool children. J. Prevent. Dent. 4:28, 1977.

122. Wiatrowski, E., et al.: Dietary fluoride intake of infants. Pediatrics 55:517, 1975.

123. Stamm, J. W., and Kuo, H. C.: Fluoride concentration in prepared infant foods (Abstract #628). J. Dent. Res. 56(Special Issue B): B209, 1977.

124. Singer, L., and Ophaug, R. H.: Fluoride content of foods and beverages. In Wei, S. H. Y. (ed.): National Symposium on Dental Nutrition. Iowa City, University of Iowa 1979, p. 47.

125. Russell, A. L.: The differential diagnosis of fluoride and nonfluoride enamel opacities. Public Health Rep. 21:143, 1961.

126. Margolis, F. J., et al.: Fluoride: Ten-year prospective study of deciduous and permanent dentition. Am. J. Dis. Child. 129:794, 1975.

127. Food and Drug Administration: Statements of general policy or interpretation, oral prenatal drugs containing fluorides for human use. Federal Register, Oct. 20, 1966.

128. Blayney, J. R., and Hill, I. N.: Evanston dental caries study. XXIV. Prenatal fluorides — value of waterborne fluorides during pregnancy. J. Am. Dent. Assoc. 69:291, 1964.

129. Tank, G., and Storvick, C. A.: Caries experience of children one to six years old in two Oregon communities (Corvallis and Albany). I. Effect of fluoride on caries experience and eruption of teeth. J. Am. Dent. Assoc. 69:749, 1964.

130. Carlos, J. P., Gittelsohn, A. M., and Haddon, W., Jr.: Caries in deciduous teeth in relation to maternal ingestion of fluoride. Public Health Rep. 77:658, 1962.

131. Horowitz, H. S., and Heifetz, S. B.: Effects of prenatal exposure to fluoridation on dental caries. Public Health Rep. 82:297, 1967.

132. Katz, S., and Muhler, J. C.: Prenatal and postnatal fluoride and dental caries experience in deciduous teeth. J. Am. Dent. Assoc. 76:305. 1968.

133. Lemke, C. W., Doherty, J. M., and Arra, M. C.: Controlled fluoridation: The dental effects of discontinuation in Antigo, Wisconsin. J. Am. Dent. Assoc. 80:782, 1970.

134. Lewis, D. W., et al.: Initial dental care time, cost and treatment requirements under changing exposure to fluoride during tooth development. J. Canad. Dent. Assoc. 38:140, 1970.

135. Feltman, R., and Kosel, G.: Prenatal and postnatal ingestion of fluorides — fourteen years of investigation — final report. J. Dent. Med. 16:190, 1961.

136. Hoskova, M.: Fluoride tablets in the prevention of tooth decay. Cesk. Pediatr. 23:438, 1968.

137. Kailis, D. G., et al.: Fluoride and caries: Observations on the effects of prenatal and postnatal fluoride on some Perth pre-school children. Med. J. Austral. 2:1037, 1968.

138. Prichard, J. L.: The prenatal and postnatal effects of fluoride supplements on West Australian school children, aged 6, 7 and 8, Perth, 1967. Austral. Dent. J. 14:335, 1969.

139. Schützmannsky, G.: Fluorine tablet application in pregnant females. Dtsch. Stomatol. 21:122, 1971.

140. Glenn, F. B.: Immunity conveyed by a fluoride supplement during pregnancy. J. Dent. Child. 44:391, 1977.

141. Glenn, F. B.: Immunity conveyed by sodium fluoride supplement during pregnancy. Part II. J. Dent. Child. 46:17, 1979.

142. Driscoll, W. S.: A review of clinical research on the use of prenatal fluoride administration for prevention of dental caries. J. Dent. Child. 48:109, 1981.

143. Aasenden, R., DePaola, P. F., and Brudevold, F.: Effects of daily rinsing and ingestion of fluoride solutions upon dental caries and enamel fluoride. Arch. Oral Biol. 17:1705, 1972.

144. DePaola. P. F., and Lax, M.: The caries-inhibiting effect of acidulated phosphate-fluoride chewable tablets: A two-year double-blind study. J. Am. Dent. Assoc. 76:554, 1968.

145. Driscoll, W. S., Heifetz, S. B., and Brunelle, J. A.: Treatment and posttreatment effects of chewable fluoride tablets on dental caries: Findings after 7½ years. J. Am. Dent. Assoc. 99:817, 1979.

146. Marthaler, T. M.: Caries-inhibiting effect of fluoride tablets. Helv. Odont. Acta 13:1, 1969.

147. Ekstrand, J., and Ehrnebo, M.: Influence of dietary calcium on the bioavailability of sodium fluoride tablets (Abstract #1043). J. Dent. Res. 57(Special Issue A):335, 1978.

148. Patterson, C., and Ekstrand, J.: The state of fluoride in milk (Abstract #1045). J. Dent. Res. 57(Special Issue A):336, 1978.

149. Hamberg, L.: Controlled trial of fluoride in vitamin drops for prevention of caries in children. Lancet 1:441, 1971.

150. Hennon, D. K., Stookey, G. K., and Muhler, J. C.: The clinical anticariogenic effectiveness of supplementary fluoride-vitamin preparations. Results at the end of five and a half years. J. Pharm. Ther. Dent. 1:1, 1970.

151. Hennon, D. K., Stookey, G. K., and Muhler, J. C.: Prophylaxis of dental caries: Relative effective-

ness of chewable fluoride preparations with and without added vitamins. J. Pediatr. *80*:1018, 1972.

152. Binder, K., Driscoll, W. S., and Schützmannsky, G.: Caries-preventive fluoride tablet programs. Caries Res. *12*(Suppl. 1):22, 1978.

153. Driscoll, W. S.: The use of fluoride tablets for the prevention of dental caries. *In* Forrester, D. J., and Schulz, E. M., Jr. (eds.): International Workshop on Fluorides and Dental Caries Reductions. Baltimore, Univ. of Maryland, 1974, p. 25.

154. Grissom, D. K., et al.: A comparative study of systemic sodium fluoride and topical stannous fluoride applications in preventive dentistry. J. Dent. Child. *31*:314, 1964.

155. Stephen, K. W., and Campbell, D.: Caries reduction and cost: benefit after three years of sucking fluoride tablets at school. Br. Dent. J. *144*:202, 1978.

156. Wespi, H. J.: Experiences and problems of fluoridated cooking salt in Switzerland. Arch. Oral Biol. *6*:33, 1961.

157. Marthaler, T. M., and Schenardi, C.: Inhibition of caries in children after 5½ years use of fluoridated table salt. Helv. Odont. Acta *6*:1, 1962.

158. Mejia, R., et al.: Use of fluoridated salt in four Colombian communities. VIII. Results

achieved from 1964 to 1972 (summary). Boletin Oficina Sanitaria Panamericana *80*:67, 1976.

159. Toth, K. :A study of 8 years domestic salt fluoridation for prevention of caries. Community Dent. Oral Epidemiol. *4*:106, 1976.

160. Mühlemann, H. R.: Fluoridated domestic salt. A discussion of dosage. Internat. Dent. J. *17*:10, 1967.

161. Wespi, H. J., and Burgi, W.: Salt-fluoridation and urinary fluoride excretion. Caries Res. *5*:89, 1971.

162. Marthaler, T. M., et al: Caries-preventive salt fluoridation. Caries Res. *12*(Suppl. 1):15, 1978.

163. Rusoff, L. L., et al: Fluoride addition to milk and its effect on dental caries in school children. J. Clin. Nutr. *11*:94, 1962.

164. Wirz, R.: Ergebnisse des Grossversuches mit fluoridierter Milch in Winterthur von 1958 bis 1964. Schweiz. Mschr. Zahnheilk *74*:767, 1964.

165. Ericsson, Y.: The state of fluorine in milk and its absorption and retention when administered in milk. Investigations with radioactive fluorine. Acta Odont. Scand. *16*:51, 1958.

166. Hellström, I., and Ericsson, Y.: Fluoride reactions with the dental enamel following different forms of fluoride supply. Scand. J. Dent. Res. *84*:255, 1976.

CHAPTER TEN
Dentifrices and Mouth Rinses

Anthony R. Volpe, D.D.S., M.S.

Part One   DENTIFRICES

RELATIONSHIP OF DENTIFRICES TO A PREVENTIVE DENTISTRY PROGRAM

A successful dental office preventive dentistry program consists of at least two important elements. First, the dental practitioner should provide the patient with the most advanced and efficiently administered treatment in the areas of restorative dentistry and preventive dentistry. Additionally, he should educate the patient in respect to the nature of proper oral hygiene procedures and stress the importance of the continuous and habitual home use of these procedures.

The most important aspect of a patient's home-care oral hygiene program involves the efficient and thorough cleaning of the dentition. In order to achieve this objective, the patient requires both a cleaning substance (dentifrice) and a cleaning device (toothbrush).

DEFINITION AND FUNCTIONS OF A DENTIFRICE

Traditionally, a dentifrice has been defined as a substance used with a toothbrush for the purpose of cleaning the accessible surfaces of the teeth.[84, 85] This definition primarily concerned the cosmetic functionality of a dentifrice and involved the removal of *materia alba*, "film," food debris, and stain from the tooth surfaces. Thus, one obtained a cosmetically clean dentition and a fresher breath.

It was further indicated that the use of a dentifrice also provided "secondary beneficial effects" upon the incidence of dental caries and gingival disease. These secondary beneficial effects, in contradistinction to an actual therapeutic effect obtainable by the incorporation of a drug substance into a dentifrice, were based primarily upon two considerations. The first consideration was the axiom that "a clean tooth does not decay," which was extensively expounded. The second factor was the results obtained from a two-year clinical study that indicated that brushing the teeth with a neutral (nontherapeutic) dentifrice immediately after the ingestion of food provided a substantial reduction (approximately 50 per cent) in the incidence of dental caries.[71]

Knowledge concerning the important role of dental plaque in the onset of oral disease has provided substantiation for these secondary beneficial effects. Dental plaque, which is a deposit that is primarily composed of microorganisms and which forms rapidly on tooth surfaces, has been shown to be the primary etiologic factor in the initiation of dental caries, dental calculus, and gingival disease. In addition to the classic animal experiments that established a definite cause-effect relationship between caries and specific microorganisms,[64, 138] direct clinical evidence also has been obtained by numerous investigators regarding the relationship between plaque, calculus, and gingivitis.

170

In one clinical study,[169] it was shown that the withdrawal of toothbrushing in young persons with excellent oral hygiene and clinically normal gingiva resulted in the accumulation of plaque on the teeth. Clinical gingivitis developed after 10 to 21 days and was closely correlated with the degree of plaque accumulation. When toothbrushing was reinstituted, clinically normal conditions were reestablished in about one week. Another clinical study[291] has indicated that the rate of early calculus formation on lower central incisor teeth was about 50 per cent lower in persons performing their habitual and individual toothbrushing than in persons who were instructed not to brush this area of the dentition.

Thus, a cosmetic dentifrice can be considered to be providing a "therapeutic effect" to the oral cavity when it is utilized in the efficient and thorough physical-mechanical removal of dental plaque from the tooth surfaces.

Additionally, there is now substantiation for the therapeutic (or actual drug) effect that can be chemically or pharmacologically provided by a dentifrice. A variety of clinical studies conducted in many areas of the world and by many different investigators has confirmed the caries-reducing therapeutic effect of some dentifrices containing various fluoride compounds in compatible and stable formulations.

Thus, the functions of a dentifrice can be threefold (cosmetic, cosmetic-therapeutic and therapeutic) and described as follows:

1. Cosmetic. This function involves the use of a cosmetic dentifrice (not containing a drug substance) in a routine, nonspecific manner in an attempt to remove materials such as *materia alba*, film (pellicle and plaque), food debris, and stain from the tooth surfaces. The net effect of this dentifrice function would be to provide a "cosmetically clean and healthy dentition" and a fresher breath.

2. Cosmetic-Therapeutic. This function involves the use of a cosmetic dentifrice (not containing a drug substance) in such a manner as to provide for the efficient and thorough physical-mechanical removal of dental plaque. The net effect of this denti-

frice function would include, in addition to those already associated with the use of a cosmetic dentifrice, a "therapeutic" effect upon the incidence of caries, calculus, and gingival disease.

3. Therapeutic. This function involves the use of a therapeutic dentifrice (containing a drug substance) so as to transport the drug substance to the tooth surface or the tooth environment (plaque, saliva, gingival tissues, and so on). Thus, the net effect of this dentifrice function would be the providing of the specific chemical or pharmacologic action of the drug substance, as manifested clinically by a reduction in the incidence of plaque, calculus, caries, or gingival disease. Additionally, depending upon the efficiency of the toothbrushing procedure, secondary cosmetic or cosmetic-therapeutic effects could be provided.

The previous discussion has been utilized as a basis for an expanded definition of a dentifrice. The revised definition is as follows:

A dentifrice is a substance used with a toothbrush to clean the accessible surfaces of the teeth so as to provide one or more of the following effects: (1) primarily cosmetic, including cleaning, polishing, and breath freshening; (2) cosmetic-therapeutic, through the efficient and thorough physical-mechanical removal of dental plaque; and (3) therapeutic or pharmacologic, by means of conveying a drug substance to the tooth surfaces or the tooth environment.

INGREDIENTS AND COMPOSITION OF DENTIFRICES

Although dentifrices are available in various physical forms (paste, powder, and liquid) throughout the world, the predominant physical form is the paste. This is especially true in the United States; thus this discussion of the ingredients and composition of dentifrices basically concerns dentifrices that are in a paste form (commonly referred to as toothpaste).

Dentifrices are composed of a variety of materials, each of which has a specific function. These materials include cleaning and polishing agents, detergents (or surface-active agents), binding agents, flavoring agents, sweetening agents, preservatives, water, and in the case of therapeutic dentifrices, a drug substance. Additionally, miscellaneous ingredients such as coloring materials, corrosion inhibitors, and whitening agents are often utilized in the dentifrice formulation. The approximate amounts of these ingredients that are present in typical dentifrice formulations are shown in Table 10–1.

Cleaning and Polishing Agents

The largest component in a dentifrice is the cleaning and polishing agent, which accounts for approximately 25 to 60 per cent of the entire formulation. Substances that clean or polish the tooth surfaces are also commonly referred to as abrasives. Dentifrice cleaning and polishing agents may be defined as solid substances that have a twofold purpose: (1) to remove debris, stain, and plaque from tooth surfaces and (2) to polish or impart a luster to the tooth surfaces.

Most persons must use a dentifrice containing a cleaning and polishing agent several times daily in order to keep their teeth reasonably clean and healthy. The cleaning and polishing agent is required to assist in the removal of the following accumulations:

1. *plaque*, which is potentially pathologic to the teeth and periodontium and which accumulates very rapidly on a clean tooth surface;

2. *debris*, which constantly accumulates on the tooth surfaces because of the ingestion and mastication of foodstuffs; and

TABLE 10–1 APPROXIMATE RANGES OF BASIC INGREDIENTS IN DENTIFRICE FORMULATIONS

INGREDIENT	APPROXIMATE PER CENT OF FORMULATION
Cleaning and Polishing Agents	25 to 60
Detergents (Surface-Active Agents)	Up to 2
Humectants	20 to 40
Binding Agents	Up to 2
Flavoring Agents	Up to 1.5
Water	15 to 50
Colors, Preservatives, Sweeteners, Stabilizers, etc.	Up to 3
Therapeutic (or Drug) Substance	Up to 2

3. *stain*, which continuously forms on the tooth surfaces of most individuals because of substances such as food, beverages, and tobacco.

Additionally, it is estimated that approximately 90 per cent of the population would form a "brown pellicle" on their teeth if they did not use a dentifrice that contained a cleaning and polishing agent. The occurrence of this cosmetically undesirable brown-black pellicle in persons using either nonabrasive dentifrices (such as the "liquid" dentifrices that do not contain conventional cleaning and polishing agents) or mildly abrasive dentifrices, has been reported by several investigators.[81, 147, 182, 289]

Ideally, cleaning and polishing agents should provide a maximum of cleaning with a minimum of abrasion, so as not to damage the tooth surfaces or the surrounding structures. Also, it is essential that the cleaning and polishing agent be chemically and physically compatible with the other dentifrice ingredients. This is especially important in formulations that contain therapeutic substances such as fluoride compounds, since it has been shown that certain cleaning and polishing agents have the capability to inactivate some fluoride compounds.

The dentifrices currently available in the United States are largely based on various grades of one or more of the following cleaning and polishing agents:

Calcium carbonate, precipitated ($CaCO_3$)
Dicalcium phosphate, dihydrate ($CaHPO_4 \cdot 2H_2O$)
Dicalcium phosphate, anhydrous ($CaHPO_4$)
Sodium metaphosphate, insoluble ($NaPO_3)_x$
Calcium pyrophosphate ($Ca_2P_2O_7$)
Silica and silicate compounds

In general, the dihydrate form of dicalcium phosphate is the least inherently abrasive compound, while the anhydrous form is the most abrasive. The remaining materials hold some intermediate position between these two extremes. Other cleaning and polishing agents that are less commonly used include tricalcium phosphate and hydrated alumina. Thermoplastic resins such as polymethylmethacrylate are currently being used as the principal cleaning and polishing agents in some European dentifrices.

Although the vast majority of currently available dentifrices are of an opaque nature, recent trends have demonstrated an increased popularity for transparent/translucent products. These are the so-called clear gel dentifrices, and they are produced by carefully matching the refractive indices of the abrasive and humectant systems. Abrasives particularly suited for this purpose include a synthetic amorphous silica zerogel and a synthetic amorphous complex aluminosilicate salt.

It should be emphasized that the cleaning and polishing characteristics of a particular substance could vary considerably depending upon such factors as the source of the material, the physical or chemical treatment that the material has received, and the particle size of the material. This is especially true in the case of calcium carbonate.

Some cleaning and polishing agents are excellent cleaning substances but have only limited polishing ability and thus tend to leave a dull finish on the tooth surfaces. Conversely, other cleaning and polishing agents have excellent polishing characteristics but are less efficient in reference to their cleaning properties. Thus, manufacturers often combine different agents in an effort to take advantage of the cleaning ability of one material and the polishing ability of another. When such a combination of materials is utilized, the dentifrice is said to contain an "abrasive system."

Many *in vitro* methods and techniques have been used to investigate the comparative cleaning and polishing abilities of various materials and formulations. These procedures are reviewed in detail in a number of excellent publications.[30, 33, 84, 85, 100, 184, 267, 272, 312] In general, abrasion is achieved in a relatively short period of time by exposing the materials to be abraded to a large number of brushing strokes with the substance or formulation under investigation. Specially constructed laboratory toothbrushing devices have been used for this purpose (Fig. 10–1).

The comparative abrasiveness of a particular substance or formulation has been estimated by the use of such techniques as determination of weight loss,[274] measurement of the cross-sectional area of loss with shadowgraphs and a planimeter,[183] determination of loss of material by use of a radioactive dentin abrasion procedure,[93] and determination of relative abrasion through use of a dentin section-shadowgraph procedure.[42] Since dental enamel is a relatively difficult substance to abrade, dentin has been the material most frequently used in these procedures.

The Council on Dental Therapeutics of the American Dental Association has conducted a series of laboratory investigations

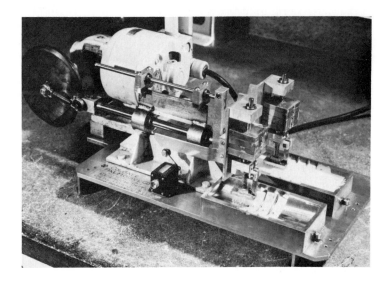

Figure 10–1 This photograph shows a two-brush model abrasion machine, which is used in *in vitro* dentifrice abrasion studies. (Reproduced from Bouchal, A. W.: Proc. Scient. Sect. TGA 45:2–5, 1966.)

to determine the comparative abrasiveness of some dentifrices commercially available in the United States. The laboratory procedure utilized to measure the abrasiveness of these dentifrices was the basic Radioactive Dentin Abrasion (RDA) procedure, slightly modified.

This procedure involves the use of the accelerated toothbrushing apparatus and dentin sections that contain radioactive phosphorus. The American Dental Association standard was set at 100, which corresponds to an RDA value of 475. The comparative abrasiveness of some representative dentifrices as determined in this evaluation are presented in Table 10–2.

Unfortunately, it is often difficult to correlate results obtained from *in vitro* techniques with the actual abrasiveness of these dentifrices on similar structures in the oral cavity. Two factors that make this correlation difficult are (1) the difference between the normal conditions of dentifrice use and employment of the accelerated toothbrushing apparatus and (2) the effect of the oral environment (saliva, pellicle, plaque, diet, and so on) on a particular tooth surface.

A number of *in vivo* techniques have been developed in an effort to evaluate the comparative cleaning and polishing ability of substances or formulations directly on the tooth surfaces. These methods, in general, were specially designed to measure one particular characteristic, such as ability to polish enamel surfaces, capacity to prevent or remove stain, ability to remove interproximal plaque, and capacity to abrade acrylic surfaces of veneer crowns.

One technique used a tooth reflectance meter to measure cleaning effectiveness of dentifrice materials.[246] The reflectance meter measures directly from the tooth surfaces (in a reproducible manner) both the diffuse and specular components of reflected light, which are believed to be related to both the degree of tooth whiteness and tooth polish (Fig. 10–2).

Another technique utilized a specially constructed intraoral photography apparatus to obtain reproducible pictures that were subsequently compared and assessed for the amount of stain that was present.[38] The camera equipment employed and some representative photographs are shown in Figure 10–3.

The effect of dentifrices on tooth stain has been evaluated *in vivo* through the use of a reproducible technique that subjectively assigns numerical values that represent equal increments of stain intensity.[162]

TABLE 10–2* COMPARATIVE ABRASIVENESS OF SOME COMMERCIALLY AVAILABLE DENTIFRICES AS DETERMINED BY A RADIOACTIVE DENTIN PROCEDURE†

DENTIFRICE	MANUFACTURER	PRINCIPAL ABRASIVE	ABRASIVITY INDEX
Sensodyne	Block Drug Co.	Silica	157
Vote	Bristol-Myers Co.	Silica	134
Plus White Plus	Bishop Industries, Inc.	Dicalcium Phosphate (anhydrous)	132
Plus White	Bishop Industries, Inc.	Dicalcium Phosphate (anhydrous)	110
Gleem II	Procter and Gamble Co.	Calcium Pyrophosphate	106
Macleans (old formulation)	Beecham Products, Inc.	Calcium Carbonate	93
Crest (Mint and Regular)	Procter and Gamble Co.	Calcium Pyrophosphate	88
Close-Up	Lever Brothers Co.	Silica	87
Pearl Drops	Carter-Wallace, Inc.	Alumina and Dicalcium Phosphate (dihydrate)	72
Macleans (new formulation)	Beecham Products, Inc.	Dicalcium Phosphate (dihydrate)	68
Ultra Brite	Colgate-Palmolive Co.	Dicalcium Phosphate (dihydrate)	64
Colgate with MFP	Colgate-Palmolive Co.	Insoluble Sodium Metaphosphate	51
Pepsodent	Lever Brothers Co.	Dicalcium Phosphate (dihydrate)	26
Thermodent	Chas. Pfizer and Co.	Magnesium Carbonate (basic) and Calcium Carbonate	24

*The data presented in this table were reproduced from Accepted Dental Therapeutics, 1971/1972 Edition.
†The American Dental Association standard is set at 100, which corresponds to a Radioactive Dentin Abrasion (RDA) value of 475. The abrasivity index values presented are averages; the lower the index value, the lower the abrasivity of the particular dentifrice, and vice versa.

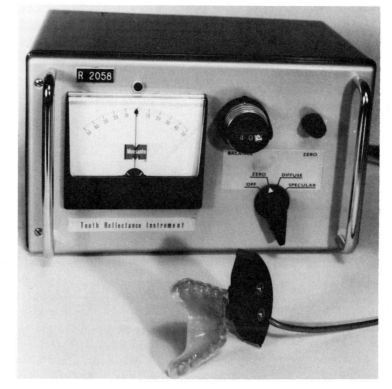

Figure 10–2 This photograph shows a tooth reflectometer and the intraoral positioning device whereby specular and diffuse readings are obtained in a reproducible manner. (Courtesy of Dr. Thomas Schiff, Monsanto Chemical Co., St. Louis, Missouri.)

The *in vivo* clearance and removal of interproximal plaque have been evaluated through the use of specially constructed removable tooth slabs inset in full gold crowns.[112, 135]

An *in vivo* technique has been recently developed to investigate the actual abrasiveness of dentifrices by determining the effect of dentifrices against acrylic surfaces of veneer crowns (Fig. 10–4). The technique consists of a tooth surface replication procedure and an evaluation of the obtained replica with a scanning electron microscope.[55]

Other *in vivo* tooth cleaning methods reported have included the use of tracer foods,[40, 226] standardized tooth surface replicas,[35] standardized photos,[308] and a modified Lobene subjective scoring system.[290]

The question constantly arises as to what is the optimal level of abrasiveness that a dentifrice should possess. This is a difficult question to answer because the abrasive needs of individuals vary to such a great extent. For example, persons who have exposed cementum and dentin or who have just undergone dental treatment procedures such as a gingivectomy have need of a very mildly abrasive dentifrice. On the other hand, persons with healthy dentitions, periodontium, and mucosal tissues can safely utilize much more abrasive dentifrices.

It is probably much more meaningful to define a minimum level of dentifrice abrasiveness rather than attempt to establish a maximum limit. The minimum dentifrice abrasive level for a particular person could be defined as that level that allows for the efficient and thorough removal of dental plaque and that does not permit "brown pellicle" (or other similar type stains) to accumulate.

Probably the most realistic and meaningful approach to dentifrice abrasiveness is that which assigns the dentist the responsibility for determining the particular level of abrasiveness that a particular person requires.[234] This approach is referred to as "individualizing dentifrices — the dentist's responsibility."

Detergents (Surface-Active Agents)

Detergents are basically cleaning agents and when present in dentifrices probably exert their cleaning effect by the following

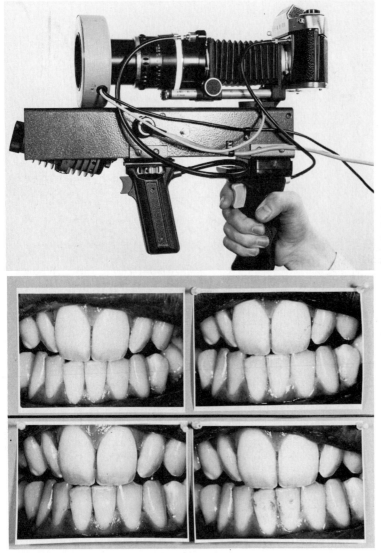

Figure 10–3 The upper portion of this photograph shows the camera that is used for intraoral photography. The lower portion depicts a representative series of photographs arranged for assessment. (Reproduced from Bull, W. H., Callendar, R. M., Pugh, B. R., and Wood, G. D.: Br. Dent. J. *124*:331–337, 1968.)

actions: (1) lowering the surface tension, (2) penetrating and loosening surface deposits, and (3) emulsifying and suspending the debris, which the dentifrice then removes from the tooth surfaces. Additionally, detergents provide dentifrices with the foaming (or sudsing) characteristic that is so popular (and expected) by almost all dentifrice purchasers.

In the early days of dentifrice manufacture, soap was the most commonly used detergent. However, soap-containing dentifrices had a relatively high alkaline pH and thus were sometimes irritating to the oral soft tissues. Also, the use of soap as a detergent greatly limited the selection of cleaning and polishing agents that could be used in the dentifrice.

All dentifrices currently available in the United States use synthetic detergents. Synthetic detergents have the following major advantages in comparison to soap: (1) compatability with many cleaning and polishing agents, thus permitting greater flexibility in the formulation of the dentifrice, (2) lack of the characteristic soapy taste, and (3) provision for the formulation of a dentifrice with a more neutral pH, resulting in no alkaline

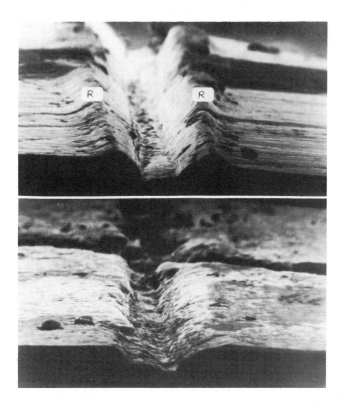

Figure 10-4 This photograph shows a cross-sectional view of the measurable arm of an indentation line in the acrylic surface of a veneer crown (500×). The upper photograph is before use of a dentifrice (R refers to the acrylic ridges created by the carving instrument). The lower photograph is after using a dentifrice for three weeks. Depth of indentation line in upper photograph is 12 microns; depth in lower photograph is 10 microns, indicating a loss of 2 microns due to the use of the dentifrice. (Reproduced from Facq, J. M., and Volpe, A. R.: J. Am. Dent. Assoc. *80*:317–323, [Feb.] 1970.)

irritation to the oral soft tissues. The three most commonly used synthetic detergents are:

Sodium lauryl sulfate

$$\left(CH_3(CH_2)_{10}\, CH_2OSO_3Na \right)$$

Sodium N-lauroyl sarcosinate

$$\left(CH_3(CH_2)_{10}CON(CH_3)CH_2COONa \right)$$

Sodium cocomonoglyceride sulfonate

$$\left(RCOOCH_2CH(OH)CH_2SO_3Na \right)$$

Sodium lauryl sulfate is probably the most widely used dentifrice detergent. In addition to its excellent detergent properties, sodium lauryl sulfate (and other detergents) possesses some antibacterial characteristics.

Sodium N-lauroyl sarcosinate, another widely used detergent, is, in addition to having excellent detergent properties, an effective enzyme inhibitor. Dentifrices containing this inhibitor have been evaluated in several human caries clinical studies that are discussed in the Therapeutic Dentifrices section of this chapter.

Humectants

The primary function of a humectant in a dentifrice is to retain moisture and thus provide for a paste that is chemically and physically stable, even if the cap on the tube is not closed and the dentifrice is exposed to air. Honey was the original humectant used, but this was gradually replaced by more satisfactory materials. The most commonly utilized dentifrice humectants are glycerin, sorbitol, and propylene glycol. Both glycerin and sorbitol have a sweet taste and thus also function to some extent as sweetening agents in the dentifrice. Since aqueous solutions of some glycols can permit bacterial or mold growth, preservatives such as sodium benzoate are often added to the humectant solution.

Binding Agents

The physical blending or mixing of the liquid and solid phases of a dentifrice may be inadequate to prevent separation, particularly during storage. The function of the binding agent in the dentifrice formulation is to prevent separation by providing a stable suspension. Basically, all binders are hydrophilic colloids that appear to dissolve but actually disperse, swell, or absorb water to form viscous liquid phases. Thus, the binder stabilizes the dentifrice against separation by increasing the consistency of the mixture of liquid and solid phases.

The first binder used in dentifrices was starch. Natural tree exudations such as gum arabic and tragacanth then became prominent as binders. Since 1940, seaweed colloids, such as Irish moss extract, and the sodium alginates have been widely used. Additionally, the synthetically prepared water-dispersible derivatives of cellulose such as sodium carboxymethylcellulose and a complex colloidal magnesium aluminum silicate are also in wide use as dentifrice binders.

The binder of choice depends upon the composition of the dentifrice and the desired ease of dispersion of the dentifrice in the oral cavity. It must also be chemically stable toward the other ingredients. As is the case with humectants, aqueous dispersions of the binders require preservation against microbial or mold contamination.

Flavoring Agents

The taste of a dentifrice is probably one of the most important factors in reference to the purchase and continuous use of a particular product. Market research and experience have shown that the majority of consumers will not re-purchase and continue to use a particular dentifrice solely because it will provide a therapeutic (or drug-related) benefit. The product must also be pleasant to use and refreshing to the taste. This may be referred to as the "cosmetic aspects of a therapeutic dentifrice" and is of great importance to the dentifrice manufacturers.

At times, some patients are advised to clean their dentition with mildly abrasive substances such as sodium chloride or sodium bicarbonate, rather than with conventional dentifrices. Although the use of these mildly abrasive substances is justifiably warranted in special situations and will be of some value in cleaning the dentition, it is extremely unlikely that a person will continuously utilize these relatively bland materials over a long period of time.

This was shown quite convincingly in a clinical study conducted to determine patients' reactions to brushing their teeth with water, a powder composed of table salt and baking soda, or a conventional dentifrice.[50] The general reaction of the participants who used either water or the salt and soda powder was most unfavorable. By contrast in the group using a conventional flavored dentifrice, the great majority of the participants stated that they preferred this method.*

The development of an acceptable flavor for a dentifrice is both an art and a science. Some of the most commonly used essential flavoring oils include spearmint, peppermint, wintergreen, cinnamon, and anise. Most dentifrices are produced by blending the various essential oils. It is interesting to note that flavor preferences vary considerably from country to country.

Miscellaneous Dentifrice Ingredients and Packaging

Water is the most important of the remaining ingredients. Deionized or distilled water is utilized. As previously mentioned, preservatives such as one of the parahydroxy benzoates are common dentifrice ingredients. In addition to naturally sweet humectants, such as glycerin and sorbitol, sodium saccharin is also used as a sweetening agent.

The dentifrice formulation may also contain tube-corrosion inhibitors such as sodium silicate, approved food colors, and traces of titanium dioxide, which is used as a whitening agent. In the case of dentifrices containing dicalcium phosphate as the principal cleaning and polishing agent, tetrasodium pyrophosphate is often used as a stabilizer to prevent hardening.

---

*A standard type toothpaste product (Peak), which has sodium bicarbonate as the principal cleaning and polishing agent and a conventional dentifrice flavor, is now available. This represents an attempt by the manufacturer to combine the mildly abrasive properties of sodium bicarbonate with conventional dentifrice characteristics, such as form, flavor, and foaming ability.

Oxygen salts such as hydrogen peroxide, sodium perborate, and magnesium peroxide are sometimes used to enhance the stain-removing properties of dentifrices. The efficacy of these materials, however, has not been established, and it has been suggested that their long-term effect on the oral soft tissues may be injurious.

In regard to packaging, most dentifrices are placed into either plain or epoxy-lined, fully collapsible aluminum tubes. One major manufacturer uses a semicollapsible polylaminate (plastic) tube.

Other Physical Forms

The previous discussion has been primarily concerned with dentifrices in their most common form, that is, toothpaste. As previously stated, other physical forms of dentifrices include powder and liquid.

Toothpowders contain essentially the same ingredients as toothpaste, with the exception of water, humectants, or binders. Their capacity to clean or polish teeth (abrasivity) would depend, to a great extent, on the degree of dilution (essentially water) that is used with them.

Liquid dentifrices, such as some "tooth polishers," also contain ingredients similar to those in toothpaste. However, they have a lesser amount of binder and thus flow more freely. Some liquid dentifrices have been formulated without detergents and thus lack conventional foaming characteristics. In general, liquid dentifrices may not be sufficiently abrasive to maintain tooth cleanliness, especially if they do not contain conventional quantities of cleaning and polishing agents.

THERAPEUTIC (DRUG-CONTAINING) DENTIFRICES

Definition and Implications

A therapeutic dentifrice may be described as one that contains a drug substance that has been incorporated into the formulation in an effort to produce a beneficial effect upon the oral tissues. This beneficial effect can be produced upon either the hard tissues (tooth surfaces) or the soft tissues (gingiva) and can be achieved by chemical, physiologic, or pharmacologic means. The two most important and beneficial oral health effects that can be attributed to a therapeutic dentifrice are (1) the prevention or reduction of the incidence of dental caries formation and (2) the prevention or reversal of gingival disease.

When a manufacturer is considering the incorporation of a drug substance into a dentifrice formulation for the purpose of obtaining a therapeutic claim, the nature of the particular drug substance to be utilized is very important. If the drug substance is one that would be generally regarded as safe and efficacious by experts (in respect to a particular formulation and a particular therapeutic claim), then the marketing of this dentifrice probably can be accomplished within a reasonable period of time and with a reasonable financial expenditure.

However, if the drug substance of interest is one that would not be generally regarded as safe and efficacious by experts, then the material is classified as a "new drug substance." As such, the manufacturer is required to comply with stringent Food and Drug Administration (FDA) regulations in an effort to establish and document the safety and efficacy of the dentifrice containing the new drug substance.

The FDA regulations require that extensive laboratory and clinical evaluations be conducted and the results submitted as part of a New Drug Application. This New Drug Application must be approved by the Food and Drug Administration prior to the marketing of the dentifrice. In the case of a therapeutic dentifrice with a caries-reducing claim (which is the major therapeutic claim utilized with current dentifrices), this could be a very long and very costly procedure. This situation occurs because caries clinical studies are usually conducted over a 2 to 3 year period of time and several such studies may be required.

Development of a Therapeutic Dentifrice

The development of a therapeutic (containing a new drug) dentifrice, in general, is a very expensive and lengthy endeavor. When a material is either obtained from a natural source or synthesized and is suspected to be of oral disease preventive value, it is generally subjected to the following evaluation sequence:

1. Laboratory *in vitro* screening procedures to determine the specific activity of the material (for example, antimicrobial, enzymatic, enamel solubility reducer).
2. Animal *in vivo* experiments to determine the ability of the material to reduce or prevent oral disease (such as caries or gingivitis) in an experimental animal model system.
3. Animal *in vivo* investigations to ascertain the relative toxicity of the material so as to determine at an early stage whether any serious problems exist or can be anticipated.
4. Short-term (carefully monitored and supervised) *in vivo* human studies to determine the pharmacologic and metabolic pattern of the material.
5. Laboratory experiments to produce an acceptable and stable formulation (for example, dentifrice, mouth rinse).
6. Short-term *in vivo* human clinical studies to evaluate a specific activity, such as the ability of the formulation to reduce dental plaque formation, to reduce the solubility of enamel, to prevent plaque pH decreases, to inhibit specific microorganisms, and so on.
7. Short-term *in vivo* human clinical studies to evaluate the effect of the formulation on a specific oral disease parameter such as gingivitis.
8. Additional (and long-term) animal *in vivo* toxicologic evaluations so as to determine whether more extensive clinical investigations can be safely conducted in humans.
9. Long-term *in vivo* human clinical studies to establish and document the safety and efficacy of the formulation.

The FDA is notified of a sponsor's intention to conduct *in vivo* human clinical investigations with a new drug substance by means of a formal submission referred to as a Notice of Claimed Investigational Exemption for a New Drug (IND). The IND contains the complete details concerning the new drug substance and the clinical study to be conducted. At the completion of each human investigation, the sponsor submits a complete report that contains the results of the study to the FDA.

The regulations concerning the components and preparations of an IND are published in the United States Code of Federal Regulation (C.F.R. 21, Part 130). This publication also includes a complete description of the FDA's classification of clinical studies (Phase I — pharmacology, Phase II — pharmacology and therapeutics, and Phase III — extensive use studies).

The laboratory and animal screening procedures currently employed in the evaluation of oral disease preventive materials are discussed in detail in an excellent article entitled Evaluation of Agents Used in the Prevention of Oral Disease.[54] The fundamentals of well-designed and well-executed human clinical studies are also discussed, to some extent, in this publication. Discussions on how to conduct caries clinical studies can be found in several other excellent reports.[6, 7, 8, 13, 122]

American Dental Association Classification*

The Council on Dental Therapeutics of the American Dental Association will consider for evaluation dentifrices and mouth rinses that make a therapeutic claim. Commercial products are examined either upon the request of the manufacturer or distributor or upon the initiative of the Council. Any firm may submit its appropriate products to the Council for consideration for acceptance. Products will be listed in Accepted Dental Therapeutics and described in suitable reports in the Journal of the American Dental Association if they meet standards of acceptance with respect to usefulness, composition, advertising, and labeling. Products are usually accepted for three years. Acceptance

---

*The material in this section has been reproduced from *Accepted Dental Therapeutics*, 1975/1976 Edition.

is renewable and may be reconsidered at any time. After consideration of a new product has been completed, the Council will classify the product as *accepted, provisionally accepted,* or *unaccepted.*

Accepted products include those for which there is adequate evidence of safety and effectiveness. They will be listed in *Accepted Dental Therapeutics* and may use the Seal of Acceptance.

Provisionally accepted includes those products for which there is reasonable evidence of usefulness and safety but which lack sufficient evidence of dental usefulness to justify being *accepted.*

Unaccepted products include those for which the Council has determined that no substantial evidence of usefulness exists and those for which a question of safety exists.

Non-Fluoride Therapeutic Dentifrices

Chlorophyll-Containing Dentifrices. The water-soluble derivatives of chlorophyll have been used in dentifrices as caries-preventive materials as well as gingival disease-preventive agents. Their use is based primarily on the ability of chlorophyll to reduce bacterial growth and to reduce the acid formed in dental plaque. The specific compound utilized is sodium copper chlorophyllin. Although human clinical caries studies have not been conducted with this compound, several animal (hamster) studies have indicated that it may have some anticaries potential.

Four clinical studies have been conduct-

ed to ascertain the effect of a dentifrice containing 0.1 per cent sodium copper chlorophyllin against gingival disease.[43, 110, 156, 189] Only one of these studies indicated that the material was of benefit against gingival disease.

The Council on Dental Therapeutics of the American Dental Association has previously indicated that the evidence available concerning chlorophyll-containing dentifrices is so limited or inconclusive that such products cannot accurately be evaluated. These dentifrices are not currently classified.

Antibiotic-Containing Dentifrices. A basic theory for the incorporation of antimicrobial substances into dentifrices is to destroy or inactivate the microorganisms that are associated with oral disease. Five clinical studies have been conducted to evaluate the anticariogenic effect of dentifrices and tooth powders containing penicillin, and one clinical study was conducted to evaluate a tyrothricin-containing dentifrice. The majority of the penicillin studies utilized a tooth powder, with the level of antibiotic ranging from 100 to 1000 units per gram of product. A summary of these clinical studies is presented in Table 10–3.

The results from these six studies (of which four provided a reduction in the incidence of caries) indicate that certain antibiotics are probably effective anticariogenic agents. However, there are two major deterrents to the routine use of antibiotics. They are as follows: (1) the possibility of allergic sensitization and (2) the possibility of the

TABLE 10–3* CLINICAL ANTICARIES STUDIES CONDUCTED UTILIZING ANTIBIOTIC-CONTAINING TOOTH POWDERS OR DENTIFRICES

INVESTIGATOR(S)	ANTIBIOTIC EVALUATED	DURATION OF STUDY	AGE RANGE	PER CENT REDUCTION IN CARIES
Hill and Kniesner, 1949	Penicillin	12 Months	8–15	None
Zander, 1950	Penicillin	24 Months	6–16	42 (DMFT) 56 (DMFS)
Walsh and Smart, 1951	Penicillin	12 Months	5–15	None
Hill, Sims, and Newman, 1953†	Penicillin	12 Months	6–12	10 (DMFT) 16 (DMFS)
Lunin and Mandel, 1955	Penicillin	18 Months	School Children	14 (DMFT)
Shiere, 1957†	Tyrothricin	24 Months	7–14	26 (DMFS)

*Adapted from Wallace, 1962.
†These studies used a conventional dentifrice (toothpaste), while the other studies utilized a tooth powder.

development of resistant or cross-resistant strains of microorganisms.

The Council on Dental Therapeutics of the American Dental Association has indicated that because of the overwhelming disadvantages of the topical application of penicillin, its use for the local treatment of oral disease is contraindicated (Accepted Dental Therapeutics, 1975/1976). The use of antibiotics is also closely regulated by the FDA, who have expressed considerable opposition to the regular use and general availability (without prescription) of all antibiotic-containing preparations.

The possibility exists that other antimicrobial agents may be able to accomplish the same purpose (destroy or inactivate microorganisms related to caries and gingival disease) and not have the undesirable characteristics of penicillin, mainly sensitization and resistance. Clinical investigations are currently being conducted in this area (discussed in the Mouth Rinse section).

Ammonium-Containing Dentifrices. Urea and dibasic ammonium phosphate have been of considerable interest as anticariogenic materials since the late 1940's. Products containing these compounds were often referred to as "ammoniated dentifrices." Initially, it had been theorized that ammonia and urea might provide an anticariogenic effect by neutralizing the acid that was produced by the bacteria in dental plaque. Also, urea could function as an enzyme inhibitor by virtue of its protein-denaturant properties.

Many clinical studies were conducted with dentifrices containing either urea, dibasic ammonium phosphate, or combinations of these substances. A summary of these clinical studies is presented in Table 10-4. As is apparent from the data, the majority of the studies, especially with the high-urea formulations, provided a beneficial anticariogenic effect. It has been indicated that a preliminary recommendation of a high urea-containing dentifrice would be consistent with the available data.[178] The Council on Dental Therapeutics of the American Dental Association has not classified preferentially any dentifrice containing urea or urea and ammonium compounds as the active ingredients, since the evidence for the usefulness of these products is so contradictory that they cannot be accurately evaluated (Accepted Dental Therapeutics, 1975/1976).

Enzyme Inhibitor-Containing Dentifrices. In the late 1940's, a theory was suggested that dental plaque might serve as a medium for the retention of enzyme inhibitors on the tooth surfaces, where they would be available to prevent the enzymatic conversion of sugar into acid. An *in vitro* procedure employing casein in a saliva-glucose medium was developed and used to screen many potential enzyme inhibitors, of which

TABLE 10-4* CLINICAL ANTICARIES STUDIES CONDUCTED UTILIZING AMMONIUM-CONTAINING DENTIFRICES

INVESTIGATOR(S)	AMMONIUM COMPOUNDS(S)	DURATION OF STUDY	AGE RANGE	PER CENT REDUCTION IN CARIES
Stephan and Miller, 1944	45% Urea (Liquid Dentifrice)	16 Months	12–25	80–100 (DMFS)
Henschel and Lieber, 1949 and 1952	22.5% Urea and 5% DBAP†	34 Months / 49 Months	17–55	38 (Lesions) / 44 (Lesions)
Kerr and Kesel, 1951	3% Urea and 5% DBAP	24 Months	10–11	11 (DMFT)
Davies and King, 1951‡	3% Urea and 5% DBAP	8 Months	12–31	None
Gale, 1951	12% Urea and 5% DBAP	21 Months	Preschool	33 (DMFT)
Lefkowitz and Venti, 1951	High Urea	18 Months	5–19	60 (DMFT)
Backer-Dirks, Winkler, and Van Aken, 1953	3% Urea and 5% DBAP	18 Months	10–14	None
Hawes and Bibby, 1953‡	12% Urea and 1% Urease	12–15 Months	7–13	None
Cohen and Donzanti, 1954	13% Urea and 3% DBAP	24 Months	9–13	25 (DMFT)
Vogel and Hess, 1957	13% Urea and 3% DBAP	14 Months	11–12	28 (Lesions)

*Adapted from Wallace, 1962 and Mandel and Cagan, 1964.

†DBAP refers to dibasic ammonium phosphate.

‡These studies used tooth powders, while the others (except Stephan and Miller) used a conventional dentifrice.

sodium N-lauroyl sarcosinate was discovered to be extremely effective.[141, 142]

A modification of this procedure (artificially developed plaque being substituted for the casein) was used to evaluate ten compounds, of which only penicillin was retained in a sufficient concentration to inhibit acid production.[73] Further investigations substantiated the sarcosinate effect and suggested that sodium dehydroacetate was also effective.[74]

The *in vivo* duration of the effectiveness of sodium N-lauroyl sarcosinate has been evaluated using various procedures to measure changes that occurred in the pH of plaque material that formed on proximal surfaces of non-carious teeth.[37, 69, 101, 111] There is general agreement that acid production is effectively inhibited immediately after use of sodium N-lauroyl sarcosinate, but results in reference to duration of effectiveness have ranged from 2 to 12 hours.

The retention of sodium N-lauroyl sarcosinate has also been demonstrated by other techniques, including the use of C^{14}-labeled sarcosinate,[5] and the use of a dentin chip placed into a removable prosthetic device.[279] Although this compound has been shown to reduce caries formation in animals, the results have not always been comparable.[139, 240, 295, 320]

One clinical study has been conducted to evaluate the caries inhibitory effect of a dentifrice containing a combination of 0.75 per cent sodium dehydroacetate and 0.5 per cent sodium oxalate.[270] The two-year results indicated approximately 50 per cent reduction in new carious lesions.

Dentifrices containing 2.0 per cent sodium N-lauroyl sarcosinate as the anti-caries agent have been evaluated in several human clinical studies. A summary of five long-term studies comparing this dentifrice to a control dentifrice is presented in Table 10-5*A*. As is apparent from the data, the sarcosinate-containing dentifrice provided a reduction in caries in a majority of the studies. Another clinical study conducted over a two-year

TABLE 10-5 CLINICAL ANTICARIES STUDIES CONDUCTED UTILIZING SODIUM N-LAUROYL SARCOSINATE-CONTAINING DENTIFRICES

A. Comparisons with a Control Dentifrice				
INVESTIGATOR(S)	DURATION OF STUDY	SPECIAL CONDITIONS	AGE RANGE	PER CENT REDUCTION IN CARIES (DMFS)
Fosdick, 1956	24 Months		17-35	47*
Frasher and Hein, 1958	27 Months	Fluoridated Water	4-12	43*
Backer-Dirks, Kwant, and Starmans, 1959	20 Months	Supervised Brushing and Controlled Diet	10-13	4
Mergele, 1968A	36 Months	Fluoridated Water	9-13	4
Zacheral, 1970	24 Months	5-10 Bite Wing X-rays	Elem. School	-15
B. Comparisons with a Stannous Fluoride–Calcium Pyrophosphate Dentifrice				
Finn and Jamison, 1963	24 Months	Supervised Brushing and Controlled Diet	8-15	-2
Frankl and Alman, 1968	36 Months		8-14	3
Mergele, 1968A	36 Months	Fluoridated Water	9-13	-10
Homan and Messer, 1969	20 Months		7 13	0 to -2 -12 to -16
Zacherl, 1970	24 Months	5-10 Bite Wing X-rays	Elem. School	-39*

*Difference is statistically significant at the 95% level of confidence.

period of time indicated that a combination of sodium N-lauroyl sarcosinate and sodium N-palmitoyl sarcosinate provided a 17 per cent reduction in caries.[52]

Five long-term clinical studies in which a dentifrice containing 2.0 per cent sodium N-lauroyl sarcosinate was compared with a positive control dentifrice (0.4 per cent stannous fluoride in a calcium pyrophosphate formulation) are summarized in Table 10–5B. In the majority of these studies, there was no statistically significant difference between the two dentifrices. A one-year clinical study has also been reported that indicates that the positive control was significantly better than the sarcosinate dentifrice.[203]

The data from the caries clinical studies evaluating a dentifrice containing 2.0 per cent sodium N-lauroyl sarcosinate indicate some effectiveness in reducing the incidence of new carious surfaces. Further evaluation of the data on an individual tooth surface basis has indicated that the dentifrice is more effective on pit and fissure surfaces than on smooth surfaces. This effect would be anticipated, since the sarcosinate is probably better retained (and not so readily washed away) in the pits and fissures as on the smooth surface areas.

The Council on Dental Therapeutics of the American Dental Association has indicated that evidence in support of anti-enzyme dentifrices is controversial and that the usefulness of these dentifrices in caries control has not been adequately established (Accepted Dental Therapeutics, 1975/1976).

Fluoride-Containing Therapeutic Dentifrices*

Sodium Fluoride Dentifrices. As a result of the success achieved in reducing the incidence of dental decay through the use of fluoride compounds in communal water supplies and as topical solutions applied to the teeth, it was only natural that fluoride compounds be incorporated into dentifrices. The

---

*Three excellent review publications are available that contain discussions concerning the subject of fluoride-containing therapeutic dentifrices (Peterson 1968; Duckworth, 1968; and Heifetz and Horowitz, 1970).

first such fluoride compound to be used in a dentifrice formulation was sodium fluoride.

The initial clinical studies conducted to evaluate dentifrices containing 0.22 per cent sodium fluoride indicated that the dentifrices were ineffective in reducing the incidence of dental caries.[24, 157, 209, 309] It has been theorized that these sodium fluoride clinical studies may have provided negative results for two reasons: (1) basic incompatibilities in the dentifrice formulations, particularly in the presence of calcium-containing cleaning and polishing agents, which rendered the fluoride compound inactive by forming insoluble calcium fluoride and (2) basic inadequacies in the design and methods of conducting the clinical studies.[94]

During the past decade, however, a number of clinical studies have been reported that indicate that dentifrices containing 0.22 per cent sodium fluoride may be effective anticaries materials when properly formulated and evaluated in properly designed and conducted clinical studies. A summary of these more recent clinical studies is presented in Table 10–6. The cleaning and polishing agents used in the different dentifrice formulations were all selected because of their compatibility with sodium fluoride.

The Council on Dental Therapeutics of the American Dental Association currently states that the early evidence to justify the inclusion of sodium fluoride in commercially available dentifrices is not convincing. They further indicate, however, that more recent reports of clinical studies with dentifrices containing sodium fluoride suggest that incompatibility is an important factor and that formulation modification can be made to provide products that will reduce the incidence of caries (Accepted Dental Therapeutics, 1975/1976).

A government notice has been issued that indicates that dentifrices containing sodium fluoride (as well as chlorophyllins, anti-enzymes, and urea) lack substantial evidence of effectiveness in reference to therapeutic claims (Federal Register, 1970). This notice was based on a review conducted by the National Academy of Sciences — National Research Council (Drug Efficacy Study Group) of certain commercially available dentifrices that were the subject of approved

TABLE 10–6   RECENT CLINICAL ANTICARIES STUDIES CONDUCTED UTILIZING
SODIUM FLUORIDE-CONTAINING DENTIFRICES

INVESTIGATOR(S)	TYPE OF FORMULATION	DURATION OF STUDY	AGE RANGE	PER CENT REDUCTION IN CARIES (DMFS)
Torell and Ericsson, 1965A	Sodium bicarbonate	24 Months	10–11	18
Brudevold and Chilton, 1966	Dicalcium phosphate Dihydrate			6
	Insoluble sodium meta-phosphate (IMP) and sodium orthophosphate	24 Months	10–19	19
Koch, 1967 and 1970*	Plastic abrasive (methacrylate polymer)	36 Months	8–10 11–12	40 48
Peterson and Williamson, 1968	IMP and sodium ortho-phosphate	36 Months	9–15	20
Zacherl, 1968	Calcium pyrophosphate	20 Months	7–14	28
Reed and King, 1970	Calcium pyrophosphate	24 Months	8–13	30
Weisenstein and Zacherl, 1972	Calcium pyrophosphate	21 Months	5–15	11–38

*Supervised brushing once per day.

New Drug Applications obtained prior to the enactment of the New Drug Regulations of 1962, which required efficacy substantiation as well as safety data.

Stannous Fluoride Dentifrices. Stannous fluoride-containing dentifrices have been subjected to extensive clinical investigation. The most well-known stannous fluoride dentifrice contains 0.4 per cent stannous fluoride and calcium pyrophosphate as the cleaning and polishing agent. Calcium pyrophosphate was selected because it was found to be more compatible with stannous fluoride; that is, it did not inactivate the stannous fluoride as readily as did commonly used polishing agents such as calcium carbonate or dicalcium phosphate dihydrate. Extensive laboratory and clinical investigations were conducted by scientists from both the manufacturing company and Indiana University in an effort to develop this dentifrice. These investigations are discussed in three excellent publications.[3, 206, 228]

Many clinical studies have been published concerning 0.4 per cent stannous fluoride-calcium pyrophosphate dentifrices. A summary of some of the longer-term clinical studies comparing stannous fluoride-calcium pyrophosphate dentifrices with a control dentifrice is presented in Table 10–7. It is readily apparent that such dentifrices are effective in reducing the incidence of new carious surfaces. The variations in the magnitude of reductions are most likely a result of different degrees of usage, different criteria of examiners, and the relative incidence between caries of smooth surfaces and pit or fissure surfaces. It is generally agreed that effectiveness is greater on smooth surfaces.

In addition to the studies listed in Table 10–7, several short-term studies (less than 18 months) have been conducted and show positive reductions compared to a control dentifrice.[208-210] There are also several clinical studies reported in which the stannous fluoride-calcium pyrophosphate dentifrice was evaluated in conjunction with other forms of fluoride therapy, such as prophylaxis pastes, topical solutions, and fluoridated water.[27, 86, 204, 211, 250] Such combined therapy has been shown to be effective, but it is generally difficult to assess the precise contribution of the fluoride dentifrice.

The Council on Dental Therapeutics of the American Dental Association classified one stannous fluoride-calcium pyrophos-

TABLE 10–7   CLINICAL ANTICARIES STUDIES CONDUCTED UTILIZING
A STANNOUS FLUORIDE-CALCIUM PYROPHOSPHATE DENTIFRICE

INVESTIGATOR(S)	DURATION OF STUDY	SPECIAL CONDITIONS	AGE RANGE	PER CENT REDUCTION IN CARIES (DMFS)
Muhler and Radike, 1957	24 Months		17–36	34
Jordan and Peterson, 1959	24 Months	Supervised School Brushing	8–12	21
Hill, 1959	24 Months		9–16	15
Peffley and Muhler, 1960	24 Months	Supervised Brushing—Military School	10–19	46
Kyes, Overton and McKean, 1961	24 Months	Naval Academy	17–24	8
Muhler, 1962	36 Months		6–18	21
Bixler and Muhler, 1962	24 Months	Supervised School Brushing	11–18	32
Henriques, Frankl, and Alman, 1964	24 Months		5–12	13
Mergele, Jennings, and Gasser, 1964	24 Months	Supervised School Brushing Fluoridated Water	8–15	9
Zacherl and McPhail, 1965	18 Months		Grades 1, 2, 7	40
Torell and Ericsson, 1965A	24 Months		10–11	23
Horowitz, Law, Thompson, and Chamberlin, 1966	36 Months	Home Use Supervised School Brushing	6–10	17 21
Thomas and Jamison, 1966	24 Months	Supervised Brushing	7–16	36
Brudevold and Chilton, 1966	24 Months		10–19	4
Bixler and Muhler, 1966A	19 Months	Oral Hygiene Motivation Military and Boarding Schools	11–23	54
Jackson and Sutcliffe, 1967	36 Months		11–12	None (Males) 18 (Females)
James and Anderson, 1967	36 Months		11–12	16–24
Slack, Berman, Martin, and Hardie, 1967	36 Months		11–13	None (Clinical) 36 (Radiographic)
Onishi, et al., 1967	24 Months		Grade 1	13 (DMFT)
Peterson and Williamson, 1968	36 Months		9–15	25
Zacherl, 1968	20 Months		7–14	28
Zacherl, 1970	24 Months		Elem. School	30
Zacherl, 1972	20 Months	Fluoridated Water High-Beta Phase Abrasive	7–14	28
Zacherl, 1972A	24 Months	Dentifrice Aged One Year at Room Temperature	Grades 2–6	22

phate dentifrice (Crest) as *provisionally accepted* in August, 1960. In 1964, this classification was changed to *accepted*, which is the present classification. Thus, this was the first therapeutic dentifrice to receive the American Dental Association's Seal of Acceptance.

Since 1960, three other stannous fluoride dentifrices have been classified as *provisionally accepted* by the Council on Dental Therapeutics of the American Dental Association (Cue, Fact, and Super Stripe). These dentifrices all contained 0.4 per cent stannous fluoride and utilized insoluble sodium metaphosphate as the principal cleaning and polishing agents. Stannous fluoride-insoluble sodium metaphosphate dentifrices are extremely stable, maintaining high soluble fluoride levels for relatively long periods of time.

Even though all three of these dentifrices were effective in regard to reducing caries and had been developed and clinically tested at considerable cost, they were removed from the market by their respective manufacturers because of an inability to promote them successfully to the consumer.

Clinical studies demonstrating the effectiveness of 0.4 per cent stannous fluoride-insoluble metaphosphate dentifrices, as compared to a control dentifrice, are summarized in Table 10–8. Also, five clinical studies have compared stannous fluoride-insoluble sodium metaphosphate dentifrices to a stannous fluoride-calcium pyrophosphate dentifrice.[36, 113, 121, 193, 277] The results suggest that the stannous fluoride-insoluble sodium metaphosphate dentifrice may be slightly more effective than the stannous fluoride-calcium pyrophosphate dentifrice.

The National Academy of Sciences — National Research Council also reviewed stannous fluoride dentifrices (with approved New Drug Applications) that were commercially available prior to the New Drug Regulations of 1962. The only such dentifrice

TABLE 10–8 CLINICAL ANTICARIES STUDIES CONDUCTED WITH STANNOUS
FLUORIDE-INSOLUBLE SODIUM METAPHOSPHATE-CONTAINING DENTIFRICES

INVESTIGATOR(S)	DURATION OF STUDY	AGE RANGE	MINOR AMOUNT OF CALCIUM COMPOUND	SPECIAL CONDITIONS	PER CENT REDUCTION IN CARIES (DMFS)
Henriques, Frankl, and Alman, 1964	24 Months	5–12	Yes		17
Mergele, Jennings, and Gasser, 1964	24 Months	8–15	Yes	Fluoridated Water/Supervised Brushing	16
Slack and Martin, 1964	24 Months	11–13	Yes	No Radiographs	None (Clinical)
Thomas and Jamison, 1966	24 Months	7–16	Yes	Supervised Brushing/ Controlled Diet	37
Brudevold and Chilton, 1966	24 Months	10–19	No		25
Segal, Stiff, George, and Picozzi, 1966	24 Months	7–12	Yes	Supervised Brushing	25 (DFS)
Fullmer, Volpe, Apperson, and Kiraly, 1966	36 Months	8–10	Yes		30
Naylor and Emslie, 1967	36 Months	11–13	Yes		15
Slack, Berman, Martin, and Young, 1967	36 Months	11–13	Yes	Supervised Brushing	None (Clinical) 28 (Radiographs)
Fanning, Gotjamanos, and Vowles, 1968	24 Months	11–13	No		22
Mergele, 1968	22 Months	7–21	No	Supervised Brushing	9

available at that time was the stannous fluoride-calcium pyrophosphate dentifrice. The government (in the same notice previously referred to — Federal Register, 1970) indicated that there is substantial evidence that a dentifrice containing 0.4 per cent stannous fluoride in a suitable formulation is effective as an aid in reducing the incidence of dental caries.

The notice further states that because the other ingredients in a stannous fluoride dentifrice may have a role in modifying the effectiveness of the products in reducing the incidence of dental caries, the usefulness of a specific formulation must be determined on the basis of adequate data. Adequate data is defined as data to assure that, in the formulation to be marketed, the fluoride ion is available for incorporation into the structure of the teeth or data that provides substantial evidence of clinical effectiveness.

Sodium Monofluorophosphate Dentifrices. Sodium monofluorophosphate-containing dentifrices have been extensively evaluated in laboratory and clinical investigations. The most well-known dentifrice contains 0.76 per cent sodium monofluorophosphate and dicalcium phosphate dihydrate as the cleaning and polishing agent.

Sodium monofluorophosphate (Na_2PO_3F) could be considered a more advantageous fluoride agent than stannous fluoride (SnF_2) because of the following factors:

1. Na_2PO_3F has a more neutral pH than SnF_2 (Na_2PO_3F dentifrices have an approximate pH range of 5.5 to 6.5, while SnF_2 dentifrices have a pH of approximately 4.8).

2. Na_2PO_3F has greater resistance to oxidation and hydrolysis than SnF_2.

3. Na_2PO_3F has greater compatibility with calcium-containing cleaning and polishing agents used in dentifrices (as indicated by the clinical studies presented in Table 10–9).

4. Na_2PO_3F-containing dentifrices do not stain teeth as do SnF_2 dentifrices.[57, 213]

5. Na_2PO_3F dentifrices have been shown to reduce the incidence of tooth hypersensitivity.[31, 104, 116, 133, 253]

6. Some clinical studies suggest that a Na_2PO_3F-insoluble sodium metaphosphate dentifrice may provide more caries protection than a SnF_2-calcium pyrophosphate dentifrice.[62, 75, 192]

Sodium monofluorophosphate is especially unique in that its calcium salt is relatively soluble as compared with calcium fluoride, which is almost completely insoluble and inert. Calcium fluoride is the insoluble and inactive salt that is found when either stannous fluoride or sodium fluoride are in the presence of calcium ions. This property

TABLE 10–9 CLINICAL ANTICARIES STUDIES CONDUCTED UTILIZING SODIUM MONOFLUOROPHOSPHATE-CONTAINING DENTIFRICES*

INVESTIGATOR(S)	CLEANING AND POLISHING AGENT	DURATION OF STUDY	AGE RANGE	PER CENT REDUCTION IN CARIES (DMFS)
Finn and Jamison, 1963†	Insoluble Sodium Metaphosphate	24 Months	8–15	27**
Torell and Ericsson, 1965B	Calcium Carbonate	24 Months	11	15
			10	6
Naylor and Emslie, 1967	Dicalcium Phosphate (dihydrate)	36 Months	11–12	18
Fanning, Gotjamanos, and Vowles, 1968	Insoluble Sodium Metaphosphate	24 Months	11–13	20
Møller, Holst, and Sørensen, 1968	Insoluble Sodium Metaphosphate	30 Months	10–12	19
Thomas and Jamison, 1968†	Insoluble Sodium Metaphosphate	24 Months	8–16	34
Mergele, 1968†	Insoluble Sodium Metaphosphate	22 Months	7–21	21
Mergele, 1968A‡	Insoluble Sodium Metaphosphate	36 Months	8–14	17
Frankl and Alman, 1968	Insoluble Sodium Metaphosphate	36 Months	6–15	11**
Takeuchi, Schimizu, Kawasaki, and Kizu, 1968	Dicalcium Phosphate (dihydrate)	12 Months	Grades 3 and 4	24
Kinkel and Stolte, 1968	Insoluble Sodium Metaphosphate	24 Months	6–13	25–33
Torell, 1969	Calcium Carbonate	20 Months	Grade 4	29
Patz and Naujoks, 1969	Insoluble Sodium Metaphosphate	24 Months	18–28	22 (Maxillary Premolars) 8 (Overall)
Onisi and Tani, 1970	Dicalcium Phosphate (dihydrate)	12 Months	Elem. School	16 (Pits and Fissures) 41 (Smooth Surfaces)
Zacherl, 1972‡	Calcium Pyrophosphate	20 Months	7–14	23
Gerdin, 1972	Calcium Carbonate	24 Months	12	5 (Compared to a NaF Dentifrice)
Kinkel and Raich, 1972 and 1974	Dicalcium Phosphate (dihydrate)	36 Months 48 Months	School Children	37–46 32–38
Lind, Møller, Von Der Fehr, and Larsen, 1974‡§	Aluminum Oxide	36 Months	8–11	32 (Clinical plus X-ray)
Hargreaves and Chester, 1973 and 1974§	Aluminum Oxide	36 Months	5 8 11	23 8 23
Kinkel, Stole, and Weststrate, 1974	Dicalcium Phosphate (dihydrate) (Also contained 2% Sodium Trimetaphosphate)	36 Months	School Children	17–38 (Unsupervised) 35–43 (Supervised)
Andlaw and Tucker, 1975	Aluminum Oxide	36 Months	11–12	19 (Overall)
Mainwaring and Naylor, 1975	Calcium Carbonate	24 Months	11–12	31 (X-ray)
Peterson and Williamson, 1975‡	Calcium Carbonate	32 Months	8–12	23
Downer, Holloway, and Davies, 1975	Calcium Carbonate (Also AFP topical and prophy paste)	36 Months	11	56 (Erupting teeth)

*Adapted from Volpe, 1968.
**These two particular reductions were obtained versus a stannous fluoride-calcium pyrophosphate dentifrice (positive control dentifrice).
†Supervised brushing and controlled diet.
‡Fluoridated water.
§These two studies evaluated 2% sodium monofluorophosphate dentifrices. All the other studies evaluated dentifrices containing approximately 0.76% of the fluoride compound.

of not being readily inactivated by calcium permits sodium monofluorophosphate to be used in a variety of dentifrice-abrasive formulations without loss of efficacy. In contrast, stannous fluoride and sodium fluoride are incompatible with such common cleaning and polishing agents as calcium carbonate and dicalcium phosphate because of the formation of insoluble and inactive calcium fluoride. A summary of the clinical studies conducted with various sodium monofluoro-

phosphate-containing dentifrices is presented in Table 10–9.

In 1969, the Council on Dental Therapeutics of the American Dental Association classified a sodium monofluorophosphate-insoluble sodium metaphosphate dentifrice (Colgate Dental Cream with MFP) as *accepted*, which is its present classification. Thus, this dentifrice, too, has received the American Dental Association's Seal of Acceptance.

Additionally, the FDA approved a New

Drug Application submitted in reference to this same sodium monofluorophosphate-insoluble sodium metaphosphate dentifrice in 1967. This approval was granted on the basis of an extensive review of the laboratory and clinical data that was submitted to the FDA to substantiate and document the safety and anti-caries efficacy of this dentifrice. Since the safety and efficacy of this particular dentifrice were established under the New Drug Regulations of 1962, it was not necessary for it to be reviewed by the National Academy of Sciences — National Research Council (as were sodium fluoride- and stannous fluoride-containing dentifrices).

Other Fluoride Dentifrices. A dentifrice containing an organic fluoride compound has been investigated in at least two clinical studies thus far. This dentifrice (Elmex) contains amine fluorides, and the principal cleaning and polishing agent is insoluble sodium metaphosphate. These fluoride compounds were selected for clinical evaluation because laboratory and animal investigations had indicated that they might provide better anticaries protection (fluoride plus antibacterial activity) than sodium fluoride. This comparison of fluoride compounds is discussed in an excellent publication.[152]

This dentifrice contains 0.125 per cent fluoride, which is provided by the following materials:

1. diethanol aminoprophyl-N-ethanol octa-decylamine-dihydrofluoride (1.51 per cent of this compound equals 0.1 per cent fluoride), and
2. cetylamine hydrofluoride (0.40 per cent of this compound equals 0.025 per cent fluoride).

The results reported thus far from two long-term clinical studies are very encouraging. In the first study, which progressed for seven years, the amine fluoride dentifrice provided a 23 to 35 per cent reduction in caries.[186] In the second study, which was a six-year investigation, the dentifrice provided a 33 per cent reduction in caries.[185]

Several recent three-year clinical studies have been reported, wherein a dentifrice

(Magnaforte) containing 0.45 per cent potassium fluoride and 0.14 per cent manganese chloride (formulated with a methacrylate abrasive) has been shown to be slightly superior to a dentifrice containing 0.22 per cent sodium fluoride.[83, 148] Further studies are necessary in order to determine the actual caries-inhibiting potential of this combination of agents.

DENTIFRICES FOR PERIODONTAL DISEASE

Thus far, the discussion of dentifrices has been primarily concerned with their effect on the incidence of caries. As stated, dentifrices can have a beneficial effect on caries, either through removal of bacterial plaque (cosmetic-therapeutic function) or through the application of drug substances such as various fluoride compounds (therapeutic function).

Since plaque accumulation is also associated with the onset of such entities as calculus and gingivitis, its thorough and efficient removal by a dentifrice (cosmetic-therapeutic function) can also have a beneficial effect on calculus formation and gingival health.

In this regard, the Council on Dental Therapeutics of the American Dental Association recognizes the importance of home care in the control of dental plaque and indicates that the brushing of the teeth and gingiva has been the home-care procedure most widely recommended to promote the cleanliness of the teeth and gingiva. The Council further states that the basic purpose of toothbrushing is to remove oral accumulations of plaque and debris, which thereby assists in the prevention of dental disease (Accepted Dental Therapeutics, 1975/1976).

At the present time, no commercially available dentifrice in the United States makes a direct drug-related (therapeutic function) claim in regard to the prevention of plaque, calculus, or gingivitis. However, many agents are currently under investigation with regard to their effect on these parameters. These agents, some of which are very promising, include quaternary ammonium compounds, antibiotics, biguanides, enzymes, organic fluorides, and others. Although these materials are evaluated to some extent in dentifrices, they are, for the most part, initially evaluated in mouth rinse formulations, since this vehicle provides the fewest problems concerning ingredient compatibility and overall product stability.

For this reason, a more complete discussion of drug substances that have been shown to affect plaque, calculus, and gingivitis is presented in the Therapeutic Mouth Rinse section of this chapter.

DENTIFRICES FOR HYPERSENSITIVE TEETH

Two dentifrices have been available that specifically claim to have a beneficial effect on hypersensitive teeth. One dentifrice (Sensodyne) contains 10 per cent strontium chloride as the active agent, and the other dentifrice (Thermodent) contains 1.4 per cent formalin as the active agent. The precise mechanism of action is not known in either product. Both of these dentifrices have been evaluated in a variety of clinical studies, many of which have indicated that they do provide a desensitizing effect.

The Council on Dental Therapeutics of the American Dental Association indicates that it has not seen adequate evidence to justify claims for dentifrices that are promoted to provide relief from hypersensitive teeth (Accepted Dental Therapeutics, 1975/1976).

It should also be mentioned that a dentifrice (Colgate Dental Cream with MFP) containing 0.76 per cent sodium monofluorophosphate has also been clinically shown to have desensitization properties in addition to its well-known anticaries effect.*

DENTIFRICES WITH SPECIALIZED FUNCTIONS

A specialized ingestible dentifrice has been developed in response to the specific

needs of astronauts while on space missions. This ingestible dentifrice, designed to assist in maintaining oral hygiene during prolonged periods of chamber confinement, was developed at the United States Air Force School of Aerospace Medicine (Brooks Air Force Base, San Antonio, Texas) under the direction and supervision of Col. Ira L. Shannon.*

The ingestible dentifrice was formulated within the following imposed limitations: (1) no volatile oils, (2) no detergent (or foaming agent), and (3) low calcium content. The ingestible dentifrice contains the following ingredients: insoluble sodium metaphosphate (40 per cent), dicalcium phosphate dihydrate (2.6 per cent), glycerin (32 per cent), carboxymethylcellulose (1.3 per cent), saccharin (0.1 per cent), and distilled water (24 per cent). The specific method of preparation of this ingestible dentifrice is provided in a separate report.[252]

A clinical study was conducted which indicated that this ingestible dentifrice was equivalent to a commercially available dentifrice in reference to patient acceptance and cleaning performance.[276] This study also indicated that the ingestible dentifrice has potential not only for isolated subjects but also for hospital patients who are physically or mentally handicapped.

DENTIFRICES AND THE ORAL TISSUES

From time to time, questions are raised concerning the possible adverse effects of dentifrices on the dentition and mucosal tissues.

Effects on Dentition

The effect of dentifrices on the dentition has been discussed to some extent in the section concerning cleaning and polishing agents. As stated previously, it is very difficult to predict with any accuracy the degree of abrasivity that a dentifrice will exhibit

---

*These clinical studies have previously been referred to in the Sodium Monofluorophosphate section of this chapter.

*Dr. Shannon is Chief, Special Laboratory for Research in Oral Physiology, Veterans Administration Hospital, 2002 Holcombe Boulevard, Houston, Texas 77031.

under actual *in vivo* conditions. This is because of the great extent of variation from person to person — especially with regard to degree of exposed cementum and dentin, frequency and method of toothbrushing, type of toothbrush, diet characteristics, masticatory forces, and other such factors.

Nor is it feasible to directly correlate laboratory data (such as RDA values) to the actual clinical situation. In one long-term clinical study (54 months), two groups of 60 subjects each used dentifrices that ranged from an RDA of 260 to an RDA of 460. The study was supervised, and each subject's dentition was exposed to his respective dentifrice for a total of approximately 45 hours during the course of the study. Careful clinical examinations at three-month intervals indicated that neither of the dentifrices caused any adverse reactions of the oral mucosal tissues and that both groups of subjects had similar patterns and levels of cervical abrasion or erosion.[300]

Also, these same two dentifrices (RDA of 260 and RDA of 460) were studied in another long-term clinical investigation (24 months) to determine their comparative effect on selected dental materials. Again, careful periodic clinical examinations indicated that neither dentifrice produced any abnormal or unusual effect on the surface characteristics of either acrylic or silicate anterior restorations or the acrylic surfaces of veneer crowns.[247]

To further complicate the matter, evidence is now coming forth that strongly suggests that the toothbrush used and the duration and method of toothbrushing employed may play as important a role in regard to tooth wear as the dentifrices themselves.[311]

As previously mentioned, this author feels that the most realistic and meaningful approach to dentifrice abrasivity is that which assigns the dentist responsibility for determining the particular level of abrasiveness that a particular person requires. At the same time, dentifrice manufacturers should continue to strive to produce more efficient products that have the least potential for producing adverse effects upon the dentition.

Effects on Mucosa

In regard to the mucosal tissues, at one time or another just about every commercially available dentifrice and mouth rinse has been reported to be associated with some type of reaction.[95, 96, 127, 154, 155, 194, 255, 262, 265]

Similarly, at one time or another almost all dentifrice ingredients (cleaning and polishing agents, detergents, flavoring oils, fluoride compounds, and so on) have been reported to be associated with some particular reaction that occurred in a particular person. In this regard, dentifrices are thus behaving in a manner identical to all other cosmetic products, including soaps, shampoos, shaving creams, deodorants, antiperspirants, facial cosmetics, and so on.

In a recent study, an exhaustive attempt was made to determine the relationship between various oral habits (for example, use of specific toothbrushes, dentifrices, mouth rinses, tobacco, alcohol, foods, and beverages) and the status of the oral mucosal tissues, as determined by clinical, microscopic, and cytologic evaluation. A population of approximately 450 persons was included in the investigation, and the results indicated that there was no association between the various factors considered and the status of the mucosal tissues.[32]

In fact, all of the ingredients used in today's dentifrices either have a substantial amount of data available concerning their utilization or they are thoroughly tested prior to use in a product. Also, it is important to indicate that the incidence of mucosal reactions to today's dentifrices is incredibly small — especially when one considers the hundreds of millions of people who use these products on a daily basis throughout their lives.

If a dentist suspects that a particular dentifrice may be associated with a mucosal reaction in a particular person, he should advise the person to discontinue the use of the present product and use another brand. In most cases, the reaction will subside and not recur with the second brand. If the person continues to experience the reaction with the new product, then a more generalized allergic-type response should be suspected, and the person should be referred to a dermatologist for further evaluation and examination. In all probability, that person will exhibit a similar response with other cosmetic products.

CURRENT TRENDS IN DENTIFRICES

Although the majority of the dentifrices are currently being sold in the United States on the basis of an anticaries therapeutic claim, it would appear that there is a definite trend toward consumer acceptance of purely cosmetic dentifrices.[217] It may be recalled that cosmetic dentifrices were defined as dentifrices that did not contain a drug substance or make a therapeutic claim. When used in a routine, non-specific manner, cosmetic dentifrices will provide a "cosmetically clean and healthy dentition and a fresher breath."

The success of five particular dentifrices (Ultra Brite, Close-Up, Macleans, Pearl Drops* and Gleem II), all of which are pri-

_____
*A tooth polish in liquid form.

marily cosmetic in nature, has substantiated this trend. In general, the cosmetic dentifrices that are commercially available are all utilizing similar types of approaches to the consumer, including "whiter teeth," "brighter teeth," "extra-strength cleaning," high-impact flavors, a combination of dentifrice and mouth rinse properties, and a combination of cosmetic and therapeutic properties.

In regard to cosmetic-therapeutic combinations, Gleem II contains sodium fluoride, and Aim toothpaste, a clear gel product similar to Close-Up, contains sodium monofluorophosphate. Macleans contains sodium monofluorophosphate.

It would appear that although efforts to develop dentifrices with therapeutic claims (prevention or reduction of the formation of dental plaque, caries, calculus, gingivitis, and so on) will continue, the manufacturers will also be very interested in the development of cosmetic dentifrices that in addition to appealing to the consumer make no therapeutic claims, so that they do not require extensive clinical testing prior to marketing.

Part Two   MOUTH RINSES

DEFINITION OF A MOUTH RINSE

A mouth rinse may be defined simply as a substance that is swished around the oral cavity and then expectorated in order to freshen the mouth and breath. Thus, its purpose is primarily cosmetic. The most popular form is a liquid, although mouth rinse troches, lozenges, concentrates, and sprays are also available. In the case of the liquid mouth rinses, the material may be introduced into the oral cavity in either a full-strength or a diluted form.

By these criteria, water and saline solution could be considered to be the simplest mouth rinses. However, the most widely purchased and utilized mouth rinses in the United States are flavored formulations that contain a variety of specialized ingredients

and characteristic flavors, such as cinnamon, clove, peppermint, and wintergreen. Mouth rinses are also often referred to by other names, such as mouthwashes, oral antiseptics, and gargles.

COMPOSITION OF MOUTH RINSES

The basic ingredients in a liquid mouth rinse formulation are water, alcohol, flavoring oils, and coloring materials. Other components may include humectants, astringents, emulsifiers, antimicrobial agents, sweeteners, and therapeutic substances. These ingredients are described in detail in three excellent publications.[44, 238, 239]

Although water makes up the greatest part of any mouth rinse formulation, ethyl alcohol is also present in fairly high concentrations (approximately 15 to 30 per cent). Alcohol is primarily present to enhance the solubility of flavoring oils and other compounds of low solubility in water.

The humectants utilized include glycerin and sorbitol, and the astringents, when present, are usually either zinc or aluminum salts. Emulsifiers, such as polyoxyethylene sorbitan fatty acid esters and block copolymers consisting of polyoxyethylene and polyoxypropylene, are used to reduce surface tension and assist in the stabilization of other ingredients. Saccharin is a widely used sweetening agent. Common anesthetics (used mainly in the troches or lozenges) are benzocaine and benzyl alcohol.

An important ingredient in the mouth rinse formulation is the antimicrobial agent. This is due to the fact that one of the means by which mouth rinses can exert their "deodorizing" effect is by inhibiting bacterial activity in the oral cavity. Although such materials as certain flavoring oils and alcohol can exert some antimicrobial effect, their action is minor compared to that of the specific antimicrobial ingredients.

The most commonly used antimicrobial agents are the quaternary ammonium compounds such as cetylpyridinium chloride, benzethonium chloride, and domiphen bromide and the phenolic compounds such as phenol, thymol, betanaphthol, and hexylresorcinol. Miscellaneous antimicrobial agents include povidone-iodine, hexetidine, and certain organic mercurial compounds.

At one time, hexachlorophene was a widely used antimicrobial agent in many cosmetic products, including mouth rinses. However, federal regulations now prohibit its use in any such formulations, except possibly in trace amounts as a preservative.

Oxygen liberating agents such as sodium perborate and urea peroxide have also been used to some extent, even though they have limited capabilities as antimicrobial agents.

Some newer and very promising antimicrobial mouth rinse ingredients are currently being subjected to clinical investigation and are discussed in detail in the Therapeutic Mouth Rinse section of this chapter.

FUNCTIONS OF A MOUTH RINSE

Cosmetic Function

As previously mentioned, the primary objective in using a mouth rinse is a cosmetic one whereby the mouth and breath are freshened. In this respect, mouth rinses could be considered to serve a social function.

Substantiation of the effect of mouth rinses on the incidence of objectionable breath odor (and other oral parameters) has generally been obtained through the use of four types of investigations, which may be described as follows:

1. *In vitro* microbiological evaluations, whereby the antimicrobial spectrum of the mouth rinse has been determined. These laboratory tests are described in three excellent publications.[97, 238, 304]

2. *In vivo* clinical microbiological sampling procedures (such as the "buccal scrapings" obtained from the inside of the cheeks), which indicate the reduction in microorganisms that occurs as a result of using the mouth rinse for specific periods of time.[4, 180, 181, 235, 292]

3. *In vivo* clinical investigations, which have determined the beneficial effect of certain mouth rinses on such specific parameters as high-speed drill bacterial aerosol contamination[160, 196, 197] and oral debris clearance.[179] Also, the use of mouth rinses (containing such materials as iodine, hexetidine, and phenol) in the area of presurgical and post-surgical care has been investigated and found to be of some value.[15, 17, 29, 136, 227, 243, 258]

4. *In vivo* clinical investigations that measure the direct effect of mouth rinses on objectionable breath odor, either through the use of organoleptic procedures (direct nose-mouth evaluation) employing the Fair-Wells osmoscope[200] or through the use of recently developed microcoulometric-chromatographic instrumental procedures.[263, 280]

Some mouth rinses, in addition to performing a cosmetic function, also claim to provide relief for sore throats and to reduce the occurrence of the common cold. These claims have been, for the most part, substantiated by *in vitro* microbiological data, although in some instances human clinical studies have been conducted. However, claims of this nature are considered to be therapeutic, and regulatory agencies have indicated their concern in reference to the adequacy of the substantiating data.

Indeed, the FDA, based on a review of mouth rinse data that was conducted by the National Academy of Sciences — National Research Council, has questioned the effectiveness of mouth rinses in regard to preventive or therapeutic claims (Federal Register, 1970A).

The Council on Dental Therapeutics of the American Dental Association refers to mouth rinses as liquids with pleasant taste and odor, used to rinse the mouth. The Council further states:

"Unfortunately, mouth rinses are often advertised to the public with claims or implications of value in preventing or treating diseases of the mouth and upper respiratory tract. The Council on Dental Therapeutics does not presently recognize any substantial contribution to oral health in the unsupervised use of medicated mouthwashes by the general public. The need for a truly therapeutic mouthwash and the degree of its usefulness must be ascertained by a dentist or physician."*

The Council on Dental Therapeutics of the American Dental Association has classified as unacceptable medicated mouth rinses that are marketed for unsupervised use by the public (Accepted Dental Therapeutics, 1975/1976).

Therapeutic Function

As was the case with dentifrices, a therapeutic mouth rinse can be defined as a formulation containing a drug substance and used to transfer this drug substance to the hard and soft tissues of the oral cavity. This drug substance then imparts a chemical, physiologic, or pharmacologic action that is manifested clinically as a reduction in the incidence of plaque, caries, calculus, and gingival disease.

As previously mentioned, claims in reference to the relief of sore throats and the prevention of the common cold would also be considered therapeutic, but primarily from a medical aspect, rather than a dental aspect.

Many therapeutic mouth rinse formulations (containing drug substances) have been evaluated with regard to their effect on plaque, calculus, caries, or gingival disease. These clinical investigations are summarized in the paragraphs that follow.

Fluoride-Containing Mouth Rinses.* In the early 1940's it was shown that fluoride treatment could make the teeth more resistant to caries formation.[294, 296] A clinical study conducted with a 0.1 per cent acidulated sodium fluoride mouth rinse did not produce a caries reduction in a group of 31 dental students.[25] The authors indicated that the small number of subjects and their age were the probable causes of failure to obtain a significant caries reduction.

However, three subsequent studies did result in significant caries reductions with a neutral 0.2 per cent sodium fluoride mouth rinse.[65, 285, 307]

Since that time, many clinical studies have been conducted with fluoride mouth rinses. For the most part, sodium fluoride has been the most widely utilized and investigated substance. A summary of some of these clinical studies is presented in Table 10–10. The data indicate that mouth rinses containing sodium fluoride (at various concentrations and frequencies of use) are safe and effective with regard to reducing the incidence of caries.

This conclusion was also substantiated at an International Workshop on Fluorides and Dental Caries Reductions (1974), where the recommendations indicated that sodium fluoride rinses, in either neutral or acidulated form, were safe and efficacious. Furthermore, the committee stated that sodium fluoride rinses should be used by individuals of age six and above who reside in either water-fluoridated or nonfluoridated areas. The

---

*Accepted Dental Therapeutics, 1975/1976.

*The subject of fluoride-containing mouth rinses is reviewed in several excellent publications (McCormick, 1968; Horowitz, 1973; and Torell and Ericsson, 1974).

TABLE 10–10   CLINICAL INVESTIGATIONS CONDUCTED WITH MOUTH RINSES CONTAINING FLUORIDES

INVESTIGATOR(S)	MATERIAL UTILIZED°	CONCLUSIONS
McCormick and Koulourides, 1965	NaF (3–40 ppm F⁻) plus calcium and phosphate	Daily rinsing for one year produced significantly less interproximal caries in Grade 1 and 2 children
Torell and Ericsson, 1965A	NaF (226 ppm F⁻)	Daily rinsing for two years produced a 50% DMFS caries reduction in 10-year-old children
	NaF (904 ppm F⁻)	Rinsing every two weeks for two years produced a 21% DMFS caries reduction in 10-year-old children
Kasakura, 1966	NaF (452 ppm F⁻)	Daily rinsing for two years produced a 60% DMFT caries reduction in Grade 4 children
Koch, 1967	NaF (2260 ppm F⁻)	Rinsing every two weeks for three years produced a 23% DMFS caries reduction in 10-year-old children
Torell, 1969	NaF (904 ppm F⁻) plus CaCO₃/0.8% sodium monofluorophosphate dentifrice used daily at home	Rinsing every two weeks for 2½ years in conjunction with daily use of the fluoride dentifrice produced significantly less caries than use of the fluoride rinse alone
Gerdin and Torell, 1969	0.2% KF + Mn Cl₂ 0.2% NaF + Mn Cl₂ 0.2% NaF	Weekly rinsing for four years indicated that the KF + Mn Cl₂ rinse produced significantly less caries than the other two rinses in 9- to 13-year-old children
Swerdloff and Shannon, 1967	0.1% SnF₂ (250 ppm F⁻)	Daily rinsing for five months established the feasibility of using this rinse and produced a non-significant DMFT caries reduction in school children
Horowitz, Creighton, and McClendon, 1971	NaF (904 ppm F⁻)	Weekly rinsing for 20 months produced a 44% DMFS caries reduction in Grade 5 children and a 16% reduction in Grade 1 children
Frankl, Fleisch, and Diodati, 1972	NaF (200 ppm F⁻) pH 4.0	Daily rinsing for two years produced a 25% DMFS caries reduction in 14-year-old children
Aasenden, DePaola, and Brudevold, 1972	NaF (200 ppm F⁻) NaF (200 ppm F⁻) pH 4.0	Daily rinsing for three years produced a 27% DMFS caries reduction (neutral rinse) and a 30% reduction (acidulated rinse) in 8- to 10-year-old children
Brandt, Slack, and Waller, 1972	NaF (904 ppm F⁻)	Twice weekly rinsing for two years produced a 36% DMFS caries reduction in 11-year-old children
Moreira and Tumang, 1972	NaF (452 ppm F⁻)	Weekly rinsing for two years produced a 35% DMFS caries reduction and three times weekly rinsing produced a 36% reduction in 7-year-old children
Radike, Gish, Peterson, King, and Segreto, 1973	0.1% SnF₂ (250 ppm F⁻) Fluoridated Water	Daily rinsing for two years produced a 33-43% DMFS caries reduction in 8- to 13-year-old children
Rugg-Gunn, Holloway, and Davies, 1973	NaF (226 ppm F⁻)	Daily rinsing for three years produced a 35% DMFS caries reduction in 11- to 12-year-old children
Gallagher, Glassgow, and Caldwell, 1973	NaF (1808 ppm F⁻)	Weekly rinsing for two years produced a 27% DMFT caries reduction in 11- to 13-year-old children
Heifetz, Driscoll, and Creighton, 1973	NaF (0.3% F⁻) NaF (0.3% F⁻) pH 4.0	Weekly rinsing for two years produced a 38% DMFS caries reduction (neutral rinse) and a 27% reduction (acidulated rinse) in Grade 7 and 9 children
Forsman, 1974	NaF (113 ppm F⁻) NaF (904 ppm F⁻)	Weekly rinsing for two years produced significant caries reductions for both rinse groups, with the lower level of fluoride providing a somewhat better effect

°All rinses are essentially neutral, unless otherwise indicated.

committee indicated that the recommendation of mouth rinses containing other fluoride compounds, such as stannous fluoride, potassium fluoride, ferric fluoride, and potassium and sodium fluoride with manganese would not be in order until further clinical data becomes available, even though, in some cases, the data already available is encouraging.

A government notice also attests to the safety and effectiveness of sodium fluoride mouth rinses (Federal Register, 1974). The notice indicates that:

1. Aqueous solutions of 0.2 per cent sodium fluoride with a pH of approximately 7.0 are safe and effective in reducing the incidence of dental caries when applied to the teeth as a rinse once a week or once every two weeks.

2. Aqueous solutions of 0.05 per cent sodium fluoride with a pH of approximately 7.0 are safe and effective in reducing the incidence of dental caries when applied to the teeth once daily as a rinse.

3. Aqueous solutions of acidulated phosphate sodium fluoride with a pH of approximately 4.0 that yield a fluoride ion concentration of approximately 0.02 per cent are safe and effective in reducing the incidence of dental caries when applied to the teeth once daily as a rinse.

Also, the Council on Dental Therapeutics of the American Dental Association has classified as "Accepted" both neutral sodium fluoride and phosphate acidulated fluoride solutions as effective agents for use in reducing the incidence of dental decay. The Council announcement also lists the specific sodium fluoride mouth rinse products that are classified as "Accepted" (Report of Councils and Bureaus, American Dental Association, 1975).

Antimicrobial-Containing Mouth Rinses. As previously mentioned, quaternary ammonium compounds are common mouth rinse ingredients and have been included primarily because of their antimicrobial properties. Several clinical studies have been conducted that indicate that substances such as benzethonium chloride, cetylpyridinium chloride, and the combination of cetylpyridinium chloride and domiphen bromide have a moderate effect (about 30 to 40 per cent reduction) on the formation of dental plaque.[10, 18, 22, 268, 299]

Other compounds with antimicrobial properties that have shown a moderate degree of effectiveness in mouth rinses with regard to plaque, calculus, and gingivitis include thymol and eucalyptol,[92] hexetidine,[23] alexidine,[163] various peroxides,[242, 257] zinc phenolsulfonate and zinc tribromsalan,[63] sodium hypochlorite,[166] and amine fluoride.[164]

Antibiotic compounds that have also shown effectiveness in clinical investigations include vancomycin,[195] erythromycin,[165] and kanamycin.[171]

In recent years, two antimicrobial substances have been subjected to clinical evaluation and have been shown to have a marked effect on the incidence of plaque, calculus, and gingival disease.

The first substance is chlorhexidine, which is effective against gram-positive and gram-negative microorganisms as well as yeasts. Initial clinical investigations indicated that a mouth rinse containing 0.1 per cent chlorhexidine (numerically coded as Z7y) was an effective calculus-preventive material.[231, 249] This material has been subjected to many clinical investigations, and it has been shown that a mouth rinse containing 0.2 per cent chlorhexidine is very effective against plaque and calculus formation as well as gingival disease.[46, 67, 88, 89, 90, 167, 168, 170, 237]

Chlorhexidine continues to be the subject of extensive laboratory and clinical investigations and still appears to be a very promising agent. One problem that has emerged concerns the formation of a brown-black extrinsic tooth stain that occurs with the continuous use of chlorhexidine dentifrices or mouth rinses.[66] Although this stain is readily removed by an oral prophylaxis, attempts are being made to prevent its formation.

The second antimicrobial substance is a macrolide antibiotic, numerically designated as CC 10232.* It is the natural product ob-

---

*This antibiotic was provided by Abbott Laboratories, North Chicago, Illinois and is the subject of U.S. Patent No. 3,342,687 (Colgate-Palmolive Co.).

tained from the fermentation of a novel strain of *Streptomyces caelestis*, NRRL-2821. CC 10232 shows strong activity against a variety of gram-positive microorganisms, including staphylococci, streptococci, enterococci, corynebacteria, and bacilli. Gram-negative bacteria, yeasts, and molds are not readily inhibited.

A series of clinical investigations have been conducted with a mouth rinse containing 0.01 per cent CC 10232. This mouth rinse has been shown to be effective against plaque and calculus formation (supragingival as well as subgingival) and gingival disease. A summary of some of these studies is presented in Table 10–11. Although these results are extremely encouraging, it should be emphasized that this substance is an antibiotic and thus must be subjected to further evaluation to determine whether its utilization causes the development of resistant microorganisms or allergic hypersensitivity reactions.

Miscellaneous Therapeutic Mouth Rinses. A variety of other substances (in mouth rinses) have been clinically evaluated for their effect on plaque, calculus, or gingivitis formation. These substances include sodium ricinoleate, urea, polyvinylpyrrolidone, lysozyme, Victamine C,* Ascoxal,†

---

*A surface-active organophosphorous compound.
†A mixture of ascorbic acid, sodium percarbonate, and copper sulfate.

and others. These materials all show some degree of effectiveness and are discussed in detail in several excellent publications.[21, 87, 190, 201, 218, 248 297, 305]

Several clinical studies have been conducted with a tablet mouth rinse containing a proteolytic enzyme obtained from a mutant strain of *Bacillus subtilis*.[245, 254] This enzyme-containing preparation was very effective in reducing plaque formation and is being subjected to further investigation. Conversely, mouth rinses containing the enzyme dextranase have not demonstrated a similar degree of efficacy.[39, 140, 161]

Another interesting compound is ethane-1-hydroxy-1,1 diphosphonate-hexahydrate, which has been shown to reduce calculus formation when evaluated in a mouth rinse[202] and a dentifrice.[269, 271]

FUTURE TRENDS IN MOUTH RINSES

Although a reduction in objectionable breath odor will probably always remain an important consideration in the formulation of mouth rinses, it is obvious that the future trend is toward the development of therapeutic mouth rinses. The function of these therapeutic mouth rinses will be to have a beneficial effect upon the oral hard and soft tissues, including the formation of dental plaque, calculus, caries, and gingival disease.

TABLE 10–11   CLINICAL INVESTIGATIONS CONDUCTED WITH A MOUTH RINSE CONTAINING 0.01 PER CENT OF A MACROLIDE ANTIBIOTIC (CC 10232)

INVESTIGATOR(S)	PARAMETER EVALUATED	RESULTS
Volpe, Kupczak, Brant, King, Kestenbaum, and Schlissel, 1969	Supragingival plaque and calculus	Approximately 70–77% reduction in plaque Approximately 75% reduction in calculus
Stallard, Volpe, Orban, and King, 1969	Supragingival plaque, calculus, and gingivitis	11–23% reduction in plaque 70–91% reduction in calculus 55–72% reduction in gingivitis
Volpe, Schulman, Goldman, King, and Kupczak, 1970	Supragingival calculus	38% reduction at 3 months 50% reduction at 6 months 33% reduction at 9 months
Kovaleski and Ash, 1970	Supragingival plaque, calculus, and gingivitis	Beneficial effect on plaque up to 60 days
Rokita, Hazen, Millen, and Volpe, 1975	Subgingival plaque and calculus	Less deposit, less mineralization and fewer spirochetes

FLUORIDE DENTIFRICES AND MOUTH RINSES IN A FLUORIDATED WATER AREA

Fluoride-containing dentifrices and mouth rinses are not intended to be used as substitutes for water fluoridation. First, they produce a topical effect on erupted teeth, while water fluoridation acts systemically during the pre-eruptive stage of tooth development. Second, clinical studies indicate that the cariostatic effect obtained from either fluoride dentifrices or mouth rinses is approximately one half that provided by water fluoridation.

Several clinical studies have indicated, however, that the use of either fluoride-containing dentifrices or mouth rinses in a community with optimal water fluoridation can provide some degree of *additive* cariostatic benefit over and above that which is provided by the water fluoridation itself.

Since there are no known contraindications to the use of fluoride-containing dentifrices and mouth rinses in a fluoridated water community, their use should be recommended and encouraged.

ADULT USE OF FLUORIDE DENTIFRICES AND MOUTH RINSES

Although the majority of the caries clinical studies conducted with fluoride-containing dentifrices and mouth rinses have utilized children and teen-age populations because of the greater incidence of the disease in these groups, there is no evidence to indicate that these products would not also be beneficial to an adult population.

On the contrary, there are two factors that would indicate that fluoride-containing dentifrices and mouth rinses should be recommended for use by adults. First, fluoride-containing products have been shown in many clinical studies to have a beneficial effect on tooth hypersensitivity, which is a condition most prevalent in adults. Second, there is evidence[103] that adults, although not very prone to conventional pit and fissure caries, are very susceptible to a special phenomenon called "root surface" caries.

Part Three: 1982 CLINICAL FLUORIDE UPDATE

Stannous Fluoride Dentifrices

A summary of recent clinical studies (supplemental to Table 10–7) that evaluated dentifrices containing 0.4 per cent stannous fluoride is presented in Table 10–12.

Two studies[2, 68] showed that a 0.4 per cent stannous fluoride dentifrice with silica as the cleaning and polishing agent was comparable in caries reducing efficacy to a 0.4 per cent stannous fluoride dentifrice with calcium pyrophosphate as the cleaning and polishing agent. A 0.4 per cent stannous fluoride–calcium pyrophosphate dentifrice was also shown to be additive in caries reducing efficacy to an acidulated-phosphate–fluoride (APF) topical gel application[19] and effective in an adult population.[172]

Sodium Fluoride Dentifrices

A summary of recent clinical studies (supplemental to Table 10–6) that evaluated dentifrices containing 0.22 per cent sodium fluoride is presented in Table 10–13.

One study showed that there was no difference in caries reducing efficacy between an alkaline and a neutral 0.22 per cent sodium fluoride dentifrice with calcium pyrophosphate as the cleaning and polishing agent.[53]

Two studies showed that a 0.243 per cent sodium fluoride dentifrice with silica as the cleaning and polishing agent was superior in caries reducing efficacy to a 0.4 per cent stannous fluoride dentifrice with calcium pyrophosphate as the cleaning and polishing agent.[20, 318] This would be in harmony with

TABLE 10-12 CLINICAL ANTICARIES STUDIES CONDUCTED UTILIZING 0.4 PER CENT STANNOUS FLUORIDE CONTAINING DENTIFRICES

INVESTIGATOR(S)	CLEANING AND POLISHING AGENT	DURATION OF STUDY	AGE RANGE	PER CENT REDUCTION IN CARIES
Fogels, Alman, Meade, and O'Donnell, 1979	Silica	36 Months	5–13	Significant reductions vs. negative control ranged from 15–25%. Also was comparable to a SnF_2/calcium pyrophosphate positive control
Abrams and Chambers, 1980	Silica	36 Months	5–12	Significant reductions vs. negative control ranged from 10–19%. Also was comparable to a SnF_2/calcium pyrophosphate positive control
Beiswanger, Billings, Sturzenberger, and Bollmer, 1978	Calcium Pyrophosphate (+ APF Topical Treatment)	24 Months	7–14	19% significant reduction for SnF_2 dentifrice and APF topical vs. the APF topical alone
Lu, Hanna, and Peterson, 1980	Calcium Pyrophosphate (adult population)	12 Months	18–78	33% significant reduction vs. control

TABLE 10-13 CLINICAL ANTICARIES STUDIES CONDUCTED UTILIZING SODIUM FLUORIDE-CONTAINING DENTIFRICES

INVESTIGATOR(S)	CLEANING AND POLISHING AGENT	DURATION OF STUDY	AGE RANGE	PER CENT REDUCTION IN CARIES
Ennever, Peterson, Hester, Segreto, and Radike, 1980	Calcium Pyrophosphate (0.22% NaF Neutral and 0.22% NaF Alkaline)	28 Months	Grades 2–6	Both NaF dentifrices significantly better than control (32–39%) but not different from each other.
Zacherl, 1981	0.243% NaF/Silica 0.4% SnF_2/Calcium Pyrophosphate	36 Months	6–13	NaF dentifrice significantly better than both negative control (40%) and SnF_2/calcium pyrophosphate dentifrice (22–24%). SnF_2/calcium pyrophosphate dentifrice significantly better than control (21–23%).
Beiswanger, Gish, and Mallatt, 1981	0.243% NaF/Silica 0.4% SnF_2/Calcium Pyrophosphate	36 Months	6–14	NaF dentifrice significantly better 11–13%, 15–16%) than the SnF_2/calcium pyrophosphate dentifrice. Negative control not used.
Koch, Peterson, Kling, and Kling, 1981	0.055% NaF (0.025% F) 0.22% NaF (0.1% F) 0.76% MFP° (0.1% F) (NaF dentifrices had insoluble sodium metaphosphate cleaning/polishing agent; MFP dentifrice had dicalcium phosphate dihydrate cleaning/polishing agent	36 Months	12–13	All three dentifrices (low NaF, 0.22% NaF and 0.76% MFP) equivalent over three years for caries increments

°MFP is the registered trademark of the Colgate-Palmolive Co. for sodium monofluorophosphate.

previous clinical data from three clinical studies (Table 10–9) wherein a 0.76 per cent sodium monofluorophosphate dentifrice was also shown to be superior to this same 0.4 per cent stannous fluoride–calcium pyrophosphate dentifrice.[62, 75, 192]

Another study has shown that there is no difference in caries reducing efficacy among a 0.055 per cent sodium fluoride dentifrice, a 0.22 per cent sodium fluoride dentifrice, and a 0.76 per cent sodium monofluorophosphate dentifrice.[151]

Sodium Monofluorophosphate Dentifrices

A summary of recent clinical studies (supplemental to Table 10–9) that evaluated dentifrices containing between 0.76 to 2.0 per cent sodium monofluorophosphate is presented in Table 10–14.

Dentifrices containing 0.76 per cent sodium monofluorophosphate with calcium carbonate have been shown to be efficacious in reducing caries both in a non-fluoridated area[91] and a fluoridated area.[222] Also, this dentifrice was not shown to be additive to an APF topical gel application.[175]

Results from studies evaluating dentifrices containing a combination of 0.76 per cent sodium monofluorophosphate and 0.13 per cent calcium glycerophosphate are conflicting. In one study,[214] there was no significant additive effect for the combination, and in another study[176, 177] there was a significant additive effect for the combination.

A study has shown that a dentifrice containing a mixture of 0.76 per cent sodium monofluorophosphate and 0.1 per cent sodium fluoride (total of 1450 ppm fluoride) is superior to a dentifrice containing 0.76 per cent sodium monofluorophosphate.[120] Another study has shown that a dentifrice containing 1.2 per cent sodium monofluorophosphate is superior to a dentifrice containing 0.76 per cent sodium monofluorophosphate.[16]

A low abrasive (RDA 60) dentifrice containing 0.8 per cent sodium monofluorophosphate was shown to be comparable in caries reduction to a regular abrasive (RDA 110) dentifrice containing 0.8 per cent sodium monofluorophosphate.[212]

A dentifrice containing 0.76 per cent sodium monofluorophosphate with a silica cleaning and polishing agent was shown to be superior to a non-fluoride dentifrice[126] and comparable to a dentifrice containing 0.76 per cent sodium monofluorophosphate with an insoluble sodium metaphosphate cleaning and polishing agent.[287]

Dentifrice Cleaning and Polishing Agents

The American Dental Association, under the direction of Dr. John Hefferren, has initiated a Laboratory and Clinical Dentifrice Abrasivity Committee. This ADA Committee has convened scientists from both industry and academia throughout the world and attempted to develop standards for the assessment of dentifrice abrasivity and tooth cleaning function. Two excellent reports have been completed thus far. The first report provides a recommendation for laboratory procedures to determine dentifrice abrasivity. This procedure was developed in major collaborative studies with six participating laboratories.[105] The other report describes the results obtained from a major collaborative clinical program conducted to compare three tooth stain grading procedures among subjects who brushed their teeth with three specially formulated calcium phosphate dentifrices differing in dentin abrasivity.[106] The data from this study indicate a linear correlation between dentin abrasivity as measured by laboratory procedures and observed clinical cleaning. A similar relationship has recently been reported by other investigators.[244]

Sodium Fluoride Mouth Rinses

A summary of recent clinical studies (supplemental to Table 10–10) evaluating mouth rinses containing sodium fluoride is presented in Table 10–15. The results from these studies show conclusively that a 0.05 per cent sodium fluoride mouth rinse used daily provides caries reduction benefits that

TABLE 10-14 CLINICAL ANTICARIES STUDIES CONDUCTED UTILIZING SODIUM MONOFLUOROPHOSPHATE CONTAINING DENTIFRICES

INVESTIGATOR(S)	CLEANING AND POLISHING AGENT	DURATION OF STUDY	AGE RANGE	PER CENT REDUCTION IN CARIES
Glass and Shiere, 1978	Calcium Carbonate (0.76% MFP°)	24 Months	6–13	MFP dentifrice produced a 23% significant reduction in caries vs. control
Peterson, 1979	Calcium Carbonate (0.76% MFP) (Fluoridated area)	31 Months	8–12	MFP dentifrice produced a 23.1% significant reduction in caries vs. control
Mainwaring and Naylor, 1978	Calcium Carbonate (0.76% MFP) (+ an APF Topical Gel)	36 Months	11–12	MFP dentifrice alone and APF Gel alone significantly reduced caries formation. Combination was not superior to individual treatments
Edlund and Koch, 1977	Dicalcium Phosphate (0.76% MFP) Silicon Dioxide (0.22% NaF)	36 Months	9–11	Both NaF and MFP dentifrices equivalent over three years for new carious teeth. NaF better than MFP in third year in new carious surfaces. (Children showed unexpectedly low caries rate in this study.)
Howat, Holloway, and Davies, 1978	Silica (0.76% MFP)	36 Months	14–15	MFP dentifrice produced a 26–36% significant reduction in caries vs. control
James, Anderson, Beal, and Bradnock, 1977	Aluminum Oxide (2% MFP)	36 Months	11–12	2% MFP dentifrice produced a 24–39% significant reduction in caries vs. control
Naylor and Glass, 1979	Calcium Carbonate (0.76% MFP) (and 0.13% Calcium Glycero-phosphate-CGP)	36 Months	11–12	Both MFP (22%) and MFP + CGP (25%) dentifrices significantly better than control. No difference between dentifrices

Author	Product	Duration	Age/Grade	Results
Mainwaring and Naylor, 1980(A) and 1980(B)	Calcium Carbonate (0.76% MFP) (and 0.13% Calcium Glycerophosphate-CGP)	36 Months	11–12	Three-year results show significant reductions vs. control for both MFP (16%) and MFP + CGP (24%) dentifrices. No significant difference between dentifrices Four-year results show significant reductions vs. control for both MFP (15.5%) and MFP + CGP (25.7%) dentifrice. MFP + CGP significantly better than MFP dentifrice
Barlage, Buhe, and Büttner, 1980	Insoluble Sodium Metaphosphate (0.8% MFP and 1.2% MFP)	36 Months	12	Both 0.8% MFP (19%) and 1.2% MFP (26%) produced significant reductions vs. control. 1.2% MFP dentifrice significantly better than 0.8% MFP dentifrice
Hodge, Holloway, Davies, and Worthington, 1980	Dicalcium Phosphate Dihydrate (0.76% MFP + 0.1% NaF) Aluminum Oxide (0.76% MFP + 0.1% NaF) Aluminum Oxide (0.76% MFP)	36 Months	14–15	DMT data show both mixed fluoride dentifrices significantly better than negative control (26% and 27%) and positive control (12.2% and 14.2%). Positive control significantly better than negative control (13.8%) DFS data show both mixed fluoride dentifrices significantly better than negative control (22.4% and 24.1%) and positive control (15.8% and 18.1%). Positive control not significantly better than negative control (6.6%)
Murray and Shaw, 1980	Low Abrasive Dentifrice (RDA 60) (0.8% MFP) Regular Abrasive Dentifrice (RDA 110) (0.8% MFP)			Low abrasive MFP dentifrice produced significant 34% reduction. Regular abrasive MFP dentifrice produced significant 27% reduction. No difference between the MFP dentifrices
Triol, Wilson, and Volpe, 1981	Insoluble Sodium Metaphosphate (0.76% MFP) Silica (0.76% MFP)	31 Months	Grades 4,5,6	Both MFP dentifrices equivalent in caries reducing activity. Negative control not used

*MFP is the registered trademark of the Colgate-Palmolive Co. for sodium monofluorophosphate.

TABLE 10–15   CLINICAL ANTICARIES STUDIES CONDUCTED UTILIZING SODIUM FLUORIDE MOUTH RINSES

INVESTIGATORS	MATERIALS UTILIZED	CONCLUSIONS
Triol, Kranz, Volpe, Frankl, Alman, and Allard, 1980	0.025, 0.05, or 0.1% NaF rinse + use of 0.76% MFP° dentifrice in non-fluoridated area (30-month study)	Use of all NaF rinses produced a significant additive effect to MFP dentifrice, especially in interproximal areas *F Concentration* *Caries Reductions* 0.025% 26.4% 0.05% 35.6% 0.1% 37.4%
Wilson, Triol, and Volpe, 1978	0.1% NaF rinse + use of 0.76% MFP dentifrice in fluoridated area (30-month study)	Combined use of NaF rinse and MFP dentifrice produced 35% significant reduction in caries in addition to that produced by use of fluoridated water and a fluoride dentifrice
Ashley, Mainwaring, Emslie, and Naylor, 1977	0.02% acidulated NaF rinse + use of 0.76% MFP dentifrice in non-fluoridated area (24-month study)	0.02% acidulated rinse alone produced significant 17.5% caries reduction. MFP dentifrice alone produced significant 20.8% caries reduction. Combined use of rinse + dentifrice produced significant 25.7% caries reduction
Driscoll, Swango, Horowitz, and Kingman, 1981	0.05% (daily) and 0.2% (weekly) NaF rinses in fluoridated area. Subjects used their regular fluoride-containing dentifrices (30-month study)	Results after 18 months show that NaF rinses produce a significant additive effect to fluoridated water. 39.8% greater reduction in caries for 0.05% NaF daily rinse and 30.7% greater reduction for 0.2% NaF weekly rinse
Heifetz, Meyers, and Kingman, 1981	0.05% (daily) and 0.2% (weekly) NaF rinses in non-fluoridated area. Subjects used their regular fluoride-containing dentifrices (36-month study)	Both rinses produced significant caries reductions. Daily (0.05% NaF) rinse produced 47.4% caries reduction and weekly (0.2% NaF) rinse produced 37.7% caries reduction
Ringelberg, Conti, Ward, Clark, and Lotzbar, 1981	0.05% NaF rinse daily 0.05% NaF rinse weekly 0.2% NaF rinse daily 0.2% NaF rinse weekly	*Caries Reduction After 24 Months* *All Surfaces* *Interproximal* 28.2% 48.7% 16.6% 34.6% 22.8% 14.1% 20.3% 41.0%

°MFP is the registered trademark of the Colgate-Palmolive Co. for sodium monofluorophosphate.

TABLE 10–16   FLUORIDE DENTIFRICES AND FLUORIDE MOUTH RINSES APPROVED BY THE COUNCIL ON DENTAL THERAPEUTICS OF THE AMERICAN DENTAL ASSOCIATION

DENTIFRICES

COLGATE MFP (Colgate-Palmolive)	0.76%	sodium monofluorophosphate
AIM (Lever Bros.)	0.76%	sodium monofluorophosphate
MACLEANS (Beecham)	0.76%	sodium monofluorophosphate
CREST (Procter & Gamble)	0.243%	sodium fluoride
AQUAFRESH (Beecham)	0.76%	sodium monofluorophosphate

MOUTH RINSES

FLUORIGARD (Colgate-Palmolive)	0.05%	sodium fluoride (daily use)
STAN CARE (Block Drug)	0.1%	stannous fluoride (daily use)

are additive to the effect of fluoride dentifrices[109, 286] and to the effect of both fluoride dentifrices and fluoridated water.[48] These studies also confirm the efficacy of weekly use of a 0.2 per cent sodium fluoride mouth rinse by school children.

Dentifrices and Mouth Rinses Approved by the American Dental Association (Council on Dental Therapeutics)

The Council on Dental Therapeutics of the American Dental Association has classified as *accepted* and authorized the appropriate use of its *Seal of Acceptance* for the fluoride dentifrice and fluoride mouth rinse products listed in Table 10–16. These (as well as other) accepted products are described more fully in the current issue of Accepted Dental Therapeutics. This is published every two years and is the official publication of the Council on Dental Therapeutics of the American Dental Association.

Anticaries Drug Products Approved by the Food and Drug Administration

The FDA recently published a Monograph on Anticaries Drug Products for Over-The-Counter (OTC) Human Use (Federal Register, March 28, 1980). This proposed rulemaking document was based on a report of its Advisory Review Panel on OTC Dentifrice and Dental Care Products. In this Monograph, the FDA states the following concerning anticaries active ingredients:

The following ingredients are generally recognized as safe and effective for use in OTC anticaries drug products when marketed within the dosage limits forms established for each ingredient:

Dentifrices

Sodium fluoride, 0.22 per cent.
Sodium monofluorophosphate, 0.76 per cent.
Stannous fluoride, 0.4 per cent.

Dental Rinses

Sodium fluoride, 0.05 per cent aqueous solution.
Stannous fluoride, marketed in a stable form and containing adequate directions for mixing with water immediately before use to result in a 0.1 per cent solution.

REFERENCES

1. Aasenden, R., DePaola, P. F., and Brudevold, F.: Effects of daily rinsing and ingestion of fluoride solutions upon dental caries and enamel fluoride. Arch. Oral Biol. 17:1705–1714, 1972.
2. Abrams, R. G., and Chambers, D. W.: Caries-inhibiting effect of a stannous fluoride silica gel dentifrice. Clin. Prev. Dent. 2:22–26, 1980.
3. Accepted Dental Therapeutics, 34th Ed., 1971/1972; 36th Ed., 1975/1976; published by the American Dental Association, 211 East Chicago Avenue, Chicago, Illinois, 60611.
4. Alderman, E. J.: An *in vivo* study of the effect of prolonged use of a specific mouthwash on the oral flora. Chron. Omaha Dist. Dent. Soc. Vol. 28, pp. 284–289, 1965.
5. Allison, J. B., and Nelson, M. F.: The distribution of C^{14} from sodium n-lauroyl sarcosinate in the rat (unpublished data), Bureau of Biological Research, Rutgers University, and Colgate-Palmolive Company Radioisotope Laboratory, 1958.
6. American Dental Association, Clinical testing of dental caries preventives — Report of a conference to develop uniform standards and procedures in clinical studies of dental caries, published by the American Dental Association, 1955.
7. American Dental Association, Conference on clinical trials of drugs used in dentistry, published by the American Dental Association, 1960.
8. American Dental Association, Proceedings of the conference on the clinical testing of cariostatic agents, published by the American Dental Association, 1968.
9. Andlaw, R. J., and Tucker, G. J.: A three-year clinical trial of a dentifrice containing 0.8 per cent sodium monofluorophosphate in an aluminum oxide trihydrate base. Brit. Dent. J. 138:426–432, 1975.
10. Arnim, S. S.: The use of disclosing agents for measuring tooth cleanliness. J. Periodontol. 34:227–245, 1963.
11. Ashley, F. P., Mainwaring, P. J., Emslie, R. D., and Naylor, M. N.: Clinical testing of a mouthrinse and a dentifrice containing fluoride. A two-year supervised study in school children. Brit. Dent. J. 143:333–338, 1977.
12. Backer-Dirks, O., Winkler, R. C., and Van Aken, J. A.: A reproducible method for caries evaluation, III. Test in a therapeutic experiment with an ammoniated dentifrice. J. Dent. Res. 32:18–26, 1953.
13. Backer-Dirks, O., Baume, L. J., Davies, G. N., and Slack, G. L.: Principal requirements for controlled clinical trials. Int. Dent. J. 17:93–103, 1967.
14. Backer-Dirks, O., Swant, G. W., and Starmans, J. L.: Effect of a sodium lauroyl sarcosinate dentifrice: A clinical investigation. J. Dent. Belge. 50:163–175, 1959.
15. Ball, D. M., and Ball, E. L.: Comparative effectiveness of two mouthwashes used after gingivectomy. J. Periodontol. 38:395–397, 1967.
16. Barlage, B., Buhe, H., and Büttner, W.: A 3-year clinical dentifrice trial using different fluoride levels: 0.8 and 1.2 per cent sodium mon-

ofluorophosphate. ORCA (European Organization for Caries Research) (Marburg) Preprinted Abstract No. 18, 1980.

17. Batten, J. R., and Collings, C. K.: The evaluation of an anesthetic mouthrinse on four hundred periodontal surgery patients. J. Periodontol. 41:654–656, 1970.

18. Beiswanger, B. B., Sturzenberger, O. P., and Bollmer, W.: Clinical effect of an antibacterial mouthwash on dental plaque and gingivitis. International Association for Dental Research. Preprinted Abstract No. 367, p. 146, 1974.

19. Beiswanger, B. B., Billings, R. J., Sturzenberger, O. P., and Bollmer, B. W.: The additive anticariogenic effect of an SnF_2-$Ca_2P_2O_7$ dentifrice and APF topical Applications. J. Dent. Child. 45:137, 1978.

20. Beiswanger, B. B., Gish, C. W., and Mallatt, M. E.: Effect of a sodium fluoride-silica abrasive dentifrice upon caries. Pharm. Therap. Dent. 4:9–16, 1981.

21. Belting, C. M.: Design of clinical studies on dental calculus. Ann. N.Y. Acad. Sci. (Evaluation of agents used in the prevention of oral disease). 153:(Art. 1) 307–313, Dec. 23, 1968.

22. Bergenholtz, A., Hugoson, A., Lundgren, D., and Ostgren, A.: The plaque-inhibiting property of some mouthwashes and their effect on the oral mucosa, Sven. Tandlak, Tidskr. 62:7–14, 1969.

23. Bergenholtz, A., and Hänström, L.: The plaque-inhibiting effect of hexitidine (Oraldene) mouthwash compared to that of chlorhexidine. Community Dent. Oral Epidemiol. 2:70–74, 1974.

24. Bibby, B. G.: Test of the effect of fluoride-containing dentifrices on dental caries. J. Dent. Res. 24:297–303, 1945.

25. Bibby, B. G., Zander, H. A., McKelleget, M., and Labunsky, B.: Preliminary reports on the effect on dental caries of the use of sodium fluoride in a prophylactic cleaning mixture and in a mouthwash. J. Dent. Res., 25:207–211, 1946.

26. Bixler, D., and Muhler, J. C.: Experimental clinical human caries test design and interpretation. J. Am. Dent. Assoc. 65:482–490, 1962.

27. Bixler, D., and Muhler, J. C.: Effect on dental caries in children in a nonfluoride area of combined use of three agents containing stannous fluoride: A prophylactic paste, a solution, and a dentifrice, II: Results at the end of 24 and 36 months. J. Am. Dent. Assoc. 72:392–396, 1966.

28. Bixler, D. and Muhler, J. C.: Effectiveness of a stannous fluoride-containing dentifrice in reducing dental caries in children in a boarding school environment. J. Am. Dent. Assoc. 72:653–658, 1966A.

29. Blum, B.: Clinical evaluation of an anesthetic mouthwash. N.Y. Dent. J. 26:419–421, 1960.

30. Bogle, G. C.: Abrasivity of dentifrices and toothbrushes. Periodontal Abstracts 22:7–13, 1974.

31. Bolden, T. E., Volpe, A. R., and King, W. J.: The desensitizing effect of a sodium monofluorophosphate dentifrice. Periodontics, 6:112–114, 1968.

32. Bolden, T. E., Lemeh, D., Stewart, E. B., and Volpe, A. R.: A comparison of oral soft tissue cytologic findings and oral habits. Quart. Nat. Dent. Assoc. 33:4–17, 1974.

33. Bouchal, A. W.: The abrasiveness of dentifrices. Proceedings of the Scientific Section of the Toilet Goods Association. No. 45, pp. 2–5, 1966.

34. Brandt, R. S., Slack, G. L., and Waller, D. F.: The use of a sodium fluoride mouthwash in reducing the dental caries increment in eleven-year-old English school children. Proc. Brit. Paedodont. Soc. 2:23–25, 1972.

35. Brasch, S. V., Lazarou, J. A., Van Abbé, N. J., and Forrest, J. O.: The assessment of dentifrice abrasivity in vivo. Brit. Dent. J. pp. 119–124, 1969.

36. Brudevold, F., and Chilton, N. W.: Comparative study of a fluoride dentifrice containing soluble phosphate and a calcium-free abrasive: Second year report. J. Am. Dent. Assoc. 72:889–894, 1966.

37. Brudevold, F., Little, M. F., and Rowley, J.: Acid reducing effects of "antienzymes" in the mouth. J. Am. Dent. Assoc. 50:18–22, 1955.

38. Bull, W. H., Callender, R. M., Pugh, B. R., and Wood, G. D.: The abrasion and cleaning properties of dentifrices. Br. Dent. J. 124:331–337, 1968.

39. Caldwell, R. C., Sandham, H. J., Mann, W. V., Finn, S. S., and Formicola, A. J.: The effect of a dextranase mouthwash on dental plaque in young adults and children. J. Am. Dent. Assoc. 82:124–131, 1971.

40. Cobb, A. B., Hay, D. I., and Schram, C. J.: A method of measuring tooth-cleaning. Brit. Dent. J. pp. 249–253, 1961.

41. Cohen, A., and Donzanti, A.: Two-year clinical study of caries control with high-urea ammoniated dentifrice. J. Am. Dent. Assoc. 49:185–190, 1954.

42. Cordon, M.: A method for measuring the abrasion of dentin by dentifrices. J. Dent. Res. 50:491–497, 1971.

43. Costich, E. R., and Hein, J. W.: Clinical study of the effect of a tooth paste containing sodium copper chlorophyllin on oral bacteria and gingival disease. J. Dent. Res. 31:474 (Abstract), 1952.

44. Darlington, R. C.: O-T-C topical oral antiseptics and mouthwashes. J. Am. Pharm. Assoc. NS8:484–496, 1968.

45. Davies, G. N., and King, R. M.: The effectiveness of an ammonium ion tooth powder in the control of dental caries. J. Dent. Res. 30:645–655, 1951.

46. Davies, R. M., Jensen, S. B., Schiött, C. R., and Löe, H.: The effect of topical application of chlorhexidine on the bacterial colonization of the teeth and gingiva. J. Periodont. Res. 5:96–101, 1970.

47. Downer, M. C., Holloway, P. J., and Davies, T. G. H.: Clinical testing of a multiple therapeutic agent caries preventive program. International Association for Dental Research, Preprinted Abstract L303, p. L76, 1975.

48. Driscoll, W. S., Swango, P. A., Horowitz, A. M., and Kingman, A.: Caries-preventive effects of daily and weekly fluoride mouthrinsing in a fluoridated community: Findings after 18 months. International Association for Dental Research. Preprinted Abstract No. 647, p. 471, 1981.

49. Duckworth, R.: Fluoride dentifrices, a review of

clinical trials in the United Kingdom. Br. Dent. J. 124:505–509, 1968.

50. Dudding, N. J., Dahl, L. O., and Muhler, J. C.: Patient reactions to brushing teeth with water, dentifrice, or salt and soda. J. Periodontol. 31:386–392, 1960.

51. Edlund, K., and Koch, G.: Effect on caries of daily supervised toothbrushing with sodium monofluorophosphate and sodium fluoride dentifrices after 3 years. Scand. J. Dent. Res. 85:41–45, 1977.

52. Emslie, R. D.: Clinical trial of a toothpaste containing sarcosinate. J. Dent. Res. 42:1079–1086, 1963.

53. Ennever, J., Peterson, J. K., Hester, W. R., Segreto, V. A., and Radike, A. W.: Influence of alkaline pH on sodium fluoride dentifrices. J. Dent. Res. 50:658–661, 1980.

54. Evaluation of agents used in the prevention of oral disease. Ann. N.Y. Acad. Sci. (Ward Pigman, Consulting Ed.) 153:1–388, Dec. 23, 1968.

55. Facq, J. M., and Volpe, A. R.: In vivo abrasiveness of three dentifrices against acrylic surfaces of veneer crowns. J. Am. Dent. Assoc. 80:317–323, 1970.

56. Fanning, E. A., Gotjamanos, R., and Vowles, N. J.: The use of fluoride dentifrices in the control of dental caries: Methodology and results of a clinical trial. Aust. Dent. J. 13:201–206, 1968.

57. Fanning, E. A., Gotjamanos, T., Vowles, N. J., and Van Der Weilen, I.: The effects of fluoride dentifrices on the incidence and distribution of stained tooth surfaces in children. Arch. Oral Biol., 13:467–469, 1968A.

58. Federal Register, Tues., July 21, 1970, Vol. 25, No. 140, pp. 11643–11645, Notice from the Dept. of Health, Education and Welfare (Food and Drug Administration) in Reference to the Efficacy of Certain Dentifrices.

59. Federal Register, Tues., Aug. 4, 1970 (A), Vol. 35, No. 150, pp. 12411–12412 and 12423–12424, Notice from the Department of Health, Education and Welfare (Food and Drug Administration) in Reference to the Efficacy of Certain Mouthwash and Gargle Preparations.

60. Federal Register, Tuesday, May 14, 1974. Vol. 39, No. 94, p. 17245, Notice from the Department of Health, Education and Welfare (Food and Drug Administration) in reference to Topical Fluoride Preparations for Reducing Incidence of Dental Caries. (A correction to this notice appears in the Federal Register, Wednesday, June 26, 1974. Vol. 39, No. 124, p. 23081; an amendment to this notice appears in the Federal Register, Thursday, November 7, 1974. Vol. 39, No. 216, p. 39488).

61. Federal Register, Friday, March 28, 1980, Vol. 45, No. 62, pp. 20666–20691, Notice from the Department of Health, Education and Welfare (Food and Drug Administration). Establishment of a Monograph on Anticaries Drug Products for Over-The-Counter Human Use; Proposed Rulemaking.

62. Finn, S. B., and Jamison, H. C.: A comparative clinical study of three dentifrices. J. Dent. Child. 30:17–25, 1963.

63. Fischman, S. L., Picozzi, A., Cancro, L. P., and Pader, M.: The inhibition of plaque in humans by two experimental oral rinses. J. Periodontol. 44:100–102, 1973.

64. Fitzgerald, R. J., and Keyes, P. H.: Demonstration of the etiologic role of streptococci in experimental caries in the hamster. J. Am. Dent. Assoc. 61:9–19, 1960.

65. Fjaestad-Seger, M., Norstedt-Larsson, K., and Torell, P.: Forsok Med Enkla Metoder for Klinisk Fluorapplication. Sver. Tandlakarforb. Tidn. 53:169–178, 1961.

66. Flötra, L., Gjermo, P., Rölla, G., and Waerhang, J.: Side effects of chlorhexidine mouthwashes. Scand. J. Dent. Res. 79:119–125, 1971.

67. Flötra, L., Gjermo, P., Rölla, G., and Waerhang, J.: A four-month study on the effect of chlorhexidine mouthwashes on 50 soldiers. Scand. J. Dent. Res. 80:10–17, 1972.

68. Fogels, H. R., Alman, J. E., Meade, J. J., and O'Donnell, J. P.: The relative caries-inhibiting effects of a stannous fluoride dentifrice in a silica gel base. J. Am. Dent. Assoc. 99:456–459, 1979.

69. Forscher, B. K., and Hess, W. C.: The validity of plaque pH measurements as a method of evaluating therapeutic agents. J. Am. Dent. Assoc. 48:134–139, 1954.

70. Forsman, B.: The caries preventing effect of mouth rinsing with an 0.025% sodium fluoride solution in Swedish children. Community Dent. Oral Epidemiol. 2:58–65, 1974.

71. Fosdick, L. S.: The reduction of the incidence of dental caries. I. Immediate toothbrushing with a neutral dentifrice. J. Am. Dent. Assoc. 40:133–143, 1950.

72. Fosdick, L. S.: Clinical experiment on the use of sodium n-lauroyl sarcosinate in the control of dental caries. Science 123:988–989, 1956. (A more detailed description of this study has also been written by L. S. Fosdick and published as a report from Northwestern University Dental School. It is entitled: A Report of Some Clinical Experiments on the Use of Sodium N-Lauroyl Sarcosinate in the Control of Dental Caries.)

73. Fosdick, L. S., Ludwick, W. E., and Schantz, C. W.: Absorption of enzyme inhibitors and antibiotics on dental plaque. J. Am. Dent. Assoc. 43:26–31, 1951.

74. Fosdick, L. S., Calandra, J. C., Blackwell, R. W., and Burrill, J. H.: A new approach to the problem of dental caries control. J. Dent. Res. 32:486–496, 1953.

75. Frankl, S. N., and Alman, J. E.: Report of a three-year clinical trial comparing a toothpaste containing sodium monofluorophosphate with two marketed products. J. Oral Therap. Pharm. 4:443–450, 1968.

76. Frankl, S. N., Fleisch, S., and Diodati, R. R.: The topical anticariogenic effect of daily rinsing with an acidulated phosphate fluoride solution. J. Am. Dent. Assoc. 85:882–886, 1972.

77. Frasher, L. A., and Hein, J. W.: Sodium n-lauroyl sarcosinate dentifrice: Effect on dental caries in children. J. Dent. Res. 37:75 (Abstract), 1958.

78. Fullmer, J., Volpe, A. R., Apperson, L. D., and Kiraly, J.: Unpublished data, Colgate-Palmolive Company, 1966.

79. Gale, J.A.: A controlled experiment on pre-school children with an ammoniated dentifrice. Dent. Rec. 71:184–185, 1951.

80. Gallagher, S. J., Glassgow, I., and Caldwell, R.: Self-application of fluoride by rinsing. J. Pub. Health Dent. 34:13–21, 1973.

81. Gerdin, P.: Studies in dentifrices. I. Abrasiveness of dentifrices and removal of discoloured stains. Swed. Dent. J. 63:275–282, 1970.

82. Gerdin, P. O., and Torell, P.: Mouth rinses with potassium fluoride solutions containing manganase. Caries Res. 3:90–107, 1969.

83. Gerdin, P.: Studies in dentifrices, VI: The inhibiting effect of some grinding and nongrinding fluoride dentifrices on dental caries. Swed. Dent. J. 65:521–532, 1972.

84. Gershon, S. D., and Pader, M.: Dentifrices, Cosmetics-Science and Technology. (M. Balsam and E. Sagarin, Eds.) New York, John Wiley and Sons, pp. 423–531, 1972.

85. Gershon, S. D., Pokras, H. H., and Rider, T. H.: Dentifrices (Chapter 15), Cosmetics-Science and Technology. (E. Sagarin, Ed.) New York: Interscience Publishers, Inc., pp. 296–360, 1957.

86. Gish, C. W., and Muhler, J. C.: Effectiveness of a SnF$_2$-Ca$_2$P$_2$O$_7$ dentifrice on dental caries in children whose teeth calcified in a natural fluoride area, II. Results at the end of the 24 months. J. Am. Dent. Assoc. 73:853–855, 1966.

87. Gjermo, P.: Some aspects of drug dynamics related to oral soft tissues. Presented at Sixth International Conference on Oral Biology, Toronto, 1974, J. Dent. Res. 54 Spec. No. B: B44–56, 1975.

88. Gjermo, P., and Eriksen, H. M.: Unchanged plaque inhibiting effect of chlorhexidine in human subjects after two years of continuous use. Arch. Oral. Biol. 19:317–319, 1974.

89. Gjermo, P., and Rölla, G.: The plaque-inhibiting effect of chlorhexidine-containing dentifrices. Scand. J. Dent. Res. 79:126–132, 1971.

90. Gjermo, P., Rölla, G., and Arskang, L.: E53ct on dental plaque formation and some in vitro properties of 12 bis-biguanides. J. Periodont. Res. 12:81–88, 1973.

91. Glass, R. L., and Shiere, F. R.: A clinical trial of a calcium carbonate base dentifrice containing 0.76% sodium monofluorophosphate. Caries Res. 12:284–289, 1978.

92. Gomer, R. M., Holroyd, S. V., Fedi, P. F., and Ferrigno, P. D.: The effects of oral rinses on the accumulation of dental plaque. J. Am. Soc. Preventive Dent., pp. 6–9, March-April, 1972.

93. Grabenstetter, R. J., Broge, R. W., Jackson, F. L., and Radike, A. W.: The measurement of the abrasion of human teeth by dentifrice abrasion: A test utilizing radioactive teeth. J. Dent. Res. 37:1060–1068, 1958.

94. Grøn, P., and Brudevold, F.: The effectiveness of NaF dentifrices. J. Dent. Child. 34:122–127, 1967.

95. Guarnieri, L. J.: Effect of dentifrice components on guinea pig oral tissue. International Association for Dental Research. Preprinted Abstract No. 661, p. 220, 1974.

96. Guarnieri, L. J.: The effect of dentifrice components on the oral tissues of humans and guinea pigs. Thesis, University of Indiana, 1970.

97. Gucklhorn, I. R.: Antimicrobials in cosmetics. Toilet Goods Assoc. Cosmetic J. 1:15–32, Fall, 1969.

98. Hargreaves, J. A., and Chester, C. G.: Clinical trial among Scottish children of an anticaries dentifrice containing 2% sodium monofluorophosphate. Community Dent. Oral Epidemiol. 1:47–57, 1973.

99. Hargreaves, J. A., Chester, C. G., and Wagg, B. J.: Assessment of children in active and placebo groups, one year after termination of a clinical trial of a 2% sodium monofluorophosphate dentifrice. ORCA (European Organization for Caries Research). Preprinted Abstract, 1974.

100. Harry, R. G.: The tooth and oral hygiene (chap. 15) and dentifrices (chap. 16), The principles and practice of modern cosmetics. Modern Cosmeticology, Chemical Publishing Company, New York, 1:239–290, 1962.

101. Hassell, T. M., and Mühlemann, H. R.: Effects of sodium n-lauroyl sarcosinate on plaque pH in vivo. Helv. Odontol. Acta. 15:52–53, 1971.

102. Hawes, R. R., and Bibby, B. B.: Evaluation of a dentifrice-containing carbamide and urease. J. Am. Dent. Assoc. 46:280–286, 1953.

103. Hazen, S. P., Chilton, N. W., Mumma, R. D.: The problem of root caries. I. Literature review and clinical description. J. Am. Dent. Assoc. 86:137–144, 1973.

104. Hazen, S. P., Volpe, A. R., and King, W. J.: Comparative desensitizing effect of dentifrices containing sodium monofluorophosphate, stannous fluoride and formalin. Periodontics 6:230–233, 1968.

105. Hefferren, J. J.: A laboratory method for the assessment of dentifrice abrasivity. J. Dent. Res. 55:563–573, 1976.

106. Hefferren, J. A.: American Dental Association Collaborative Study of Clinical Methodology: Methods to Assess Dentifrice Cleaning Function, ADA Monograph, 1977.

107. Heifetz, S. B., and Horowitz, H. S.: An appraisal of therapeutic dentifrices. J. Public Health Dent., 30:206–211, 1970.

108. Heifetz, S. B., Driscoll, W. S., and Creighton, W. E.: The effect on dental caries of weekly rinsing with a neutral sodium fluoride or an acidulated phosphate-fluoride mouthwash. J. Am. Dent. Assoc. 87:364–368, 1973.

109. Heifetz, S. B., Meyers, R. J., and Kingman, A.: A comparison of the anticaries effectiveness of daily and weekly rinsing with sodium fluoride solutions: Final results after 3 years. International Association for Dental Research. Preprinted Abstract No. 645, p. 471, 1981.

110. Hein, J. W.: Present status of chlorophyll derivatives as dental therapeutic agents. J. Am. Dent. Assoc. 48:14–20, 1954.

111. Hein, J. W.: Effect of sodium n-lauroyl sarcosinate on the fall of pH of tooth surface films and plaques. J. Dent. Res. 34:755 (Abstract No. T21), 1955.

112. Hendon, G. E., Keller, S. E., and Manson-Hing, L. R.: Clearance studies of proximal tooth surfaces — Part I. Ala. J. Med. Sci. 6:213–227, 1969.

113. Henriques, B. L., Frankl, S. N., and Alman, J. E.: Cited in evaluation of Cue tooth paste. J. Am. Dent. Assoc. 71:197–198, 1964.

114. Henschel, C. J., and Lieber, L.: Caries incidence reduction by unsupervised use of a 27.5 per cent ammonium therapy dentifrice. J. Dent. Res. 28:248–257, 1949.

115. Henschel, C. J., and Lieber, L.: High urea ammoniated dentifrice: Caries reduction through four years home use. Oral Surg. 5:155–169, 1952.

116. Hernandez, F., Mohammed, C., Shannon, I., Volpe, A. R., and King, W. J.: Clinical study evaluating the desensitizing effect and duration of two commercially available dentifrices. J. Periodontol., 43:367–372, 1972.

117. Hill, T. J.: Fluoride dentifrices. J. Am. Dent. Assoc. 59:1121–1127, 1959.

118. Hill, T. J., and Kniesner, A. H.: Penicillin dentifrice and dental caries experience in children. J. Dent. Res. 28:263–266, 1949.

119. Hill, T. J., Sims, J., and Newman, M.: The effect of penicillin dentifrice on the control of dental caries. J. Dent. Res. 32:696–702, 1953.

120. Hodge, H. C., Holloway, P. J., Davies, T. G. H., and Worthington, H. V.: Caries prevention by dentifrices containing a combination of sodium monofluorophosphate and sodium fluoride. Brit. Dent. J. 149:201–204, 1980.

121. Homan, B. T., and Messer, H. H.: The comparative effect of three fluoride dentifrices on clinical caries in Brisbane school children — Preliminary report. J. Dent. Res. 48:1094 (Abstract), 1969.

122. Horowitz, H. S.: Clinical trials of preventives for dental caries. J. Pub. Health Dent. 32:229–233, 1972.

123. Horowitz, H. S.: The prevention of dental caries by mouth rinsing with solutions of neutral sodium fluoride. Int. Dent. J. 23:585–590, 1973.

124. Horowitz, H. S., Creighton, W. E., and McClendon, B. J.: The effect on human dental caries of weekly oral rinsing with a sodium fluoride mouthwash. A final report. Arch. Oral Biol. 16:609–616, 1971.

125. Horowitz, H. S., Law, F. E., Thompson, M. B., and Chamberlin, S. R.: Evaluation of a stannous fluoride dentifrice for use in dental public health programs, I. Basic findings. J. Am. Dent. Assoc. 72:408–422, 1966.

126. Howat, A. P., Holloway, P. J., and Davies, T. G. H.: Caries prevention by daily supervised use of a MFP gel dentifrice. Report of a 3-year clinical trial. Brit. Dent. J. 145:233–235, 1978.

127. Hutchins, D. W., Whitehurst, V. E., and Barnes, G. P.: Evaluation of tissue response to commercially available dentifrices: Clinical and laboratory results. International Association for Dental Research. Preprinted Abstract No. 280, p. 122, 1971.

128. International workshop on fluorides and dental caries reductions, University of Maryland School of Dentistry (Chairman: Dr. Donald Forrester), 1974.

129. Jackson, D., and Sutcliffe, P.: Clinical testing of a stannous-fluoride-calcium pyrophosphate dentifrice in Yorkshire school children. Br. Dent. J. 123:40–48, 1967.

130. James, P. M. C., and Anderson, R. J.: Clinical testing of a stannous fluoride-calcium pyrophosphate dentifrice in Buckinghamshire school children. Br. Dent. J. 123:33–39, 1967.

131. James, P. M. C., Anderson, R. J., Beal, J. F., and Bradnock, G.: A 3-year clinical trial of the effect on dental caries of a dentifrice containing 2% sodium monofluorophosphate. Comm. Dent. Oral Epidem. 5:67–72, 1977.

132. Jordan W. A., and Peterson, J. K.: Caries-inhibiting value of a dentifrice containing stannous fluoride: Final report of a two-year study. J. Am. Dent. Assoc. 58:42–46, 1959.

133. Kanouse, M. C., and Ash, M. M.: The effectiveness of a sodium monofluorophosphate dentifrice on dental hypersensitivity. J. Periodontol. 40:38–39, 1969.

134. Kasakura, T.: Dental observation on school feeding. Part 3 — Effect of dental caries prevention by oral rinsing with a sodium fluoride solution. Shigaker Odontology. 54:22–39, 1966.

135. Keller, S. E., and Manson-Hing, L. R.: Clearance studies on proximal tooth surfaces, Parts III and IV. *In vivo* removal of interproximal plaque. Ala. J. Med. Sci. 6:399–405, 1969.

136. Keosian, J., Weinman, I., and Rafel, S.: The effect of aqueous diatomic iodine mouthwashes on the incidence of postextraction bacteremia. Oral Surg. 9:1337–1341, 1956.

137. Kerr, D. W., and Kesel, R. G.: Two-year caries control study utilizing oral hygiene and an ammoniated dentifrice. J. Am. Dent. Assoc. 42:180–188, 1951.

138. Keyes, P. H.: The infectious and transmissable nature of experimental dental caries — Findings and implications. Arch. Oral Biol., 1:304–320, 1960.

139. Keyes, P. H., and White, C. L.: Dental caries in the molar teeth of rats, III. Bio-assay of sodium fluoride and sodium lauroyl sarcosinate as caries-inhibiting agents. J. Am. Dent. Assoc. 58:43–55, 1959.

140. Keyes, P. H., Hicks, M. A., Goldman, B. M., McCabe, R. M., and Fitzgerald, R. J.: Dispersion of dextranous bacterial plaques on teeth with dextranase. J. Am. Dent. Assoc. 82:136–141, 1971.

141. King, W. J.: Unpublished data, Colgate-Palmolive Company, 1950.

142. King, W. J., Manahan, R. D., and Russell, K. L.: Laboratory methods for screening possible inhibitors of dental caries. J. Dent. Res. 36:307–313, 1957.

143. Kinkel, H. J., and Raich, R.: Die Karieshemmung einer Na$_2$FPO$_3$-Zahnpaste nach 3 Jahren Applikation. Schweiz. Mschr. Zahnheilk. 82:1240–1244, 1972.

144. Kinkel, H. J., and Raich, R.: Die Karieshemmung einer Na$_2$FPO$_3$-Zahnpaste nach 4 Jahren Applikation. Schweiz. Mschr. Zahnheilk. 84:226–229, 1974.

145. Kinkel, H. J., and Stolte, G.: On the effect of a sodium monofluorophosphate- and bromochlorophene-containing toothpaste in a chronic animal experiment and on caries in children during a two-year period of unsupervised use. Dtsch. Zahnaerstb. 22:455–460, 1968.

146. Kinkel, H. J., Stolte, G., and Westrate, J.: Etude de l'efficacite d'une pâte dentifrice au fluorophosphate sur la denture des enfants. Schweiz. Mschr. Zahnheilk. 84:577–589, 1974.

147. Kitchin, P. C., and Robinson, H. B.: How abrasive

210 DENTIFRICES AND MOUTH RINSES

need a dentifrice be? J. Dent. Res. 27:501–505, 1948.

148. Koch, G.: Comparison and estimation of effect on caries of daily supervised toothbrushing with a dentifrice containing potassium fluoride and manganese chloride. Odont. Revy 23:341–354, 1972.

149. Koch, G.: Effect of sodium fluoride in dentifrice and mouthwash on incidence of dental caries in school children. Odont. Revy 18: (Suppl. 12) 1–125, 1967.

150. Koch, G.: Long-term study of effect of supervised toothbrushing with a sodium fluoride dentifrice. Caries Res. 4:149–157, 1970.

151. Koch, G., Peterson, L. G., Kling, E., and Kling, L.: Three-year clinical test of low fluoride (0.025%) dentifrice. International Association for Dental Research. Abstract No. 1070, p. 577, 1981.

152. König, K. G., and Mühlemann, H. R.: Caries-inhibiting effect of amine fluoride-containing dentifrices tested in an animal experiment and in a clinical study. Caries Symposium Zürich, The present status of caries prevention by fluoride-containing dentifrices. Hans Huber Publishers, Berne, Switzerland, pp. 126–132, 1961.

153. Kovaleski, W. C., and Ash, M. M.: Clinical evaluation of a macrolide antibiotic as a plaque preventing agent. Thesis, University of Michigan, 1970.

154. Kowitz, G., Lucatorto, F., and Bennett, W.: Effects of dentifrices on soft tissues of the oral cavity. J. Oral Med. 28:36–40, 1973.

155. Kowitz, G., Lucatorto, F., and Cherrick, H.: Effect of mouthwashes on the oral soft tissues. International Association for Dental Research. Preprinted Abstract No. 660, p. 219, 1974.

156. Kutcher, A. H., and Chilton, N. W.: Observations on the clinical use of a chlorophyll dentifrice. J. Am. Dent. Assoc. 46:420–429, 1953.

157. Kyes, F. M., Overton, N. J., and McKean, T. W.: Clinical trials of caries-inhibitory dentifrices. J. Am. Dent. Assoc. 63:189–193, 1961.

158. Lefkowitz, W., and Venti, V. I.: A preliminary clinical report on caries control with a high urea ammoniated dentifrice. Oral Surg. 4:1576–1580, 1951.

159. Lind, O. P., Möller, I. J., von der Fehr, F. R., and Larsen, M. J.: Caries-preventive effect of a dentifrice containing 2% sodium monofluorophosphate in a natural fluoride area in Denmark. Community Dent. Oral Epidemiol. 2:104–113, 1974.

160. Litsky, B. Y., Mascis, J. D., and Litsky, W.: Use of an antimicrobial mouthwash to minimize the bacterial aerosol contamination generated by the high-speed drill. Oral Surg. 29:25–30, 1970.

161. Lobene, R. R.: A clinical study of the effect of dextranase on human dental plaque. J. Am. Dent. Assoc. 82:132–135, 1971.

162. Lobene, R. R.: Effect of dentifrices on tooth stain with controlled brushing. J. Am. Dent. Assoc. 77:849–855, 1968.

163. Lobene, R. R., and Soparkar, P. M.: The effect of an alexidine mouthwash on human plaque and gingivitis. J. Am. Dent. Assoc. 87:848–851, 1973.

164. Lobene, R. R., and Soparkar, P. M.: The effect of amine fluorides on human plaque and gingivitis. International Association for Dental Research. Preprinted Abstract No. 369, p. 147, 1974.

165. Lobene, R. R., Brion, M., and Socransky, S. S.: Effect of erythromycin on dental plaque and plaque forming microorganisms in man. J. Periodont. 40:287–291, 1969.

166. Lobene, R. R., Soparkar, P. M., Hein, J. W., and Quigley, G. A.: A study of the effects of antiseptic agents and a pulsating irrigating device on plaque and gingivitis. J. Periodont. 43:564–568, 1972.

167. Löe, H., and Schiött, C. R.: The Effect of Suppression of the Oral Microflora Upon the Development of Dental Plaque and Gingivitis. In McHugh, W. D. (ed.): Dental Plaque. Dundee, Scotland, D. C. Thomson and Company, Ltd., pp. 247–256, 1970.

168. Löe, H., and Schiött, C. R.: The effect of mouthrinses and topical applications of chlorhexidine on the development of dental plaque and gingivitis in man. J. Periodont. Res. 5:79–83, 1970A.

169. Löe, H., Theilade, E., and Jensen, S. B.: Experimental gingivitis in man. J. Periodont. Res. 36:177–189, 1965.

170. Löe, H., Mandell, M., Derry, A. W., and Schiött, C. R.: The effect of mouthrinses and topical application of chlorhexidine on calculus formation in man. J. Periodont. Res. 6:312–314, 1971.

171. Loesche, W. J., Green, E., Kenney, E. B., and Nafe, D.: Effect of topical kanamycin sulfate on plaque accumulation. J. Am. Dent. Assoc. 83:1063–1069, 1971.

172. Lu, K. H., Hanna, J. D., and Peterson, J. K.: Effect on dental caries of a stannous fluoride-calcium pyrophosphate dentifrice in an adult population: One-year results. Pharmacol. Ther. Dent. 5:11–16, 1980.

173. Lunin, M., and Mandel, I. D.: Clinical evaluation of a penicillin dentifrice. J. Am. Dent. Assoc. 51:696–702, 1955.

174. Mainwaring, P., and Naylor, M. N.: The clinical testing of an MFP toothpaste and A.P.F. gel. International Association for Dental Research. Preprinted Abstract No. L304, p. L76, 1975.

175. Mainwaring, P. J., and Naylor, M. N.: A three-year clinical study to determine the separate and combined caries-inhibiting effects of a sodium monofluorophosphate toothpaste and an acidulated phosphate-fluoride gel. Caries Res. 12:202–212, 1978.

176. Mainwaring, P. J., and Naylor, M. N.: The anti-caries effect of CaCO_3-based sodium MFP dentifrices with CaGP or NaF additives. American Association for Dental Research. Preprinted Abstract No. 563, p. 408, 1980(A).

177. Mainwaring, P. J., and Naylor, M. N.: Anti-caries effects of NaMFP/CaCO_3 toothpastes containing calcium glycerophosphate (CaGP) or sodium fluoride (NaF): A 4-year clinical study. British Division International Association for Dental Research, Abstract No. 56, 1980(B).

178. Mandel, I. D., and Cagan, R. S.: Pharmaceutical agents for preventing caries — A review, Part I. Dentifrices. J. Oral Therap. Pharm. 1:218–227, 1964.

179. Manhold, B. A., Manhold, J. H., and Weisinger, E. A.: A study of total oral debris clearance, J. N.J. State Dent. Soc. pp. 1–14, 1967.

180. Manhold, J. H., and Manhold, B. A.: Further *in vivo* study of commercial mouth wash efficacy. N.Y. J. Dent. *33*:383–386, 1963.

181. Manhold, J. H., Parker, L. A., and Manhold, B. A.: Efficacy of a commercial mouth wash: *In vivo* study. N.Y. J. Dent. *32*:165–171, 1962.

182. Manly, R. S.: A structureless recurrent deposit on teeth. J. Dent. Res. *22*:479–486, 1943.

183. Manly, R. S.: Factors influencing tests on the abrasion of dentin by brushing with dentifrices. J. Dent. Res. *23*:59–72, 1944.

184. Manly, R. S., Wiren, J., Manly, P. J., and Keene, R. C.: A method for measurement of abrasion of dentin by toothbrush and dentifrice. J. Dent. Res. *44*:533–540, 1965.

185. Marthaler, T. M.: Caries-inhibition by an amine fluoride dentifrice — Results after six years in children with low caries activity. Helv. Odont. Acta *18*:35–44, 1974.

186. Marthaler, T. M.: Karieshemmung durch Amin-fluoridzahnpasten nach sieben jähriger Studiendauer (Results after seven years' use of an amine fluoride dentifrice). Schweiz. Monatsschr. Zahnheilkd. *78*:134–147, 1968.

187. McCormick, J.: A critical review of the literature on mouthwashes. Ann. N.Y. Acad. Sci. (Evaluation of agents used in the prevention of oral disease). *153*:374–385, Dec. 23, 1968.

188. McCormick, J., and Koulourides, T.: A study of neutral calcium, phosphate, and fluoride remineralizing mouthwashes. International Association for Dental Research, Abstract No. 402, p. 138, 1965.

189. McDonnell, C. H., and Domalakes, E. F.: The effects of toothbrushing with dentifrices containing chlorophyllin on gingivitis. J. Periodont. *23*:219–236, 1952.

190. McNeal, D. R.: Anticalculus agents for the treatment, control and prevention of periodontal disease. J. Public Health Dent. *29*:138–152, 1969.

191. Mergele, M.: Report I. A supervised brushing study in state institution schools. Bull. Acad. Med. N.J. *14*:247–250, 1968.

192. Mergele, M.: Report II. An unsupervised brushing study on subjects residing in a community with fluoride in the water. Bull. Acad. Med. N.J. *14*:251–255, 1968A.

193. Mergele, M., Jennings, R. E., and Gasser, E. B.: Cited in evaluation of Cue tooth paste. J. Am. Dent. Assoc. *69*:197–198, 1964.

194. Millard, L.: Acute contact sensitivity to a new toothpaste. J. Dentistry *1*:168–170, 1973.

195. Mitchell, D. F., Holmes, L. A., Martin, P. W., and Sakurai, E.: Topical antibiotic maintenance of oral health. J. Oral. Ther. Pharm. *4*:83–92, 1967.

196. Mohammed, C. I., and Monserrate, V.: Preoperative oral rinsing as a means of reducing air contamination during use of air turbine handpieces. Oral Surg. *20*:291–294, 1970.

197. Mohammed, C. I., Manhold, J. H., and Manhold, B. A. Efficacy of preoperative oral rinsing to reduce air contamination during use of air turbine handpieces. J. Am. Dent. Assoc. *69*:715–718, 1964.

198. Möller, I. J., Holst, J. J., and Sörensen, E.: Caries-reducing effect of a sodium monofluorophosphate dentifrice. Br. Dent. J. *124*:209–213, 1968.

199. Moreira, B. W., and Tumang, A. J.: Prevencão da cárie dentária através de bochechos com solucões de fluoreto de sodio a 0.1% — Resultados após dois anos de estudos. Rev. Bras. Odont. Nr. *173*:37–42, 1972.

200. Morris, P. P., and Read, R. R.: Halitosis: Variations in mouth and total breath odor intensity resulting from prophylaxis and antisepsis. J. Dent. Res. *28*:324–331, 1949.

201. Mühlemann, H. R.: *In vivo* measurements of calculus. Ann. N.Y. Acad. Sci. (Evaluation of agents used in the prevention of oral disease) *153*:164–196, Dec. 23, 1968.

202. Mühlemann, H. R., Bowles, D., Schaitt, A., and Bernimoulin, J. P.: Effect of diphosphonate on human supragingival calculus. Helv. Odontol. Acta *14*:31–35, 1970.

203. Muhler, J. C.: A clinical comparison of fluoride and antienzyme dentifrices. J. Dent. Child. *37*:501–514, 1970.

204. Muhler, J. C.: The combined anticariogenic effect of a single stannous fluoride treatment and the unsupervised use of a stannous fluoride dentifrice. J. Dent. Res. *38*:994–1007, 1959.

205. Muhler, J. C.: Effect of a stannous fluoride dentifrice on caries reduction in children during a three-year study period. J. Am. Dent. Assoc. *64*:216–224, 1962.

206. Muhler, J. C.: Fifty-two pearls and their environment (Chapter 12 — Dentifrices and Oral Hygiene). Bloomington, Indiana University Press, pp. 124–143, 1965.

207. Muhler, J. C., and Radike, A. W.: Effect of a dentifrice containing stannous fluoride on dental caries in adults, II. Results at the end of two years of unsupervised use. J. Am. Dent. Assoc. *55*:196–198, 1957.

208. Muhler, J. C., Radike, A. W., Nebergall, W. H., and Day, H. G.: The effect of a stannous fluoride-containing dentifrice on caries reduction in children. J. Dent. Res. *33*:606–612, 1954.

209. Muhler, J. C., Radike, A. W., Nebergall, W. H., and Day, H. G.: A comparison between the anticariogenic effect of dentifrices containing stannous fluoride and sodium fluoride. J. Am. Dent. Assoc. *51*:556–559, 1955.

210. Muhler, J. C., Radike, A. W., Nebergall, W. H., and Day, H. G.: The effect of a stannous fluoride-containing dentifrice on adults. J. Dent. Res. *35*:49–53, 1956.

211. Muhler, J. C., Spear, L. B., Bixler, D., and Stookey, G. K.: The arrestment of incipient dental caries in adults after the use of three different forms of SnF_2 therapy: Results after 30 months. J. Am. Dent. Assoc. *75*:1402–1408, 1967.

212. Murray, J. J., and Shaw, L.: A 3-year clinical trial into the effect of fluoride content and toothpaste abrasivity on the caries inhibitory properties of a dentifrice. Comm. Dent. Oral Epidem. *8*:46–51, 1980.

213. Naylor, M. N., and Emslie, R. D.: Clinical testing of stannous fluoride and sodium monofluorophosphate dentifrices in London school children. Br. Dent. J. *123*:17–23, 1967.

214. Naylor, M. N., and Glass, R. L.: A 3-year clinical trial of calcium carbonate dentifrice containing calcium glycerophosphate and sodium monofluorophosphate. Caries Res. *13*:39–46, 1979.

215. Onisi, M., and Tani, H.: Clinical test on the caries-preventive effect of two kinds of fluoride dentifrices. Jap. J. Dent. Health *20*:105–111, 1970.

216. Onishi, E., Okada, S., Hinoide, M., Akada, H., Kon, K., Sugano, N., Sakakibara, Y., Morita, J., and Imamura, Y.: Effect of stannous fluoride dentifrice on the reduction of dental caries in school children. Jap. J. Dent. Health, *17*:68–74, 1967.

217. Pader, N.: Dentifrices: Problems of growth. Drug and cosmetic industry *108*: Part I (from p. 36), June, 1971, and *109*: Part II (from p. 36), July, 1971.

218. Parsons, J. C.: Chemotherapy of dental plaque — A review. J. Periodont. *45*:177–186, 1974.

219. Patz, J., and Naujoks, R.: Clinical investigation of a fluoride-containing dentifrice in adults. Results of a two-year unsupervised study. Dtsch. Zahnaerztl. Z. *7*:614–621, 1969.

220. Peffley, G. E., and Muhler, J. C.: The effect of a commercially available stannous fluoride dentifrice under controlled brushing habits on dental caries incidence in children: Preliminary report. J. Dent. Res. *39*:871–875, 1960.

221. Peterson, J. K.: The current status of therapeutic dentifrices. Ann. N.Y. Acad. Sci. (Evaluation of Agents Used in the Prevention of Oral Disease) *153*:334–349, Dec. 23, 1968.

222. Peterson, J. K.: A supervised brushing trial of sodium monofluorophosphate dentifrices in a fluoridated area. Caries Res. *13*:68–72, 1979.

223. Peterson, J. K., and Williamson, L.: Three-year caries inhibition of a sodium fluoride acid orthophosphate dentifrice compared with a stannous fluoride and a non-fluoride dentifrice. International Association for Dental Research, Preprinted Abstract No. 255, p. 101, 1968.

224. Peterson, J., and Williamson, L. D.: Caries inhibition with MFP-calcium carbonate dentifrice in fluoridated area. International Association for Dental Research, Preprinted Abstract No. L 338, p. L 85, 1975.

225. Pigman, Ward (ed.): Evaluation of agents used in the prevention of oral disease. Ann. N.Y. Acad. Sci. *153*:1–388, Dec. 23, 1968.

226. Pinsent, B. R. W.: Methods of assessing the efficiency of tooth-cleaning products. Cosmetic Science. (A. W. Milleton, ed.) 1962.

227. Pinson, T. J., and Stanback, J.: Evaluation of chloraseptic solution as an anesthetic mouth wash. Q. Natl. Dent. Assoc. *22*:49–52, 1964.

228. Radike, A. W.: Current status of research on the use of a stannous fluoride dentifrice. J. Indiana Dent. Assoc. *39*:82–92, 1960.

229. Radike, A. W., Gish, C. W., Peterson, J. K., King, J. D., and Segreto, V. A.: Clinical evaluation of stannous fluoride as an anticaries mouth rinse. J. Am. Dent. Assoc. *86*:404–408, 1973.

230. Reed, M. W., and King, A. D.: A clinical evaluation of a sodium fluoride dentifrice. International Association for Dental Research, Preprinted Abstract No. 340, p. 133, 1970.

231. Renggli, H.: Zahnbelage und Gingivale Entzündung unter dem Einfluss eines antibakteriellen Mundspülmittels (Effect of antimicrobial mouthwash on dental deposits and gingival inflammation). Medical Thesis, University of Zürich, Zürich, Switzerland, 1966.

232. Report on Councils and Bureaus — Council on Dental Therapeutics. Council classifies fluoride mouthrinses. J. Am. Dent. Assoc.*91*:1250–1252, Dec. 1975.

233. Ringelberg, M. L., Conti, A. J., Ward, C. B., Clark, B., and Lotzbar, S.: Effectiveness of different concentrations and frequencies of sodium fluoride mouthrinse. International Association for Dental Research. Abstract No. 649, p. 472, 1981.

234. Robinson, H. B. G.: Individualizing dentifrices: The dentist's responsibility. J. Am. Dent. Assoc. *79*:633–636, 1969.

235. Robinson, R. G.: The effect of a quaternary ammonium compound on oral bacteria: An *in vivo* study using cetylpyridinium chloride. J. Dent. Assoc. S. Afr. *25*:68–74, 1970.

236. Rokita, J. R., Hazen, S. P., Millen, D., and Volpe, A. R.: An *in vivo* study of an antimicrobial mouth rinse on supragingival and subgingival plaque and calculus formation. Pharmacol. Ther. Dent. *2*:1–11, 1975.

237. Rölla, G., Löe, H., and Schiött, C. R.: The affinity of chlorhexidine for hydroxyapatite and salivary mucins. J. Periodont. Res. *5*:90–95, 1970.

238. Rosenthal, M. W.: Mouthwashes (Chapter 16), Cosmetics-Science and Technology. (E. Sagarin, ed.) New York, Interscience Publishers, Inc., pp. 361–379, 1957.

239. Rosenthal, M. W.: Mouthwashes, Cosmetics-Science and Technology. (M. Balsam and E. Sagarin, eds.) New York, John Wiley and Sons, pp. 533–563, 1972.

240. Rosenthal, M. W., Marson, L. M., and Abriss, A.: Some laboratory observations on the chemical, bacterial and enzymatic properties of sodium n-lauroyl sarcosinate. J. Dent. Child. *21*:194–199, 1954.

241. Rugg-Gunn, A. J., Holloway, P. J., and Davies, T. G. H.: Caries prevention by daily fluoride mouth rinsing. Brit. Dent. J. *135*:353–360, 1973.

242. Rundegren, J., Fornell, J., and Ericson, T.: In vivo and in vitro studies on a new peroxide-containing toothpaste. Scand. J. Dent. Res. *81*:543–547, 1973.

243. Sackler, A. M., Rockoff, S. C., and Rockoff, H. S.: Evaluation of chlorpactin WCS 60 as an adjunct in periodontal therapy. N.Y. J. Dent. *26*:199–201, 1956.

244. Saxton, C. A., and Cowell, C. R.: Clinical investigation of the effects of dentifrices on dentin wear at the cementoenamel function. J. Am. Dent. Assoc. *102*:38–43, 1981.

245. Schiff, T.: Clinical study to evaluate a proteolytic enzyme in plaque retardation. International Association for Dental Research, Preprinted Abstract No. 706, p. 225, 1970.

246. Schiff, T., and Shaver, K.: The comparative effect of two commercially available dentifrices on tooth surfaces as determined by a tooth reflectance meter. J. Oral Med. *26*:127–133, 1971.

247. Schiff, T., and Volpe, A. R.: A two-year clinical study comparing the effect of dentifrices on selected dental materials. J. Oral Rehab. *2*:407–412, 1975.

248. Schroeder, H. E.: Formation and Inhibition of

Dental Calculus. Berne, Switzerland, Hans Huber Publishers, 1969 (available in the U.S.A. from International Medical Press, 130 East 59th Street, New York, N.Y.).

249. Schroeder, H. E., Marthaler, T. M., and Mühlemann, H. R.: Effect of some potential inhibitors on early calculus formation. Helv. Odontol. Acta 6:6–9, 1962.

250. Scola, F. P., and Ostrom, C. A.: Clinical evaluation of stannous fluoride when used as a constituent of a compatible prophylactic paste, as a topical solution, and in a dentifrice in naval personnel, II. Report of findings after two years. J. Am. Dent. Assoc. 77:594–597, 1968.

251. Segal, A. H., Stiff, R. H., George, W. A., and Picozzi, A.: Caries-inhibiting effectiveness of a stannous fluoride-insoluble sodium metaphosphate (IMP) dentifrice in children, Two-year results. International Association for Dental Research, Preprinted Abstract No. 250, p. 101, 1966.

252. Shannon, I. L.: Preparation and use of stannous fluoride solutions and ingestible dentifrice. Aeromedical Reviews (USAF School of Aerospace Medicine, Aerospace Medical Division, Brooks Air Force Base, Texas), Review 2–66, pp. 1–11, May, 1966.

253. Shapiro, W. B., Kaslick, R. S., Chasens, A. I., and Weinstein, D.: Controlled clinical comparison between a strontium chloride and a sodium monofluorophosphate toothpaste in diminishing root hypersensitivity. J. Periodontol. 41:523–525, 1970.

254. Shaver, K. J., and Schiff, T.: Oral clinical functionality of enzyme AP used as a mouthwash. J. Periodontol. 41:333–336, 1970.

255. Shea, J. J.: Allergy to fluoride. Ann. Allergy 25:388–391, 1967.

256. Shiere, F. R.: The effectiveness of tyrothrycin dentifrice in the control of dental caries. J. Dent. Res. 36:237–244, 1957.

257. Shipman, B., Cohen, E., and Kaslick, R. S.: The effect of a urea peroxide gel on plaque deposits and gingival status. J. Periodontol. 42:283–285, 1971.

258. Simring, M.: Deodorization and healing: Hexetidine in periodontal surgery. Oral Surg. 16:1432–1442, 1963.

259. Slack, G. L., and Martin, W. J.: The use of a dentifrice containing stannous fluoride in the control of dental caries. Br. Dent. J. 117:275–280, 1964.

260. Slack, G. L., Berman, D. S., Martin, W. J., and Young, J.: Clinical testing of a stannous fluoride-insoluble metaphosphate dentifrice in Kent school girls. Br. Dent. J. 123:9–16, 1967.

261. Slack, G. L., Berman, D. S., Martin, W. J., and Hardie, J. M.: Clinical testing of a stannous fluoride-calcium pyrophosphate dentifrice in Essex school girls. Br. Dent. J. 123:26–33, 1967.

262. Smith, I. L. F.: Acute allergic reaction following the use of toothpaste. Brit. Dent. J. 33:304–305, 1968.

263. Solis, M. C., and Volpe, A. R.: Determination of sulfur volatiles in putrefied saliva by a gas chromatography-microcoulometric system. J. Periodontol. 44:775–778, 1973.

264. Stallard, R. E., Volpe, A. R., Orban, J. E., and King, W. J.: The effect of an antimicrobial mouth rinse on dental plaque, calculus and gingivitis. J. Periodontol. 40:683–694, 1969.

265. Stec, I. P.: A possible relationship between desquamation and dentifrices — A clinical study. J. Am. Dent. Hygienists Assoc. 46:42–45, 1972.

266. Stephan, R. M., and Miller, B. F.: Effectiveness of urea and synthetic detergents in reducing activity of human dental caries. Proc. Soc. Exp. Biol. Med., 55:101–104, 1944.

267. Stookey, G. K., and Muhler, J. C.: Laboratory studies concerning the enamel and dentin abrasion properties of common dentifrice polishing agents. J. Dent. Res. 47:524–532, 1968.

268. Sturzenberger, O. P., and Leonard, G. J.: The effect of a mouthwash as an adjunct in tooth cleaning. J. Periodontol., 40:299–302, 1969.

269. Sturzenberger, O. P., Swancar, J. R., and Reiter, G.: Reduction of dental calculus in humans through use of a dentifrice containing a crystal-growth inhibitor. J. Periodontol. 42:416–519, 1971.

270. Sulser, G. F., Fosket, R. R., and Fosdick, L. S.: Use of sodium dehydroacetate-sodium oxalate dentifrice in the control of dental caries. J. Am. Dent. Assoc. 56:368–375, 1958.

271. Suomi, S. D., Horowitz, H. S., Barbano, J. P., Spolsky, V. W., and Heifetz, S. B.: A clinical trial of a calculus inhibitory dentifrice. J. Periodontol. 45:139–145, 1974.

272. Swartz, M. L., and Phillips, R. W.: Cleansing, polishing and abrasion techniques (in vitro). Ann. N.Y. Acad. of Sci. (Evaluation of Agents Used in the Prevention of Oral Disease) 153:120–136, 1968.

273. Swerdloff, G., and Shannon, I. L.: A feasibility study of the use of a stannous fluoride mouthwash in a school preventive dentistry program. SAM-TR-67-52. U.S. Air Force Sch. Aerospace Med. 1–10, June, 1967.

274. Tainter, M. L., and Epstein, S.: Use of metal plates for testing the abrasiveness of dentifrices. J. Dent. Res. 22:381–387, 1943.

275. Takeuchi, M., Schimizu, T., Kawasaki, T., and Kizu, T.: A field study on the effect of a dentifrice containing sodium monofluorophosphate in caries prevention. J. Soc. Oral Hygiene 18:26–57, 1968.

276. Terry, J. M., and Shannon, I. L.: Clinical evaluation of an ingestible dentifrice. J. Oral Ther. 4:426–430, 1968.

277. Thomas, A. E., and Jamison, H. C.: Effect of SnF_2 dentifrices on caries in children: Two-year clinical study of supervised brushing in children's homes. J. Am. Dent. Assoc. 73:844–852, 1966.

278. Thomas, A. E., and Jamison, H. C.: Effect of a combination of two cariostatic agents on caries in children: Two-year clinical study of supervised brushing in children's homes. Bull. Acad. Med. N.J. pp. 241–246, 1968. (Also published in J. Am. Dent. Assoc. 81:118–124, 1970.)

279. Tomlinson, K., and Davies, T. G. H.: Unpublished data, Colgate-Palmolive Company, 1962.

280. Tonzetich, J.: Direct gas chromatographic analysis of sulphur compounds in mouth air in man. Arch. Oral Biol. 16:587–597, 1971.

281. Torell, P.: Bruk av fluortandkräm i samband nud fluorsköloljning varannan vecka. (The use of fluoride toothpaste combined with fluoride rinsing every two weeks.) Sveriges Tandläk. Tidning. 61:873–875, 1969.

282. Torell, P., and Ericsson, Y.: Two-year clinical tests with different methods of local caries-preventive fluorine application in Swedish school-children (Part I: The Göteberg study). Acta Odontol. Scand. 23:287–312, 1965A.

283. Torell, P., and Ericsson, Y.: Two-year clinical tests with different methods of local caries-preventive fluorine application in Swedish school-children (Part II: The Södertälje study). Acta Odontol. Scand., 23:313–321, 1965B.

284. Torell, P., and Ericsson, Y.: The potential benefits to be derived from fluoride mouth rinses. International workshop on fluorides and dental caries reductions, University of Maryland School of Dentistry, 1974.

285. Torell, P., and Siberg, A.: Mouthwash with sodium fluoride and potassium fluoride. Odont. Revy 13:62–72, 1962.

286. Triol, C. W., Kranz, S. M., Volpe, A. R., Frankl, S. N., Alman, J. E., and Allard, R. L.: Anticaries effect of a sodium fluoride rinse and an MFP dentifrice in a nonfluoridated water area: A thirty-month study. J. Clin. Prev. Dent. 2:13–15, 1980.

287. Triol, C. W., Wilson, C. J., and Volpe, A. R.: Effect on caries of two monofluorophosphate dentifrices in a nonfluoridated water area: A thirty-one month study. J. Clin. Prev. Dent. 3:5–7, 1981.

288. United States Code of Federal Regulations, Title 21, Part 130.

289. Vallotton, C. F.: An acquired pigmented pellicle of the enamel surface I. Review of the literature. J. Dent. Res. 24:161–169, 1945.

290. Van Abbé, N. J., Bridge, A. J., Ribbons, J. W., Dean, P. M., and Lazarou, J. A.: The effect of dentifrices on extrinsic tooth stain. J. Soc. Cosmetic Chemists 22:457–476, 1971.

291. Villa, P.: Degree of calculus inhibition by habitual toothbrushing. Helv. Odontol. Acta 12:31–36, 1968.

292. Vinson, L. J., and Bennett, H. G.: Evaluation of oral antiseptic products on buccal epithelial tissue. J. Am. Pharm. Assoc. (Scientific Ed.). 47:635–639, 1958.

293. Vogel, P., and Hess, W.: Clinical evaluation of caries-reducing effect of a dentifrice containing 13% carbamide and 3% dibasic ammonium phosphate. J. Dent. Child. 24:237–242, 1957.

294. Volker, J. F., Sognnaes, R. F., and Bibby, B. G.: Studies on the distribution of radioactive fluoride in the bones and teeth of experimental animals. Am. J. Physiol. 132:707–712, 1941.

295. Volker, J. F., Apperson, L. D., and King, W. J.: The influence of certain protein adsorbed agents on hamster caries. Antibiot. Chemother. 6:56–62, 1956.

296. Volker, J. F., Hodge, H. C., Wilson, H. J., and Van Voochis, S. M.: The adsorption of fluorides by enamel, dentin, bone and hydroxyapatite as shown by the radioactive isotope. J. Biol. Chem. 134:543–548, 1940.

297. Volpe, A. R.: Indices for the measurement of hard deposits in clinical studies of oral hygiene and periodontal disease. J. Periodontol. Res. 9:31–60, 1974.

298. Volpe, A. R.: Summary of clinical findings with a monofluorophosphate dentifrice. Bull. Acad. Med. N.J. 14:256–260, 1968.

299. Volpe, A. R., Kupczak, L. J., Brant, J. H., King, W. J., Kestenbaum, R. C., and Schlissel, H. J.: Antimicrobial control of bacterial plaque and calculus and the effects of these agents on the oral flora. J. Dent. Res. 48:832–841, 1969.

300. Volpe, A. R., Mooney, R., Zumbrunnen, C., Stahl, D., and Goldman, H. M.: A long-term clinical study evaluating the effect of two dentifrices on oral tissues. J. Peridontol. 46:113–118, 1975.

301. Volpe, A. R., Schulman, S. M., Goldman, H. M., King, W. J., and Kupczak, L. J.: The long-term effect of an antimicrobial formulation on dental calculus formation. J. Periodontol. 41:464–467, 1970.

302. Wallace, D. A.: Therapeutic dentifrices. A review of the literature on clinical investigations. Dent. Prog. 2:242–248, 1962.

303. Walsh, J. P., and Smart, R. S.: Clinical trial of a penicillin tooth powder. N.Z. Dent. J. 47:118–122, 1951.

304. Wedderburn, D. L.: The Use of Antiseptics and Germicides in Toilet Preparations (Chap. XXI). In Hibbott, H. W. (ed.): Handbook of Cosmetic Science. Fairlawn, N.J., Oxford University Press, 1963, p. 445–472.

305. Weinstein, E., and Mandel, I. D.: The present status of anticalculus agents. J. Oral Therap. Pharm. 1:327–343, 1964.

306. Weisenstein, P. R., and Zacherl, W. A.: A multiple-examiner clinical evaluation of a sodium fluoride dentifrice. J. Am. Dent. Assoc. 84:621–623, 1972.

307. Weisz, W. S.: The reduction of dental caries through use of a sodium fluoride mouthwash. J. Am. Dent. Assoc. 60:438–443, 1960.

308. Wilkinson, J. B., and Pugh, B. R.: Toothpastes — Cleaning and abrasion. J. Soc. Cosmetic Chemists 21:595–605, 1970.

309. Winkler, K. C., Backer-Dirks, O., and Van Amerongen, J.: Reproducible method for caries evaluation. Test in a therapeutic experiment with a fluorinated dentifrice. Br. Dent. J. 95:119–127, 1953.

310. Wilson, C. J., Triol, C. W., and Volpe, A. R.: The clinical anticaries effect of a fluoride dentifrice and mouthrinse. International Association for Dental Research. Preprinted Abstract No. 808, 1978.

311. Workshop conference on the physical functionality of dentifrices (abrasion-cleaning-polishing). American Dental Association (Chairman: Dr. John Hefferen), 1974.

312. Wright, K. H. R., and Stevenson, J. I.: The measurement and interpretation of dentifrice abrasiveness. J. Soc. Cosmetic Chemists 18:387–411, 1967.

313. Zacherl, W. A.: A clinical evaluation of sodium fluoride and stannous fluoride dentifrices. International Association for Dental Research, Preprinted Abstract No. 253, p. 101, 1968.

314. Zacherl, W. A.: Clinical evaluation of a sarcosinate dentifrice. International Association for Dental Research, Preprinted Abstract No. 339, p. 133, 1970.

315. Zacherl, W. A. and McPhail, C. W. B.: Evaluation of a stannous fluoride-calcium pyrophosphate dentifrice. J. Can. Dent. Assoc. 31:174–180, 1965.

316. Zacherl, W. A.: Clinical evaluation of neutral sodium fluoride, stannous fluoride, sodium monofluorophosphate and acidulated fluoride-phosphate dentifrices. J. Can. Dent. Assoc. 1:35–38, 1972.

317. Zacherl, W. A.: Clinical evaluation of an aged stannous fluoride-calcium pyrophosphate dentifrice. J. Can. Dent. Assoc. 4:155–157, 1972A.

318. Zacherl, W. A.: Clinical evaluation of a sodium fluoride-silica abrasive dentifrice. Pharm. Therap. Dent. 6:1–7, 1981.

319. Zander, H. A.: Effect of a penicillin dentifrice on caries incidence in school children, J. Am. Dent. Assoc. 40:569–574, 1950.

320. Zipkin, I., and McClure, F. J.: The effect of sodium lauroyl sarcosinate, sodium lauryl sulfate and dehydroacetic acid on occlusal and smooth surface caries in the rat. J. Dent. Res. 34:768–773, 1955.

RECOMMENDED READING

COMPOSITION OF DENTIFRICES AND CLEANING AND POLISHING ASPECTS

Accepted Dental Therapeutics, 38th Edition, 1979/1980; published by the American Dental Association, 211 East Chicago Avenue, Chicago, Illinois 60611.

Bouchal, A. W.: The abrasiveness of dentifrices. Proc. of the Scient. Section of the Toilet Goods Assoc. No. 45, pp. 2–5, 1966.

Gershon, S. D., and Pader, M.: Dentifrices, Cosmetics-Science and Technology. Vol. 1, 2nd ed. (M. Balsam and E. Sagarin, eds.) New York, John Wiley and Sons, pp. 423–531, 1972.

Gershon, S. D., Pokras, H. H., and Rider, T. H.: Dentifrices (Chapter 15), Cosmetics-Science and Technology. (E. Sagarin, ed.) New York, Interscience Publishers, Inc., pp. 296–360, 1957.

Harry, R. G.: The tooth and oral hygiene and dentifrices. The principles and practice of modern cosmetics. (Vol. 1). Modern Cosmetology, New York, Chemical Publishing Co., pp. 239–290, 1962.

Hefferren, J. J.: A laboratory method for assessment of dentifrice abrasivity. J. Dent. Res. 55:563–573, 1976.

Hendon, G. E., Keller, S. E., and Manson-Hing, L. R.: Clearance studies of proximal tooth surfaces, Part I. Ala. J. Med. Sci. 6:213–227, 1969.

Jefopoulos, T.: Dentifrices, 1970. Published by Noyes Data Corporation, Park Ridge, New Jersey (also Zug, Switzerland and London, England).

Manly, R. S., Wiren, J., Manly, P. J., and Keene, R. C.: A method for measurement of abrasion of dentin by toothbrush and dentifrice. J. Dent. Res. 44:533–540, 1965.

Naylor, M. N., and Pindborg, J. J. (eds.): Contribution of Dentifrices to Oral Health. Comm. Dent. and Oral Epidem. 8:217–285, 1980.

Robinson, H. B. G.: Individualizing dentifrices: The dentist's responsibility. J. Am. Dent. Assoc. 79:633–636, 1969.

Stookey, G. K., and Muhler, J. C.: Laboratory studies concerning the enamel and dentin abrasion properties of common dentifrice polishing agents. J. Dent. Res. 47:524–532, 1968.

Swartz, M. L., and Phillips, R. W.: Cleansing, polishing and abrasion techniques (in vitro). Ann. N.Y. Acad. Sci. (Evaluation of agents used in the prevention of oral disease) 153:120–136, 1968.

Wilkinson, J. B., and Pugh, B. R.: Toothpastes — Cleaning and abrasion. J. Soc. Cosmetic Chemists 21:595–605, 1970.

Workshop conference on the physical functionality of dentifrices (abrasion-cleaning-polishing). American Dental Association (Chairman: Dr. John Hefferren), 1974.

Wright, K. H. K., and Stevenson, J. I.: The measurement and interpretation of dentifrice abrasiveness. J. Soc. Cosmetic Chemists 18:387–411, 1967.

THERAPEUTIC DENTIFRICES

Accepted Dental Therapeutics, 38th Ed. 1979/1980. Published by the American Dental Association, 211 East Chicago Avenue, Chicago, Illinois 60611.

American Dental Association, Clinical testing of dental caries preventatives — Report of a conference to develop uniform standards and procedures in clinical studies of dental caries. Published by the American Dental Association, 1955.

American Dental Association, Conference on clinical trials of drugs used in dentistry. Published by the American Dental Association, 1960.

American Dental Association, Proceedings of the conference on the clinical testing of cariostatic agents. Published by the American Dental Association, 1968.

Backer-Dirks, O., Baume, L. J., Davies, G. N., and Slack, G. L.: Principal requirements for controlled clinical trials. Int. Dent. J. 17:93–103, 1967.

Bartelstone, H. J., Mandel, I. D., and Chilton, N. W.: Critical evaluation of clinical studies with stannous fluoride dentifrices. N.Y. State Dent. J. 28:147–156, 1962.

Bibby, B. G.: Caries: Preventive effects of topical fluoride applications: A review of recent clinical trials in North America. Bull. Acad. Med. N.J. 14:210–226, 1968.

Duckworth, R.: Fluoride dentifrices. A review of clinical trials in the United Kingdom. Br. Dent. J. 124:505–509, 1968.

Duckworth, R.: Review of recent clinical trials outside North America. Bull. Acad. Med. N.J. 14:226–239, 1968.

Establishment of a Monograph on Anticaries Drug Products for Over-The-Counter Use; Proposed Rulemaking. Federal Register (U.S. Government Food and Drug Administration), Friday, March 28, 1980, p. 20666–20691.

Evaluation of agents used in the prevention of oral disease. Ann. N.Y. Acad. Sci. (Ward Pigman, Consulting ed.) 153:1–388, Dec. 23, 1968.

Fluorides in the control of caries. A symposium on recent clinical advances in the use of fluorides for controlling caries. Bull. Acad. Med. N.J. 14:201–265, Dec., 1968.

Gish, C. W., and Mercer, V. H.: "Doctor, which tooth-paste do you recommend?" Consumer Bull., pp. 12–16, May, 1968.

Grøn, P., and Brudevold, F.: The effectiveness of NaF dentifrices. J. Dent. Child. *34*:122–127, 1967.

Hartles, R. L.: Toothpaste as anticaries agents. Am. Perfumer. *77*:53–55, 1962.

Heifetz, S. B., and Horowitz, H. S.: An appraisal of therapeutic dentifrices. J. Public Health Dent. *30*:206–211, 1970.

Hill, T. J.: Fluoride dentifrices. J. Am. Dent. Assoc. *59*:1121–1127, 1959.

Horowitz, H. S.: Clinical trials of preventives for dental caries. J. Pub. Health Dent. *32*:229–233, 1972.

Mandel, I. D., and Cagan, R. S.: Pharmaceutical agents for preventing caries — A review. Part I — Dentifrices. J. Oral Therap. Pharm. *1*:218–227, 1964.

Mühlemann, H. R., and König, K. G. (eds.): Caries Symposium Zürich: The present status of caries prevention by fluoride-containing dentifrices. Berne, Switzerland, Hans Huber Publishers, 1961.

Muhler, J. C.: Fifty-two pearls and their environment. Chapter 12 — Dentifrices and Oral Hygiene. Bloomington, Indiana University Press, pp. 124–143, 1965.

Pader, N.: Dentifrices: Problems of growth. Drug and Cosmetic Industry *108*: Part I (from p. 36) June, 1971; *109*: Part II (from p. 36) July, 1971.

Peterson, J. K.: The current status of therapeutic dentifrices. Ann. N.Y. Acad. Sci. (Evaluation of agents used in the prevention of oral disease) *153*:334–349, Dec. 23, 1968.

Radike, A. E.: Current status of research on the use of a stannous fluoride dentifrice. J. Indiana Dent. Assoc. *39*:82–92, 1960.

Rapoport, S.: Toothpaste — Should it whiten and brighten? Can it give you the breath of springtime? Consumer Bull., pp. 7–9, Aug., 1971.

United States Code of Federal Regulations, Title 21, Part 130.

Volpe, A. R.: Summary of clinical findings with a monofluorophosphate dentifrice. Bull. Acad. Med. N.J. *14*:256–260, 1968.

Von der Fehr, F. R., and Møller, I. J.: Caries-preventive fluoride dentifrices. Caries Res. *12*:(Suppl. 1): 31–37, 1978.

Wallace, D. A.: Therapeutic dentifrices. A review of the literature on clinical investigations. Dent. Prog. *2*:242–248, 1962.

Ware, A. L.: A review of dentifrices as therapeutic agents. Aust. Dent. J. *9*:203–208, 1964.

MOUTH RINSES

Birkeland, J. M., and Torell, P.: Caries-preventive fluoride mouthrinses. Caries Res. *12* (Suppl. 1): 38–51, 1978.

Darlington, R. C.: O-T-C topical oral antiseptics and mouthwashes. J. Am. Pharm. Assoc. *NS8*:484–496, 1968.

Gjermo, P.: Some aspects of drug dynamics related to oral soft tissues. Presented at Sixth International Conference on Oral Biology, Toronto, 1974, J. Dent. Res. *54*:B44–B56, 1975.

Gucklhorn, I. R.: Antimicrobials in cosmetics, Toilet Goods Assoc. Cosmetic J. *1*:15–32, Fall, 1969.

Horowitz, H. S.: The prevention of dental caries by mouth rinsing with solutions of neutral sodium fluoride. Int. Dent. J. *23*:585–590, 1973.

International workshop on fluorides and dental caries reductions, University of Maryland School of Dentistry (Chairman: Dr. Donald Forrester), 1974.

McCormick, J.: A critical review of the literature on mouthwashes. Ann. N. Y. Acad. Sci. (Evaluation of agents used in the prevention of oral disease) *153*:374–385, Dec. 23, 1968.

Parsons, J. C.: Chemotherapy of dental plaque — A review. J. Periodontol. *45*:177–186, 1974.

Rosenthal, M. W.: Mouthwashes (Chapter 16), Cosmetics-Science and Technology. (E. Sagarin, ed.) New York, Interscience Publishers, Inc., pp. 361–379, 1957.

Rosenthal, M. W.: Mouthwashes, Cosmetics-Science and Technology. (M. Balsam and E. Sagarin, eds.) Vol. 1, 2nd Ed. New York, John Wiley and Sons, pp. 533–563, 1972.

Torell, P., and Ericsson, Y.: The potential benefits to be derived from fluoride mouth rinses. International workshop on fluorides and dental caries reductions, University of Maryland School of Dentistry, 1974.

Volpe, A. R.: Indices for the measurement of hard deposits in clinical studies of oral hygiene and periodontal disease. J. Periodont. Res. *9*:31–60, 1974.

Wedderburn, D. L.: The Use of Antiseptics and Germicides in Toilet Preparations (Chap. XX1). In Hibbott, H. W. (ed.): Handbook of Cosmetic Science. Fairlawn, N.J., Oxford University Press, 1963, pp. 445–472.

CHAPTER ELEVEN

Oral Hygiene Techniques and Home Care

R. Anthony Adams, B.D.S., M.S.
Wallace V. Mann, D.M.D., M.S.

Why do so many Americans eventually lose their teeth from the effects of periodontal disease and caries? Why is it that one third of all Americans are edentulous by age 67?[2] Is it because they do not care to keep their teeth or because they did not know how to care for them? The answer is probably an admixture.

Many patients faithfully follow the advice of their dentist and seek annual or semi-annual check-ups. At these appointments, carious teeth may be repaired, teeth weakened by previous disease crowned, pulpal disease successfully treated, and periodontal problems managed by scaling and polishing. Yet, despite regular dental treatment and patient cooperation many dentitions succumb to the ravages of uncontrolled dental disease. It is as though many patients are maintained in a state of quasi-health or overt disease. The "final" solutions are often either referral to a specialist for "oral rehabilitation" or extractions of teeth and eventual denture construction. It is not surprising that our profession and our patients seem to have little confidence in the possibility of long-lasting oral health.

The purpose of this chapter is to discuss some constructive ideas and techniques aimed at providing and maintaining long-term oral health in our patients. As members of the dental profession, we must fulfill our basic purpose, namely, returning the patient to a state of optimal oral health that can be maintained by the patient.

One of our most important roles is that of teacher. While we may have the task of returning a patient to health, the patient must bear a large share of the responsibility for maintenance of health. In dentistry, we refer to patient responsibility and functions directed toward health maintenance as "home care" and the techniques used for this end as "oral hygiene procedures." The term "oral hygiene" has different meanings for different people. Nevertheless, most agree that the phrase implies oral cleanliness. Some use it to designate the condition or state of cleanliness that is present at a given point in time, while others use it to designate the procedures or practices that are used to establish the state of cleanliness. We define "oral hygiene" as those measures necessary to attain and maintain oral health, including practices required to cleanse the teeth, the periodontal tissues, and the mouth, thereby contributing to a state of cleanliness of the oral cavity.

There are many reasons patients may want oral cleanliness. They can be broadly categorized into two main groups. The first group comprises those who desire the achievement of oral cleanliness for the sake of being healthy. The patient desires a healthy, functioning dentition as a component of total body health. Those with this inherent, strong motivation need the dental clinician for direction and guidance in establishing a healthy lifestyle, with habit patterns directed toward the person as a whole and specifically, toward the oral structures.

The second major reason for patients

desiring such cleanliness is derived from peer and social pressures. The patient may want clean, white teeth and a fresh breath. But, regardless of the reason, methods and habits must be established such that a state of oral hygiene that is compatible with health and cleanliness is reached.

THE RELATIONSHIP OF ORAL HYGIENE TO CARIES AND PERIODONTAL DISEASE

Caries and the inflammatory periodontal diseases are among the most prevalent chronic diseases in the world. Both share important common characteristics; for instance, both require colonization of bacteria on exposed tooth surfaces. They are distinctly different, complex host-parasite diseases, but they have similar multifactorial etiologies. It is well established that the degree of oral cleanliness determines the absence or presence of dental disease.[3, 12, 26] Neither gingivitis nor caries can develop in the absence of microbial plaque on the tooth surface. Health will prevail as long as the host is able to effectively combat antagonistic forces, namely, microbial plaque.

The intrinsic systems of host defenses are referred to as host resistance. Some people have a naturally high resistance to dental disease and, consequently, low disease susceptibility. Such people have a low risk of acquiring dental disease. In their lives they may develop few carious lesions and only mild periodontal inflammation.

At the opposite end of the spectrum are the "high risk" people, those with low host resistance and high disease susceptibility. Examples include children with rampant caries and those with the disease juvenile periodontitis. These young people develop severe and rapid tissue destruction, seemingly disproportionate to their level of oral hygiene.

The vast majority of the population lie between these extremes, their degree of oral cleanliness approximating the magnitude of disease in their mouths. For all patients, our aim is to educate and motivate them to a level of oral hygiene sufficient to attain and preserve oral health.

Three factors are important in the development of dental disease:

1. The intrinsic balance between host resistance and susceptibility to oral disease.
2. The nature of the microflora adherent to the tooth surface (termed "dental plaque").
3. The specific substrate required by the microflora to survive and multiply.

The substrate is directly related to the host's diet. A high intake of fermentable carbohydrates, especially sucrose, results in a substrate that is suitable for the development of caries. The pathogenic bacteria associated with periodontal disease are more complex, and their nutritional requirements are incompletely understood. It is known that the dentogingival plaques associated with both gingivitis and periodontitis are affected by sugar intake. An absence or reduction in sucrose will not prevent plaque formation. However, a sucrose-rich diet causes an increase in the amount of plaque.[16]

The patient's crucial role in hygienic home care involves actions against these three previously mentioned factors. The reduction or elimination of the microflora from the tooth surface is very important. This can be achieved by mechanical or chemical means. The patient must also understand the reasons for disease and the rational basis for regular supra- and subgingival debridement with proper home care measures. Obviously, he or she must be properly trained in effective methods of cleaning all surfaces of each tooth. Although several techniques of tooth cleaning are discussed in this chapter, it is pertinent to note that most dental diseases occur interproximally, that is, between teeth.[29, 39] Whereas the toothbrush is extremely effective in removing plaque from the labial, lingual, and occlusal surfaces of teeth, it is relatively ineffective interproximally. Clearly, the goal of oral health can only be met if devices aimed at interproximal tooth surface cleaning are also utilized.

Another objective of home care is to increase the resistance of the tooth and gingival tissues to pathogenic microorganisms. For example, fluorides are commonly administered to dentitions vulnerable to caries. If the water supply has less than an optimal level of fluoride, appropriate home care would include the use of fluoride-containing toothpaste and carefully prescribed fluoride supplements.

Dietary modification must be emphasized to the patient. This is aimed at depriving the potentially pathogenic bacteria of necessary substrates. For caries control, the carbohydrate-dependent bacteria can be greatly reduced or even eliminated by not eating sugar-rich foods at and between meals.[3, 13, 28]

In summary, it is clear that we can positively affect our patients' oral health by increasing their awareness and appreciation of health, by helping them develop appropriate methods of plaque removal, by increasing the resistance of the oral cavity to attack, and by realistically modifying the diet. Generally, there is a lower prevalence of caries and periodontal disease in those who practice good oral hygiene procedures than in those who do not.[12, 22]

THE ROLE OF HOME CARE IN CARIES PREVENTION

The purpose of tooth cleaning can be stated as those techniques performed by the patient that are directed at maximum elimination of plaque. The interrelationship between poor home care and oral disease susceptibility has been well documented. If all oral hygiene measures are withdrawn, caries develops within a few weeks.[12, 29] It is clear that patients must be well educated and motivated in a wide range of home-care principles for the maintenance of dental health. To cooperate, they must perceive its necessity.

Mansbridge[28] examined 426 children between the ages of 12 and 14 and rated the oral hygiene in each child as "good" or "neglected." He concluded that there was a significantly lower prevalence of caries in individuals with good oral hygiene. This and other studies suggest a cause and effect relationship between caries and oral hygiene.

However, there are conflicting reports on this question. Some studies have shown that there is no difference in caries activities among individuals with good and poor oral hygiene. Davies[13] has commented on this conflicting conclusion and has suggested that the measurement of all oral hygiene at a given point in time might be misleading, since the caries that is present reflects an accumulation of disease over a long time. Thus, the state of oral hygiene at a given point may not represent the true condition of cleanliness over the period it took to develop the caries.

In most societies the dentate mouth requires regular chemical or physical auxiliary help if it is to sustain a level of cleanliness compatible with health. Quite simply, man's dentition has evolved in such a fashion that it cannot look after itself. The dental structures are only partially "self-cleansing." Tissues such as the tongue, lips, and cheeks are quite effective at removing food and debris from prominently exposed areas such as cusp tips but are completely unable to render pits and fissures and interproximal and dento-gingival areas plaque-free. Thus, it is not surprising to find interproximal and occlusal caries and generalized periodontal disease in people who do not routinely undertake effective home care.

Likewise, a diet low in fermentable carbohydrates and enriched in hard fibrous foods such as apples, vegetables, and grains is often recommended by clinicians. Although this is sensible advice in terms of reducing the intake of carbohydrates and of helping the patient avoid caries and such systemic problems as obesity, these so-called "detergent foods" are not truly dental detergents. The same "high risk" areas left unclean by the physiologic activities of the mouth are similarly unaffected by food consistency.

It is most important to realize that in man, self-cleansing of teeth by food or oral function does not play a meaningful role in disease prevention. Auxiliary help is required, including the toothbrush for cleaning occlusal, buccal, and lingual tooth surfaces, and devices such as floss, interproximal brushes, and wooden toothpicks for cleaning interproximal areas.

Those surfaces routinely rendered plaque-free by the toothbrush will be caries-free. Interproximal areas, usually inaccessible to the brush, will not benefit from this aspect of home care. Teeth that are regularly rendered plaque-free do not develop caries, while those that are infrequently cleaned can become carious. If oral health is to be maintained, it is quite clear that an effective cleaning regimen is necessary each day. Patients tend to "forget" the importance of interproximal cleaning and are satisfied to merely brush the visible surfaces of their teeth. Easily accessible prominent areas are usually brushed, such as the labial surfaces of anterior teeth, but posterior and interproximal areas are frequently neglected.

A major home-care consideration is the diet and the effect of specific foods on the tooth surface. Although it is not the purpose of this chapter to study disease etiology in detail, it is pertinent to recognize that the ingestion of easily fermentable carbohydrates results in rapid acid production by microorganisms in plaque. A marked plaque acidity reaches its peak within ten minutes after eating. From the caries standpoint, the host is most susceptible to attack at this time. This has important ramifications. After an extensive review of the literature, Davies[13] concluded that cleaning the teeth markedly reduces caries only if carried out immediately after eating. This supported the earlier observations of Fosdick,[18] who examined approximately 700 young adults over a period of two years. He showed that an experimental group who brushed within ten minutes after food ingestion had 41 per cent fewer cavities than the control group who cleaned their teeth independent of meal times.

The relationship between caries incidence and the time of day oral hygiene is undertaken can be summarized as follows: If oral hygiene is performed after each meal, the caries reducing effect is significantly more pronounced than if the time of brushing is not related to meals. However, tooth cleaning in itself does not provide a complete caries reducing effect if the cleaning is aimed merely at removing food debris. Carious lesions will still occur if plaque is left on the teeth, the incidence of caries being highest if cleaning is not undertaken immediately after eating.

THE RELATIONSHIP BETWEEN ORAL HYGIENE AND PERIODONTAL DISEASE

The relationship between the presence of plaque microorganisms at the dentogingival area and inflammatory periodontal disease has been well documented.[26, 34, 37] It is quite clear that the degree of oral cleanliness determines the degree of periodontal health in individual dentitions. If the dentogingival area is rendered completely plaque-free, any existing disease activity will cease and the periodontium will become healthy.[26]

Perhaps the first major study implicating the role of poor oral hygiene in periodontal disease etiology was published by Arno in 1958.[5] He determined that the prevalence and severity of gingivitis in Oslo factory laborers was significantly greater than in administrative personnel. This was attributed to a generally poor level of oral hygiene in the former group. The administrators were more effective in their home-care methods.

It has been shown that the degree of periodontal disease is directly proportional to the amount of debris left on the tooth surface. A study was undertaken by Brandtzaeg[12] in 1964, who showed that when comprehensive instructions in oral hygiene methods were given to patients, there was a 40 per cent improvement in oral hygiene with a concurrent 45 per cent improvement in periodontal health. This established a positive relationship between the degree of oral cleanliness and the periodontal health status. At about this time, Greene[22] published a thorough review of the literature on oral hygiene as it relates to periodontal disease. In the summary of his review he wrote, "The one consistent factor associated with the prevalence and severity of periodontal disease is the status of oral cleanliness."

Several other well-controlled clinical studies have shown that the degree of gingival inflammation is related to the level of oral hygiene. Loe and coworkers[26] and Thielade and coworkers[37] studied the development of experimental gingivitis in young adults. Students with completely healthy gingivae abstained from cleaning their teeth for 21 days, then re-instituted cleaning. The degree of gingival disease and the subgingival microflora were studied throughout the experimental period. In summary, the findings were:

1. In healthy persons with excellent oral hygiene and healthy gingivae, abstention of all oral hygiene leads to rapid accumulation of dentogingival plaque.

2. Gingivitis develops within 21 days.

3. When oral hygiene is reintroduced, the plaque reduces, and the gingiva returns to its former healthy state.

4. Cessation of oral hygiene leads to characteristic bacterial changes in subgingival plaque as gingivitis progresses. However, when oral hygiene is resumed, the bacterial flora revert to that which existed in the healthy gingival sulcus prior to the withdrawal of oral hygiene.

Such experiments confirm that poor oral hygiene is directly related to the development of periodontal disease and that if subgingival plaque is absent, inflammatory periodontal disease will not occur.

Another very important study consisted of young Swedish school children between the ages of 7 and 14.[6] They were recalled for re-education in the rationale of home care and motivation every second week for two years. In addition, clinicians thoroughly cleaned their teeth with a sodium fluoride–containing toothpaste. By these procedures, all children attained and maintained optimal periodontal health and developed very few carious lesions. Once again this study confirmed the fact that the major dental diseases cannot exist in the absence of plaque.

Recently, further weight has been added to this philosophy by Scandinavian investigators Rosling and coworkers,[33] who studied 50 adult patients between 28 and 62 years of age. The patients presented with moderate to advanced periodontitis and had all disease eliminated by conventional treatment techniques. Post-operatively, they were seen every two weeks for reinforcement in plaque control, re-education in home-care tech-

niques, and thorough polishing of their teeth. After two years, they were virtually plaque-free and had almost no gingivitis or periodontitis. In other words, their dentition had been returned to and maintained in health. This was entirely a result of the excellence of their plaque control. Such studies show that periodontal health can be achieved and maintained only when patients regularly undertake subgingival plaque control.

The dentogingival area around the entire tooth circumference must be routinely cleaned. As mentioned previously, interproximal regions are the areas most neglected by the patient, and buccal areas are the most accessible. This explains the fact that destructive periodontal disease occurs most frequently and with the greatest severity in interproximal areas. The least diseased sites are buccal, with lingual areas falling in between. This has led to the erroneous belief that interproximal tissues are intrinsically more susceptible to inflammatory periodontal diseases than buccal or lingual areas. The differences in distribution of periodontal disease are simply caused by varying efficiency in home care of the different tooth surfaces.

From a positive point of view, periodontal health can be attained when patients regularly remove all subgingival plaque. The home-care aids used to control caries are also the ones used against the periodontal disease-producing plaque. For buccal and lingual surfaces, the toothbrush is most effective. To reach the subgingival tooth surfaces, its bristles must be angled into the sulcus, as will be discussed later in this chapter. Floss or wooden toothpicks are most commonly recommended for interproximal subgingival cleaning, particularly when the papilla fills the embrasure space. If the embrasure is "open," that is, some papillary recession has occurred, specially designed toothbrushes can be used for interproximal subgingival cleaning. All hygienic procedures used as part of a daily regime can clean the tooth surface to about 3 mm subgingivally. This is usually the maximum depth of gingival sulcus in health. When the gingival tissue becomes enlarged and inflamed, the probable sulcus deepens beyond 3 mm and becomes a periodontal pocket. When this occurs, normal cleaning to the base of the sulcus is impossible. The intervention of the clinician is then required, primarily to institute treatments aimed at establishing a high level of patient motivation and home care and at reducing the pockets to their original "physiologic depth" of 1 to 3 mm or less. It is very important to remember that it is the clinician's job to re-create a gingival morphology and sulcus depth that is compatible with good home-care procedures. At the outset, it must be made quite clear to the patient that it is his responsibility to maintain periodontal health with proper, daily hygiene measures. A crucial part of therapy also includes regularly recalling the patient to monitor and reinforce home-care efforts.

Although much work still needs to be done to determine the best methods of motivating a patient toward achieving a high level of subgingival plaque control and to determine how frequently the patients should be recalled, it is quite clear that the effectiveness of home care determines the level of periodontal health. A poorly motivated patient requires special attention. There is no point in comprehensively treating such people until they can become motivated enough to undertake proper home care, pre- and post-operatively.

Earlier it was pointed out that the consistency of the diet had little effect in reducing caries. Obviously, if the forces of mastication do not clean the dentogingival area, they will not favorably influence periodontal health. While the nature of the diet is undoubtedly important in affecting systemic health, it does not appear to influence human periodontal health. Diet by itself initiates neither plaque formation nor gingivitis.[16] It seems that regardless of the patient's diet, if the teeth are kept clean, periodontal health prevails.

Much research is currently being directed toward the role of mouth rinses as part of an effective home-care plan. While solutions such as chlorhexidine, and oxygen-liberating agents help reduce plaque and gingivitis,[27, 40] they seem to have little influence on the subgingival microflora. Such differences seem to be quantitative rather than qualitative. It has never been shown that solutions such as those that reduce but do not completely eliminate gingivitis or plaque on a long-term basis are of any clinical value in preventing eventual periodontitis. It appears that it is the *presence* of pathogenic subgingival plaque that is crucial for disease onset, not *quantity*. Similarly, it is not at all clear that mildly inflamed gingivae are any less likely to develop periodontitis than more inflamed areas.

One may conclude that, at present, the most practical way to prevent oral disease is to develop specific procedures for each patient. This will enable the patient to maintain an optimal level of oral hygiene. Currently, the maintenance of cleanliness is primarily achieved by mechanical dispersion and removal of adherent microorganisms from the tooth surfaces.

These views are expressed by Loe,[27] who has written a succinct review of the methods through which plaque may be prevented and controlled. He discussed the three major categories of cleaning described above, namely, natural, mechanical, and chemical cleaning. His conclusions were as follows:

Available data from research seems to justify the clinical hypothesis that bacterial plaque is the direct cause of marginal periodontal disease and that caries will not develop in the absence of plaque. Consequently, the control of plaque represents the essential measure in the prevention of the two main dental diseases.

Since natural cleansing of the dental-gingival area is inadequate, plaque control can only be achieved through its active removal at regular intervals. The addition of various enzymes, theoretically capable of interfering with plaque development . . . has not as yet been promising. Prevention of plaque adhesion by changing the surface charge of the teeth is also at the experimental stage. Tests of various antibiotic substances have confirmed that complete prevention of plaque is possible [in animals]. However, the problems inherent to continuous use of antibiotics suggest that they will not be acceptable to the lifelong control of plaque. Experiments with antibacterial agents other than antibiotics have demonstrated that bacterial colonization of teeth can be inhibited by suppressing the oral flora. More knowledge of the effect of such ecological shifts and possible side effects is needed before antibacterial substances can be introduced for clinical use.

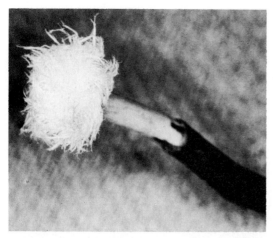

Figure 11–1 A twig from a black gum tree found in the southeastern United States. The bark is removed and the end chewed until it is frayed. (Courtesy of Dr. T. Weatherford, University of Alabama.)

It is with this in mind that the following portion of this chapter discusses the equipment necessary for the removal of plaque and the various methods by which this equipment can be used.

THE PREVENTIVE EQUIPMENT

Before beginning a detailed description of specific preventive measures, it is useful to gain an historic perspective of dental hygienic concepts and procedures. Oral cleanliness was advocated by the Sumerians around 3000 B.C. Golden toothpicks unearthed at Ur in Mesopotamia indicate a significant awareness of dental health. The Babylonians described elaborate oral hygiene measures, including gingival massage and herbal mouth rinses.

The "chew sticks" apparently were first used by ancient Chinese civilizations and are still in use by certain people as illustrated in Figures 11–1 and 11–2. The patient had excellent oral hygiene, which was achieved by cleaning with the frayed ends of a small twig. This emphasizes the point that motivation and habitual patterns of optimal plaque control, not the device itself, are the important factors in disease prevention.

As dentistry evolved into a professional entity, specific preventive concepts began to become established. In 1917 Hill[23] wrote: "Modern dentistry is devoting much effort toward preventing and removing the cause of disease, as well as repairing the damage after bad habits. . . . The way to avoid decay and pyorrhea (periodontitis) is to keep the mouth scrupulously cleaned, preventing deposits from forming on the teeth." He recommended such oral hygiene aids as toothbrushes, wooden toothpicks, and floss.

Sixty-two years later, in 1979, Axelsson and Lindhe[6] made similar conclusions fol-

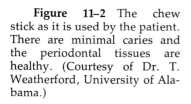

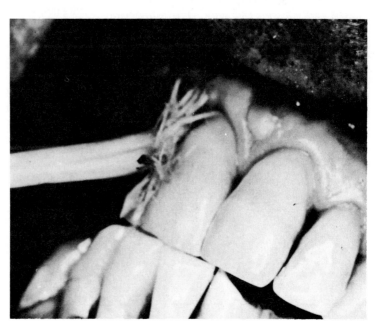

Figure 11–2 The chew stick as it is used by the patient. There are minimal caries and the periodontal tissues are healthy. (Courtesy of Dr. T. Weatherford, University of Alabama.)

lowing a study that showed that good oral hygiene could eliminate caries and periodontal disease. The home-care aids used by their patients were disclosing tablets, the toothbrush, floss, and toothpicks. They concluded that "dental treatment is a highly ineffective means of curing caries and periodontal disease." It is the dispersion of plaque from an infected tooth surface that is important.

The techniques employed toward this end must fulfill the following criteria:

1. The technique must be simple and easily learned.
2. It must not be injurious.
3. It must be able to render all accessible supra- and subgingival tooth surfaces plaque-free.

Generally, no single technique meets these criteria. Proper home care incorporates several techniques. Those most commonly recommended include: disclosing solution to stain plaque and make it obvious to the patient; a lighted mouth mirror with which to see the stained plaque; and the toothbrush, floss, or other devices to remove the plaque. These are illustrated in Figure 11–3. This approach to the problem of plaque control was largely developed by Bass[8] and Arnim,[3] who directed attention toward preventive care by stressing the need to control the disease onset. However, it is humbling to note that although dental disease prevention has been taught and advocated since antiquity, the dental diseases are still among the most common in the world. It seems as though each generation acknowledges the importance of dental preventive care but fails to adhere strongly to its concepts.

PLAQUE DETECTION AND DISCLOSING AGENTS

A cleaned tooth surface rapidly accumulates plaque when cleaning routines are stopped. The top part of Fig. 11–4 illustrates tooth surfaces that have been cleaned and polished by a hygienist. A solution containing a vegetable-derived dye, erythrosin, was applied to the teeth. This dye stains bacterial

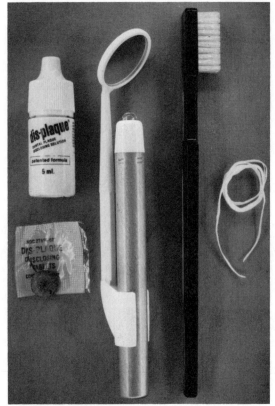

Figure 11–3 The essential equipment for plaque control: disclosing solution or tablets and lighted mouth mirror to see the plaque; brush and floss for plaque removal.

deposits and can be used to locate bacterial plaque. In this instance, because the teeth had been cleaned recently, they were free of bacterial deposits. When plaque is allowed to accumulate over 24 hours, it accumulates both interproximally and at the dentogingival area (Fig. 11–5). In Figure 11–4 also notice the plaque in the depressions on the mid-labial tooth surfaces, "protected" from tongue and lip actions. Plaque-infected tooth surfaces and the adjacent gingival tissues are now "at risk" areas. After six days of plaque accumulation (bottom part of Figure 11–4), note that the deposits stain intensely, indicating their thickness and that they cover most of the surfaces of all teeth. These examples also illustrate the inability of the mouth to "self-cleanse."

The relationship of continued plaque apposition to periodontal disease is illustrated in the photomicrograph in Figure 11–6. Mature subgingival plaque has caused ulcer-

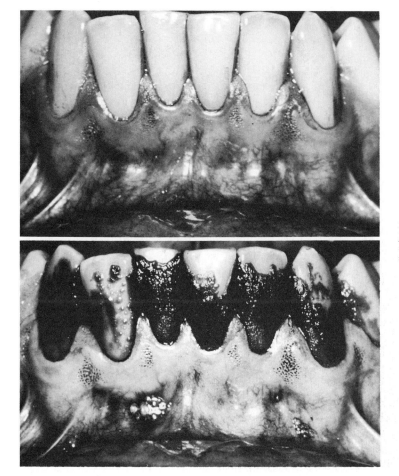

Figure 11–4 *Top:* Staining immediately after prophylaxis. *Bottom:* Plaque accumulation pattern in a patient who has not brushed for six days.

Figure 11–5 Plaque accumulation pattern in a patient who has not brushed for 24 hours.

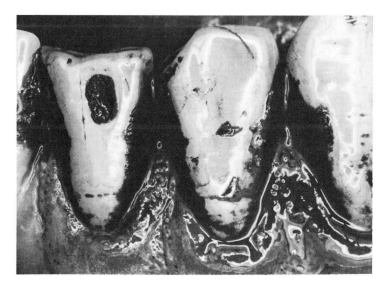

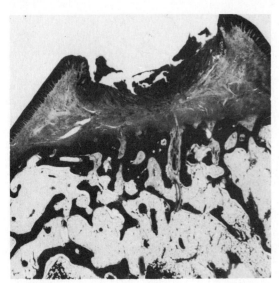

Figure 11–6 Interdental gingiva with plaque in close proximity to ulcerated epithelium. There is characteristic chronic inflammatory reaction in this area. (Courtesy of Dr. S. Hazen, University of Connecticut.)

ations of the sulcular epithelium and marked inflammation in the gingival connective tissues. If plaque build-up is allowed to continue, the inflammation will spread to the alveolar bone, causing resorption of the alveolar bone and destruction of the periodontal ligament fibers. These are the features of advancing periodontitis. The clinical relation of plaque to gingival inflammation is illustrated in Figure 11–7. Regular use of a disclosing solution by the patient after thoroughly cleaning the teeth is strongly advocated.[4] This enables the patient to see all areas that he or she has missed. Any cleaning mistakes can then be corrected.

When a papilla fills the interproximal area, the patient is unable to see the plaque between the papilla and the tooth surface. But, most periodontal disease and caries begin in this crucial, interproximal subgingival area. Perhaps the best way for the patient to determine the efficiency of the interproximal cleaning is to establish the habit of routinely observing the floss, or toothpick for signs of blood. Diseased or inflamed gingivae bleed easily. This is because the gingival lining is ulcerated, as mentioned previously. If a patient notices blood on the floss, this should immediately alert him to the presence of subgingival plaque and associated gingival disease. The patient, know-

ing that he has allowed disease to develop in this area, must then pay particular attention to cleanliness in the future.

The chief value of a disclosing agent is to enable both the patient and the dentist or hygienist to evaluate the efficiency of home care, which is the crucial part of a preventive program. A variety of dyes in either tablet or solution form have been used for many years. The two types most commonly used now are F.D.C. Red No. 3 (erythrosin) and a metachromatic, two-color dye.

A problem with erythrosin is that the red-stained dentogingival plaque is similar in color to the adjacent gingivae. This can be confusing to patients in such difficult-to-see areas as embrasure spaces and around posterior teeth. Plaque stained blue by the metachromatic dye is better visualized. Another advantage of the metachromatic dye is that it differentially stains "new" and "old" plaque. The blue-stained older plaque has the following characteristics:

1. It is thick and densely populated with many bacteria.
2. The microorganisms are arranged in specific patterns: the colonies are in parallel rows, perpendicular to the tooth surface.
3. Numerous rods, cocci, and filaments are seen.
4. Spirochetes are plentiful. These organisms are characteristic of pathogenic plaque associated with gingivitis and periodontitis.

The red staining plaque, which is immature, demonstrates the following features:

1. The plaque is extremely thin and not densely populated with bacteria.
2. There is no orderly arrangement of bacteria.
3. No spirochetes are present.

In commenting on the value of two-toned agents over erythrosin, Block and coworkers[10] stated: "The two-toned dye test provides the patient and dentist with a color guide to quickly determine where the patient consistently fails to remove plaque efficiently." The advantages of a plaque disclosant to a patient are obvious, and all conscientious

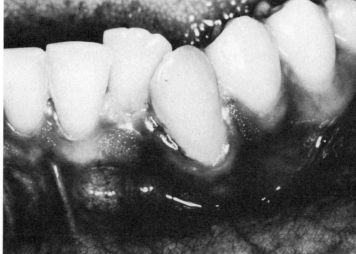
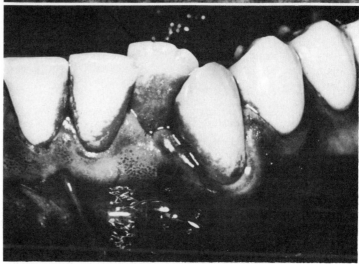

Figure 11–7 *Top:* Plaque that is not evident. *Bottom:* Plaque stained with a disclosing solution. Notice the amount of gingival inflammation in the areas of heavy plaque accumulation and minimal inflammation where there is little or no plaque.

home-care programs should include this routine.

TOOTHBRUSH

In Western societies, the toothbrush has been described as "the classic and often principal method employed in oral hygiene procedures."[38] Toothbrush design has been widely studied, yet there is no convincing evidence to support the idea that one type is better than another in terms of plaque-removing efficiency. The Council on Dental Therapeutics of the American Dental Association[1] clearly stated this position and concluded that "the method and toothbrush of choice depend upon the patient's oral health, manual dexterity, personal preference, and his ability and desire to learn and follow prescribed procedures." No definite superiority has been shown for either natural or synthetic bristles.

In the past, hard-bristle brushes were recommended. These days, most authorities generally suggest the use of a multitufted brush either identical or similar in design to that recommended by Bass.[7] The specifications of such brushes are as follows:

A. *General form and shape*
   1. Plain, straight handle about 6″ long and ⁷/₁₆″ wide.
   2. Three rows of tufts; six tufts per row; each row evenly spaced.
B. *Filaments*
   1. Made of high quality nylon.
   2. Width of bristles: .007 inch wide.

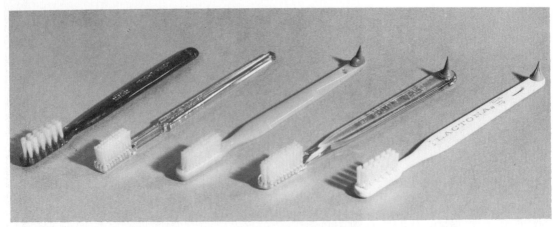

Figure 11–8 Various types of multitufted brushes with nylon bristles. From left to right: Bass "Right Kind," Oral B-40, Pycopay Softex, Butler GUM-411, Lactona S-19.

3. Length of bristles: $^{13}/_{32}$ inch.
4. Ends of bristles should be rounded and polished.
C. *Tufts*
1. 80 to 86 filaments per tuft.

This type of brush is shown in Figure 11–8 on the extreme left. It is an example of the original multitufted brush design that has now been modified. The modifications were necessary because the original design deteriorated rapidly. The newer design, exemplified by the other brushes, provides more rigidity and lasts longer under normal conditions. The head of the newer brush is shown in Figure 11–9.

The bristles are perhaps the most important consideration in selecting a good toothbrush. It is generally agreed that rounded, polished bristle tips are more effective and the least damaging to tissues. An excellent report on different bristles has been published by Gilson and coworkers.[20] He examined the ends of the bristles of twelve different multitufted hand brushes and six brushes used in electric toothbrushes. Wide variation in the ends of the bristles was found. It was concluded that only one (Butler GUM) had ends that were polished and smooth to "a high degree of roundness." Figure 11–10 is an enlargement of rounded, polished bristles; Figure 11–11 shows a magnification of three different bristle types.

Repeated traumatic toothbrushing can gradually lead to irreversible defects in the form of gingival recession and cervical tooth abrasion. Researchers have found that it is the toothpaste that is largely responsible for most cervical tooth abrasion.[32] Gingival damage is usually caused by trauma from bristle ends.[14] It has been shown that most acute gingival injuries occur when patients begin using a new toothbrush.[21] Up to 80 per cent of new toothbrushes have bristles with sharp, cut ends rather than polished tips. This is important to the patient, because the

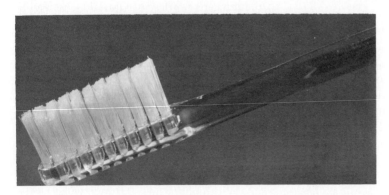

Figure 11–9 Butler GUM-411. A multitufted brush with filaments longer toward the center of the brush. There are 42 tufts, 34 bristles per tuft; .007 inch bristle diameter; bristle length: 11/32 to 14/32 inch.

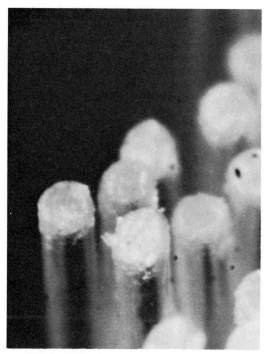

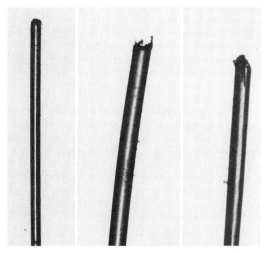

Figure 11–11 Bristle ends. From left to right: round nylon polished bristle from a multitufted brush; nylon bristle from a brush labeled "extra hard"; a bristle from a hard, natural-bristled brush.

Figure 11–10 Magnification of rounded polished ends of the proper type of bristle.

incidence of traumatic gingival injuries is 30 per cent higher when the bristle ends are unpolished.[14]

The potential danger of the hard-bristled brush is shown in Figure 11–12. This patient was a twenty-eight-year-old woman who was given the brush just one week previously. Notice the amount of splaying of the tufts and how jagged the edges of the bristles

became. This patient was a compulsive brusher who used a lot of force in her strokes. The amount of recession was probably directly related to this toothbrush trauma.

Unfortunately, the brush most frequently recommended by the clinician may not be the one used by the patient. The brushes with multitufted, soft bristles are most desirable. However, O'Connor[30] studied the toothbrushes in Lancaster County, Pennsylvania and found that only one fourth of them were satisfactory in bristle design. Fanning

Figure 11–12 Localized moderate gingival recession associated with hard bristles and excessive brushing.

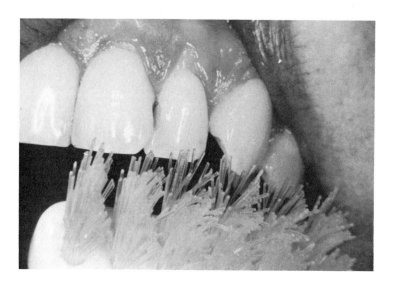

and Henning[17] in Australia showed that of 51 brushes only 5 were acceptable in design and bristle characteristics. Of eight brushes available for children, none were acceptable.

A question that frequently arises is the relative efficiency of the hand versus the powered brush. The advantages of the powered brush are that more strokes can be applied in a shorter period and that it can be used for a longer time because there is less arm fatigue. It is suggested that the hand brush may be more versatile, but in the final analysis it is the motivation of the patient that determines the degree of cleanliness. There are no essential differences between the ability of hand and powered brushes in terms of plaque removal. When used correctly, both are equally effective. Obviously, the opposite is also true. When improperly used,

TABLE 11–1 SUMMARY OF METHODS OF BRUSHING

METHOD	BRISTLE AND PLACEMENT	MOTION	ADVANTAGES AND DISADVANTAGES
Bass	apically, toward gingiva into the gingival sulcus at a 45-degree angle to the tooth surface	very short back and front vibratory; bristle ends remain in the sulcus	removes plaque from cervical area and sulcus, small area covered at one time, good gingival stimulation, easily learned
Charters	coronally, with sides of bristles half on teeth and half on gingiva at a 45-degree angle to tooth surface	small circular, with bristle ends remaining stationary	cleans interproximal areas, but bristle ends do not go into sulcus, hard to learn, hard to position brush in some areas of the mouth, excellent gingival stimulation
Fones	perpendicular to tooth surface	on buccal surfaces, a wide circular movement to include gingiva and tooth surfaces; on lingual surfaces, a back-and-forth horizontal motion	interproximal areas not cleaned, easy to learn, possible trauma to gingiva
"Physiologic"	coronally and then along an arc over the tooth surfaces and gingiva	gentle sweeping starting on teeth and progressing over gingiva	is "physiologic," mimics the passage of food over the gingiva, does not emphasize the interproximal or sulcus areas
Roll	apically, nearly parallel to the tooth surface, then in an arc over tooth surfaces	on buccal and lingual surfaces slight inward pressure at first, then a rolling of the head to sweep bristles over the gingiva and tooth surfaces; occlusal surfaces cleaned with horizontal stroke	does not clean sulcus area, easy to learn, requires moderate dexterity, good gingival stimulation
Stillman	on buccal and lingual surfaces, apically at an oblique angle to the long axis of the tooth; ends rest on gingiva and cervical portion of tooth; on occlusal surfaces, perpendicular to occlusal surface	on buccal and lingual surfaces, slight rotary with bristle ends stationary; on occlusal surfaces, horizontal	excellent gingival stimulation, bristles do not enter sulcus, interproximal area is cleaned when occlusal surfaces are brushed, moderate dexterity required
Intrasulcular	apically, towards gingiva into gingival sulcus at a 45-degree angle to the tooth surface or towards gingiva almost parallel to long axis of the teeth	on buccal and lingual surfaces, a very short back-and-forth vibratory or very small circular motion with bristle tips remaining in the sulcus, then the brush head is rolled toward the occlusal surface; occlusal surfaces cleaned with horizontal stroke	good interproximal and gingival cleaning, good gingival stimulation, requires moderate dexterity

both are ineffective. At present one may conclude that the powered brush is useful for patients with such physical handicaps as paralysis or arthritis or for patients with limited manual dexterity.

Methods of Brushing

There are almost as many methods of brushing as there are types of brushes. The rationale and directions for the Bass technique are presented in detail here. The most common methods are summarized in Table 11–1. There are two basic ways a brush can be used to clean the teeth. The first is as a broom would be used, with the sides of the bristles moving in a sweeping motion. The other is a scrubbing action whereby the ends of the bristles scrub the tooth surfaces clean.

The requirements of any method are that it be easily learned and that it not injure the periodontal tissues. The scrub technique is the most popular method of brushing and requires the least time. In the 1977 International Conference on Research in the Biology of Periodontal Disease,[24] scrubbing was recommended as the basic method of choice. The best techniques involve brushing and the use of unwaxed floss. The position of the brush in relation to the gingiva is shown in Figure 11–13. The bristles actually displace

the marginal gingiva and reach the base of a healthy sulcus (Fig. 11–14). A recent study has shown that this technique is superior to the roll technique in removing dentogingival plaque.[19] In terms of periodontal disease prevention, this technique is most useful. The angulation of the brush also allows the bristles to reach into and clean the embrasure spaces. This is illustrated in Figure 11–15. The top half of the photograph shows the bristles incorrectly placed at a right angle to the tooth surface. With this angulation, the patient can clean the prominences of each tooth surface, but the subgingival and embrasure areas cannot be reached. The bottom half of the photograph shows the results of placing the bristles at a 45° angle to the tooth. In this position the cervical and embrasure areas can be cleaned effectively.

Even with this placement, however, the entire interproximal area is not reached. Consequently, Bass[9] suggested that dental floss be used to remove this plaque. Although waxed floss was popular at the time, Bass believed that unwaxed floss would be superior by entrapping the plaque in its many fine filaments. Some people suggest that unwaxed floss is superior to waxed. Studies do not reveal significant differences between them. Recently, another floss, "Super Floss," has been introduced into the market. It is illustrated with the other floss

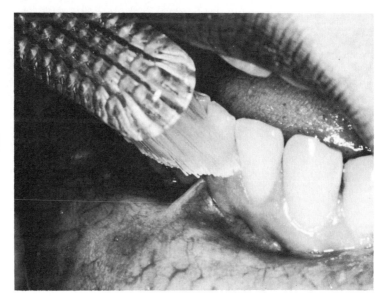

Figure 11–13 Angulation of bristles in the Bass method of brushing.

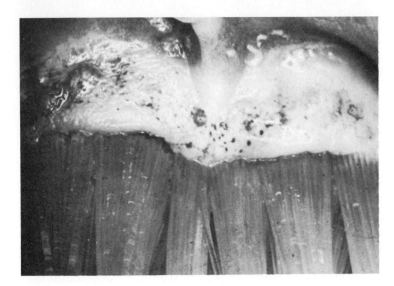

Figure 11–14 Bristles placed into the gingival sulcus. (Courtesy of Dr. G. J. Parfitt, University of British Columbia.)

Figure 11–15 *Top:* Angulation of bristles at a right angle to tooth surface fails to reach interproximal areas. *Bottom:* Angulation of bristles at a 45 degree angle to tooth surface causes bristles to reach the interproximal area.

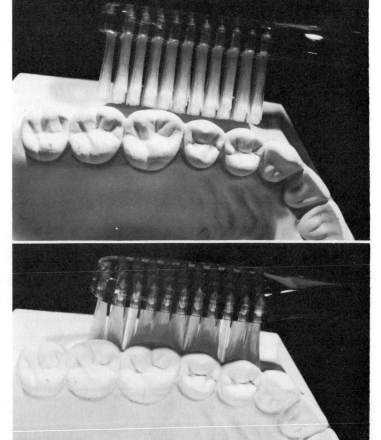

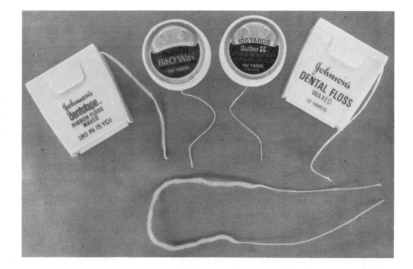

Figure 11–16 Different types of dental floss. *Bottom:* Super Floss. *Left to right:* Dental tape, lightly waxed, shred-resistant unwaxed, waxed.

types in Figures 11–16 and 11–17. The broadened, "Fluffy" area supposedly cleans the interproximal surfaces better than conventional floss, but no studies have been undertaken to test this contention.

Each of the different flosses has its advantages, but the thinner unwaxed floss is generally preferred by most patients. It does have a tendency to shred but can be passed through the contact area with less separation of teeth than waxed floss. People who have tight contacts or large, rough restorations often find waxed floss easier to use. All floss should be used with care. It can injure the gingival tissue if passed through contact areas with too much force.

The technique of flossing is important. The method is illustrated in Figure 11–18. Floss is wound around the index finger of each hand and then placed through the contact area by gentle pressure with the thumbs. It is then guided between the gingival margin into the sulcus and gently flattened against the tooth surface, as shown in Figures 11–18 and 11–19. The flattened floss is then moved in an apico-coronal direction. The tooth surface above and below the gingival margin is cleaned in this manner. The floss is then moved across the interproximal tissue to the adjacent tooth surface, which is cleaned in a similar fashion. When the floss is removed from between the two teeth, the

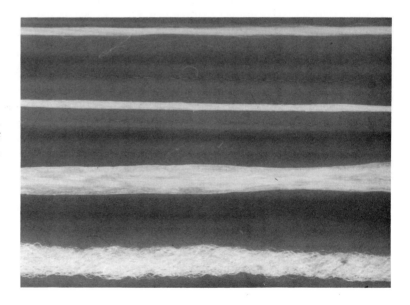

Figure 11–17 Magnification of different types of floss. *Top to bottom:* unwaxed floss; lightly waxed floss; dental tape; Super Floss.

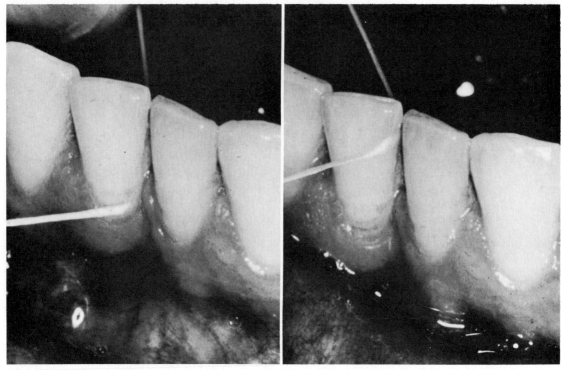

Figure 11-18 Placement of floss in the interproximal areas.

patient must remember to check it for signs of gingival bleeding. Such bleeding indicates the presence of inflamed gingivae caused by chronic build-up of subgingival plaque. When it is not possible to place floss through a contact area, for example, under bridgework, a floss threader must be used to thread the floss under the pontic (Fig. 11–20). A specially designed brush, such as the Proxa-

brush, is also useful in such situations (see Fig. 11–20).

The value of meticulous subgingival plaque removal in periodontal disease control is illustrated by the following case:

A twelve-year-old female presented with heavy supra- and subgingival plaque accumulations (Fig. 11–21). A disclosing solution was used (middle part of figure) and

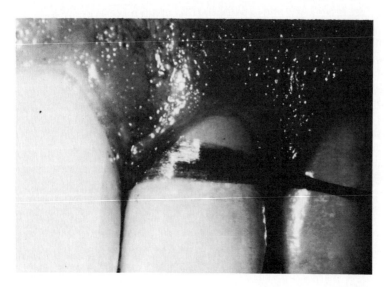

Figure 11–19 Flattening of the unwaxed floss against the surface of the tooth in the gingival sulcus. (Courtesy of Butler Brush Company and Dr. J. Seibert.)

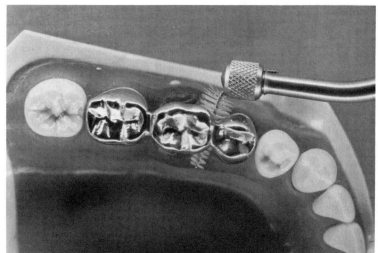

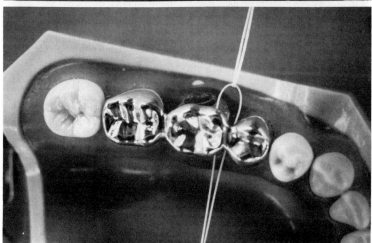

Figure 11–20 Home care of bridgework. *Top:* Interproximal brush. *Bottom:* Floss threader and floss.

the patient was instructed in the use of a multitufted brush and floss, using the method described by Bass. No other treatment was given. At the end of the week, the patient was re-examined and a disclosing solution was again used. The results are shown in the bottom part of Figure 11–21. Plaque-control had improved considerably. There was some plaque in the interproximal area, which showed that reinforcement of the technique of floss use was needed. Notice that the improved home care had caused a marked decrease in gingival inflammation over this time.

It may be concluded that tooth-cleaning methods are subject to much variation. Many techniques are based on empiricism, clinical experience, and personal preference. To be effective, any brushing program should be simple, easily learned, and require minimal reinforcement and dexterity. It must remove the plaque from the gingival sulcus and the interproximal area, where periodontal disease and caries most commonly occur. For these reasons the technique suggested by Bass is the one that is recommended.

THE AUXILIARY AIDS IN ORAL HYGIENE

The previous sections have stressed the importance of mechanical plaque removal by brushing and flossing. There are many other types of mechanical devices available. Only two types are discussed here: devices for interproximal cleaning and devices using forced water irrigation.

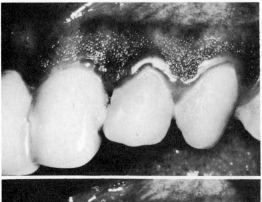

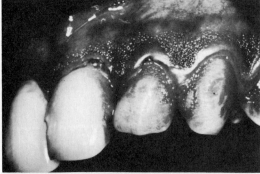

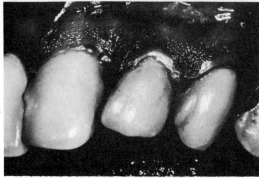

Figure 11–21 *Top:* Patient at initial visit with heavy plaque accumulation. *Middle:* Patient at initial visit with disclosing solution applied to reveal heavy plaque. *Bottom:* Patient seven days later with disclosing solution applied. Treatment has consisted of oral hygiene instruction with Bass technique. There is much less plaque and the gingival inflammation has been reduced.

Water Irrigating Devices

As in the case of the powered brushes, there has been a flurry of discussion in recent years on the usefulness of water irrigating devices. It is not a new idea; it was suggested by G. V. Black in 1915 as a possibly useful method of cleaning the subgingival area. These devices supposedly flush the gingival sulcus free of bacteria, their products, and other debris. However, they have been shown to be only minimally effective in these functions. Although they may have some effect on supragingival plaque, they do not appear to have any significant effects on subgingival plaque.[11, 31] Of course, it is subgingival plaque control that is so important in maintaining periodontal health, and these devices are not effective in this regard.

A very serious possible consequence of water irrigating devices must be discussed. It has been shown that it can cause bacteremia in patients with periodontitis.[36] More significantly, some case reports[15, 25] have suggested that the use of water irrigation may have contributed to the onset of a severe cardiac disease, infective endocarditis. It is for this reason as well as its ineffectiveness in subgingival plaque control that we cannot recommend the routine use of such devices. If they are ineffective, they only frustrate conscientious patients and waste their time. Patients would be better off concentrating on the use of conventional cleaning techniques.

Miscellaneous Interproximal Cleaning Aids

Generally, devices other than floss are limited to use by adult patients. In children and adolescents, the interdental space is filled with the papilla and there is inadequate room for anything but floss. This is also the case with many adults. However, adults who have gingival recession or who have undergone periodontal treatment usually have adequate space for the placement of interdental devices. The cleaners are usually wooden toothpicks of varying shapes and sizes or specially devised brushes such as the Proxabrush. A multitude of other aids, including rubber tips on the ends of toothbrushes and pipe cleaners have been recommended. Some of these are illustrated in Figure 11–22. If used correctly, all seem to have a role in periodontal health maintenance. Perhaps the most widely used cleaners are the interdental brushes and the wooden toothpicks. These are extremely useful for patients with fixed bridgework. Although floss has been shown to be most

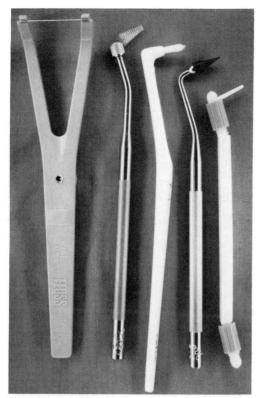

Figure 11–22 Home-care aids for interproximal cleaning. *From left to right:* Floss holder, interproximal brush, single-tufted toothbrush, rubber "stimulator," toothpick and handle.

effective in removing plaque from the interproximal and embrasure spaces, there is little difference in the effectiveness of any interproximal device when used correctly.

CHEMOTHERAPEUTIC AGENTS IN HOME CARE

Investigators have long been interested in the possibilities of utilizing chemicals in the control of dental diseases. Fluoride is a dramatic example of success in this field. It is not the purpose of this chapter to embark upon a lengthy dissertation on chemotherapy, since this is adequately covered elsewhere in the book.

In the field of periodontics, many attempts have been made to devise an antiplaque solution that could replace the types of mechanical techniques discussed previously. Ideally, such a chemical must remain in the mouth and on the tooth long enough to destroy the bacteria or matrix of the plaque. Such a chemical must also prevent the re-formation of plaque. Most antiplaque agents tested so far have been ineffective, since they do not remain on the tooth surface long enough, or have poor penetration into the crucial subgingival area.

Many different mouth rinses have been developed, but the only one with promising results is chlorhexidine. Its effectiveness seems to result from its ability to be retained in the mouth for long periods. However, animal and human studies indicate that it may only be of limited, short-term benefit.[24, 27] It reduces but does not eliminate plaque and gingivitis. It also seems to have poor penetration into the sulcus and has several side effects such as an unpleasant taste and adverse effects on taste sensation. It also tends to discolor anterior restorations.

It must be remembered that plaque bacteria are part of the total oral and body microbiologic ecosystem. Long-term attempts at the chemical destruction of selected bacterial populations could adversely affect this entire ecology. This has already been demonstrated by the use of antibiotic administrations, which upset this delicate balance, leading to overpopulation of certain oral fungi and sometimes resulting in the disease moniliasis or "thrush." This ecologic factor must be considered when evaluating new mouth rinses.

SUMMARY

In summary, the underlying theme of this chapter is that prevention of disease onset is the only effective way of resolving the major dental diseases, caries and periodontitis. For this to be efficient, both clinician and patient must have a strong, positive attitude toward the desirability of oral health. This may be no problem for the clinician, but appropriate patient counseling may be necessary. Generally, the public is painfully unaware that they are in a diseased state.

Many ways have been proposed to make the teeth clean. A few of these have been discussed in this chapter, while others have not. Perhaps a method of reviewing some of

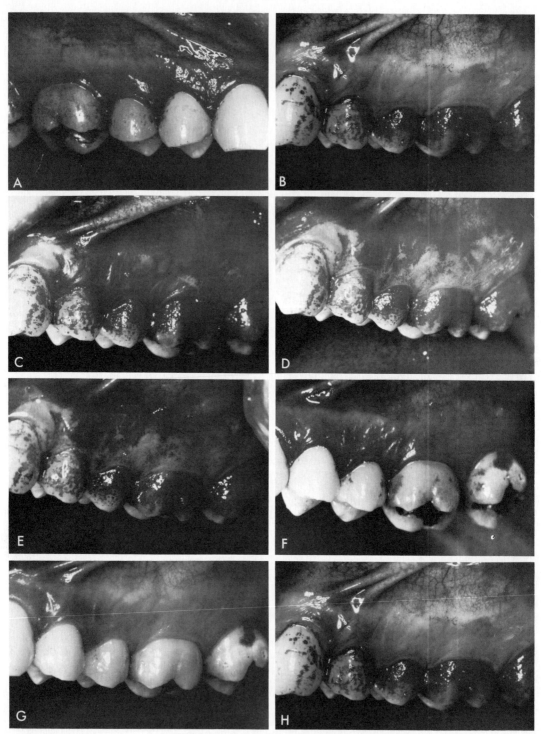

Figure 11–23 Plaque accumulation over a three-day period and a series of procedures to remove plaque. Each procedure followed in order listed: *A,* Regular brushing on left side. *B,* No brushing for three days on right side. *C,* Effect of rinsing for two minutes with a mouth rinse. *D,* Effect of chewing a carrot for two minutes. Plaque is removed primarily from the attached gingiva. *E,* Effect of two minutes' irrigation with a water irrigating device. *F,* Effect of brushing for two minutes: Bass technique with a dentifrice. *G,* Effect of using floss for two minutes and a final water rinse. Even though extensive cleaning has been done, plaque remains in the carious lesion. *H,* Contrast of cleaned versus non-cleaned tooth surfaces.

the ways would be to look at Figure 11–23. This is a technique suggested by Arnim to show the relative effectiveness of various agents in removing plaque. It is also an excellent teaching and learning device for students. This photograph shows a dental student who was given hard candy to eat and was told not to brush the right side of his mouth for three days. He was allowed to brush the left side. The contrast between the brushed and nonbrushed sides is evident in parts *A* and *B*. After the plaque was stained the student was told to perform a number of procedures in the following order for a two-minute period: rinse with a commercial mouth rinse (Fig. 11–23*C*), chew a carrot (Fig. 11–23*D*), use a water irrigating device (Fig. 11–23*E*), brush according to the Bass technique with a dentifrice (Fig. 11–23*F*), and use dental floss (Fig. 11–23*G*). The teeth were stained after each procedure. Slight differences can be detected depending on the procedure. However, the most obvious changes are seen when the brush is used and the final interproximal areas are cleaned with the floss. It is interesting to see the plaque retention in the carious lesion on the buccal surface of the second molar.

The frequent removal of plaque from all exposed tooth surfaces is the mandatory first step in disease prevention. This is usually by physical means, utilizing such aids as tooth brushes, floss, and wooden toothpicks. It is also important to remember that interproximal cleaning is usually the most inefficient part of the prevention program of most people. It is here that disease occurs most frequently and with greatest severity. We cannot recommend lavage by pulsating water devices for plaque removal. It is generally a useless device, with possible serious systemic consequences. Chemotherapeutic plaque control is still not available, although the search continues. Most of all, the chief determinants in successful preventive practice are the patient's attitude toward and desire to undertake the necessary oral hygiene measures.

REFERENCES

1. Accepted Dental Therapeutics 1971/1972, 34th ed. Chicago, American Dental Association, p. 241.
2. American Dental Association, Bureau of Economic Research Statistics, Utilization of Dental Services by the Elderly Population. 1979.
3. Arnim, S. S.: An effective program of oral hygiene for the arrestment of dental caries and the control of periodontal disease. J. South. Calif. Dent. Assoc. 35:264, 1967.
4. Arnim, S. S.: The use of disclosing agents for measuring tooth cleanliness. J. Periodontol. 34:277, 1963.
5. Arno, S., et al.: Incidence of gingivitis as related to sex, occupation, tobacco consumption, toothbrushing, and age. Oral Surg. 11:587, 1958.
6. Axelsson, P., and Lindhe, J.: The effect of a preventive programme on dental plaque, gingivitis and caries in school children. J. Clin. Periodontol. 1:126, 1979.
7. Bass, C. C.: The optimum characteristics of toothbrushes for personal oral hygiene. Dent. Items Int. 70:967, 1948.
8. Bass, C. C.: An effective method of personal hygiene (Part II). J. La. Med. Soc. 106:100, 1954.
9. Bass, C. C.: The optimum characteristics of dental floss for personal oral hygiene. Dent. Items Int. 70:921, 1948.
10. Block, P., Lobene, R., and Derdivanis, J.: A two-tone dye test for dental plaque. J. Periodontol. 43:423, 1972.
11. Brady, J. M., Gray, W., and Bhaskar, S.: Electron microscopic study of the effect of water jet lavage devices on dental plaque. J. Periodont. Res. 52:1310, 1973.
12. Brandtzaeg, P.: The significance of oral hygiene in the prevention of dental diseases. Odontol. Tidskr. 72:460, 1964.
13. Davies, G. N.: Social customs and habits and their effect on oral disease. J. Dent. Res. 42 (Suppl.) 1:209, 1963.
14. Breitenmoser, J., Mormann, W., and Muhlemann, H. R.: Damaging effects of toothbrush bristle end form on gingiva. J. Periodont. 50:212, 1979.
15. Drapkin, M. S.: Endocarditis after the use of an oral irrigation device. Ann. Int. Med. 87:454, 1977.
16. Egelbert, J.: Local effect of diet on plaque formation and development of gingivitis in dogs. Odont. Rev. 16:50, 1965.
17. Fanning, E. A., and Henning, F. R.: Toothbrush design and its relation to oral health. Aust. Dent. J. 12:464, 1967.
18. Fosdick, L. S.: The reduction of the incidence of dental caries. Immediate toothbrushing with a neutral dentifrice. J. Am. Dent. Assoc. 40:133, 1950.
19. Gibson, J. S., and Wade, A. B.: Plaque removal by the Bass and Roll brushing techniques. J. Periodont. 48:456, 1977.
20. Gilson, C. M., et al.: A comparison of physical properties of several soft toothbrushes. J. Mich. Dent. Assoc. 51:347, 1969.
21. Glickman, J.: Clinical Periodontology. Philadelphia, W. B. Saunders, 1972.
22. Greene, J. C.: Oral health care for the prevention and control of periodontal disease. *In* World Workshop in Periodontics. Ann Arbor, University of Michigan Press, 1966, pp. 399–443.
23. Hill, D. S.: Dental Physiology and Oral Hygiene (Chapter 6). Effingham, Illinois, LeCrone Press, 1917.
24. International Conference on Research in the Biology

of Periodontal Disease. Chicago, Illinois, American Academy of Periodontology, 1977.

25. Kaplan, E. L., and Anderson, R. C.: Infective endocarditis after use of dental irrigation device. Lancet 2:610, 1977.

26. Loe, H., Theilade, E., and Jensen, S. B.: Experimental gingivitis in man. J. Periodont. 36:177, 1965.

27. Loe, H.: A review of the prevention and control of plaque. In McHugh, W. D. (ed.): Dental Plaque. London, E. and S. Livingstone, Ltd., 1970, pp. 259–270.

28. Mansbridge, J. N.: The effects of oral hygiene and sweet consumption on the prevalence of dental caries. Br. Dent. J. 109:343, 1960.

29. Miller, J., and Hobson, P.: The relationship between malocclusion, oral cleanliness, gingival conditions and dental caries in school children. Br. Dent. J. 111:43, 1961.

30. O'Connor, N. J.: Brands, bristles and tufts. The Dental Assistant. 17:22, 1977.

31. O'Leary, T. J., et al.: Possible penetration of crevicular tissue from oral hygiene procedures: 1. Use of oral irrigating devices. J. Periodont. 41:33, 1970.

32. Reisstein, J., Lustman, I., Hershkovitz, J., and Gedalia, J.: Abrasion of enamel and cementum in human teeth due to toothbrushing estimated by S.E.M. J. Dent. Res. 57:42, 1978.

33. Rosling, B., Nyman, S., Lindhe, J., and Jern, B.: The healing potential of the periodontal tissues following different techniques of periodontal surgery in plaque-free dentitions. J. Clin. Periodontol. 3:233, 1976.

34. Saxe, S. R., et al.: Oral debris, calculus and periodontal disease in the beagle dog. Periodontics 5:271, 1967.

35. Suomi, J. D., et al.: The effect of controlled oral hygiene procedures on the progression of periodontal disease in adults: Results after two years. J. Periodontol. 40:416, 1969.

36. Tamini, H. A., et al.: Bacteremia study using a water irrigating device. J. Periodont. 40:424, 1969.

37. Theilade, E., et al.: Experimental gingivitis in man. II. A longitudinal, clinical and bacteriological investigation. J. Periodont. Res. 1:1, 1966.

38. Town, G.: The role of oral hygiene in prevention of periodontal disease and dental caries. N. Z. Dent. J. 75:29, 1979.

39. Waerhaug, J.: Current basis for prevention of periodontal disease. Int. Dent. J. 17:267, 1967.

40. Wennstrom, J., and Lindhe, J.: Effect of hydrogen peroxide on developing plaque and gingivitis in man. J. Clin. Periodontol. 6:115, 1979.

CHAPTER TWELVE

Dental Caries: Prevention and Control

Charles F. Schachtele, M.S., Ph.D.

It has been clearly documented that the formation of dental caries in humans may be completely prevented by the systematic application of measures currently available to the dental profession. As discussed elsewhere in this textbook, disease reduction can result from utilization of fluoride in a manner that optimizes its effectiveness, through application of appropriate oral hygiene procedures, and via alterations in the patterns of ingestion of foodstuffs containing fermentable carbohydrate. Unfortunately, as we are fully aware, these control measures require either changes in individual habits, development of adequate dexterity and skills, or strong motivation. Few individuals have a lifestyle that supports these types of measures, especially for control of a chronic problem that is not life threatening. In addition, the disease primarily affects children and young adults who are unaware of the importance of good oral hygiene. In light of these problems dental scientists have attempted to develop means for caries prevention that require minimal effort and cooperation by the individual.

The current approaches to preventing caries formation in humans are all based on attempts to disrupt the interactions among the etiologic factors known to be responsible for the disease. In this chapter, a selected overview of some of the more exciting nascent approaches to caries prevention are analyzed. An attempt is made to evaluate the efficacy of each approach and to place it into perspective relative to the known multifactorial etiology of the disease.

COMBATING CARIOGENIC BACTERIA

Oral Bacteria and the Human Diet

Scherp[24] clearly described caries as an interaction of bacteria, diet, and host. This simple procedure has provided the basis for efforts to delineate the exact etiology of caries. Much of the progress in this pursuit has resulted from research in oral microbiology. This particular area of investigation has entered a logarithmic phase of growth, and the current literature is presenting new information on this subject at a remarkable rate. As our knowledge of oral bacteria has expanded, we have gained insight into the role of specific oral microorganisms in oral health and disease. In order to appreciate several of the current approaches to caries prevention, it must be clearly emphasized that dental caries is an infectious disease resulting from specific interactions between cariogenic oral bacteria and the fermentable carbohydrates found in the diet. To put this discussion into a proper perspective, we must look first of all at the ecology of the bacteria found in the mouth.

The human oral cavity contains a complex bacterial flora. There are representatives of at least 22 genera of bacteria, and greater than 60 individual strains have been classified into species. This latter number is increasing as previously unisolatable or unidentifiable strains succumb to sophisticated microbiologic methodology. Each type of oral bacteria has characteristics that allow it to survive in the mouth and elude both the flushing and antibacterial influences of saliva as well as competition from other members of this microbial community. It is important that we consider the members of our indigenous oral flora as friends and realize that the symbiotic relationship we have with them may be critical to our health. Members of our oral flora have the potential to contribute to our nutrition, to induce the production of protective antibodies, and to influence the development of various organs and tissues.[9] We are just beginning to appreciate the developmental and immunologic consequences of the several grams of oral bacteria that we swallow each day.

Analysis of the distribution and concentration of the oral flora has demonstrated consistent localization and high population densities. For example, whole human saliva contains approximately 1×10^8 viable bacterial cells per ml. These microbes represent cells dislodged from the different oral surfaces and primarily reflect the composition of the flora attached to the epithelial cells of the tongue. In contrast to mucosal surfaces, which undergo continuous desquamation and recolonization by oral bacteria, the surfaces of human teeth are relatively permanent and consequently accumulate dental plaque with a density of approximately 2×10^{11} bacterial cells per g of wet material. Although the predominant bacteria that make up typical coronal tooth surface plaque are streptococci and gram-positive filaments, a number of other types of bacteria can be isolated from such plaque. By analyzing the composition of plaque collected from adjacent sites on teeth it can be demonstrated that this material consists of a heterogeneous collection of superimposed microcolonies of bacteria. Indeed, the complexity of plaque is emphasized by the statement "the microbial composition of a dental plaque on a single tooth is unique to that site at that time."[26] With this in mind, it is easy to appreciate the problems dental scientists have encountered

in their attempts to associate the bacterial content of plaque samples with the development of dental caries in distinct sites.

Another relevant concept concerning the indigenous flora relates to its nutrition. If we compare the oral cavity to other microbial niches in nature, it would appear that the mouth is a nutritionally rich environment. Substrates capable of supporting a complex and fastidious mixture of bacteria are obtained from the host, other oral bacteria, and the diet. The localized entry into the mouth of various host fluids has a significant influence on the composition and metabolic activity of bacteria at different sites in the oral cavity. Saliva and gingival crevicular fluid contain many potential bacterial substrates, and *in vitro* growth in these fluids has been demonstrated. Support for the nutritional contribution of the host is obtained from data that show (1) that a complex bacterial flora exists and (2) that plaque accumulates on the teeth of human subjects who receive all of their food by stomach tube. It is important to note that the plaque that accumulates under such conditions has diminished acid-producing potential when supplied with fermentable carbohydrate. These types of experiments emphasize the contribution of the host to the nutrition of the oral flora and indicate that the diet may significantly influence the bacteria residing on the various surfaces of the mouth. Although diet may affect the oral flora by altering the ability of the host to provide an acceptable environment, at this time we are primarily concerned with local effects that can occur when substrates are directly supplied as foodstuffs. Surprisingly, with one exceptional case, this is an area that has received minimal attention. Little information is available on the effect of diets with varying levels of nutrients on the oral flora. Dental researchers have obviously missed ideal opportunities to collaborate with investigators involved in past human nutrition studies in which diet control was carefully maintained.

The one aspect of the potential effect of diet on oral bacteria that has received significant study involves investigations on the functioning of carbohydrate. This is not surprising in light of our previous statements on the etiology of caries. It is known that alterations in the ingested levels of carbohydrate can dramatically influence the oral concentrations of certain types of bacteria. Specifically, we know that *Streptococcus mutans* levels in the mouth can be markedly elevated by increasing the quantity of sucrose in the diet. Reduced ingestion of sucrose or replacement of this disaccharide with other carbohydrates causes a decrease in the numbers of *S. mutans* on the teeth.[29] These observations on the response of *S. mutans* to dietary sucrose have been discussed by many scientists and clinicians and are the focal point for much of the controversy concerning the role of dietary components in caries etiology. The exact contribution of various fermentable carbohydrates to dental caries formation in man cannot be properly evaluated without considering what we know about the cariogenicity of *S. mutans* and its interactions with various carbohydrate substrates.

S. MUTANS AS A CARIOGENIC BACTERIUM

The great progress in oral microbiology that we alluded to previously can best be illustrated by evaluating some of the information we have obtained about *S. mutans*. Since the literature on these bacteria is massive and continuously growing, we will focus on aspects of *S. mutans* that are directly related to caries formation.

S. mutans is a bacterium whose rise to prominence required time and insight. In the early 1920's, Clark[4] was attempting to evaluate the etiology of caries by analyzing the microbial content of plaque from human carious lesions. A streptococcal bacterium was isolated consistently from the samples, and its pleomorphic nature (ranging from cocci to rods, depending upon the culture conditions) caused it to be named *Streptococcus mutans*. After this initial report, there were sporadic publications on bacteria with similar characteristics, but it was not until nearly four decades later that intense investigations on *S. mutans* were initiated. The impetus for this work was supplied by investigations performed at the National Institute of Dental Research in the 1960's. In

an expansion of the pioneering studies of Orland and his coworkers,[22] who had conclusively demonstrated that microorganisms were required for the initiation of dental caries, Keyes[13] and Fitzgerald and Keyes[8] showed that, in the animal model, caries is an infectious and transmissible disease and that specific streptococci from carious lesions in animals could induce extensive decay in hamsters. Streptococci that had characteristics very similar to the animal strains were subsequently isolated from human mouths and shown to be capable of causing caries when implanted in animals. The bacteria used in these initial studies were designated *S. mutans* because of their expression of traits that we now use to identify these microorganisms. In general, *S. mutans* is recognized by its ability (1) to produce a distinct colonial morphology when grown under standardized conditions on a sucrose-containing selective medium called mitis salivarius agar, (2) to synthesize extracellular polysaccharide from sucrose, (3) to undergo cell-to-cell aggregation when mixed with sucrose or the polymer of glucose called dextran, and to ferment the polyols mannitol and sorbitol. As we will see, these characteristics may be related to the cariogenic potential of this bacterium.

A great deal of effort has been put into studies attempting to demonstrate the role of *S. mutans* in human caries formation. Although the data from cross-sectional, association-type studies clearly indicate that *S. mutans* can be a significant factor in the development of carious lesions, researchers have been unable to obtain unequivocal evidence concerning the direct involvement of this bacterium in disease initiation or progression. Longitudinal studies evaluating the appearance and increase in levels of *S. mutans* coincident with caries development at a particular site have been attempted, but these provided equivocal results. Because of the multifactorial etiology of caries and the difficulties encountered in longitudinal studies, we may never be able to utilize this method for quantitating the contribution of *S. mutans* to human caries. However, if we were able to eliminate *S. mutans* from the mouths of a group of subjects, we would learn a great deal about the role of this microbe in the disease. This might allow us to evaluate the relative contribution to caries of other members of the oral flora. This is surely a worthwhile goal. Arguments for treating caries as an infectious disease caused by a specific pathogen have been clearly presented by Loesche[14-16] and others. As we will see, this may be achievable through proper application of current theories and technology.

ECOLOGY OF *S. MUTANS*

In order to appreciate the focus of attempts to eradicate *S. mutans* from the oral cavity, the ecology of this bacterium must be considered. The only natural habitat of *S. mutans* appears to be the mouth of humans and some animals. Specifically, this bacterium requires a non-desquamating surface for colonization and consequently is found primarily in plaque on the surfaces of teeth. *S. mutans* does not colonize the mouth of predentate infants but appears shortly after teeth have erupted. This bacterium disappears from the human mouth after the loss of the teeth and will return if dentures are provided.

Our current knowledge concerning acquisition of *S. mutans* by children indicates that maternal transfer is a likely possibility. Parental reservoirs of *S. mutans* are a potential source of bacterial infection in infants whose erupting teeth are being colonized for the first time. In adults, the situation is more complicated, and it has been shown to be difficult to establish experimentally characterized strains of *S. mutans* in the mouths of individuals with a well established oral flora. Rinsing the mouth with cultures of *S. mutans* does not usually lead to implantation, and the bacterium is quickly cleared from the oral cavity. Interestingly, one of the best ways to implant strains of *S. mutans* on human adult teeth is to place a drop of a culture of this bacterium onto a piece of waxed dental floss and work the floss at an approximal site on successive days.[7] Intense localization of high densities of *S. mutans* at specific sites appears to overcome some of the suppressors of colonization. The floss implantation technique has significant implications for the proper use of this material during an individual's routine hygiene procedures. Studies by several groups of investigators have shown that the factors that can regulate the interoral spreading of *S. mutans* would appear to include (1) the frequency of exposure to the bacterium, (2) the dose received during each exposure, (3) the nature and quantity of antibacterial substances present in saliva at the time of exposure, (4) the flow rate of the saliva, (5) the nature of the indigenous flora at the sites of initial contact, (6) and other factors related to the specific adherence mechanisms of *S. mutans*.

One of the key concepts related to *S. mutans* infections and caries involves the results that clearly indicate that this bacterium colonizes teeth in a very localized manner and that the sites that harbor high concentrations of *S. mutans* are those sites that most readily become diseased. In humans, *S. mutans* is isolated with greatest frequency from occlusal surface pits and fissures, approximal areas, and close to the gingival margin. It is well documented that fissure decay is the most prevalent form of human dental caries and that the smooth surfaces of teeth are attacked less effectively. One study has implicated *S. mutans* in fissure caries,[16] and work by Duchin and van Houte[6] strongly supports a role for *S. mutans* in the formation of incipient white spot lesions on buccal tooth surfaces.

It is also important that we appreciate the limited intraoral spread of *S. mutans*. In the dental floss implantation studies it was noted that the established *S. mutans* strains could rarely be subsequently isolated from plaque obtained from teeth on the opposite side of the mouth. Confirmation of the limited intraoral movement of *S. mutans* has been made by placement of *S. mutans* "seeded" artificial fissures into the mouths of human volunteers.[27, 28] In these studies, streptomycin-resistant strains of *S. mutans* were shown to spread very slowly to adjacent and antagonistic teeth and only on the side of the mouth where the fissure was placed. There are clearly strong inhibitors that prevent *S. mutans* from spreading in a manner analogous to more rapidly disseminating bacterial infections. This limited movement of *S. mutans* has direct implications for clini-

Figure 12–1 Extracellular sucrose metabolism by *Streptococcus mutans*. The disaccharide is cleaved, releasing the hexoses glucose and fructose and forming the polysaccharides fructan (Step 1) and glucan (Step 3). The fructan can be degraded to free fructose (Step 2), which is available for cell metabolism. Formation of glucan by *S. mutans* enhances this bacterium's ability to colonize tooth surfaces.

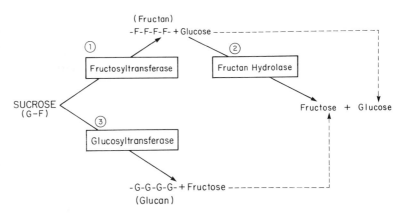

cal dentistry when we consider the possible effects of various techniques routinely used by the dentist. The most striking finding is the demonstration that by probing with a dental explorer *S. mutans* can be transferred with high frequency from a fissure on one side of the mouth to a fissure on the opposite side.[15] Alteration of the microbial content of caries-prone sites on human teeth with a dental explorer is an event whose incidence and significance is probably worthy of additional study.

S. MUTANS AND SUCROSE

S. mutans has the ability to metabolize the disaccharide sucrose by several pathways. Figure 12–1 illustrates how sucrose can be modified by extracellular enzymes to form the polysaccharides fructan (step 1) and glucan (step 3). These reactions allow *S. mutans* to take advantage of the energy contained in the bond between the glucosyl and fructosyl moieties of sucrose. The fructan can be catabolized by a hydrolase (step 2) produced

by several plaque bacteria and this polysaccharide can be considered an extracellular storage material to be utilized when needed. The production of glucans by *S. mutans* is considered to be the critical reaction in the oral accumulation and cariogenicity of this bacterium. Figure 12–2 illustrates the reaction involved in the conversion of sucrose to (1-6) linked glucan with the release of free fructose. Dextransucrase or glucosyltransferase (GTF) is of great interest, since mutants of *S. mutans* that produce elevated or reduced levels of this enzyme initiate correspondingly higher or lower levels of caries when tested in animal model systems. Consequently, this enzyme has been proposed as the prime candidate antigen in the development of an anti-caries vaccine. Blockage of glucan formation from dietary sucrose by secretory antibody inhibition of dextransucrase is an approach to caries prevention that is discussed later in this chapter.

Although intensive research has failed to provide a complete understanding of glucan formation by *S. mutans*, several impor-

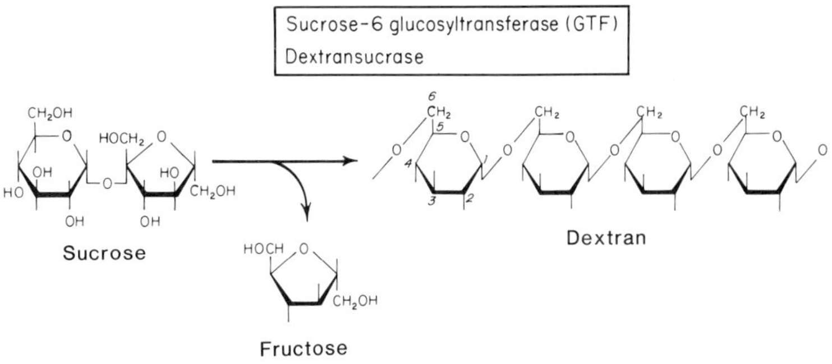

Figure 12–2 Schematic drawing of the conversion of the glucosyl moiety of sucrose to dextran by the enzyme glucosyltransferase (dextransucrase). This enzyme is essential for the production of extracellular glucans by *S. mutans* and is the prime candidate antigen for immunization against *S. mutans*-dependent dental caries.

tant concepts must be emphasized. First, part of the glucan produced by S. mutans contains high proportions of (1-3) linkages. These bonds make the polysaccharide less soluble in water, and this property may add unique physical characteristics to colonies of S. mutans within dental plaque. Second, in contrast to several other plaque bacteria, S. mutans appears to form discrete, compact colonies on the surfaces of teeth. Localized, glucan-coated colonies of S. mutans adjacent to the enamel surface might limit access to buffering entities from saliva and block diffusion of acid away from the teeth. Finally, the aggregated and compact colonies of S. mutans might be less susceptible to disruption and removal for analysis. This could affect the efficiency of certain oral hygiene procedures and complicate attempts to perform the longitudinal caries studies discussed previously. Greater problems can be envisioned when S. mutans colonizes retentive areas with limited accessibility.

Figure 12–3 illustrates the uptake of various carbohydrates by S. mutans. It is important that this bacterium uses the intracellular metabolite phosphoenolpyruvate (PEP) to facilitate uptake of substrates. This mechanism conserves energy in that transport is directly linked to phosphorylation and entry into the cells' catabolic pathways. Fluoride is capable of inhibiting transport by blocking PEP production via an interaction with the enzyme enolase. In addition to the transport of glu-

cose and fructose, it is now known that sucrose, lactose, and polyols are taken up by S. mutans by means of the phosphotransferase system. S. mutans clearly has the ability to efficiently transport and metabolize various dietary carbohydrates when they become available. This may give S. mutans a selective advantage over other plaque bacteria with more limited metabolic capabilities.

Another aspect of intracellular sugar metabolism that may be important to S. mutans and caries formation involves the synthesis and degradation of intracellular polysaccharide (see Fig. 12–3). The ability to store carbohydrate and to degrade this material to acid would allow a bacterium such as S. mutans to produce acid over an extended period of time and thus maintain a low pH in plaque. This process would also provide a source of energy for cell maintenance or proliferation within plaque.

A logical prediction based on our brief survey of sucrose metabolism by S. mutans would be that samples of dental plaque enriched for this bacterium should metabolize the disaccharide in a definable manner. Studies by Minah and Loesche[20] have demonstrated that there is a marked difference in sucrose metabolism by plaque taken from an approximal lesion of a primary first molar and plaque removed from a non-carious surface on the same tooth. In comparison to the non-cariogenic plaque, the cariogenic plaque

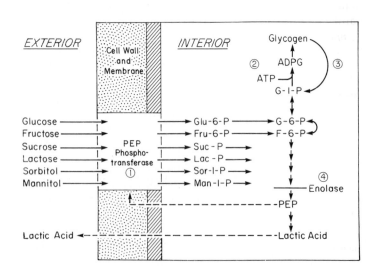

Figure 12–3 Schematic drawing of fermentable carbohydrate metabolism by *Streptococcus mutans*. Carbohydrates are transported into the cell by a PEP-dependent phosphotransferase system (Step 1) and can be stored in the form of glycogen (Pathway 2), which can be degraded subsequently (Step 3). Carbohydrates can also be metabolized to lactic acid (Pathway 4). Enolase is an enzyme in the glycolytic pathway that can be inhibited with fluoride. When this enzyme is inhibited, carbohydrate transport is reduced because of a lack of PEP.

samples contained high levels of *S. mutans* and metabolized sucrose to lactic acid at a faster rate. In addition, the plaque from the carious lesions produced more extracellular glucan and intracellular storage polysaccharide and yielded significantly more lactic acid by catabolism of the latter polysaccharide. These results imply that *S. mutans* may be metabolically dominant in plaque associated with carious lesions and strengthen the argument for a key role for this bacterium and sugar metabolism in human caries formation.

SUPPRESSION OF *S. MUTANS* INFECTIONS

We have discussed evidence that indicates that dental caries in humans is associated with *S. mutans* and that sucrose is utilized by this bacterium to promote its colonization of the oral cavity. Many dental scientists feel that great progress in caries control could be made by specifically suppressing or blocking *S. mutans* infections of tooth surfaces. Success in such endeavors would greatly clarify the microbial specificity of human caries and possibly open the door to complete disease eradication.

Based on evidence that colonization of the human mouth by *S. mutans* could be reduced by using a topically applied iodine solution and that this bacterium might be selectively sensitive to this halide, Caufield and Gibbons[3] performed a study of great potential significance. It was demonstrated that a prophylaxis of the teeth followed by three topical applications of an iodine-potassium iodide solution could significantly reduce the levels of *S. mutans* in plaque from fissures and approximal surfaces and in saliva. Reductions in the levels of *S. mutans* persisted for 20 to 24 weeks after treatment. These findings are consistent with our previous discussion concerning the problems that *S. mutans* has in colonizing teeth and being transmitted from one intraoral site to another. It is readily apparent that his technique could be very useful for both the short-term reduction and possibly the long-term elimination of *S. mutans* from the surfaces of human teeth. Used in conjunction with fluoride and sealants, solutions of iodine might effectively be used to minimize the challenge to the teeth from *S. mutans*. Clinical caries studies utilizing iodine are in progress.

Evidence has been presented in several systems that certain bacterial infections may be controlled by allowing the host to be colonized with non-virulent variants of bacteria with disease-producing potential. Hillman[12] has obtained mutants of *S. mutans* that lack the enzyme lactate dehydrogenase. Although these isolates produce less acid than their parents when supplied with glucose, they appear to be capable of colonizing the oral cavity to high levels. Replacement therapy would involve supplying the mutants to the mouths of subjects either prior to colonization of the teeth by wild-type strains of *S. mutans* or after reduction in the levels of *S. mutans* by various methods (for example, iodine). It is possible that the mutant strains could occupy the sites normally colonized by *S. mutans*, and, consequently, there would be a reduction in the cariogenic challenge to the teeth. The mutants would be expected to reduce the ability of superinfecting acid-producing strains of *S. mutans* to become established in the oral cavity.

An additional and related approach would involve the creation of unique oral bacteria using recently developed genetic engineering techniques.[5, 10] Gene splicing with recombinant deoxyribonucleic acid (DNA) methods could be used to selectively remove from or add to oral bacteria specific genetic traits that would alter the microorganisms' cariogenic or anti-cariogenic properties. Because of the amazing progress being made in this area of science and our increasing knowledge of oral bacteria, it seems reasonable that new approaches to caries prevention will evolve in the near future. A practical application of this technology is presented in the following discussion.

An approach to caries prevention that has received considerable publicity and elicited great interest from the public is the development of an anti-caries vaccine. The reason for much of the optimism and work in this area is our increased understanding of the microbial etiology of human caries and man's secretory immunologic system. Since enhanced colonization of teeth by *S. mutans* involves production of glucans from dietary sucrose, it is possible that inhibition by antibodies of the enzyme involved in glucan synthesis could prevent *S. mutans*–induced caries. Indeed, the *S. mutans* dextransucrase is a primary candidate for the antigen to be used in a caries vaccine. When crude preparations of the enzyme are injected in the salivary gland region of rats and hamsters a local protective secretory immune response is induced. There are several groups of scientists using genetic engineering to isolate and manipulate the *S. mutans* DNA that codes for the production of dextransucrase. Large quantities of antigen will become available when this DNA is placed into appropriate bacteria. Pure antigen will accelerate studies on development of the appropriate vaccine.

Caries immunization studies have clearly suggested a role for secretory immunoglobulin A (sIgA) antibodies in protection against caries. The secretory immune system is being studied with increasing intensity. Briefly, the external secretions of the body, including saliva, contain sIgA as their predominant immunoglobulin. These fluids bathe the mucous membrane surfaces of the body, and their immunoglobulins are involved in "first-line defenses" such as the trapping of microorganisms at mucous surfaces, coating of bacteria and inhibition of their adherence, viral and toxic neutralization, lysis of bacteria, and opsonization. In regard to caries, it has been shown that local injection of *S. mutans* followed by direct instillation of antigen into the parotid duct of monkeys induced the production of sIgA, which reduced the levels of *S. mutans* on the animals' teeth. Recent excitement in caries immunization stems from the observation that oral or intragastric administration of antigens results in the appearance of sIgA antibodies in saliva and other external secretions. It has been proposed that the antibody-producing lymphoid cells originate and are stimulated in the gut-associated lymphoid tissue. The cells then migrate through the lymphatics via the mesenteric lymph nodes into the blood stream. They then home to secretory tissues located in various parts of the body. When they are in the environment of these tissues, the lymphocytes differentiate into mature IgA-secreting plasma cells with antibody specifically directed to the ingested antigen.

Our advancing knowledge of secretory immunity stimulated a pioneering study by investigators at the University of Alabama in Birmingham.[17] Four adult volunteers ingested gelatin capsules filled with 100 mg of formalin-killed *S. mutans* cells for 14 consecutive days. Antibodies to the strain of *S. mutans* used in the capsules could be detected in samples of saliva and tears within one week of immunization. A second cycle of antigen ingestion in capsules produced a more rapid and pronounced increase in antibody levels. The immunoglobulins were shown to be sIgA and were not present in the subjects' serum. The data are consistent with the concept that the ingested antigen stimulated precursor IgA cells in the gut-associated lymphoid tissue and that homing of cells to the salivary glands resulted in the localized production of specific antibodies. This approach to immunization eliminates some of the many problems previously encountered during attempts to immunize against caries.

Another facet of caries immunization involves the passive transfer or direct supplying to the oral cavity of antibodies specific for *S. mutans*. It has been demonstrated that rat dams immunized by various methods to *S. mutans* have high levels of antibody to this bacterium in colostrum, milk, and serum. When offspring suckling these dams were challenged with *S. mutans* it was observed that fewer carious lesions developed in the pups.[18] Passive transfer and immunity could be important to man, since caries primarily affects children at a time when they may be consuming large quantities of milk. It is not inconceivable that bovine milk supplemented with antibody or milk from cows immunized with the appropriate cariogenic bacteria could be used as part of a caries prevention program. What is exciting about this approach to suppression of *S. mutans* infections is that breakthroughs in the area of monoclonal antibody production[19] will make available large quantities of human antibodies specific for *S. mutans*. The supplying of such molecules to the human oral cavity at appropriate times could markedly suppress *S. mutans* infections and possibly eliminate this bacterium as a member of the human oral flora. Sequestering of other oral bacteria with cariogenic potential might also be accomplished.

It seems likely that in the near future the application of high technology molecular research will have a profound effect on our understanding and treatment of oral disease.

DIET MODIFICATION

Role of Fermentable Carbohydrate

Research with animals and epidemiologic analyses have strongly implicated fermentable carbohydrate, and sugars in particular, in human dental caries formation. It has been concluded that decay in humans is associated with both the frequency of ingestion of readily fermentable carbohydrates and the duration of time the substrate is retained in the mouth. It is unfortunate that few clinical trials designed to determine the cariogenicity of various sugars in humans have been performed. One of the most significant studies to date was performed in Turku, Finland.[23] One group of subjects was supplied with a diet containing a normal level of sucrose. Another group received a diet that had similar products made with fructose in place of the sucrose. A third group consumed a similar diet with xylitol in place of sucrose. This carefully controlled study provided unequivocal support for the role of fermentable sugar in human caries formation. After two years on the various diets, it was determined that the group consuming sucrose had a mean increment in the number of decayed, missing, and filled tooth surfaces (DMFS) of 7.2. The DMFS index of the group consuming the fructose diet was 3.8, while the xylitol group had an index of 0.0.

Sucrose Replacement

As a consequence of accumulating evidence, it has been proposed that caries could be prevented by altering the diet through replacement of sucrose with a less potent substrate. Replacement of sucrose by some acceptable sweetener seems reasonable. However, problems in this area are great. Briefly, sucrose has many properties that have caused it to be used in many foodstuffs. In addition to considerations such as cost, sucrose increases the sweetness, osmotic pressure, viscosity, boiling point, and moisture retention of foods. Sucrose also enhances flavor and appearance by improving clarity, lustre, and gloss. Finally, the disaccharide provides calories, affects the solubility of other ingredients, imparts plasticity, provides bulk and body, and assists emulsification and color development. These properties make attempts to substitute other agents extremely difficult. Artificial sweeteners and other sugar substitutes have been extensively discussed at two recent meetings.[11, 25] It is clear that in order to evolve an appropriate substance we have to consider such things as the absorption, metabolism, and safety of the substitute, practical problems in using the compound in various foodstuffs, and the legal and regulatory aspects of its utilization. Evaluation of the cariogenic potential of a possible substitute is in many instances upstaged by an evaluation of its carcinogenicity. This subject may be viewed by some as a reasonable approach to caries control, but the scientific problems, which are many, may actually be irrelevant when compared with regulatory and acceptance complications.

There is one sugar substitute that is worthy of additional discussion at this time. Sorbitol is a sugar alcohol that meets many of the criteria for a sugar substitute. Although there are some problems in its utilization in a wide range of foodstuffs, it has been generally accepted in chewing gums, and a significant portion of the gum sold in this country is of the sugarless type. Some producers have labeled their gums as non-cariogenic. It is true that if one does an animal model study and compares sorbitol with sucrose, there is little question that the latter is more cariogenic. If one supplies sorbitol to dental plaque either *in vivo* or *in vitro*, there is a minimal pH drop caused by limited production of acid. There are few bacteria in the oral cavity capable of utilizing sorbitol as a primary source of energy. However, as illustrated in Figure 12–3, *S. mutans* has the ability to transport sorbitol and metabolize it for energy and possibly to produce acid. Based on our discussion about the complexity of the oral flora and competition between oral bacteria, it would appear to be important that we consider the possibility that by utilizing polyols in increasing concentrations we will be giving *S. mutans* a selective advantage over other oral bacteria. Since individuals chewing sorbitol-containing gum or ingesting this compound in other forms are probably also obtaining sucrose in their diet it would appear that *S. mutans* colonization might be further enhanced under these conditions. It has been argued that the enzymes needed to metabolize sorbitol must be induced for production by the bacterium and that this would reduce the utilization of sorbitol by *S. mutans* within plaque. The truth is that we have no idea of the metabolic capabilities of this bacterium when it is in the mouth, and it may be fully derepressed to metabolize sorbitol under conditions where more readily fermentable carbohydrates are not available. Although dentistry may recommend certain sorbitol-containing products, we have to question whether all the answers are available concerning the rationale for this support. Supplying sorbitol between meals in significant concentrations might be aiding a bacterium with documented cariogenic potential.

Decreasing Sucrose in the Diet

One of the dietary guidelines from the United States Department of Agriculture and the Department of Health, Education and Welfare suggests a reduction in the consumption of refined and other processed sugars including foods high in sugars such as soft drinks, cereal, and bakery products and confections. If this goal is achieved it would reduce simple sugar consumption

from about 13 million tons to six million tons per year in the United States. This rather staggering decrease might have some helpful effects on the population. However, with regard to dental caries, it is difficult to project any change in disease level. There is no experimental support for a direct correlation between the total intake of sugar and the incidence of dental caries. As discussed previously, the frequency of ingestion and the form of the carbohydrate are the most critical parameters regarding caries enhancement by food consumption. Indeed, a strong controversy exists concerning the relative cariogenicity of different carbohydrates. In general, it appears that monosaccharides and disaccharides are more cariogenic than starch, and sucrose is considered the most cariogenic sugar. However, there are conflicting data on this subject and some animal studies indicate that there is little difference in the cariogenicity of sucrose, glucose, and fructose. It cannot be too strongly emphasized that one must carefully monitor which surfaces of the teeth are being attacked in such studies and also the type of bacterial flora present on the teeth before, during, and at the termination of the experiment. The level of *S. mutans* in the subjects under study is of great importance, since high levels of this bacterium can be associated with elevated decay on the smooth surfaces of teeth. As illustrated in Figure 12–3, *S. mutans* can readily transport the predominant sugars found in the typical human diet. Thus, a great deal of caution should be used when attempting to evaluate studies in which multiple types of fermentable carbohydrate are available. Another problem would be in diet shifting studies. A subject with high or moderate levels of *S. mutans* might develop significant caries after shifting to a diet free of sucrose if the new diet contained quantities of a carbohydrate that this bacterium could still ferment. It is clear that there are no simple answers when discussing the cariogenicity of various fermentable carbohydrates.

Cariogenicity of Foods

Current interest in the role of nutrition in human disease and the documented relationship between diet and dental caries has placed the dental profession in a difficult situation. Ideally, the clinician would like to be able to recommend to patients a diet that is compatible with both oral and total health. Unfortunately, because of the complex interactions involved in human caries formation, this ideal situation will not be approached without a great deal of work and subsequent insight. For example, based on our increased understanding of the etiology of dental caries, the practitioner might suggest a reduction or elimination of between-meal snacking. Unfortunately, in modern society snacking is becoming more prevalent, and recommendations contrary to this trend are unlikely to be effective. This situation consequently has caused a marked increase in pressure on the clinician to recommend foods that can be eaten with minimum risk to the teeth. Since we have previously expressed problems with pinpointing the contribution of specific carbohydrates to caries and the difficulties involved in altering the carbohydrate content of foods, it is important to look at the status of current attempts to evaluate the cariogenicity of individual foodstuffs. The intimate relationship

between diet and caries indicates that accomplishments in this area might have a profound influence on the magnitude of the caries problem.

Table 12–1 presents a brief summary of the various factors that may contribute to the cariogenic potential of a food when it is ingested. Since the relative contribution of each of the factors could vary depending on the food in question, it is clear that a formidable task confronts the scientist attempting to study food cariogenicity.

Practical and ethical considerations have limited the researcher's capacity to evaluate the cariogenicity of individual foods through human clinical trials. A variety of non-clinical procedures have been used to obtain data on particular food items. These procedures include chemical analysis of foods, measurement of oral retention, quantitation of buffering capacity, evaluation of enamel decalcification potential, plaque pH responses, and *in vitro* caries formation. The large number of factors involved in evaluating a food (see Table 12–1) emphasize that no single procedure is adequate for all types of food items.

Emphasis in recent years has been

TABLE 12–1 FACTORS CAPABLE OF INFLUENCING THE CARIOGENIC POTENTIAL OF A FOOD AT THE TIME OF INGESTION

HOST FACTORS	Buffering capacity of saliva
	Calcium and phosphate concentration of saliva
	Flow rate and viscosity of saliva
	Presence and age of plaque at caries-prone sites
	Composition of the plaque matrix
	Anatomy of the dentition
	Microstructure of the enamel
	Fluoride content of enamel and plaque
	Pattern of mastication, sucking, rinsing, and swallowing
	Breathing by mouth
	Frequency of food ingestion
MICROBIAL FACTORS	Concentration of acidogenic bacteria at specific sites on the teeth
	Acidogenic potential of bacteria on mucosal surfaces and in saliva
	Concentration of acid-utilizing bacteria in plaque
SUBSTRATE FACTORS	Total fermentable carbohydrate
	Concentration of mono-, di-, oligo-, and polysaccharides
	Concentration and types of proteins and fats
	Physical form, including factors that effect oral retention
	Presence of fluoride, calcium, phosphate, and trace elements
	Total buffering capacity
	Presence and quantity of sialogogues, metabolic inhibitors, flavors, and organic phosphates
	Acidity of the food
	Sequence of ingestion relative to other foods

placed on three approaches to the problem of food cariogenicity. First, *in vitro* models involving construction of artificial mouths have provided some data. Second, animal model systems using rodents have been developed and employed to provide data on a wide range of foods.[1] Finally, plaque pH measurements after ingestion of foods by human volunteers have been extensively utilized by various groups of investigators. This latter approach, in which plaque acid production in the mouth can be accurately monitored, appears to hold great promise as a means of comparing the acidogenic potential of many foodstuffs. Unfortunately, the actual level of acid needed to cause damage to teeth *in situ* is not known at this time.

Various methods have been used to measure plaque pH. A technique usually referred to as "plaque sampling" has been used with considerable success by a number of scientists. In this method, plaque is removed from teeth at intervals following test food ingestion, and the pH is measured after dispersion of the sample in diluent. In a second method, microelectrodes are placed within plaque on the tooth surface at intervals after food ingestion. Such "touch electrode" techniques allow direct readings of pH on the plaque surface. In general, this method provides information similar to that obtained by plaque sampling. In a more complex technique, plaque is allowed to accumulate on glass electrodes that have been fixed within the dentition. After food ingestion, pH readings can be made continuously from the "indwelling electrode" by either wire or radiotelemetry. This technique has been used extensively in Switzerland, and the Swiss health authorities have issued regulations that sweets could be advertised as "zahnschonend" (that is, friendly to teeth) when studies showed that telemetric measurements did not drop below 5.7 within 30 minutes after ingestion.

It is conceivable that if appropriate input can be obtained from individuals in the food industry, dental scientists, food science and nutrition researchers, the dental profession, and various regulatory and professional agencies, collaborative investigations could be performed that would eventually allow the development of reasonable and acceptable means for evaluating the cariogenicity of foods. This would open the door for the food industry to develop non-cariogenic new foods and possibly modify existing products to reduce their challenge to the teeth.

PROTECTING THE TEETH

Fluoride

Fluoride has been effectively used to inhibit caries formation in humans. Water fluoridation, salt fluoridation, and fluoride-containing tablets, dentifrices, mouth rinses, and gels have all been shown to be capable of preventing caries in populations and selected subjects. What is surprising about the use of fluoride is that we do not know exactly how it functions in disease reduction.

Three new approaches to delivering fluoride more effectively are being developed.[21] The technology being used takes advantage of recent advances in controlled drug release. Uses of controlled delivery devices in human therapy include the supplying of pilocarpine to the eyes of glaucoma patients, progesterone delivery by an intrauterine device, and the delivery of insulin to diabetics. This technology is based on the need to ensure that an agent gets to the correct site at a concentration and for a period of time that allows it to exert its maximal effect. An agent can be delivered *in vivo* at a constant or slowly declining rate if it is encased in a protective polymeric sheath that allows release by either diffusion or erosion. Sodium fluoride has been incorporated into capsules that when chewed or sucked in the mouth release 10 to 15 per cent of the encased ion. When the capsule is swallowed, the remaining fluoride is released in the gastrointestinal tract over a two-day period. The net effect of the capsules is that fluoride is immediately available for local oral interactions and then for a prolonged interval through elevated levels in blood and saliva. A related approach involves attempts to develop an oral aerosol delivery system that would cause fluoride-containing microcapsules to adhere directly to the teeth. Sodium fluoride is encapsulated in carboxymethyl cellulose and mixed with guar gum as an adhesive. It is envisioned that the adhered capsules would enhance fluoride intake by plaque and enamel over a prolonged interval. Probably the most advanced utilization of time-release technology is in the development of fluoride-containing "sandwiches." A small trilaminate device consisting of an inner core of fluoride-containing copolymer surrounded by a copolymer membrane can be made and attached on or near the teeth. Fluoride is slowly released from the biocompatible device at a constant predetermined linear rate for at least six months. Studies with humans will be performed in the near future. It is envisioned that utilization of means to supply increased levels of fluoride to caries-prone sites will reduce caries formation by suppressing fermentable sugar metabolism by cariogenic bacteria, by making the enamel more resistant to dissolution, and by stimulating remineralization of the tooth surface. Recent attempts to stimulate the latter effect by utilization of "artificial saliva" containing fluoride and appropriate minerals have been successful in some clinical trials. This approach would appear to be promising in light of what is now known about the repair capacity of saliva-enamel interactions.

SEALANTS

It is important that fluoride is most effective in reducing caries on the smooth surfaces of teeth, that is, the approximal, buccal, and lingual surfaces. However, fluoride used at the concentration normally available is much less effective in reducing caries that develop on the occlusal surfaces. Unfortunately, occlusal caries accounts for approximately 40 per cent of all carious surfaces in six- and seven-year-old children. This probably reflects the normally inaccessible pits and fissures that are found on these surfaces and that can accumulate oral debris and bacteria. Consequently, efforts have been made to develop materials that can be used to seal and protect these surfaces. Excellent materials have become available and have been shown to firmly adhere to the enamel surfaces of teeth and block caries formation. Although the sealing of occlusal tooth surfaces is utilized as part of some preventive dentistry programs, these materials are surely underused by the dental profession. Since virtually every criticism raised against the use of sealants has been refuted by sound clinical data and since materials are now available that can be retained on teeth for many years, it may be necessary to stimulate consumer demand for these products and encourage dental schools to train students more thoroughly in the proper use of these protective polymers. If we consider our previous discussion on the oral ecology of *S. mutans*, it becomes apparent that sealants will remove one of the niches in the mouth that can harbor high concentrations of this bacterium. One can predict that sealing decreases the overall cariogenic challenge to the teeth by reducing the number of sites capable of harboring the infection.

CONCLUSIONS

This has been a brief and selected overview of some of the current approaches to prevention of human dental caries. Each of the avenues has some merit, and in every case we are learning a great deal about man and his interactions with his indigenous microbial flora. A critical complicating factor in dental caries formation is that man's diet causes certain indigenous oral bacteria to express detrimental traits. In order to eliminate the microbial oral diseases we must learn to control these activities. Attempts to prevent caries must take into account the multifactorial etiology of the disease and what is known about the specific bacteria and dietary factors that initiate and extend carious lesions. One must be optimistic and realize that the complexity of the problem means that there are many points from which to approach prevention. Biomedical research is rapidly progressing in numerous areas. Sophisticated theories and technologies are having a profound effect on man's health. It is essential that dental scientists appreciate and attempt to apply this progress to oral disease. Some examples of this have been presented in this chapter. It is hoped that there will be many more examples in the near future.

REFERENCES

1. Bowen, W. H., Amsbaugh, S. M., Monell-Torrens, S., et al.: A method to assess cariogenic potential of foodstuffs. J. Am. Dent. Assoc. *100*:677–681, 1980.
2. Bowden, G. H. W., Elwood, D. C., and Hamilton, I. R.: Microbial ecology of the oral cavity. *In* Alexander, M. (ed.): Advances in Microbial Ecology, Vol. 3, New York, Plenum Press, 1979.
3. Caufield, P. W., and Gibbons, R. J.: Suppression of *Streptococcus mutans* in the mouths of humans by a dental prophylaxis and topically-applied iodine. J. Dent. Res. *58*:1317–1326, 1979.
4. Clark, J. K.: On the bacterial factor in the aetiology of dental caries. Br. J. Exptl. Pathol. *5*:141–147, 1924.
5. Cohen, S. N.: The manipulation of genes. Sci. Am. *233*:24–33, 1975.
6. Duchin, S., and van Houte, J.: Relationship of *Streptococcus mutans* and lactobacilli to incipient smooth surface dental caries in man. Arch. Oral Biol. *23*:779–786, 1978.
7. Edman, D. C., Keene, H. J., Shklair, I. L., and Hoerman, K. C.: Dental floss for implantation and sampling of *Streptococcus mutans* from approximal surfaces of human teeth. Arch. Oral Biol. *20*:145–148, 1975.
8. Fitzgerald, R. J., and Keyes, P. H.: Demonstration of the etiologic role of streptococci in experimental caries in the hamster. J. Am. Dent. Assoc. *61*:9–19, 1960.
9. Gibbons, R. J.: Significance of the bacterial flora indigenous to man. Amer. Inst. Oral Biol. Symp. *26*:27–39, 1969.
10. Gilbert, W., and Villa-Komanoff, L.: Useful proteins from recombinant bacteria. Sci. Am. *242*:74–94, 1980.
11. Guggenheim, B.: Health and sugar substitutes. Basel, S. Karger, 1979.
12. Hillman, J. D.: Lactate dehydrogenase mutants of *Streptococcus mutans*: Isolation and preliminary characterization. Infect. Immun. *21*:206–212, 1978.
13. Keyes, P. H.: The infectious and transmissible nature of experimental dental caries. Arch. Oral Biol. *13*:304–320, 1960.
14. Loesche, W. J.: Clinical and microbiological aspects of chemotherapeutic agents used according to the specific plaque hypothesis. J. Dent. Res. *58*:2404–2412, 1979.
15. Loesche, W. J., Svanberg, M. L., and Pape, H. R.: Intraoral transmission of *Streptococcus mutans* by a dental explorer. J. Dent. Res. *58*:1765–1770, 1979.
16. Loesche, W. J., and Straffon, L. H.: Longitudinal investigation of the role of *Streptococcus mutans* in human fissure decay. Infect. Immun. *26*:498–507, 1979.
17. McGhee, J. R., Mestecky, J., Arnold, R. R., et al.: Induction of secretory antibodies in humans following ingestion of *Streptococcus mutans*. Advan. Exp. Med. Biol. *107*:177–184, 1978.
18. Michalek, S. M., and McGhee, J. R.: Effective immunity to dental caries: Passive transfer to rats of antibodies to *Streptococcus mutans* elicits protection. Infect. Immun. *17*:644–650, 1977.
19. Milstein, C.: Monoclonal antibodies. Sci. Am. *243*:66–74, 1980.
20. Minah, G. E., and Loesche, W. J.: Sucrose metabolism in resting-cell suspensions of caries-associated and non-caries–associated dental plaque. Infect. Immun. *17*:43–54, 1977.
21. Mirth, D. B., and Bowen, W. H.: Chemotherapy: Antimicrobials and methods of delivery. *In* Stiles, H. M., Loesche, W. J., and O'Brien, T. C. (eds.): Microbial Aspects of Dental Caries, Vol. 1. Wash. D.C., Information Retrieval, 1976, pp. 249–262.
22. Orland, F. J., Blayney, J. R., Harrison, R. W., et al.: Experimental caries in germ free rats inoculated with enterococci. J. Am. Dent. Assoc. *50*:259–272, 1955.
23. Scheinin, A., and Makinen, K. K.: Turku sugar studies I–XXI. Acta Odont. Scand. *33*:1–348, 1975.
24. Scherp, H. W.: Dental caries: Prospects for prevention. Science *173*:1199–1205, 1971.
25. Shaw, J. H., and Roussos, G. G.: Sweeteners and dental caries. Wash. D.C., Information Retrieval, 1977.
26. Socransky, S. S., and Manganiello, A. D.: The oral microbiota of man from birth to senility. J. Periodontol. *42*:485–497, 1971.
27. Svanberg, M. L., and Loesche, W. J.: Implantation of *Streptococcus mutans* on tooth surfaces in man. Arch. Oral Biol. *23*:551–556, 1978.
28. Svanberg, M. L., and Loesche, W. J.: Intraoral spread of *Streptococcus mutans* in man. Arch. Oral Biol. *23*:557–561, 1978.
29. van Houte, J.: Carbohydrates, sugar substitutes and oral bacterial colonization. *In* Guggenheim, B. (ed.): Health and Sugar Substitutes. Basel, S. Karger, 1979, pp. 199–204.

CHAPTER THIRTEEN

Periodontal Disease: Prevention and Control

Leonard Shapiro, D.M.D., M.S.

The practice of dentistry is changing from one of treatment and repair of previous damage to one of prevention of disease. The patient's role is being altered from that of passive bystander to one of an active participant in disease prevention. The dental office also is becoming less of a repair-oriented facility and is assuming a teaching role in the prevention of pathology. A need will always exist for excellence in restorative therapy, but dentistry can no longer be practiced without patient education and motivation for prevention of these lesions.

Motivation on the part of both the teacher and the student is the key factor for the success of a plaque control program. Chronic lesions, such as those associated with the inflammatory periodontal lesion, are not usually sufficient to bring a patient to the office seeking care. One of the main motivating factors in dental disease — pain — is absent. Past experience of relief from noxious stimuli, rather than the prevention and elimination of future painful experiences, may be the only reference the patient has for seeking dental care.

The behavior of the patient must be modified to seek early preventive care rather than relief from pain. The drive to seek dental care must come from within the patient, and then usually only after he has been exposed to the benefits of preventive rather than reparative care. The patient is not motivated by an adequate zone of attached gingiva or knife-edged papillae, but rather by selfish drives, for example, improving his appearance, improving social acceptability, and finally, maintaining his dentition. These

TABLE 13-1 PATIENT EDUCATION AND MOTIVATION FOR ORAL HYGIENE*

AGE	SEX	OHI-S†	PRETREATMENT Expect to Retain Their Teeth	Brush to Improve Gum Health	AGE	SEX	OHI-S	ONE YEAR POSTTREATMENT Expect to Retain Their Teeth	Brush to Improve Gum Health
30–39	Male	1.83	59%	15%	30–39	Male	1.45	66%	50%
	Female	1.55	61%	36%		Female	1.30	58%	66%
40–49	Male	2.17	35%	12%	40–49	Male	2.70	40%	60%
	Female	1.78	58%	40%		Female	1.82	62%	75%
50–59	Male	1.92	30%	21%	50–59	Male	1.81	25%	100%
	Female	1.30	63%	38%		Female	1.10	75%	83%
60 + over	Male	1.72	42%	25%	60 + over	Male	1.32	62%	75%
	Female	1.32	74%	51%		Female	1.55	80%	66%
Means	Male	1.91	42%	18%	Means	Male	1.82	48%	71%
	Female	1.48	64%	41%		Female	1.44	69%	67%
	Overall	1.70	53%	30%		Overall	1.63	59%	69%
Total N = 100					Total N = 89				

*From Awwa, I., and Stallard, R. E.: Periodontal prognosis: Educational and psychological implications. J. Periodontol. *41*:55–57, 1970.
†Oral Hygiene Index Simplified.

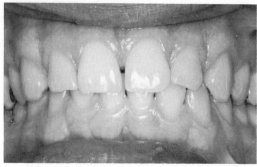

Figure 13–1 The primary objective of complete elimination of dental plaque from all surfaces of teeth can be seen in this clinical photograph. The patient is free of dental plaque and accompanying gingival disease.

needs or drives will lead to action on the part of the patient to achieve the goal of oral health (Table 13–1).

It may well be that the patient who presents in the dental office is sufficiently motivated, but this may not be sufficient to make him accept preventive therapy. It is then necessary to establish an educational rapport with the patient to make him aware of oral disease and the means by which the disease and repair cycle can be stopped. Once rapport has been established, communication between the patient and dentist is easy, provided that the common language is commensurate with the patient's ability to understand. Failure to achieve this common language will negate the previously established rapport and make communication as well as motivation impossible.

PLAQUE CONTROL PROGRAMS

Once the rapport has been established, mechanisms must be instituted to carry out an adequate plaque control program. Office procedures for preventive dentistry vary from office to office. A dentist, control therapist, or hygienist may be the teacher. Regardless of who the teacher is, however, the motivation that brought the patient to seek preventive care must be carried over to this phase of the learning experience. Before the patient can accept preventive therapy, he must be taught the rationale for this phase of treatment and, more important, the cause of this problem. If the patient is taught the cause of his disease, he can better appreciate practicing the techniques necessary for its prevention. It is not necessary to delve into the esoteric aspects of the controversy about whether sulcular fluid is an exudate or a transudate, but rather the teacher should go into the development of dental plaque and the effects of bacterial products on the hard and soft tissues of the oral cavity.

The primary objective of oral hygiene procedures is the elimination of dental plaque from all tooth surfaces (Figs. 13–1 and 13–2). In the past, patients have been presented with a myriad of items that required an inordinate amount of time and a degree of dexterity that many patients lacked. In addition, little or no instruction was given concerning the etiology of the lesion.

This is particularly true in adolescents

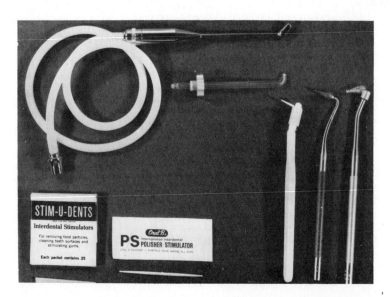

Figure 13–2 The market is flooded with numerous devices claiming to be superior in the elimination of dental plaque. A few such devices can be seen in this illustration. To date none of these has been shown to be superior to routine tooth brushing, flossing, or other interproximal cleaning.

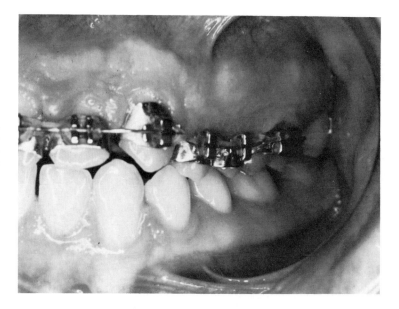

Figure 13-3 13-year-old orthodontic patient with generalized marginal inflammation. (Courtesy of Dr. Sumner M. Sapiro.)

undergoing orthodontic treatment. While preventive periodontal home care is paramount in the success of the orthodontic treatment, the individual patient perceives the orthodontic treatment as having greater importance. Figures 13–3 and 13–4 show a 13-year-old orthodontic patient with generalized marginal inflammation, which was controlled entirely by effective oral hygiene procedures.

Armamentarium

The basic armamentarium for effective plaque control should consist of a disclosing agent, a toothbrush, and a method for interproximal cleaning (Fig. 13–5).

Disclosing Agents. Disclosing agents are used so that the patient can better visualize the dental plaque, the cause of his problem. Basically, the following three types of disclosing solutions are available: a red dye (FDC #3) in either a tablet or liquid, which colors the plaque relatively uniformly; a fluorescing dye, which must be activated by an incandescent light and has the advantage of being relatively invisible when the light is not used; and a temporal agent, which selectively stains plaque by its age rather than by

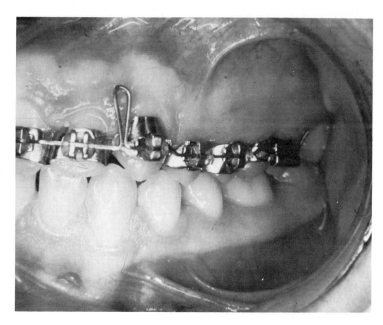

Figure 13-4 In the same patient seen in Figure 13–3, a significant reduction of the marginal inflammatory response occurred following two months of plaque control. (Courtesy of Dr. Sumner M. Sapiro.)

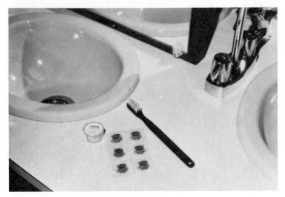

Figure 13–5 The basic armamentarium for a preventive and control program in periodontal disease consists of the toothbrush, disclosing tablets, and dental floss.

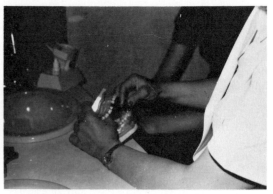

Figure 13–7 For the patient's first exposure to presentation of oral hygiene procedures, demonstration on a model has proved to be the most effective teaching method.

amount. With the temporal dye, newer plaque is red, while older plaque is blue (Fig. 13–6). It has the advantage of allowing the patient to visualize more easily the problem areas of his dentition, which he may have had difficulty in cleaning.

In addition to being a guide to areas to be cleaned, the disclosing solution also acts as an efficient method for evaluating plaque control once all the procedures have been performed.

Toothbrush. Once the presence of plaque has been shown on the teeth, it must be removed. Plaque is removed by mechanical methods. The toothbrush is an aid in the removal of soft accumulated debris that has

collected on the tooth. The method to be used is demonstrated first on a model (Fig. 13–7), next in the patient's mouth, and third by the patient himself (Fig. 13–8). Recent studies have indicated that a modification of the Bass technique, the use of a soft multituft nylon brush with the bristles inclined into the gingival sulcus, is the most efficient technique for removal of plaque from the sulcular area. The brush is moved from one area of the dentition to the adjacent area until the facial and lingual surfaces of all teeth have been cleaned. Unfortunately, a single technique cannot be used by all patients, and modifications of a basic technique are necessary to adapt to the individual situation. The most important part, however, is the thoroughness with which the technique is performed.

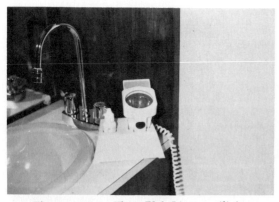

Figure 13–6 The Plak-Lite, utilizing a fluorescing dye and an incandescent light, offers an innovative method of disclosing the presence of dental plaque. One of its principal advantages is with the adult patient, who looks somewhat askance at leaving the dental office with a red mouth.

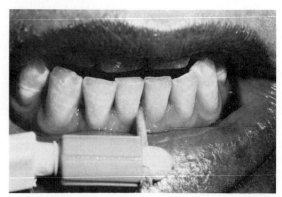

Figure 13–8 After model presentation, demonstration in the patient's own mouth, followed by utilization of the toothbrush or other device by the patient, is essential.

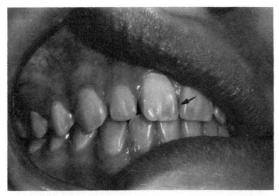

Figure 13–9 Note the plaque remaining in interproximal areas after thorough brushing. This can only be removed by the use of an interproximal cleaning aid such as dental floss.

The toothbrush has the disadvantage of being unable to cleanse the proximal surfaces of the teeth. Even after the most thorough brushing, plaque remains interproximally (Fig. 13–9). Various modalities have been developed for interproximal plaque control, ranging from dental floss to plastic stimulators. The most efficient method of interproximal plaque control appears to be dental floss. The floss is gently eased through the contact area and rubbed along the proximal surfaces until they are plaque-free (Fig. 13–10). As is the case with the toothbrush, modifications must be made to compensate for dexterity, fixed splinting, and anatomic variations. To this end other modalities such as soft balsa wood and rounded tooth picks, as well as interproximal brushes, have been developed to reach areas that the patient is unable to reach with the dental floss.

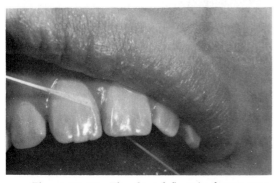

Figure 13–10 The dental floss is drawn taut across the surface of the tooth so that it can rub gently on the tooth surface, eliminating dental plaque both supra- and subgingivally.

Other instruments such as the electric toothbrush and water pressure devices have been introduced into the plaque control armamentarium. There are no available data to indicate that a powered toothbrush is any more efficient in plaque removal than the manual brush. Initial success with the electric brush may be due more to a novelty effect than to increased efficiency. Water pressure devices have been advocated for removal of sulcular debris. Again, there are no available data to indicate they have any efficiency in plaque removal.

CHEMICAL AND CHEMOTHERAPEUTIC PLAQUE CONTROL

From past experience it is apparent that mechanical means alone are not sufficient to prevent dental disease. Recent investigations have dealt with chemical control of disease, which would eliminate the dexterity now necessary to practice adequate plaque control. The chlorhexidine group of compounds has shown promise as a means of preventing plaque formation without eliminating entirely the resident bacterial population of the oral cavity. However, much more investigation along this line is needed to develop a substance that is both nontoxic to the host, yet capable of preventing new plaque formation.

In addition to topical medications, much emphasis lately has been placed on chemotherapeutic means of plaque control.

It is well recognized that periodontal inflammation does not occur in a direct linear fashion but rather as a series of exacerbations and remissions. It has been postulated that it is during the period of exacerbation that the resident bacterial flora are most pathogenic and thus most destructive. In theory, if this time frame could be ascertained, then antibiotic therapy could be utilized when it would be the most beneficial.

Attempts have been made experimentally to introduce the antibiotic locally by means of a strip around the tooth and systemically, resulting in its excretion through the sulcular exudate.

On a short term basis of three months,

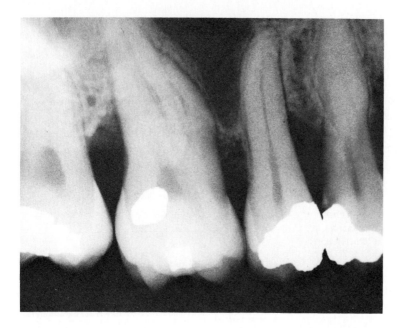

Figure 13–11 Preoperative radiograph of 31-year-old female with a generalized periodontitis.

daily use of a broad-spectrum antibiotic, tetracycline, did not have any significant effect on the gingival index, debris index, or papillary bleeding index.

While no long-term studies are available to determine the efficacy of antibiotics as sole measures to control periodontal disease, they are probably of relatively little value. Indiscriminate use of antibiotics will arrest bacterial growth and allow the propagation of non-bacterial species or resistant organisms.

Until it can be determined exactly when exacerbation of the inflammatory process occurs and which specific bacterial species are involved, antibiotic therapy should be reserved as an adjunctive measure along with local debridement in non-refractory cases.

In unique situations such as periodontosis the utilization of tetracycline has proved to be an effective adjunctive therapy to suppress the bacterial growth when used in conjunction with the appropriate surgical and non-surgical modalities of periodontal treatment (Figs. 13–11 and 13–12).

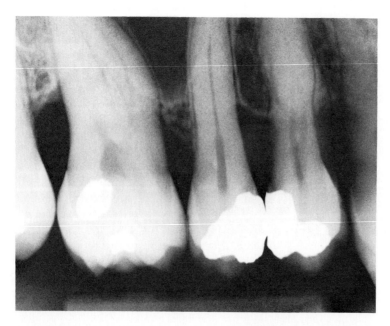

Figure 13–12 One-year postoperative radiograph after patient had been treated surgically. In addition, tetracycline was used as adjunctive therapy in an attempt to suppress the microbiota associated with the disease process.

PATIENT RECALL

Once the patient has been instructed in the methods of disease control in his mouth, he must be sufficiently motivated to carry on these procedures in his home. It is not enough that he demonstrate a complete understanding in the office. The instruction must also be integrated into a daily habit pattern in order to prevent a recurrence of disease. Closely integrated with good home care is a carefully planned recall sequence.

Not all patients are compulsive personality types; therefore, most patients do not exhibit perfect plaque control, and it is probably also true that most patients are incapable of maintaining a satisfactory level of plaque control over a long period of time without some assistance. The recall visit provides opportunity to re-orient and re-educate the patient in the rationale and methods of plaque control.

Without this continuous reinforcement to remain highly motivated, patients may relapse into old comfortable habits.

The prevention of periodontal disease requires a sufficiently motivated patient practicing adequate plaque control. With an understanding of the disease process the patient can better appreciate the methods used to control disease in his mouth. At present only mechanical methods are available for disease control, but current research has shown promise for a chemical means of individual plaque control.

ADDITIONAL READING

1. Anderson, J.: Integration of plaque control into the practice of dentistry. Dent. Clin. North Am. *16*:621, 1972.

2. Arnim, S. S.: The use of disclosing agents for measuring tooth cleanliness. J. Periodontol. *34*:227, 1963.
3. Awwa, I., and Stallard, R. E.: Periodontal prognosis: Education and psychological implications. J. Periodontol. *41*:55–57, 1970.
4. Bass, C. C.: An effective method of personal oral hygiene. J. La. State Med. Soc. *106*:100, 1954.
5. Bass, C. C.: The optimum characteristics of toothbrushes for personal oral hygiene. Dental Items of Interest *70*:697, 1948.
6. Cohen, D. W., Stoller, N. H., Chace, R., and Laster, L.: A comparison of bacterial plaque disclosants in periodontal disease. J. Periodontol. *43*:333, 1972.
7. Hill, H. C., Levi, P. P., and Glickman, I.: The effects of waxed and unwaxed dental floss on interdental plaque accumulation and interdental gingival health. J. Periodontol. *44*:411, 1973.
8. Less, W.: Mechanics of teaching plaque control. Dent. Clin. North Am. *16*:647, 1972.
9. Lifer, L.: Motivation of the patient by the dentist. Dent. Clin. North Am. *16*:609, 1972.
10. Loe, H., Theilade, E., and Jensen, S. B.: Gingivitis in man. J. Periodontol. *36*:177, 1965.
11. Loe, H., Schiott, C. R., Glavind, L., and Karring, T.: Two Years of Oral Use of Chlorhexidine in Man. I. General Design and Clinical Effects. J. Periodont. Res. *11*:135, 1976.
12. Radentz, W. G., Barnes, G., Carter, H., Ailor, J., and Johnson, R.: An evaluation of two techniques for teaching proper dental flossing procedures. J. Periodontol. *44*:177, 1973.
13. Schiott, C. R., Briner, W. W., and Loe, H.: Two year oral use of chlorhexidine in man. II. The effect on the salivary bacterial flora. J. Periodont. Res. *11*:145, 1976.
14. Schiott, C. R., Briner, W. W., Kirkland, J. J., and Loe, H.: Two years oral use of chlorhexidine in man. III. changes in sensitivity of the salivary flora. J. Periodont. Res. *11*:153, 1976.
15. Schiott, C. R., Loe, H., and Briner, W. W.: Two year oral use of chlorhexidine in man. IV. Effect on various medical parameters. J. Periodont. Res. *11*:158, 1976.
16. Scopp, I. W., Froum, S. J., Sullivan, M., Kazandjian, G., Wank, D., and Fine, A.: Tetracycline: A clinical study to determine its effectiveness as a long-term adjuvant. J. Periodontol. *51*:328, 1980.
17. Van de Voorde, H. E.: A movie versus chairside instruction to present preliminary oral hygiene information. J. Periodontol. *43*:277, 1972.

CHAPTER FOURTEEN
Preventive Dental Radiology

Arthur H. Wuehrmann, D.M.D.

Concepts of prevention related to dental radiology take at least two forms. The appropriate use of radiologic procedures can assist in preventing advanced dental disease through the early recognition and treatment of various pathologic entities. Alternatively, preventive radiology can, through the implementation of good radiologic health principles, reduce somatic and genetic alterations that could result from using ionizing radiation.* Preventive dental radiology encompasses both concepts, and this chapter touches on salient features related to both.

Of maximum importance in understanding the concepts of preventive radiology is an appreciation of the term *diagnostic yield*. Human exposure to ionizing radiation has a deleterious effect, regardless of the type of ionizing radiation. From a purely biological standpoint, it would be best if humans were not subjected to man-made ionizing radiation. This statement is true until the balance between risk and gain is examined. Man's longevity has increased materially in civilized countries during the 20th century because of the many advances in health care. Among these advances must be included the diagnostic use of x-radiation. Thus, the undesirable effects of x-radiation exposure are offset but not eliminated by health benefits. Since the use of x-radiation is potentially harmful, each exposure should result in the greatest amount of diagnostic information possible per unit of x-radiation used. Diagnostic yield can be defined as the amount of diagnostic information made available per unit of x-radiation absorbed by the patient.

It becomes immediately obvious that diagnostic yield is related directly to three aspects of x-radiation use: 1) radiation reduction methods employed by the dentist, 2) adequacy of chairside and darkroom radiographic techniques, and 3) competency in interpreting the diagnostic information available on radiographic films. Weakness in one or more of these three facets of the science lowers the diagnostic yield either by causing the patient to receive more radiation than is necessary in order to attain the desired diagnostic end product or by causing the patient to be exposed unnecessarily because of the non-use of available diagnostic information.

A complete discussion of the above-mentioned three factors that interrelate in producing diagnostic yield would require a textbook on dental radiology rather than a chapter in a preventive dentistry text. Accordingly, the material to follow is not complete, and the reader is encouraged to study in considerably greater detail all matters that relate to dental radiology. Although interpretation and chairside radiographic techniques are mentioned, emphasis is given to radiation reduction methods in the dental office.

---

*Ionizing radiation is any particulate or electromagnetic energy that causes atoms or molecules to ionize. Except in research endeavors, the dental profession uses, with few exceptions, only x-radiation. Therefore, the terms ionizing radiation and x-radiation (and x-rays) are synonymous in this text.

Prior to such discussion, attention is given to certain general considerations for the purpose of clarifying issues to follow.

GENERAL CONSIDERATIONS

It must be recognized by the health science professions that the use of ionizing radiation constitutes a public health problem. No facet of dental practice other than the use of x-radiation represents anything other than an interpersonal relationship between dentist and patient. Perhaps with the advent of more state and federally sponsored dental programs, government agencies will be considered a third party, but the interrelationship still will be basically between doctor and patient. An unsatisfactory denture is immediately recognizable and can be remedied or destroyed without loss except in terms of time and money. Similarly, a restoration that is dislodged or has a rough margin can be noted and corrected. Other examples are obvious. Ionizing radiation, on the other hand, can create somatic effects that are not recognizable immediately and that may not become obvious at any time during an individual's lifetime. In addition to somatic effects in the exposed individual, genetic changes can occur that may affect progeny. Much has yet to be learned by radiation biologists about the effects of low-level radiation exposures on individuals and their offspring. Because the situation is so intangible, the health professions must accept professional responsibility beyond that ordinarily recognized in the course of practice.

X-radiation effects on vital tissue are fundamentally those of ionization and excitation of atoms within molecules. The result of ionization (the creation of electrical instability in an atom or molecule) is the recombination of the affected molecule with other unlike charged atoms or molecules to form incompatible substances not intended to exist in the human body. This statement, of necessity, is a gross generalization and oversimplification (textbooks have been written on the subject). It will serve for purposes of understanding certain terms that should be in the vocabulary of all practicing dentists.

X-radiation *exposure* is stated in terms of roentgens, abbreviated R. The roentgen* can be thought of as that amount of X- or gamma radiation that will create a known amount of ionization in air under certain conditions. The roentgen can be considered in the same vein as other devices for measuring quantities, such as the meter, the gram, or the liter. The roentgen is a measure of x-radiation made in air and is used to state the amount of radiation emanating from the x-ray machine.

X-radiation *dosage* is stated in terms of rads. The rad,† which relates directly to the roentgen, is a measure of *absorbed radiation* in tissue or in any other substance. Although an understanding of radiation output (R) is important, an understanding of the amount of radiation absorbed by the body is even more so. For example, if 100 R were produced at the radiation source, but the radiation were of such a character as to penetrate the human body without being absorbed, the amount of radiation would have little importance in terms of biological effect.

Directly allied to the concept of the rad is the idea of gram-rads. It is obvious that if only one gram of tissue were to receive a given amount of radiation, the effect would be far less deleterious than if 1000 grams of tissue each received one rad. These concepts will be used in discussing radiation reduction methods, but, for purposes of understanding, it will be helpful to give a suitable example. Under certain conditions, the output of the modern dental x-ray machine at eight inches from the source of radiation (x-ray tube anode) is approximately 1 R per second. Since for x-radiation, the roentgen and the rad are approximately equivalent, each exposed gram of tissue near the skin surface will absorb approximately one rad. (This assumes an approximately eight-inch source to skin distance.) However, if one x-ray beam is well confined in comparison to

---

*The roentgen (R) is a special unit of exposure. It can be defined as that amount of X- or gamma radiation that will produce in 1 cc of air (at standard temperature and pressure) one electrostatic unit of either sign. One electrostatic unit equals 2.08×10^9 ion pairs.

†The rad is a special unit of absorbed dose equal to 100 ergs per g of absorbing material.

another beam that has a larger diameter, the amount of tissue exposed in the first instance will be less than that of the second, and the gram-rads for the second individual will be greater than for the first. This is one reason why dentists are encouraged to use an x-ray beam collimated to just cover the film to be exposed. With these general considerations in mind, it is appropriate to think in terms of radiation reduction methods in the dental office.

RADIATION REDUCTION METHODS IN THE DENTAL OFFICE

Radiation protection methods used in the dental office should relate to two categories of individuals: patients and dental office staff. Patients may be further subdivided into those actually being exposed and those being treated in other operatories or waiting in the reception room for treatment. Similarly, the staff may be separated into persons actually operating the x-ray equipment and those working in contiguous rooms. Reference will be made later in this chapter to structural shielding; these comments will relate primarily to the protection of patients not being exposed to x-radiation and to personnel other than those actually using the x-ray equipment. For the present, reference to the patient implies the patient actually being exposed and reference to the operator implies the individual operating the x-ray equipment.

Patient Protection

Patient protection can be accomplished by suitable alterations, when necessary, in x-ray machine design, by the use of fast films of appropriate size, and by the employment of satisfactory x-ray techniques. Each of these will be discussed in detail.

X-Ray Machine Alterations

Although currently produced dental x-ray equipment conforms to desirable standards, verification of conformity should be made when the machine is installed.

Older machines often need modification. The changes that are more frequently needed are in x-ray beam collimation, filtration, and tube head (or tube housing) leakage.

X-ray Beam Collimation. The x-ray beam emanates from a small area on the surface of the x-ray tube anode. For present purposes, this can be considered a point source. The beam ordinarily passes through a round aperture in the x-ray tube housing, thus giving the beam a rounded shape, the diameter of which can be determined. The remainder of the tube housing fully absorbs the radiation unless it leaks (see tube head leakage). Federal standards require that the x-ray field (the greatest dimension of an x-ray beam at or beyond the end of a collimating device, that is, at skin surface) for a minimum source-to-skin distance of 18 cm (7 in) or greater be limited to 2¾ in and that the x-ray field for minimum source-to-skin distances less than 18 cm be limited to 2⅓ in. If the beam is excessively large, it can be further reduced by the insertion of a suitable lead diaphragm (often called a lead washer) into the tube head housing where the x-ray beam emanates from the housing (Fig. 14–1). In addition to suitable collimation by this means, the dentist should use an open-end cylinder that is lined with a heavy metal (a lead foil of approximately 0.3 millimeter in thickness is usually recommended) or one that has been lead impregnated during manufacture (Fig. 14–2). The frequently used plastic pointed cone should be discarded because primary radiation striking the cone

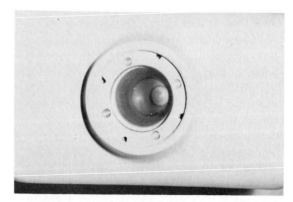

Figure 14–1 Aperture through which the x-ray beam emerges from the tube head. Cylinder with appropriate lead diaphragm is not shown. It attaches over the opening.

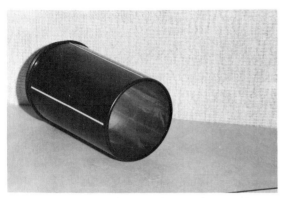

Figure 14–2 Open-ended lead-lined dental x-ray cylinder. The open end and lead lining are essential in reducing scatter radiation.

creates secondary radiation, which scatters in directions other than that of the primary beam, causing exposures of the patient and the operator that do not contribute in any way to high diagnostic yield. The lining of a plastic cylinder is simple and has been described in the literature.

An x-ray beam diameter greater than 2.75 in is frequently needed for various types of extraoral film. Consequently, different size lead collimators and different lengths of lined cylinders may be needed depending on whether or not the dentist makes extraoral film exposures. Extraoral films, particularly the lateral oblique projection of the maxilla and mandible, should be used frequently by the dentist in an effort to obtain a high diagnostic yield.

Filtration. Commercially pure aluminum is commonly used for the filtration of x-ray beams using kilovoltages ordinarily employed in dentistry. The purpose of the filtration is to absorb or attenuate long wavelength x-ray photons that have little likelihood of penetrating the patient's tissue and reaching the film. Such photons are absorbed in the tissue between the outside of the face and the film and cause tissue destruction but no diagnostic yield.

Federal standards related to minimum total filtration (the inherent filtration built into the x-ray tube plus added filtration) changed as of December 1, 1980. Machines operating at 70 kVp and below must now have a minimum half-value layer of 1.5 mm of aluminum (Al). Whereas formerly, low kilovoltage machines were required to have only 0.5 mm total Al filtration, machines operating at 50 kVp now are required to have slightly greater than 2.0 mm Al filtration. The amount of filtration required decreases to 1.5 mm Al at 65 kVp and then increases with increasing kilovoltage. Filtration specifications for machines operating at 70 kVp and above were not changed. Recently manufactured machines ordinarily will conform to these specifications except for the low kilovoltage machines, especially those of foreign manufacture. The new standard will likely remove some machines from the market because increased exposure times necessary to compensate for the added filtration will not be practicable. In most cases, the dentist can add the needed thicknesses of chemically pure aluminum, or he can have this done by qualified personnel who are usually available through the state health department.

The dentist frequently does not know whether the total filtration in his machine is adequate, but a very simple test is available. Preferably using a phantom,* although the use of a patient over the reproductive age is permissible, the dentist makes a conventional intraoral exposure using an exposure time he knows will produce a diagnostic film of suitable density (density is defined as the degree of blackness of a radiographic film). An additional 0.5 mm Al is then inserted in the x-ray beam by removing the cylinder, placing an aluminum disc of appropriate size in the x-ray tube head opening, and replacing the cylinder. Another exposure is made of the same phantom or patient, using exactly the same exposure technique. Both films are processed simultaneously on the same processing rack. If the original filtration was adequate, the insertion of the additional filtration will produce a noticeably lighter film, and the added thickness of aluminum should be removed. If the density of the second film is not visibly reduced, additional 0.5 mm thicknesses of chemically pure aluminum should be sequentially added until the film density is definitely altered. The last thick-

*A substance of thickness and density comparable to human tissue through which the x-ray beam is passed.

ness of aluminum that causes a reduction in density should then be removed. The rationale for this test is based on a desire to filter nonuseful radiation but not to attenuate x-ray photons that can reach the film.

It must be recognized that public health authorities oppose the use of human beings for making such determinations, and their opposition has considerable merit. They feel that humans should be exposed only when the exposure is expected to have benefit for that patient. However, the average dentist does not ordinarily have a suitable phantom at his disposal, and in the author's opinion, a modest excessive exposure of one person in order to minimize exposure in many other people also has merit. The best solution is to consult with trained city or state health department personnel if they are available.

Tube Head Leakage. Modern dental x-ray machines are ordinarily examined during manufacture for tube head leakage and generally can be considered safe for dental office use. On occasion, however, new tube heads have been found to leak x-radiation, and older tube heads frequently show some degree of leakage. To determine leakage, the aperture in the x-ray tube head through which the x-ray beam emanates must be completely obliterated with an approximately ¼ in thick lead disc and the tube head surveyed while the machine is activated, using suitable monitoring equipment that ordinarily is not available in the dental office. State or city health departments often have appropriate personnel and equipment for this type of survey at little or no cost.

Radiation leakage sometimes occurs when the usual lead collimator (or lead washer) does not have a sufficiently large outside diameter. This leakage may not be discovered using ordinary monitoring procedures. It can be detected by using an 8 × 10 in or larger film. The open end of the cylinder is placed in contact with the center of the film surface, and an exposure of relatively long duration is made. When processed, the exposed portion of the film should be totally black, and the surrounding area should be clear. Film blackening beyond the exposed circle indicates a need for modification that can be done by the dentist or a suitable

technician. The use of a pointed plastic cone instead of an open-end lined cylinder will cause film blackening beyond the exposure circle. This is not tube head leakage; it can be remedied by discarding the pointed cone.

Film Speed and Size

The sensitivity of intraoral film emulsions used in dentistry varies widely. Film speeds have been characterized by the American National Standards Institute* using alphabetical speed designations wherein A is the slowest (least sensitive) film. The fastest practical film presently available is the D speed. A and B speed films are no longer available on the American market. Each alphabetical speed designation contains a speed range, but, in general, a C speed film is considered only half as fast (as sensitive) as a D speed. There is a strong likelihood that the Eastman Kodak Co. will market an E speed intraoral film in the near future. Although not required by regulation, most American film manufacturers indicate speed of their product on the outside of the paper package containing approximately a gross of film.

The American National Standards Institute also has classified film according to size. It is suggested that the 1.00 and the 1.0 film, the very small film generally used for children, not be employed because of its small size and the lack of information that can be recorded on it. It is true that the small film is more easily inserted into the child's mouth, but the 1.1 film, a size smaller than the customarily employed 1.2 film, is ordinarily quite suitable even for small children. Tables showing the American National Standards Institute speed and size groupings for dental film are available by writing to the address given in the footnote.

It also is pertinent that the 2.3 bite-wing film (the long, narrow film frequently used by dentists) is inadequate. It is too narrow to

*American National Standards Institute, 1430 Broadway, New York, N.Y. For the most current information about intraoral dental radiographic film standards, contact the American Dental Association's Council on Dental Materials, Instruments, and Equipment, 211 East Chicago Avenue, Chicago, Illinois 60611.

show both maxillary and mandibular structures adequately, and the inclusion of all posterior teeth on one side increases the likelihood of tooth overlap. For these reasons diagnostic yield decreases when 2.3 film is used.

The use of high speed film in older machines having mechanical timers often is difficult because of timer deficiencies. Most mechanical timers will not time below ½ second and not accurately below approximately ¾ of a second. Electronic timers can be purchased for use with most older machines, but there are three other alternatives that may be useful. 1) The inverse square law states that the intensity of x-radiation varies inversely with the square of the distance. Thus, if a dentist is using an 8-in radiation source (x-ray tube anode) to film distance, an increase of this distance to approximately 12 in will require twice the exposure time (assuming all other exposure factors are constant) required at 8 in. Therefore, if a dentist using a C speed film changed to a D speed film, he could use the same exposure time for the D speed film as for the C speed film by increasing his source to film distance by approximately 4 in. 2) Alternatively, the milliamperage of the dental machine, which ordinarily is 10 on the older machines, could be reduced to 5 mA by the insertion of suitable resistors in the wiring of the machine. This can be done inexpensively by a knowledgeable service man. Exposure ordinarily is the product of the mA multiplied by the seconds used. If a dentist employed 10 mA and used a one second exposure for a C speed film, he could use 5 mA and one second for a D speed film; the exposure can be kept constant by decreasing the mA. 3) The third alternative available to the dentist is the use of additional filtration. Added filtration hardens the beam (increases the relative proportion of short wavelength x-ray photons and decreases the proportion of usable but longer wavelength x-ray photons) and reduces the x-ray beam intensity (number of x-ray photons per unit of time). Some experimentation is necessary to determine the amount of added filtration necessary to make the mechanical timer useful with the high speed film. A combination of in-

creased distance, decreased milliamperage, and increased filtration could be used. Film exposure determinations would have to be used and will be considered below.

Determination of Exposure Time. Suitable exposure times using exposure factors predetermined by the dentist should be made regardless of whether alterations in distance, milliamperage, or filtration have been employed to accommodate to mechanical timers. The principle involved is based on the fact that all films should be fully exposed but never overexposed. An underexposed film will always be light (appear underdeveloped) because film processing procedures can be effective only on emulsion grains that have been adequately exposed. Overexposed emulsions will be excessively dark unless darkroom procedures are modified (developing time reduced) to prevent excessive film darkening. Such procedures are contraindicated in view of previously discussed attitudes relating to diagnostic yield. Radiation exposure that is not diagnostically useful should be avoided. Failure to minimize exposure could be classified as an act of malpractice. The darkroom should be used in an entirely standardized fashion according to recommendations of solution manufacturers. The darkroom will be considered at greater length later in this chapter.

Although suitable exposure determinations are best accomplished by using a phantom, the dentist ordinarily will have to use a patient beyond the reproductive age.* A series of approximately six films ordinarily are used. The dentist first determines all the exposure factors he plans to use except exposure time. These factors include kilovoltage, milliamperage, x-ray source to film distance, collimation, filtration, and film type (speed). The first exposure is made for the purpose of producing a film the dentist believes will be objectionably light but at least sufficiently dense to show an image. The remaining films are exposed so that each subsequent film exposure represents a 50 per cent in-

---

*Refer to the section on "Filtration," wherein the objections of public health authorities about the use of patients in lieu of phantoms are made. The author's feelings are also expressed.

crease over the exposure time used for the previous one. For example, if the first, rather light film was exposed for ½ second, the second film would be exposed for ¾ second and the third film would be exposed for 1⅛ seconds. The films are exposed sequentially and are then processed simultaneously on the same film holder using the time-temperature processing directions of the solution manufacturer. Prior to processing, the processing solutions should have been changed, the solution tanks thoroughly cleaned, and all precautions taken to ensure that the darkroom is functionally adequate (see section on darkroom). After the films have been appropriately washed and dried, they are examined, and the dentist determines the most suitable density for his use. Often the dentist will select an exposure time between two of those used for experimental purposes.

The patient employed for this type of procedure should be an adult of average structure. Exposures will have to be increased for heavy boned or obese individuals and decreased for children. The mandibular molar area is ordinarily used for this examination because it requires an average exposure in comparison to the mandibular anterior and the maxillary posterior segments of the dental arches. An exposure for the mandibular anterior area is ordinarily ½ that of the mandibular molar area, and exposure for the maxillary molar region utilizes about a ⅓ increase over that of the mandibular molar region. Exposure values for children and elderly persons may have to be decreased as much as 50 per cent, and for heavy-boned or obese individuals it may have to be doubled. If high kilovoltage techniques in the region of 90 to 100 kVp are employed (with a commensurate decrease in mAs), the need for material changes in exposure time is reduced both for exposure area in the same individual and for people of varying bodily structures.

Technique

Excellence in the performance of all mechanical dental radiologic procedures is essential if high quality films are desired. Pa-tient protection can be accomplished by avoiding repetitious exposure as a result of poor technique and by increasing the diagnostic yield through the availability of optimum quality films.

Radiographic technique is ordinarily divided into chairside and darkroom procedures, and the former is subdivided into intra- and extraoral methods. Space does not permit adequate discussion of these procedures. Extraoral technique will not be mentioned, and only a few salient features of intraoral and darkroom methods will be discussed. The reader should recognize his responsibilities and take adequate steps to ensure the delivery of highly diagnostic radiographic film.

Intraoral Technique. Intraoral techniques ordinarily used in dentistry include the bisecting angle technique and the right angle–paralleling technique. The former ordinarily employs the use of an eight-inch source-to-film distance, while the latter requires an extended distance of 16 inches minimum. The techniques themselves will not be discussed in this chapter. It is pertinent that the right angle or paralleling technique (the film and the object are placed parallel with each other and the x-ray beam is directed at right angles to both the film and the object) will produce a superior intraoral radiograph to one produced using the bisecting procedure. However, both techniques are capable of producing acceptable film, particularly when bite-wing films are used in conjunction with a complete radiographic series made using the bisecting angle procedure. Of considerably greater importance than a discussion of the pros and cons of one technique versus another is the essentiality of using the selected technique with care to produce the best possible intraoral film without the need for re-exposing the patient or being satisfied with less than satisfactory films. Although the use of an increased radiation source to film distance as well as the use of higher kilovoltages (90 or 100 kVp as compared with 50 to 70 kVp) does result in some decreased patient radiation exposure, the difference in absorbed x-radiation using long versus short distances and/or high versus low kilovoltages is too small to recom-

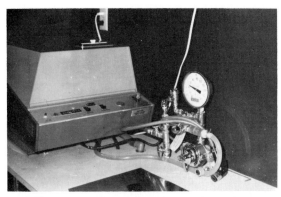

Figure 14-3 Cleanliness and the utilization of proper techniques are essential in the darkroom to achieve the greatest diagnostic yield from the image recorded on the x-ray film.

mend technique changes entirely on this basis. However, increased radiation source to object distance does improve the film definition and reduces film distortion, and kilovoltage alterations do change the contrast of the radiographic film. The dentist may also wish to alter distance and kilovoltage for purposes other than patient protection.

Darkroom. As was mentioned earlier, the darkroom should be used for standardized processing of radiographic film using a strict time-temperature method according to the manufacturer's directions. Adequate technique requires a clean darkroom (Fig. 14–3) and the careful scrubbing of solution tanks with bland soap and a non-abrasive cloth or sponge prior to solution replacement. After the use of soap, all tanks should be carefully rinsed with water. Flushing the fixing tank with dilute acetic acid to insure the complete removal of all alkali before replacing the fixing solution is also advisable. Developing and fixing tanks and covers should not be used interchangeably. Solutions should be used within temperature ranges of 60 to 75 degrees; a developer temperature of 65 to 68 degrees is usually recommended. (Higher temperatures are used in automatic processing units according to the manufacturer's directions.) Maintenance of solution temperature often requires the use of refrigerated water and always requires adequate plumbing, the details of which will not be described in this chapter.

Film fogging is often the result of inade-quate facilities or poor darkroom technique. Fogging is the overall addition to the film surface of varying degrees of blackness caused by factors other than x-radiation exposure. Fogging reduces film quality and minimizes diagnostic yield. Film fogging in the darkroom is ordinarily caused by extraneous light, excessive darkroom safelighting, or contaminated or exhausted processing solutions. The darkroom should be carefully examined for extraneous light by turning off *all* lights and standing in the darkroom for a minimum of five minutes in order to allow for eye accommodation. Chalk or other suitable marking materials should be available. Light leaks can be noted, marked, and subsequently remedied by taping, puttying, or plastering. The most usual locations of light leaks are keyholes and cracks around the darkroom door, but leaks are not limited to these areas.

The use of not more than a 10-watt bulb behind a suitable filter, both contained in a metal housing and placed not closer than four feet from the darkroom counter top, can be recommended for most dental office darkrooms. As with x-radiation, the intensity of visible light varies inversely as the square of the distance. Bringing the darkroom light closer to the counter top increases the intensity of the darkroom lighting and may cause film fogging.

Safelight filters vary with different film. The Kodak ML-2 filter can be used with intraoral film, but it cannot be used with blue- or green-sensitive extraoral film. The Kodak GBX filter can be used with all of these films. The ML-2 filter gives the greatest amount of darkroom light using a constant wattage bulb.

A question often asked is, "How often should x-ray processing solutions be changed?" A very practical answer is, "As often as is necessary." Solutions that are kept covered and at the recommended temperature will last a long time. Obviously, the use of the solutions gradually exhausts the chemicals. Rather than suggest a specific time when solutions should be changed, it seems preferable to advocate placing a control radiograph on the view box ordinarily found in the darkroom. (If a view box is not available in the darkroom, the control film can be put on a view box in the operatory.) This control radiograph should be of optimal quality. When subsequent radiographs do not demonstrate this quality, the dentist should investigate. Under ordinary circumstances, the reason will be exhausted processing solutions, and at this time the solutions should be changed. The replenishment of processing solutions because the level is low can be done either by adding solution replenisher or by adding ordinary developer or fixer. Replenisher is somewhat stronger, but it must be purchased separately and is not generally available through dental supply houses. Because of the small quantities of solution used in dental tanks, it is customary to discard used solutions rather than to attempt to increase solution strength.

Booklets specifically describing darkroom care and utilization can be obtained from leading film and solution manufacturers. The darkroom should be an area of absolute standardization. Failure to standardize darkroom procedures results in an inability to adequately vary chairside exposure techniques in the interest of producing highly diagnostic radiographs.

Lead-Impregnated Aprons. The biological effects of low level x-radiation are not well understood and are, for the most part, extrapolated from experiments using radiation levels far in excess of that acquired in a dental office. Experimental evidence suggests that in most instances almost no adverse effects can be anticipated from exposure to very small quantities of x-radiation. However, some x-radiation absorption effects, particularly those related to blood dyscrasias and genetic alterations, appear to be linearly related to dosage. Strictly as a preventive measure and recognizing that the need may be minimal, it is advocated that lead-impregnated aprons (a minimum of 0.25 millimeter lead equivalent) be used when radiographing children and adults through their reproductive years. It is a well established radiobiological fact that the more embryonic and the more metabolically active cells are most susceptible to ionizing radiation; for this reason and others, children should be protected.

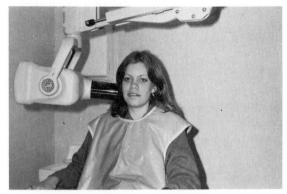

Figure 14–4 Protection against primary and secondary radiation is provided to the patient by both safety factors built into the equipment and the use of a lead apron.

It is frequently stated that the use of the apron provokes unnecessary conversation and possibly promotes apprehension. This may be true. On the other hand, radiation is hazardous, and patients are entitled to be adequately protected. If they are apprehensive, they are deserving of assurance and of explanation as needed. Failure to use adequate preventive measures because of possibly creating obstacles, which subsequently will have to be overcome, is no excuse for neglect (Fig. 14–4).

Structural Shielding. Suitable radiation barriers of a structural nature (permanently fixed) should be incorporated in any new structure and should be added to present structures. However, the amount of barrier material designed to protect people, both patients and employees, in rooms adjoining the radiation exposure area will depend greatly on the workload,* the occupancy factor,† and the use factor.‡ Lead is usually the structural shielding material of choice, but other materials such as ceramic tile, glass, stainless steel, and certain types of plaster, in addition to the distance between the radiation source and the individual who might be

---

*Workload is expressed in milliampere seconds per week.

†Occupancy factor is the factor by which the workload should be multiplied to correct for the degree of occupancy of the area in question while the x-ray machine is "ON."

‡Use factor (or beam direction factor) is the fraction of the workload during which the useful x-ray beam is directed at the barrier under consideration.

exposed, can be suitable barriers depending on a variety of considerations. These matters will not be discussed in detail; rather, the reader is referred to the report of the National Council on Radiation Protection and Measurements No. 35, entitled "Dental X-Ray Protection," which can be secured at a modest cost from NCRP Publications, P. O. Box 4867, Washington, D.C. 20008. This report as it relates to structural shielding design is excellent; however, the report as it relates to *General Considerations* and to *X-ray Equipment* is excessively permissive and in the opinion of this author is not in the best interests of the public. Similarly, certain portions of the section entitled *Operating Procedures* are weak. Appendix A, which includes definitions of radiologic terms, is excellent. The shortcomings as well as the strong points of this report are mentioned for reader guidance.

Operator Protection

The operator, unless he stands directly in the path of the primary radiation beam (the useful beam as it emanates from the x-ray tube head), is exposed primarily to secondary or scattered radiation from the patient. Accordingly, everything that the operator does to minimize the radiation received by the patient in turn reduces the amount of radiation received by him (unless he is standing behind a barrier designed specifically for his protection) (Fig. 14–5).

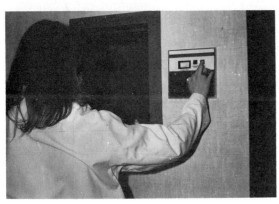

Figure 14–5 The operator is protected from radiation by structural shielding. Federal standards have been set to protect against both primary and secondary radiation. Here the operator is standing behind a lead-lined wall with a lead-glass window.

The use of barriers in the dental office is advocated but may not be necessary unless x-radiation is used frequently. For example, it is essential to have a barrier for operator protection in a clinic where radiographs are being taken almost constantly as part of the clinic's diagnostic procedure. Conversely, the need for a barrier simply does not exist in an office where very minimal usage is made of x-radiation. Thus, in the average dental office, barriers probably should be placed in the "nice to have" category. Barriers for operator protection should not be confused with structural shielding for non-occupationally exposed individuals.

Of considerably greater importance than barriers in the average situation is distance and position. These factors will be discussed in some detail.

Distance. As has been mentioned several times earlier, the intensity of x-radiation varies inversely with the square of the distance. If a dentist foolishly stands one foot from the patient during exposure, he receives "x" amount of scattered radiation, and he will receive one fourth of that amount if he moves two feet away from the patient. It is ordinarily recommended that the dentist stand a minimum of five feet from the patient and from the x-ray tube head and that he definitely not stand in the primary x-ray beam. If the operatory situation makes this impossible, the need for a suitable x-ray barrier must be considered; in all probability a barrier will no longer be in the "nice to have" category, but rather it will be needed. However, other factors, particularly the workload, enter into these deliberations. Naturally, the existence of any leakage radiation (which definitely should not exist) is an important consideration.

Operator Position. When exposing the anterior part of the face, the operator should stand on either side of the patient, toward the back of the patient's head, in a position between 90 and 135 degrees to the x-ray beam. Secondary and scattered radiation produced at the anterior part of the face is well filtered by the head, and little of it emanates from the side of the head near the occipital region. When an exposure is made of the side of the face, the operator is advised to stand in a position from 90 to 135 degrees to the x-ray beam in back of the patient's head. The advantages of this position are identical with those above. It is preferable that the operator not stand 90 to 135 degrees to the x-ray beam in front of the patient's face because more secondary and scattered radiation can emanate out of the soft tissues of the patient's face than through the denser portions of the patient's skull.

Maximum Permissible Dose. Radiation protection standards permit users of x-radiation, namely the operators, to absorb substantially more whole body exposure than that allowed the average individual in the population. This is not because the operator has or acquires more resistance to the radiation. The percentage of individuals in the population who are using radiation is extremely small in comparison with those who are exposed to x-radiation for diagnostic purposes, and, from a genetic standpoint, the accumulation of genetic alterations in the entire population (the genetic mutation pool) is affected very minimally by x-radiation users.

While the concept of a maximum permissible dose (MPD) for operators generally is not publicized because it tends to produce a false sense of security, a formula does exist that states that radiation workers may receive an accumulated dose to critical organs (hence whole body radiation) of $(N-18) \times 5$ rem (roentgen equivalent man). For dental purposes, the rem can be thought of as equivalent to the roentgen or rad. The N in this formula is the present age of the patient. The product of this formula indicates the amount of whole body radiation that a radiation worker can accumulate through any given age, with the important stipulation that the radiation dose in any 13 consecutive weeks must not exceed 3 rem. An analysis of this formula indicates that individuals 18 years of age and younger should not be using x-radiation. It is also important to emphasize that a weekly accumulation in excess of 25 milliroentgens of whole body radiation (approximately ¼ of the average weekly permissible accumulation using the above formula) should be considered maximum, and means should be taken to greatly reduce total exposure. The MPD for users has no direct relationship to the exposure of users for diagnostic purposes. There is no maximum permissible dose for non-users.

DIAGNOSTIC YIELD IN RELATION TO TECHNIQUE AND INTERPRETATION

It was emphasized in the opening paragraphs of this chapter that "diagnostic yield" is a measurement of the effectiveness with which x-radiation is used. It was pointed out that diagnostic yield is heavily interrelated with radiation protection methods, chairside technique, and radiographic interpretation. Radiation protection methods in the dental office have been discussed, and certain aspects of chairside and darkroom technique have been incorporated into radiation reduction methods. Space does not permit more detailed discussion of these topics. The reader is encouraged to use appropriate dental radiology texts to become more informed.

It is equally impossible to discuss radiographic interpretation adequately within the space permitted. However, a chapter of this nature must include certain pertinent matters related to interpretation if the concepts of preventive dentistry as related to radiology are to be even reasonably complete. Discussion will be limited to a description of 1) what constitutes an adequate single film or complete mouth radiographic survey, and 2) what are the most frequently made radiographic interpretive errors related to preventive dentistry.

Criteria of an Adequate Intraoral Radiographic Survey

Radiographs should be taken for specific purposes (Fig. 14–6). Single films or complete radiographic surveys ordinarily are taken to examine crowns, periodontal structures, and periapical regions of the dentition. Accordingly, the apices of all teeth should be observed at least once in a complete survey. This does not mean that all radiographic films of a region must demonstrate the apical portion of the tooth adequately in all films,

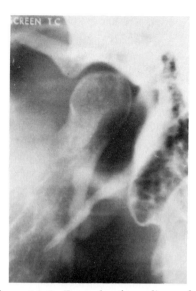

Figure 14–6 Example of a radiograph taken with an S. S. White Panorex unit utilizing appropriate techniques for visualization of the temporomandibular joint and surrounding structures.

but the apex of each tooth root must be clearly observable at least one time in the survey. This criterion is necessary in order to detect apical pathology. Additionally, the interproximal contacting surfaces of abutting teeth must be observable at least once without any overlapping of contiguous teeth and, in the case of the posterior teeth, with the buccal cusps superimposed on the lingual or palatal cusps. The detection of incipient caries and incipient periodontal bone changes definitely requires a lack of interproximal surface superimposition and an angulation technique that neither distorts the height of the periodontal bone level nor hides small carious lesions in the bulk of remaining enamel in the contact point region. To fulfill these criteria, it becomes absolutely necessary to utilize the principles of the right angle–paralleling technique, either through employing the technique itself or through the use of bite-wing films. If bite-wing films are used, it is strongly advocated that two 2.2 films be used on each side (or alternatively two 1.2 films can be used if the dentist chooses to place his own bite-wing tabs) rather than one 2.3 bite-wing film (through age approximately 12 years only, one 2.2 film per side is necessary).

American National Standards Institute classification of intraoral film and the reasons for the above recommendations were stated earlier in this chapter.

Frequent Interpretive Errors Related to Preventive Dentistry

Radiographic interpretation of hard tissue abnormalities is an essential aspect of oral diagnosis. Detection of a diseased state usually prevents progress of pathologic conditions; within this concept all radiographic interpretation is a part of preventive dentistry. There are, however, a few interpretive errors related to caries, periodontal disease, and apical pathology that are very commonly made. Because of space limitations, only these will be discussed.

Interpretive Errors Related to Dental Caries. Among numerous errors in the interpretation of dental caries that are made frequently are two that must be mentioned in this chapter. It is essential to emphasize that a dental caries lesion observed radiographically *always* appears smaller than the carious lesion actually is when observed either clinically or microscopically. Consequently, there is no such thing as a radiographically "small" lesion. The statement: "That carious area is small. Let's leave it and watch it," if made with respect to children and young adults, is synonymous with neglect unless there are other extenuating circumstances that suggest a need for delaying treatment. The location of these "small" lesions is usually interproximal, just below the contact area, but it may be occlusal, at the dentoenamel junction. The latter, however, is usually detected clinically. In a patient over approximately 30 years of age, a small-appearing lesion is probably arrested caries and often will not need treatment.

The second frequently made error is in the interpretation of pulp exposure based on observing a large carious lesion and its *apparent* continuity into the pulp chamber. The position of the lesion in relation to the pulp or angulation of the x-ray beam can easily superimpose a carious lesion onto the pulp chamber and create an erroneous interpretation. The radiograph is very useful in demonstrating the presence of the carious lesion, and it gives some idea of the lesion's extent, but clinical methods should be used to determine the actual depth of the carious lesion. Less reliance on the radiographic film may prevent tooth loss in such instances.

Interpretive Errors Related to Periodontal Disease. Probably the most neglected field of dental practice is periodontology. Similarly, one of the more important diagnostic shortcomings of dental practitioners is a failure to recognize radiographic signs of incipient periodontal disease. These manifestations include triangulation; lack of continuity (hence irregularity) of the crestal alveolar bone surface between abutting teeth; and a tendency to produce excessive bone condensation, particularly near the crest of the interproximal alveolar bone.

The other frequent error relates directly to the x-ray beam angulation used to produce the radiograph. Intraoral films taken for periodontal purposes are most useful when the film and the tooth are parallel to each other and the x-ray beam is directed at a right angle to both. The right angle–parallcling technique or a well-taken bitewing film accomplishes this purpose. Failure to follow these directions distorts the anatomic relationship of tooth and supportive bone, causing the buccal bone shadow to be cast closer to the tooth crown than it actually is. An impression is gained that more supportive bone exists than is actually the case.

Interpretive Errors Related to Apical Pathology. The periapical radiograph serves the important objective of demonstrating the presence of apical pathology when it exists in a chronic state unaccompanied by subjective patient symptoms. In doing so, it is extremely valuable. The radiograph cannot be used to differentiate between the abscess, the granuloma, and the cyst, and treatment should not be based on the dentist's efforts to do the impossible. Accordingly, endodontic and oral surgery decisions relative to the treatment of apical lesions should not be based on radiographic information. One exception seems to exist: a lesion that appears "typically" cystic is likely to be cystic. (Cysts are described radiographically as a *distinctly*

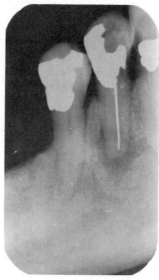

Figure 14–7 X-ray demonstrating periapical lesion. Diagnosis of a periapical granuloma was made histologically on retreatment.

radiolucent area clearly delineated by a peripheral opaque lamina that may or may not be continuous with the lamina dura of the involved tooth.) Conversely, a lesion can appear to be "typically" an abscess or granuloma (Fig. 14–7) (typical in terms of descriptions found in many textbooks and criteria used generally by the profession) and yet contain epithelial cells in lumen formation, the usual histologic criterion for a cyst. While the need for enucleating cysts is not a radiographic problem (Fig. 14–8), it is pertinent to mention that apical lesions measuring not more than approximately a centimeter in

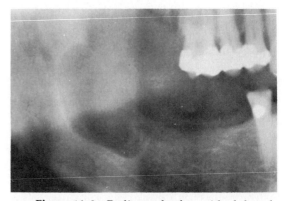

Figure 14–8 Radiograph of a residual dental cyst resulting from the incomplete removal of a third molar. The lesion was treated surgically and diagnosis confirmed histologically.

diameter, regardless of their radiographic appearance (thus regardless of whether they are abscesses, granulomas, or cysts), ordinarily will be replaced by normal bone without surgical interference if the agent causing the lesion is eliminated.

SUMMARY

This chapter has interrelated dental radiology with preventive dentistry and has emphasized the justification of x-radiation usage by the dental profession on the basis of *diagnostic yield*. It has intimated that dentists whose diagnostic yield is consistently low probably should be denied the use of x-radiation. In the interest of present and future generations, technical and interpretive competency should be determined. The adequacy of equipment should be certified by local or state agencies. Everything possible should be done to increase the balance between risk and gain in the use of x-radiation in dentistry by heavily outweighing gain as opposed to risk. This is preventive dentistry.

It now remains, not as a summary of previous material but as an additional statement of fact, to relate patient whole body (hence genetic organ) exposure to background radiation received from the cosmos and from surrounding environmental situations. Such background radiation has been in existence since man evolved and has probably contributed substantially to his evolution. A complete mouth survey of 17 periapical films and four bite-wing films can be taken using less than 5 R of exposure at skin. For each R of exposure at skin, it is estimated that the gonadal exposure is approximately 1/10,000 of an R or 0.5 mR for the full mouth survey. This amount of radiation is approximately equivalent to the background radiation received by the patient each day of his normal life if he resides at or near sea level. People in higher altitudes receive more background exposure. Such minimal exposure can be justified. However, the above stated 5 R total exposure is based on the optimal use of x-radiation by the dentist. Dental practice habits commonly in vogue frequently result in a total exposure of from 25 to 60 R instead

of the 5 R, and grossly poor technique no doubt could increase the total exposure still more. Obviously, the diagnostic yield would be materially decreased under such circumstances. These data relate entirely to x-ray machine adequacy and to technical excellence. They cannot be related to interpretive ability, but unless this ability is high, any exposure is unjustified.

It is hoped that the remarks in this chapter will encourage the reader to become more conscious of the inherent dangers of diagnostic dental radiography. The profession has needed the services of dental radiology specialists for many years, but efforts to have such a group recognized have been thwarted. The intent has never been to deny the profession use of x-radiation; rather, emphasis has been placed on making a service available to the public and the profession to the extent that these services could be helpful. The availability of such specialists could be most useful to those dentists whose technical and interpretive abilities are marginal.

ADDITIONAL READING

1. Alcox, W. A., and Jameson, W. R.: Patient exposures from intra-oral radiographic examinations. J. Am. Dent. Assoc. *88*:568, 1974.
2. American Dental Association: New American Dental Association Specification No. 26 for dental x-ray equipment. J. Am. Dent. Assoc. *89*:366, 1974.
3. American Dental Association: Recommendation in radiographic practices — January 1975. J. Am. Dent. Assoc. *90*:171, 1975.
4. American Dental Association: Advantages and disadvantages of the use of dental tomographic radiography. J. Am. Dent. Assoc. *94*:147, 1977.
5. American Dental Association: Recommendations in radiographic practices — March 1978. J. Am. Dent. Assoc. *96*:485, 1978.
6. Beideman, R. W., Johnson, O. N., and Alcox, W. A.: A study to develop a rating system and evaluate dental radiographs submitted to a third party carrier. J. Am. Dent. Assoc. *93*:1010, 1976.
7. Berkman, M. D.: Pedodontic radiographic interpretation. Dent. Radiogr. Photogr. *44*:27, 1971.
8. Cheraskin, E.: Roentgenographic manifestations of osseous changes in the jaws. Oral Surg. *12*:442, 1959.
9. Clark, D. E.: Association of irradiation with cancer of the thyroid in children and adolescents. J. Am. Dent. Assoc. *159*:1007, 1955.
10. Curby, W. A., and Wuehrmann, A. H.: Utilization

Illustrations for this chapter furnished by Richard E. Stallard, Minndent Associates, Inc., Edina, Minnesota.

of constant exposure factors for intraoral roent-genographic studies. J. Dent. Res. *32*:790, 1953.

11. Darzenta, N. C., and Giunta, J. L.: Radiographic changes of the mandible related to oral contraceptives. Oral Surg. *43*:478, 1977.

12. Duffy, B. J., Jr., and Fitzgerald, P. J.: Cancer of the thyroid in children: A report on 28 cases. J. Clin. Endocr. *10*:1296, 1950.

13. Dummett, C. O.: Review of the clinical and roentgenologic manifestations of incipient periodontal disease. Ann. Dent. *4*:47, 1945.

14. Fitzgerald, G. M.: Dental roentgenography. I. An investigation in adumbration, or the factors that control geometric unsharpness. J. Am. Dent. Assoc. *34*:1, 1947.

15. Gibbs, S. J., Crabtree, C. L., and Johnson, O. N.: An educational approach to voluntary improvement of dental radiological practices. J. Am. Dent. Assoc. *95*:562, 1977.

16. Goepp, R., et al.: The reduction of unnecessary x-ray exposure during intraoral examinations. Oral Surg. *16*:39, 1963.

17. Hurlburt, E. H., and Wuehrmann, A. H.: Comparison of interproximal carious lesion detection in panoramic and standard intraoral radiography. J. Am. Dent. Assoc. *93*:1154, 1976.

18. Johnson, O. N., and Barone, G. J.: What the federal x-ray regulations mean to the dentist. J. Am. Dent. Assoc. *95*:810, 1977.

19. Lopez, J., Jr.: Xeroradiography in dentistry. J. Am. Dent. Assoc. *92*:106, 1976.

20. Manson-Hing, L. R.: On the evaluation of radiographic techniques. Oral Surg. *27*:631–634, 1969.

21. Manson-Hing, L. R.: Kilovolt peak and the visibility of lamina dura breaks. Oral Surg. *31*:268–273, 1971.

22. Manson-Hing, L. R.: The fundamental biologic effects of x-rays in dentistry. Oral Surg. *12*:562, 1959.

23. Manson-Hing, L. R.: Vision and oral roentgenology. Oral Surg. *15*:173, 1962.

24. Menezer, L. F.: The open-ended metal column for the dental x-ray machine. J. Am. Dent. Assoc. *73*:1083, 1966.

25. National Council on Radiation Protection and Measurements: Dental x-ray protection, NCRP report no. 35, Washington, D.C., 1970, NCRP Publications.

26. Parfitt, G. J.: An investigation of the normal variations in alveolar bone trabeculation. Oral Surg. *15*:1453, 1962.

27. Prichard, J.: The role of the roentgenogram in the diagnosis and prognosis of periodontal disease. Oral Surg. *14*:182, 1961.

28. Priebe, W. A., et al.: The value of the roentgeno-graphic film in the differential diagnosis of periapical lesions. Oral Surg. *7*:979, 1954.

29. Report of the Radiation Protection Committee, American Academy of Oral Roentgenology: The effective use of x-radiation in dentistry. Oral Surg. *16*:294, 1963.

30. Richards, A. G.: Roentgen-ray doses in dental roentgenography. J. Am. Dent. Assoc. *56*:351, 1958.

31. Richards, A. G., et al.: X-ray protection in the dental office. J. Am. Dent. Assoc. *56*:514, 1958.

32. Richards, A. G.: New concepts in dental x-ray machines. J. Am. Dent. Assoc. *73*:69, 1966.

33. Richards, A. G.: Sources of x-radiation in the dental office. Dent. Radiogr. Photogr. *27*:51, 1964.

34. Richards, A. G.: Radiation barriers. Oral Surg. *25*:701, 1968.

35. Shafer, W. G., Hine, M. K., and Levy, B. M.: A Textbook of Oral Pathology. 2nd ed., Philadelphia, W. B. Saunders Co., 1963.

36. Shira, R. B.: Roentgenographic interpretation as an aid in oral surgical procedures. J. Am. Dent. Assoc. *65*:449, 1962.

37. Stafne, E. C.: Oral roentgenographic diagnosis, Philadelphia, W. B. Saunders Co., 1958.

38. Terezhalmy, G. T., and Bottomley, W. K.: General legal aspects of diagnostic dental radiography. Oral Surg. *48*:486, 1979.

39. Trout, E. D., et al.: Conventional building materials as protective barriers in dental roentgenographic installations. Oral Surg. *15*:1211, 1962.

40. White, S. C., and Weissman, D. D.: Relative discernment of lesions by intraoral and panoramic radiography. J. Am. Dent. Assoc. *95*:1117, 1977.

41. White, S. C., and Rose, T. C.: Absorbed bone marrow dose in certain dental radiographic techniques. J. Am. Dent. Assoc. *98*:553, 1979.

42. Worth, H. M.: Principles and Practice of Oral Radiologic Interpretation. Chicago, Year Book Medical Publishers, Inc., 1963.

43. Wuehrmann, A. H.: Evaluation criteria for intraoral radiographic film quality. J. Am. Dent. Assoc. *89*:345, 1974.

44. Wuehrmann, A. H.: Radiation Protection and Dentistry, St. Louis, The C. V. Mosby Co., 1960.

45. Wuehrmann, A. H.: Procedure for lining open-end dental x-ray cylinders with lead foil. Oral Surg. *30*:64–65, July 1970.

46. Wuehrmann, A. H.: The long cone technic. P.D.M., p. 1, July, 1957.

47. Wuehrmann, A. H.: Roentgenographic interpretation of dental caries. P.D.M., pp. 3–46, Sept., 1959.

48. Wuehrmann, A. H., and Manson-Hing, L. R.: Dental Radiology. 5th ed., St. Louis, The C. V. Mosby Co., 1981.

CHAPTER FIFTEEN

The Prevention and Detection of Oral Cancer

Theodore E. Bolden, D.D.S., Ph.D.

At present, total prevention of cancer before its occurrence is difficult, if not impossible. However, cancer can be prevented from causing rapid destruction of tissues and death to the patient by early diagnosis detection and treatment. Cancer can be cured and prevented from causing sequelae and complications *prior* to the appearance of the classical symptoms and signs of the disease. Therefore, in thinking in terms of prevention in its truest sense, early diagnosis detection and the use of control methods can prevent mutilation of tissues and metastasis of the disease and provide the greatest chance of survival for the patient.

THE "FACE" OF ORAL CANCER

Variability

The first step toward the prevention and detection of oral cancer in the individual patient is for the health professional to develop an awareness for the high degree of variability in the appearance, that is, in the "face," of oral cancer.

Tissues and Areas Involved

The second step is for the health professional to develop an appreciation for the fact that oral cancer may involve any of the basic tissues of the oral cavity as the "primary" site and, conversely, that any of the

tissues of the oral cavity may be involved as the "secondary" site for malignant processes primary to other parts of the body.

We define the basic tissues as epithelium, connective tissue, muscle, nerve, and blood. What the dentist "sees" when he examines the oral tissues is primarily epithelium, the mucous membrane that lines the oral cavity. For convenience, we divide the oral cavity into anatomical areas designated as lips, gingiva, jaws, floor of the mouth, tongue, buccal mucosa, palate, pulp, and para-oral tissues. These areas are readily accessible for direct observation, palpation, and inspection. A section through each one would be composed of a representative of each of the five basic tissues. Only the proportions of these would differ. For example, a section of tongue would show a preponderance of muscle, while a section through the palate would show little muscle (Figs. 15–1 and 15–2).

CANCER OF THE LIP

About one per cent of all malignant neoplasms appearing in the human are carcinoma of the lip. A 20-year survey, from 1940 to 1959, showed 4,357 cancers of the lip. Ninety-four per cent involved the lower lip, and more were observed in males than females. Most labial cancers are squamous cell carcinomas. Localization showed no sex predilection (Table 15–1).

Sixty-one cases of lip cancer were col-

277

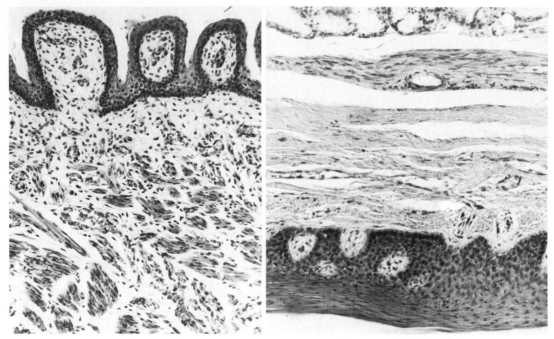

Fig. 15–1   Fig. 15–2

Figure 15–1   Photomicrograph of a normal human tongue demonstrating the stratified squamous epithelium on the surface with an underlying layer of connective tissue. Note the thick muscular layer beneath. (×120)

Figure 15–2   Compare this photomicrograph of human palate with Figure 15–1. Note the absence of muscular tissue in the section. (×120)

lected from 1962 to 1974 at the University of Florida Medical Center. Nearly 86 per cent occurred in males;[2] nearly 23 per cent involved the upper lip.[2] Therapy consisted of surgery or radiotherapy or combined therapy and in two cases chemotherapy. Death was attributable to cancer of the lip in 23 per cent of the cases. The mortality for 27 patients with recurrent lip cancer was 52 per cent.

Basal cell carcinoma presents with nearly equal frequency on the upper and lower lip

(Table 15–2). Lip cancer is associated with the use of tobacco, most frequently as a cigarette (Table 15–3).[3]

Carcinoma of the lip has also been attributed to such factors as smoking of short hot pipes, leukoplakia, chronic inflammatory fissuring of the lip, and sun exposure. The consumption of alcohol does not appear to be significant in the production of lip cancer. This is more often a disease of men whose average age is 66. The incidence of lip cancers increases with increase in age (Table 15–4). Metastasis to the submental and submandibular lymph nodes occurs in about 25 per cent of patients, often appears late, and is predominantly from the lower lip. The five-year survival rate is remarkably high, ranging from approximately 70 to 95 per cent (Table 15–5)[3] to 85 to 100 per cent, but it is lower in females than in males.[4]

It should be understood that approximately 80 per cent of carcinomatous lesions of the lip are smaller than 2 cm in diameter, have little tendency to infiltrate, present on

TABLE 15–1   ORAL CANCER°

SITE	NO. PATIENTS	SEX RATIO	PERCENTAGE LOCALIZED	
			Male	*Female*
Lip	4,357	13:1	85	86
Tongue	3,335	4:1	39	54

°Adapted from Latourette, H. B., and Myers, M. H.: End-results of treatment of oral and laryngopharyngeal cancer. Fifth National Cancer Conference Proceedings. Philadelphia, J. B. Lippincott Co., 1964.

TABLE 15–2 CELLULAR TYPES OF LIP CARCINOMAS BY ANATOMICAL
SITES AMONG NEGRO AND WHITE MALES°

| | ANATOMICAL SITES | | | | | | | |
| | LOWER LIPS | | UPPER LIPS | | BOTH LIPS | | TOTAL | |
CARCINOMAS	No.	Per Cent	No.	Per Cent	No.	Per Cent	No.	Per Cent
Squamous cell	279	88.8	12	3.8	3	1.0	294	93.6
Basal cell	6	1.9	9	2.9	1	0.3	16	5.1
Both 1 and 2			1	0.3	3	1.0	4	1.3
Total	285	90.7	22	7.0	7	2.3	314	100.0

°From Keller, A. Z.: Cellular types, survival, race, nativity, occupations, habits and associated diseases in the pathogenesis of lip cancers. Am. J. Epidemiol. *91*(5):486–499, 1970.

the lower lip as well as differentiated lesions, and develop regional metastasis late.[5] Nearly 95 per cent of these carcinomas are cured by various methods of radiotherapy.

CANCER OF THE GINGIVA

The highest incidence of gingival cancer occurs in South India where it constitutes roughly 9 per cent of all cancer cases seen. Twenty-five per cent of all oral cancers in South India and 16 per cent and 12 per cent of all oral cancers seen in Georgia and Memorial Hospital, respectively, were epidermoid cancers of the gingiva.[6] The distribution by sex of 606 patients with epidermoid cancer of the gum (1942–1961) was 77 per cent men (465) and 23 per cent women.[7] In 79 per cent of all females and 88 per cent of all males, the cancer occurred between 50 and 80 years of age. Symptoms consist of ulceration or pain or both in nearly every case. A few patients complained primarily of inability to wear previously well-fitting dentures or of bleed-

TABLE 15–3 TYPE OF TOBACCO SMOKED BY CASES OF LIP CANCERS AND
THEIR CONTROLS (WHITE MALES ONLY)°

| | CASES OF LIP CANCER | | CONTROLS | | | |
| | | | CANCER† | | GENERAL‡ | |
CLASSIFICATION	No.	Per Cent	No.	Per Cent	No.	Per Cent
Non-smokers	22	7.3[b]	16	5.3[a]	44	16.6[a,b]
Ex-smokers	7	2.3[d]	2	0.7[d]	3	1.1
Cigarettes only	181	60.2	194	64.5	140	52.8
Cigars only	7	2.3	10	3.3	10	3.8
Pipes only	18	6.0	14	4.6	9	3.4
Cigarettes and cigars	4	1.3	1	0.3	0	0.0
Cigarettes and pipes	13	4.3[c]	6	2.0	0	0.0[c]
Cigars and pipes	4	1.3	10	3.3[c]	0	0.0[c]
Cigarettes, cigars and pipes	2	0.7	2	0.7	1	0.4
Not stated	43	14.3	46	15.3	58	21.9
Total	301	100.0	301	100.0	265	100.0

°From Keller, A. Z.: Cellular types, survival, race, nativity, occupations, habits and associated diseases in the pathogenesis of lip cancers. Am. J. Epidemiol. *91*(5):486–499, 1970.
†Males with squamous cell carcinomas of the intra-oral cavity and pharynx.
‡Males from all diagnostic categories of medical and surgical patients.
[a]:p <0.00001.
[b]:p <0.001.
[c]:p <0.01.
[d]:p <0.05.

TABLE 15–4 MINIMUM ANNUAL
RATES OF CASE INCIDENCE AND THE
TOTAL DISTRIBUTION BY AGE FOR
WHITE MALES WITH LIP CANCERS*

	TOTAL CASES		ANNUAL INCIDENCE	
AGE IN YEARS	No.	Per Cent	No.†	Rate‡
25–29	2	0.6	2	0.07
30–34	3	1.0	2	0.06
35–39	23	7.4	22	0.53
40–44	26	8.4	23	0.74
45–49	24	7.7	21	1.20
50–54	24	7.7	21	1.95
55–59	15	4.8	12	1.89
60–64	45	14.5	41	3.55
65–69	94	30.2	86	9.07
70+	55	17.7	53	9.73
Total	311	100.0	283	1.43

*From Keller, A. Z.: Cellular types, survival, race, nativity, occupations, habits and associated diseases in the pathogenesis of lip cancers. Am. J. Epidemiol. 91(5):486–499, 1970.
†Newly diagnosed cases of lip cancer from 1958 through 1962.
‡Number of cases per 100,000 living veterans.

TABLE 15–5 FIVE-YEAR RATES OF
SURVIVAL FOR MALES WITH LIP
CANCERS BY STAGE, SITE AND
CELLULAR TYPE OF THE DISEASE
AND BY RACE*

CLASSIFICATION	NO.	RATE†	STANDARD ERROR‡
Total			
Cases	314	95.23	1.20
U. S. males[a]	314	86.44	0.61
Race			
Negroes[b]	3	98.69	0.00
Whites	311	95.20	1.20
Stage of disease			
Localized	283	96.61	1.12
Metastasized	31	82.34	4.58
Site of disease			
Lower lip	285	94.74	1.35
Upper lip[b]	22	100.00	0.00
Both lips[b]	7	96.99	0.00
Cellular type of disease			
Squamous cell	294	94.84	1.32
Basal cell	16	100.00	0.00
Both cell types[b]	4	97.80	0.00
Cases with skin cancers of head, face and neck			
Present	38	91.98	3.96
Absent	276	95.65	1.19

*From Keller, A. Z.: Cellular types, survival, race, nativity, occupations, habits and associated diseases in the pathogenesis of lip cancers. Am. J. Epidemiol. 91(5):486–499, 1970.
†Each rate and standard error is adjusted to the age distribution of the total cases.
‡One standard error of the rate.
[a]United States males of the case's age and race.
[b]Among each of these, there were no deaths; thus each unadjusted survival rate is 100 per cent and standard error of the rate is zero.

ing. When pain was cited as the primary symptom, 51 per cent of the patients had symptoms for less than three months, while in those with the complaint of relatively painless ulceration, 42 per cent sought care within this period.

An accurate history of smoking was obtained in 452 of the 606 cases. Thirty-four per cent of male patients were either cigar or pipe smokers.[6] The majority of gingival lesions averaged between three and five cm when first observed by the dentist (Table 15–6).

In radiologic examination of 216 of the 606 cases, 81 per cent (97 of 113 cases) proved to have histologic evidence of bone invasion, if no roentgenographic evidence of bone distribution was seen. Pathologic examination of the surgical specimen removed indicated that the epidermoid cancer extended to medial soft tissues, such as the floor of the mouth and tongue, or to lateral soft tissues, such as the gingivobuccal gutter, cheek, lip, and retromolar space, in a high proportion of patients. The use of snuff in the gingivobuccal sulcus is considered causative for gingival carcinoma.[8]

Most cancers of the gingiva require removal or destruction of the mandible be-

cause, in over 85 per cent of the cases, the bone is invaded. By contrast, in the case of cancer of the floor of the mouth, bone invasion occurs in less than 20 per cent of the patients.[9] Bone has been sacrificed in both instances in order to obtain a safe margin and to effectuate closure.

TABLE 15–6 SIZE OF PRESENTING
LESION*

SIZE	NO. OF CASES	PER CENT
Less than 2 cm.	134	22
2–3 cm.	176	29
3–5 cm.	193	32
Greater than 5 cm.	72	12
Unknown	21	

*From Cady, B., and Catlin, D.: Epidermoid carcinoma of the gum. A 20-year survey. Cancer 23: 551–564, March 1969.

TABLE 15-7   NUMBER OF PATIENTS AND PER CENT AGE DISTRIBUTION BY SEX—
CANCER OF FLOOR OF MOUTH IN CONNECTICUT, 1935–1959*

	TOTAL		MALE		FEMALE	
AGE	No.	Per Cent	No.	Per Cent	No.	Per Cent
0–49	56	11.8	49	11.3	7	16.7
50–59	129	27.1	116	26.7	13	31.0
60–69	196	30.7	137	31.6	9	21.4
70–79	106	22.3	97	22.4	9	21.4
80+	39	8.2	35	8.1	4	9.5
All Ages	476	100.0	434	100.0	42	100.0
Median Age	63		64		61	

*From Shedd, D. P., Von Essen, C. F., Ferraro, R. H., Connelly, R. R., and Eisenberg, H.: Cancer of the floor of the mouth in Connecticut, 1935–1959. Cancer 21:97–101, January, 1968.

Some 25 per cent of all oral cancers seen at the Cancer Institute, Madras, India, are cancers of the lower gingiva and are related to the habit of tobacco, betel, and nut chewing.[10]

Of 188 cases of lower gingival carcinoma, 120 were primary, and 68 were metastatic. Less than 14 per cent were confined to the gingiva; 86 per cent involved the gingiva, cheek, or floor of the mouth or all three. The mandible was involved in 69 per cent[11] of the cases. One hundred sixty-six cases already had clinical cervical lymph node metastasis, while less than 2 per cent had distant metastases (3 cases).[12]

CANCER OF THE FLOOR OF THE MOUTH

Epidermoid carcinoma is the most frequent malignant lesion of the floor of the mouth, and it is seen more often in males than in females.[13] Other malignancies that are encountered in the floor of the mouth are adenocarcinoma, transitional cell carcinoma, basal cell carcinoma, myxosarcoma, and unspecified sarcoma. The incidence in males increases with increase in age (Table 15–7). The lowest incidence for males is experienced in Sweden, and the highest figure for males and females was reported from Puerto Rico (Table 15–8). The most frequent sites of oral cancer in Puerto Rico are the tongue and the floor of the mouth. The highest incidence of carcinoma of the floor of the mouth in males is seen in the fifth decade and in females in the sixth decade.[14] The disease is usually localized at the time of original diagnosis and responds well to surgery (Table 15–9). Women tend to survive better than men (Tables 15–10 and 15–11), and localized lesions have the best five-year

TABLE 15-8   ANNUAL INCIDENCE OF CANCER OF FLOOR OF MOUTH BY
SEX AND GEOGRAPHIC AREA*

		ANNUAL INCIDENCE RATES (per 100,000)					
		NO. OF PATIENTS		CRUDE		AGE-ADJUSTED†	
GEOGRAPHIC AREA	PERIOD	Male	Female	Male	Female	Male	Female
10 U.S. Cities	1947	89	19	1.4	0.3	–	–
Sweden	1958–61	25	11	0.2	0.1	0.1	0.1
Norway	1953–61	107	61	0.7	0.4	0.6	0.3
New York‡	1958–60	160	45	1.2	0.3	1.2	0.3
Puerto Rico	1950–61	194	66	1.4	0.5	2.4	0.8
Connecticut	1935–59	434	42	1.7	0.2	1.8	0.1

*From Shedd, D. P., Von Essen, C. F., Ferraro, R. H., Connelly, R. R., and Eisenberg, H.: Cancer of the floor of the mouth in Connecticut, 1935–1959. Cancer 21:97–101, January, 1968.
†The total population of the continental United States (1950) was used as the standard.
‡Exclusive of New York City.

TABLE 15-9 NUMBER OF PATIENTS AND PER CENT STAGE DISTRIBUTION
BY TYPE OF TREATMENT—CANCER OF FLOOR OF MOUTH IN CONNECTICUT,
1935–1959*

STAGE OF DISEASE	SURGERY ALONE		RADIATION ALONE		SURGERY PLUS RADIATION		NO TREATMENT	
	No.	Per Cent	No.	Per Cent	No.	Per Cent	No.	Per Cent
Localized	62	56.4	114	47.1	25	37.9	10	31.3
Regional	33	30.0	101	41.7	34	51.5	16	50.0
Distant	3	2.7	10	4.1	3	4.5	4	12.5
Unknown	12	10.9	17	7.0	4	6.1	2	6.2
All Stages	110	100.0	242	100.0	66	100.0	32	100.0

*Live diagnoses only. Excludes cases reported only by autopsy and death certificate. (From Shedd, D. P., Von Essen, C. F., Ferraro, R. H., Connelly, R. R., and Eisenberg, H.: Cancer of the floor of the mouth in Connecticut, 1935–1959. Cancer 21:97–101, January, 1968.)

TABLE 15-10 NUMBER OF PATIENTS AND RELATIVE SURVIVAL RATES BY
TIME PERIOD OF DIAGNOSIS—CANCER OF FLOOR OF MOUTH IN
CONNECTICUT, 1935–1959*

PERIOD	NO.	RELATIVE SURVIVAL RATES (%)		
		1-year	3-year	5-year
1935–49	216	60.2	33.0	27.5
1950–59	234	70.9	48.3	42.3
All Cases	450	65.8	40.9	35.2

*Live diagnoses only. Excludes cases reported only by autopsy or death certificate. (From Shedd, D. P., Von Essen, C. F., Ferraro, R. H., Connelly, R. R., and Eisenberg, H.: Cancer of the floor of the mouth in Connecticut, 1935–1959. Cancer 21:97–101, January, 1968.)

TABLE 15-11 FIVE-YEAR RELATIVE SURVIVAL RATES BY TYPE OF TREATMENT
AND STAGE OF DISEASE—CANCER OF FLOOR OF MOUTH IN
CONNECTICUT, 1935–1959*

TYPE OF TREATMENT	FIVE-YEAR RELATIVE SURVIVAL RATES (%)		
	Total all Stages	Localized	Regional
Surgery alone	58.2	72.7	31.3
Surgery plus radiation	32.3	57.0	17.7
Radiation alone	28.5	40.1	17.8
No treatment	9.4	0.0	8.0
Treated and Not Treated	35.2	50.3	19.3

*Based on live diagnoses only. (From Shedd, D. P., Von Essen, C. F., Ferraro, R. H., Connelly, R. R., and Eisenberg, H.: Cancer of the floor of the mouth in Connecticut, 1935–1959. Cancer 21:97–101, January, 1968.)

TABLE 15-12 NUMBER OF PATIENTS AND PER CENT HISTOLOGIC TYPE
DISTRIBUTION BY SEX—CANCER OF THE TONGUE*

	TOTAL		MALE		FEMALE	
HISTOLOGIC TYPE	No.	Per Cent	No.	Per Cent	No.	Per Cent
Squamous cell carcinoma	722	74.2	590	73.1	132	79.5
Carcinoma, NOS	104	10.7	85	10.5	19	11.4
Other specified types	22	2.3	18	2.2	4	2.4
Unspecified types	125	12.8	114	14.1	11	6.6
All Types	973	100.0	807	100.0	166	100.0

*From Shedd, D. P., Von Essen, C. F., Ferraro, R. H., Connelly, R. R., and Eisenberg, H.: Cancer of the floor of the mouth in Connecticut, 1935–1959. Cancer 21:97–101, January, 1968.

survival rate.[13] As the disease progresses, the tongue and mandible are invaded and the cervical lymph nodes become permeated with cancer.

In one study of cancer of the mouth the following data were obtained: the five-year survival for the 50 patients with lesions in the anterior part of the mouth was 62 per cent; for the middle mouth group, 48 per cent; and for the posterior mouth group, 25 per cent.[15] These data demonstrate a high five-year cure rate for stage I and stage II squamous cell carcinoma, which is similar to that reported for the floor of the mouth.[16]

CANCER OF THE TONGUE

Comparative data show that squamous cell carcinoma is the most frequent malignant lesion of the tongue (Table 15–12) and involves men more frequently than women, except in Sweden (Table 15–13).

In Britain, cancer of the tongue is most often seen in men in the lower income bracket, and the mean age at diagnosis is 62. Approximately one half of the patients seen at diagnosis have a primary neoplasm still confined to the tongue; two fifths of these are two cm in size or smaller. Nodal metastasis occurs in about 40 to 50 per cent of patients at first and 20 per cent more are likely to develop it.[17]

Out of the 904 cases of cancer of the tongue studied by Flamant and coworkers between 1943 and 1959 inclusive, 87 per cent were male and 13 per cent were female (Fig. 15–2).[18] The average age was 59. The largest per cent of patients were in the 55 year age group.[19]

TABLE 15-13 CRUDE AND AGE-ADJUSTED RATES FOR INCIDENCE OF CANCER OF
TONGUE PER 100,000 POPULATION BY SEX AND GEOGRAPHIC AREA*

		INCIDENCE RATES PER 100,000			
		CRUDE		AGE-ADJUSTED†	
GEOGRAPHIC AREA	PERIOD	Male	Female	Male	Female
10 U.S. Cities	1947	4.1	1.2	4.2	0.8
Finland	1953–62	0.8	0.6	1.0	0.6
Sweden	1958–61	0.8	0.9	0.6	0.6
Norway	1953–61	1.0	0.7	0.9	0.5
New York‡	1958–60	2.6	0.8	2.4	0.7
Puerto Rico	1950–61	3.9	1.3	6.6	2.2
Denmark	1943–57	0.8	0.7	0.8	0.6
S. E. England	1960–62	1.9	1.0	1.4	0.6
Connecticut	1935–59	3.3	0.7	3.3	0.6

*From Shedd, D. P., Von Essen, C. F., Ferraro, R. H., Connelly, R. R., and Eisenberg, H.: Cancer of the floor of the mouth in Connecticut, 1935–1959. Cancer 21:97–101, January, 1968.
†The total population of the continental United States (1950) was used as the standard.
‡Exclusive of New York City.

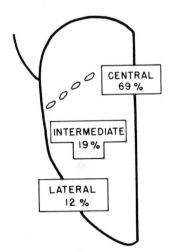

Figure 15–3   The site of origin of the primary tumors along the transverse axis. Sixty-nine per cent were centrally located. (From Flamant, R., et al.: Cancer of the tongue: A study of 904 cases. Cancer *17*:377–385, 1964.)

TABLE 15–14   CANCER OF THE TONGUE*

SITE OF ORIGIN (Where Specified)	NO. CASES	SEX RATIO	PER CENT LOCALIZED	5-YEAR RELATIVE SURVIVAL RATES (Male Cases Diagnosed 1940–1954) *All Stages*	*Localized*
Anterior 2/3 of tongue	549	3:1	49:65	31	54
Base of tongue	498	6:1	32:47	22	43

*From Latourette, H. B., and Myers, M. H.: End-results of treatment of oral and laryngopharyngeal cancer. Fifth National Cancer Conference Proceedings. Philadelphia, J. B. Lippincott Co., 1964.

TABLE 15–15   NUMBER OF PATIENTS WITH CANCER OF THE TONGUE AND PER CENT SUBSITE DISTRIBUTION BY SEX*

SUBSITE	TOTAL *No.*	*Per Cent*	MALE *No.*	*Per Cent*	FEMALE *No.*	*Per Cent*
Base plus other locations	151	15.5	124	15.4	27	16.3
Base only	203	20.9	172	21.3	31	18.7
Other than base	398	30.9	323	40.0	75	45.2
Tongue, NOS	221	22.7	188	23.3	33	19.9
All Locations	973	100.0	807	100.0	166	100.0

*From Shedd, D. P., Von Essen, C. F., Ferraro, R. H., Connelly, R. R., and Eisenberg, H.: Cancer of the floor of the mouth in Connecticut, 1935–1959. Cancer *21*:97–101, January, 1968.

TABLE 15–16   NUMBER OF PATIENTS WITH CANCER OF THE TONGUE AND PER CENT STAGE DISTRIBUTION BY SEX*

STAGES OF DISEASE	TOTAL *No.*	*Per Cent*	MALE *No.*	*Per Cent*	FEMALE *No.*	*Per Cent*
Localized	399	47.4	306	44.5	93	60.4
Regional	313	37.2	273	39.7	40	26.0
Distant	47	5.6	39	5.7	8	5.2
Other and unknown	82	9.7	69	10.0	13	8.4
All Stages	841	100.0	687	100.0	154	100.0

*From Shedd, D. P., Von Essen, C. F., Ferraro, R. H., Connelly, R. R., and Eisenberg, H.: Cancer of the floor of the mouth in Connecticut, 1935–1959. Cancer *21*:97–101, January, 1968.

Patients could be placed in three groups according to the site of origin of the cancer as follows:

Group I   mobile portion of the tongue   513 patients

Group II   base of the tongue   368 patients

Group III origin not determined because of poor anatomic description   23 cases

In Group I, 396 cases had the site of origin in the lateral border of the tongue, anterior to insertion of the anterior pillars; 37 cases in the dorsal surface, anterior to the circumvallate papillae; 16 cases in the tip of the tongue; and 64 cases on the ventral surface of the tongue, excluding the borders.

In Group II, there were 274 cases in which the site of origin of the cancer was in the posterior portions of the tongue, posterior to the circumvallate papillae. In 94 cases, there were instances of massive or total involvement of the base of the tongue. The primary tumor tended to favor the left side rather than the right. However, the majority (69 per cent) were in the central area, while 19 per cent were in the intermediate area, and only 12 per cent were situated laterally. The primary tumor was larger at the base of the tongue and smaller at the tip (Fig. 15–3).[18]

In another population, carcinoma of the tongue showed a sex ratio of 3:1, males to females, for the anterior two thirds and 6:1 for the base of the tongue. The five-year survival rate varied from 31 per cent to 54 per cent for cancer of the anterior two thirds to 22 per cent to 43 per cent for cancer of the base of the tongue (Table 15–14).[4]

In Connecticut, cancer of the tongue is more often found on the anterior two thirds of the tongue without inclusion of the base (Table 15–15). Based on a classification of localized regional spread and distant or remote spread, females have a more favorable stage distribution (Table 15–16). The tumor is localized at the time of diagnosis in 60 per cent of the female patients as compared to 45 per cent of the male patients.

Survival patterns differ greatly, depending upon the stage of the disease at the time of diagnosis, the location of the lesion, and the mode of therapy. Treatment includes surgery alone, surgery plus radiation, radiation alone, and no therapy.[13] The shortest five-year survival is experienced by patients with distant metastases (0 per cent) and the longest by those with localized tumors (45 per cent). Five-year survival is greater for patients with lesions involving the anterior two thirds of the tongue only. Surgery alone offers the best prognosis and five-year survival rate.

The case incidence rate of cancer of the tongue in California is twice that of cancer of the floor of the mouth. Mean annual deaths from cancer of the tongue are more than two times that from cancer of the floor of the mouth (Table 15–17).

TABLE 15–17 ORAL CANCER MORTALITY AND MORBIDITY BY SPECIFIC SITES*

ORAL CANCER SITE (ICD Code)	MEAN NO. OF ANNUAL DEATHS, CALIFORNIA (1960–1962)†	AGE-ADJUSTED AVERAGE ANNUAL CASE INCIDENCE RATES/100,000 POPULATION (Alameda County, California)‡
Lip (140)	10.33	4.7
Tongue (141)	106.33	3.6
Salivary (142)	26.67	0.9
Floor (143)	42.33	1.6
Other mouth (144)	50.33	1.5
Mesopharynx (145)	47.00	1.7
Nasopharynx (146)	33.00	0.7
Hypopharynx (147)	25.67	1.2
Unspecified pharynx (148)	67.00	0.7
Total (140–148)	408.66	16.6

*From Weir, J. M., Dunn, J. E., Jr., and Buell, P. E.: Smoking and oral cancer: Epidemiological data, educational responses. Am. J. Public Health 59(7): 959–966, June 1969.

†Sum of site-specific deaths for California in 1960, 1961, and 1962, divided by 3.

‡Incidence for males, from "Incidence of Cancer in Alameda County, California 1960–1964." (Table 18–15) State of California, Department of Public Health.

CANCER OF THE BUCCAL MUCOSA

Cancer of the buccal mucosa is less common than the other oral cancers and is nearly as common in females as males. Of 819 patients with cancer of the buccal mucosa, palate, or gingiva, 74 per cent were male, all patients were in the fifth to eighth decades of life, and the majority of the lesions were localized epidermoid carcinoma.[21] The incidence rate for cancer of the cheek, palate, and gingiva increases with age. The highest incidence is found in Puerto Rico. Causative agents are tobacco chewing, snuff dipping, and heavy pipe smoking.

Carcinoma of the buccal mucosa tends to be a flat plaque-like lesion often associated with long-standing leukoplakic changes.[20] The histology is divided between squamous carcinoma and adenocarcinoma, and tumors of salivary gland origin also occur. Tumors may be localized or exhibit regional involvement or distant metastases at the time of diagnosis.[21]

Localization is higher in women than in men and women have a higher survival rate than men. The response is better to surgery alone when the lesion is localized. The five-year relative survival rate is improved when the lesion is localized; it is just under 40 per cent.

CANCER OF THE PALATE

Squamous cell carcinoma is the most frequent cancer of the palatine arch (the mouth, the soft palate, the tonsil and its bed, and the tonsillar pillar) and the palate and is primarily a disease of elderly males (Table 15–18). Other cancers include transitional cell carcinoma, lymphoepithelioma, and malignant lymphoma. Sore throat, pain on swallowing, pain in ear, lump or ulcer in throat, lump in neck, or bleeding may be the primary symptom and may be present up to one year before the patient seeks relief.

The tumor varies greatly in appearance. It may be soft and fluctuant, hard and indurated, cauliflower-like, or present as an oro-antral fistula.

Reverse smoking frequently produces or is directly associated with cancers of the palate.[22]

TABLE 15–18 DISTRIBUTION BY AGE AND SEX OF CANCER OF THE PALATINE ARCH*

AGE	MALES (%)	FEMALES (%)	TOTAL
20	0	0	0
20–30	2	0	2
30–40	1	1	2
40–50	19–65	10–35	29
50–60	62–80	14–20	76
60–70	87–90	13–10	100
70–80	68–90	5–10	73
80+	19	4	23
Total	258–85	47–15	305

*From Schulz, M. D., Lintner, D. M., and Sweeney, L.: Carcinoma of the palatine arch. Am. J. Roentgenol. Radium Ther. Nuclear Med. 89(3):541–548, March, 1963.

CANCER OF THE SALIVARY GLANDS

Carcinoma of the salivary glands is predominantly adenoid cystic, acinic cell, adenocarcinoma, mucoepidermoid, or undifferentiated. The majority of salivary cancers arise from the parotid gland and occur in males.

The majority of these cancers appear to have a predilection for the Caucasian, since the highest incidence for both male and female is reported from the United Kingdom, Sweden, and the German Democratic Republic. For males, the highest incidence is in the United Kingdom, Connecticut, and Finland, and for females, the highest incidence is in Hawaii (Caucasian), Nevada, Canada, and Newfoundland. In each location cited, the annual average incidence of cancer of the salivary glands per 100,000 population by age is 85.[23]

Experience gathered from treatment of 327 cases of parotid gland tumors at the University of Zurich between 1959 and 1976 suggests that in order to prevent misdiagnosis, the total tumor mass must be available for microscopic examination.[19] Radical surgery alone plays the major therapeutic role. However, highly malignant salivary gland tumors demand the combination therapy of surgery and radiotherapy.

The survival pattern for cancer of the salivary glands is high. Nearly 53 per cent of patients with malignant tumors of the parotid gland were alive and free of the

TABLE 15-19   RESULTS AFTER FIVE YEARS OR LONGER IN 111 PATIENTS
WITH MALIGNANT TUMORS OF PAROTID GLAND*

TYPE OF TUMOR	NO. OF PATIENTS	NO EVIDENCE OF DISEASE	DIED OF DISEASE	DIED OF OTHER CAUSES
Malignant mixed	34	15	12	7
Mucoepidermoid	32	23	6	3
Squamous	8		6	2
Adenoid cystic	13	6	4	3
Acinic cell	8	8		
Adenocarcinoma	16	6	8	2
Total	111	58	36	17

*From Bardwill, J. M.: Tumors of the parotid gland. Am. J. Surg. *114*:498–502, October, 1967.

disease five or more years after therapy (Table 15–19).

CANCER OF THE PULP

Cancer has been reported in pulps of molar and cuspid teeth of Caucasians as secondary lesions only. Pulp cancer occurs predominantly in teeth on the right side. The greatest incidence occurs in male subjects who range from three to seventy years of age.[24] Primary sites include the mandible, antrum, lower lip, and the oral mucous membrane (Table 15–20). Roentgenologic examination of the affected jaw shows a general loss of lamina dura and bone architecture around the involved teeth, areas of radiolucency, and multiple lytic lesions. The principal clinical symptoms are pain or swelling or both and loosening of the

TABLE 15-20   SITE OF PRIMARY
TUMORS IN PATIENTS WHOSE TEETH
WERE EXAMINED FOR PULP
INVOLVEMENT*

NUMBER OF CASES	SITE OF ORIGIN	PERCENTAGE OF TOTAL
12	Mandible	30.8
8	Antrum	20.5
8	Lower Lip	20.5
3	Floor of Mouth	7.7
3	Tongue	7.7
2	Gingiva of Mandibular Alveolus	5.1
1	Upper Lip	2.3
1	Maxilla	2.3
1	Tibia	2.3

*Modified after Stewart and Stafine, 1955. (From Bridgewater, V. R. C., and Bolden, T. E.: Cancer of the pulp—A review of the literature—1904–1967. The Meharri-Dent. 28(2), March, 1969.)

affected teeth. Histologically, the affected pulp shows invasion by tumor cells (Fig. 15–4).

LEUKEMIA

The most frequent type of cancer in children is leukemia. The gingivae are distended by leukemic infiltrates, but frank hemorrhage, as observed in adults, seldom occurs.[25] Leukemia is a neoplastic disease originating in the blood-forming tissues of the body. Its "face" presents as an abnormal and uncontrolled proliferation of mature and immature leukocytes in the peripheral blood and the infiltration of these cells into the various tissues of the body. Leukemias are usually fatal whether acute, chronic, or subacute, or monocytic, lymphocytic, granulocytic, or myelocytic. The acute leukemias are seen predominantly in children, while the chronic leukemias occur more often in adults beyond 40 years of age. The primary cause of death in acute leukemia is hemorrhage, infection, and pulmonary edema.[26]

The presenting oral lesions include ecchymoses, ulcerations, infections, and bleeding. Spontaneous gingival bleeding, gingival hypertrophy, or petechial and submucosal hemorrhage may be the initial presenting oral findings (Fig. 15–5). There may be an associated anemia, hepatosplenomegaly, and generalized lymphadenopathy. Mucosal ulcers, cervical or submandibular lymphadenopathy, atrophy of the lingual papillae, pain, pallor of the oral tissues, and mucosal ulcers may also be observed.[27]

The white cell count may be less than 5,000/mm.[3] Hypofibrinogenemia, thrombo-

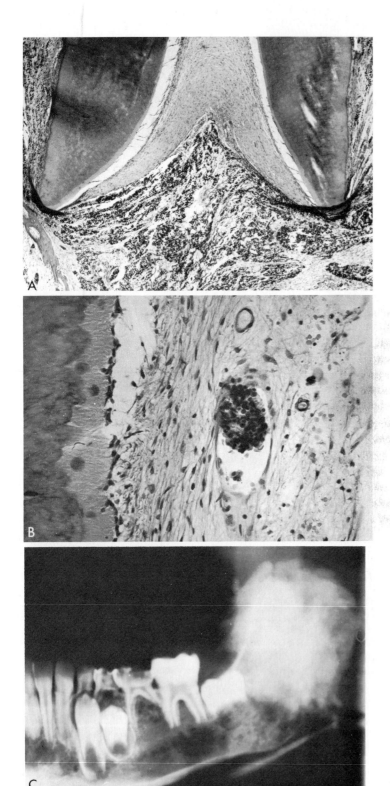

Figure 15–4 *A*, Indentation and compression of the apical pulpal tissue of the permanent first molar. (Hematoxylin and eosin stain. Original magnification, × 40). *B*, Nest of tumor cells within a pulpal blood vessel in the deciduous second molar. Compare the morphology of these tumor cells to those seen in other areas of the jaw. (Hematoxylin and eosin stain. Original magnification, × 200). *C*, Panoramic radiographic appearance of the involved portion of the jaw. Note the bulk of tumor overlying the ramus, with destruction of the condyle and coronoid process. There are also osteolytic changes in the body of the mandible. (From Snyder, M. B., and Cawson, R. A.: Jaw and pulpal metastasis of an adrenal neuroblastoma. Oral Surg. *40* (6):775–784, Dec. 1975.)

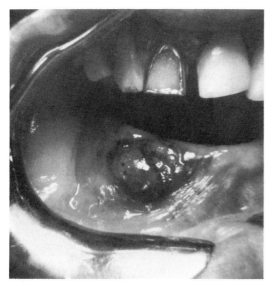

Figure 15–5 Intraoral photograph showing well demarcated nodular, bulbous, hemorrhagic lesion on alveolar ridge of 38 year old black female. Chronic myelogenous leukemia.

cytopenia, and clot degeneration may be seen, especially in acute promyelocytic leukemia.[28] The chief complaints include weakness, fever, chills, shortness of breath, nosebleeds, and abdominal, back, or leg pain.[27]

Metastases originate from adenoid cystic carcinoma, mucoepidermoid carcinoma, anaplastic carcinoma, and poorly differentiated carcinoma (Table 15–21).

Even the pleomorphic adenoma has been shown to metastasize. Some eight cases have been cited from the literature. The chief

sites of metastases are the lungs, bones, lymph nodes, and liver. Tomographs demonstrate the osteolytic nature of the tumor, while the histology highlights the varying components of the tumor, that is, chondroid, sebaceous, and epithelial.[29]

The average age of onset of metastasizing disease of the salivary glands is 40, with an average of 14 years between onset of the disease and diagnosis of the malignancy.

INCIPIENT ORAL CANCER

There is an increasing demand for the prevention of dental diseases. The present trend in the philosophy of preventive dentistry focuses on all aspects of clinical dental practice. One of the major aspects of the preventive dentistry philosophy involves the prevention of oral cancer. Moreover, lack of knowledge of definite etiology and primary preventive measures to preclude the initiation of the disease necessitates the orientation of the dentist, the dental profession, and the public toward secondary preventive measures, namely, early diagnosis and treatment of incipient oral cancer.

Since the dental office is the first place where recognition of an abnormality in the oral cavity usually occurs, the dentist's responsibility is that of recognition and identification of any oral lesion that has the potential to become cancerous, as well as referral to specialists if cancer is suspected. Therefore,

TABLE 15–21 CLINICAL AND HISTOLOGIC FEATURES OF MALIGNANT MIXED TUMORS OF THE MAJOR SALIVARY GLANDS IN NINE CASES WITH METASTASES*

| | PRIMARY TUMOR | | SITE OF METASTASIS | | | | |
CASE	Gland	Recur-rence	Lymph node Neck	Lungs	Skin	Bone	TYPE OF TUMOR
4	Parotid	X	X		X		Adenoid cystic carcinoma
6	Parotid		X	X			Adenoid cystic carcinoma
8	Parotid	X			X		Adenoid cystic carcinoma
7	Parotid	X	X	X		X	Mucoepidermoid carcinoma
11	Submandibular		X				Mucoepidermoid carcinoma
1	Parotid	X	X	X	X		Poorly differentiated carcinoma
2	Parotid	X		X	X		Anaplastic carcinoma
9	Parotid		X			X	Anaplastic carcinoma
10	Submandibular	X	X	X		X	Anaplastic carcinoma

*From Moberger, J. G., and Eneroth, C. M.: Malignant mixed tumors of the major salivary glands. Cancer *21*(6):1198–1211, June, 1968.

in order to accept his responsibility as a member of the health team for prevention of oral cancer, the dentist should have a knowledge of the natural history of oral cancer, which includes the following:

1. Description of the disease or what it looks like and what it is.

2. Ways of diagnosing or detecting the disease.

3. How to differentiate oral cancer from other diseases.

4. The most frequent locations of oral cancer.

5. What happens clinically or identifiable clinical features.

As a part of the health team that is involved in the management of oral cancer, it is extremely important that the dentist be informed and motivated so that he will be able to recognize the occurrence of oral cancer and assume the responsibility for forestalling the ravages of this disease in the incipient stage.

The purpose of early detection of oral cancer is to improve the survival rate, that is, the five- and ten-year survival rate, of the patient. The earlier the appropriate therapy is started, the better the survival rates. That therapy may include surgery, irradiation, chemotherapy,[30] or any combination of these.

Incipient oral cancer is extremely difficult to recognize clinically because the accompanying changes may be so subtle as to produce only minor alterations in function, color, texture, continuity, or consistency of the affected tissues.[31]

In 98 per cent of the cases, oral cancers are surface lesions. A high proportion of these are low-grade malignancies. Direct inspection of these surface lesions permits ready identification. Since a precancerous stage is also identifiable cytologically, smears are an important part of early detection.[32]

The primary efforts of the dental profession in the field of oral malignancy must be focused on detection and diagnosis. Unless the malignancy is controlled, the patient will die from the disease. The best hope for survival of the patient is through the early detection of the malignant process.[2, 33] Tissue analysis plays an important role in preventive dentistry, and biopsy is necessary to establish an accurate definitive diagnosis of a malignant process.[34]

Early detection is especially significant, since it has been estimated that 80 per cent of patients with untreated oral malignant disease die within 18 months as compared to two years for carcinoma of the rectum and five years for carcinoma of the breast.

In regard to the relatively high incidence of oral cancer, the practicing dentist, through the performance of a thorough oral examination, has a very important role to play in the prevention of oral cancer and the early detection of cancerous lesions. Careful attention should be paid to certain critical areas that are known to be common sites of oral cancer.

There are several clinical procedures that the dentist may employ for the early detection and prevention of oral cancer. He can listen, look, examine, take x-rays, perform simple diagnostic tests, scrape, aspirate, order clinical tests, biopsy, and educate. The ultimate weapon is the biopsy. Let us examine the various possibilities for prevention and detection of oral cancer in terms of their application and degree of reliability.

Listen. Listen to the patient! The patient probably thinks that the role of the dentist or other health professionals is to ferret out what is wrong with him. The dentist becomes an agent, 007, a professional Killmaster. This frequently means that the patient will not volunteer information. The dentist has to drag it out of him. Frequently, too, the patient will not know what kind of information is important and pertinent; hence he may respond only with a "yes" or "no" to a battery of questions. The patient frequently fails to remember bits of information until after the visit. However, the patient will talk if given the opportunity, and it behooves the astute diagnostician to listen. The dentist is also obliged to conduct the interview in such a manner that the following information may be learned: a complete history of the present complaint, previous dental complaints, previous medical complaints, previous dental and medical history and therapy, lifestyle and personal habits, oral habits, medical and dental phobias and fears, nutritional and religious background, family history, socioeconomic status, family size, and occupational pursuits. The patient talks, the dentist listens. Thus, clues are obtained upon which the dentist can draw logical conclusions. The patient knows his case better than any other person!

Look. Look at the patient! The structures of primary interest to the dentist are usually in full view, though occasionally obscured by a cosmetic veneer. But even though the lips may be red, the eyelashes long and black, the eyelids shadowed white and the cheeks a sunburst brown, it still may be possible to see the edematous ankles, the heightened respiration, the pallor to the nail bed, the vitiliginous or hyperpigmented zones, the facial asymmetry, the open bite, the cervical lymphadenopathy, the keratotic zones, or the butterfly lesions. These signs may be the first evidence of abnormality. They may already represent the advanced "face" of disease. They may, however, be the first "face," the early face of cancer. One can learn a great deal about the health of the patient and the potential for the development of oral or para-oral cancer by astute observation of the patient. The look when added to the listen may result in the early diagnosis of cancer.

Examine. Examine the patient! Every patient deserves complete examination of the oral and para-oral tissues. Techniques may differ from examiner to examiner, but the basic principles remain the same. The tissues should be examined so as to locate and to describe deviations from the normal. Consequently, when examining the external face and the oral cavity, one should look for changes in color and take particular notice of white, red, and black. White patches, erythematous zones, petechiae, and zones of hypo- and hyperpigmentation should be noted as well as the duration of such color changes. Four other features need to be evaluated:

1. Consistency — Is the tissue flaccid, fluctuant, hard, firm, or nodular?
2. Contour — Is the surface rough, asymmetric, ulcerated, or pitted? Is a sinus or fistula present?
3. Temperature — Is the tissue cold, flushed, hot, dry, or moist?
4. Function — Can the patient open his

mouth fully? Can he eat, talk, and breathe normally?

The troika "look-listen-examine" increases the possibility for detection of an abnormality and improves the diagnostic acumen of the dentist.

X-ray. Take an x-ray! Routine bitewing and periapical x-ray examinations of the teeth and jaws frequently reveal the presence of osteolytic and osteosclerotic changes in the bones of the face as unexpected findings. The complete x-ray evaluation may necessitate the taking of appropriate occlusal, anteroposterior, and lateral views of the skull and face.

The x-ray is a fairly reliable tool for the detection of changes in bone contour, bone profile, and patterns of bone growth. The x-ray points the way as a reliable indicator of changes in bone metabolism and of the presence of forces that act beyond physiologic limits or that augment bone deposition.

Simple Diagnostic Tests. Perform a test! Perhaps the two oral diagnostic tests that hold the most promise in terms of early detection of oral cancer are the sialograph and the toluidine blue test.

SIALOGRAPHY. The sialograph permits a roentgenographic evaluation of the parotid or submaxillary glands by instillation of radiopaque material such as Ethiodol. The technique requires the cannulation of Stenson's or Wharton's duct with polyethylene tubing. Using a Luer-Lok syringe and constant pressure, 1 cc of Ethiodol is slowly introduced into the duct system. X-rays are taken while the gland is full and at appropriate intervals — one hour, two hours, three hours, four hours, eight hours, and twelve hours — to measure the emptying capacity of the gland.

Parenchymal changes in the gland associated with cancer produce specific changes in the sialograph. Intrinsic lesions produce a filling defect outlined by a displaced duct system. Malignant lesions are generally infiltrative and result in the pooling of radiopaque material on filling. Retention of the contrast medium and its permeation of the surrounding parenchyma upon stimulation of the gland is also characteristic of the malignant process.[35]

TOLUIDINE BLUE TEST. The toluidine blue test permits a topographic evaluation. Toluidine blue, an acidophilic metachromatic nuclear stain, has affinity for areas of carcinoma-in-situ and invasive carcinoma but not for normal mucosa. Consequently, it affords the dentist a painless method for obtaining information quickly without evoking a de novo or pre-existing fear of cancer in the patient.

Whereas initial observations were limited to the stainability of areas of epidermoid carcinoma,[36-38] recent evidence indicates that lymphosarcoma, fibrosarcoma, and melanoma also yield positive staining.[39]

Technique of Use. Patients with suspected lesions are instructed to rinse the mouth with water and to swallow some water. Excess saliva is removed by suction. A mucolytic agent, one per cent acetic acid, is applied to the mucosa with a cotton applicator. Toluidine blue (one per cent) is then applied with a cotton applicator. The dye should cover the entire lesion and clinically normal margins. Excess toluidine blue is removed by rinsing with water. Lesions that retain the dye stain blue and are classified as positive. Negative lesions do not retain the dye. A mucolytic agent is used so that the dye will come into direct contact with the surface of the lesion. Lesions that stain should be biopsied. Negative lesions should be followed clinically for variable periods and restained. False positives have not been reported by this technique.[39]

The toluidine test holds great promise for (1) differential diagnosis of dysplastic or hyperkeratotic lesions, traumatic ulcers, and inflammatory ulcers; (2) determination of resection margins; (3) multicentric malignancies; (4) recurrences and (5) differentiation of benign from malignant lesions.

Scrape (Acquire a Surface Sample). It is estimated that 80 per cent of the deaths from oral cancer could be prevented by early detection and prompt adequate therapy.[40] Cytodetection, oral exfoliative cytology, and oral smears provide the dentist with a third diagnostic weapon that may lead to the early detection of oral malignancy. They too are painless procedures and produce no fear of cancer in the patient.[41]

Oral cytology or oral exfoliative cytology is the study of normal and abnormal desquamated cells of the oral cavity. Cells may be induced to desquamate artificially by scraping, or they may accumulate in the natural fluids of the body and be recovered by aspiration.

The normal oral living cell goes through its life cycle and drops from the surface mucosa to become part of the saliva. Those changes associated with age, that is, pyknosis of nuclei, loss of granules, parakeratosis, and keratosis, can be observed in the regular hematoxylin and eosin preparation. Individual cells are desquamated.

The surface biopsy, that is, suface scraping, usually produces sheets of cells in various stages of maturation. Depending upon how vigorously the clinician scrapes, he will probably obtain surface cells only; seldom are basal cells included.

The cytologic picture of normal human oral mucosa collected by this method demonstrates three predominant cell types, representing various stages of keratinization of the squamous epithelial cell. These include blue cells, red cells, and yellow cells when treated according to the method of Papani-

TABLE 15–22   CHARACTERISTICS OF EPITHELIAL CELLS OF THE ORAL MUCOSA*

DENOMINATION	NUCLEUS (Size)	CYTOPLASM (Amount)	(Color)
Small blue	Large	Small	Blue
Large blue	Small	Large	Blue
Large mixed	Small	Large	Blue-red
Large red	Small	Large	Red
Red-yellow	Small	Small	Red-yellow
Yellow	Absent	Small	Yellow

*From Montgomery, P. W.: A study of exfoliative cytology of normal human oral mucosa. J. Dent. Res. *30*(1): 12–18, February, 1951.

**TABLE 15–23 PERCENTAGE DISTRIBUTION OF EPITHELIAL CELLS
OF THE ORAL MUCOSA**

REGION	CELL TYPE	MEAN PERCENTAGE	STANDARD DEVIATION	CONFIDENCE INTERVALS
Soft palate	Blue	50.8	28.8	35.96–77.69
	Red	41.7	27.2	19.82–54.70
	Yellow	7.5	12.9	0.31–20.81
Cheek	Blue	51.5	26.6	37.81–62.48
	Red	43.8	23.8	25.89–60.29
	Yellow	4.7	12.3	0.0 – 9.54
Vestibule	Blue	45.0	28.9	25.29–64.74
	Red	42.9	26.8	28.77–64.01
	Yellow	12.1	21.7	0.50–30.11
Tongue (anterior)	Blue	19.7	16.7	6.93–31.74
	Red	47.3	20.7	33.01–58.33
	Yellow	33.7	21.4	19.32–47.24
Tongue (posterior)	Blue	30.9	16.8	17.77–45.34
	Red	35.5	15.9	25.20–47.19
	Yellow	33.5	15.4	23.27–42.09
Gingiva	Blue	7.3	9.1	0.0 –13.41
	Red	17.8	18.1	4.51–33.30
	Yellow	75.0	21.5	56.98–83.65

colaou. The size and stainability of the cells are shown in Table 15–22.[42]

When these cells are grouped according to the predominant types, that is, blue, red, and yellow, certain significant cytologic patterns emerge (Table 15–23). Blue cells predominate on the soft palate, cheek, and vestibular area. The tongue shows a predominance of red cells. The gingiva has a high incidence of yellow cells.[42]

No relationship between age and sex and the distribution of cell types in the oral cavity is shown. Cells may also be collected by using a moist wooden tongue blade. Scrapings taken in this manner from the dorsal and ventral aspects of the tongue and the buccal mucosa of 50 male students, aged 20 to 30, showed two cell types: large, red-staining cells with irregular outlines and pyknotic nuclei and blue-staining cells with more regular outlines and longer granular nuclei.

The gingiva released a third cell type — yellow ones with indefinite outlines and no nuclear detail. The degree of cornification was greatest, in descending order, on the gingiva, the dorsum of the tongue, the cheek, and the ventral surface of the tongue.[43] These cytologic findings agree with histologic and clinical observations.

Smears from oral leukoplakia from six areas of the oral cavity revealed no typical "leukoplakia cell" nor any abnormality in the nucleus or nucleolus. Yellow-staining cells without nuclei are found in increased number.[44]

Smears from the center of oral carcinoma lesions are more valuable than those taken from the periphery or margin of the lesion.[45] The most frequent abnormality found in a series of 15 cases or oral carcinoma was an abnormally large nucleus with a definitely altered nuclear-cytoplasmic ratio and a typical nucleolus.

In 50 selected patients with carcinoma, smears and biopsies from the same oral mucosal site were evaluated by different observers. Five types of carcinoma were identified in the material and classified as follows:

Type I	21 cases	Hornifying epidermoid carcinoma
Type II	2 cases	Well-differentiated epidermoid carcinoma with minimal hornification
Type III	10 cases	Anaplastic carcinoma
Type IVa	1 case	Transitional cell carcinoma
Type IVb	1 case	Verrucous carcinoma
Type V	15 cases	Carcinoma in situ

The cytologic characteristics of each carcinoma type and of malignant melanoma were distinctive enough to permit definitive identification of the tumor mass of the primary tumor (Table 15–24).

TABLE 15–24 CHARACTERISTICS OF ISOLATED MALIGNANT CELLS
AND TUMOR TYPE

Hornifying Epidermoid Carcinoma (21 cases)	Marked pleomorphism Chromatin—salt and pepper, thread-like, or in heavy opaque masses Nuclear membrane—thickened, irregular, or indented Nuclei—angular or cigar-shaped or round, multinucleated, and/or binucleated Excessive cornification, epithelial pearls
Well differentiated Epidermoid Carcinoma with Minimal Hornification (2 cases)	Nuclei—round or oval; nucleoli large Chromatin—granular Cytoplasm—pink or orange Tadpole or snake cells—few
Anaplastic Carcinoma (10 cases)	(1) Uniform in Size and Shape 　　Cytoplasm—scant 　　Nuclei—hyperchromatic 　　Chromatin—net-like and coarse 　　Arrangement—clumps	(2) Round or oval 　Scant or no blue 　Vesicular 　Irregularly placed 　Single/scattered
Transitional Cell Carcinoma (1 case)	Nuclei—large, elongated, vesicular; lobulated Nucleoli—multiple and prominent Cytoplasm—pale, scanty, indistinct borders
Verrucous Carcinoma (1 case)	Papillary clusters of small round squamous cells Nuclei—round or oval Cytoplasm—scant clear blue or colorless Some keratinized
Carcinoma in situ (15 cases)	Nuclei large, regular, hyperchromatic Chromatin—granular Cytoplasm (parabasal)—blue, pink, or orange with sharp cytoplasmic borders
Melanoma	Tumor cells—little or no cytoplasm and indistinct borders Cytoplasm—vacuolated stained blue, pink, or orange Nuclei—hyperchromatic; pleomorphic Nuclear membrane—delicate Chromatin—small clumps, evenly distributed Nucleoli—large irregular internal vacuoles; central densities; anastomosing filaments Granules—melanin—inside and outside the cell sometimes fused into round aggregates up to 100 μ; sometimes evenly dispersed throughout cytoplasm; orange, black, or brown

°From Medak, H., McGrew, E. A., Burlakow, P., and Tiecke, R. W.: Correlation of cell populations in smears from the oral cavity. Acta Cytol. (Balt.) *11*:279–288, July–August, 1967.

Disproportionate enlargement of the nucleus, marked nucleoli and increase in nucleoli, scant cytoplasm, and slight anisokaryosis are features of the various types of maxillo-oral sarcoma.[46]

USEFULNESS. Smears of clinically evident abnormalities yielded 45 positive smears from 1,297 smears submitted, which is a two per cent incidence of cancer. In three patients, existing cancer was not detected by oral smear.[47]

Over 3,600 smears taken over a three-year period yielded 37 oral malignancies in a Canadian population,[48] 34 of which were confirmed by biopsy. Twenty of these were not clinically diagnosed as cancer; thus, the cytologic smear provided the early detection of the disease.[48]

Cytologic examination of 1,561 cases seen between November 1956 and December 1967 revealed 312 malignant neoplasms. The correct diagnosis of carcinoma was made in 80.4 per cent (185/230) and of sarcoma in 78.5 per cent (22/28) of them.[49]

MULTIPHASIC SCREENING. Automated multiphasic health screening of 14,749 apparently healthy patients 35 years of age and older included exfoliative cytology of all lesions or abnormalities. One intraoral malignancy was found. Ten per cent, or 1,468, examinees had an intraoral lesion or abnormality for which a cytology smear was taken. All except six of these lesions clinically appeared innocuous, and all except 34 were classified as Class I (no abnormal cells) on the cytology reports. Of the six lesions that clinically appeared malignant, none were confirmed as malignant on biopsy. One lesion that clinically appeared innocuous, a 0.3 cm "keratosis" on the lateral border of the tongue of a 56-year-old female, was classified as Class IV (suggestive of cancer) and on biopsy was confirmed as squamous cell carcinoma — one malignancy in under 15,000 patients.[50]

RELIABILITY OF ORAL CYTOLOGY.
The reliability of oral cytology as a prognosticator of oral malignancy varies according to the experience of the user. One series yielded a 98 per cent reliability,[51] another 85.4 per cent[52] (Table 15–25).

The false negatives reported in those series where cytology and biopsy were performed on the same lesion vary from 0 per cent[53] to 26.15 per cent.[54]

False-negative percentages fall as one gains experience. The decrease relates directly to multiple examinations, careful collecting technique, or adoption of a different collecting technique. Fifty-two false-negatives out of 237 cases of carcinoma and sarcoma (21.9 per cent) was reduced to 20 out of 175 (12.0 per cent) and subsequently to 24 out of 268 (9.0 per cent) during the period 1956 to 1965.[49]

Correlative cytology and biopsy of 75 patients with visible oral lesions revealed 34 (45.3 per cent) malignant and 41 (54.7 per cent) non-malignant lesions. All malignant lesions were squamous cell carcinoma. Cytologically, 10 (13.3 per cent) of the lesions

diagnosed as malignant by biopsy were classified as Class I or Class II (false-negative), and one (1.3 per cent) benign lesion was classified as Class III (false-positive).[55]

Twenty-seven per cent of 22 oral malignant tumors were cytologically negative for cancer.[56] In another study of 1,500 oral biopsies and smears, from 10 to 15 per cent of oral carcinomas yielded negative cytological results.[57]

Cawson (1960) carried out a cytologic examination on 40 cases of proved or suspected oral malignant disease. In 31 cases of carcinoma of the oral mucous membrane, the correct diagnosis was made in 25 (81 per cent).[33]

RADIATION CHANGES. If the predictability of the radiosensitivity of oral carcinoma could be determined by the percentage of exfoliated epithelial cells showing radiation effects, thus good radiation response (RR) and good clinical results or survival rates, one could also predict survival rates.[58]

Twenty-two biopsy-proved cases of oral carcinoma receiving radiation therapy were followed by oral smear taken from the tumor and from the surrounding normal tissue (1) prior to therapy, (2) at intervals of four to seven days during therapy, (3) on completion of therapy, and (4) at follow-up visits. The criterion for good clinical results was regression of the primary growth.[58]

The effects of radiation on benign epithelial cells included cell enlargment, cytoplasmic vacuoles, multinucleation, nuclear

TABLE 15–25   FALSE NEGATIVES REPORTED WITH ORAL CYTOLOGY*

	NO. OF ORAL LESIONS	HISTOLOGICALLY PROVED	NEGATIVE CYTOLOGY	FALSE NEGATIVE INCIDENCE (%)
Rowe, 1967	372	Carcinomas (65)	17	26.15
Sklar, Meyer, Cataldo, Taylor, 1968	2,052 Biopsy + Cytology	Carcinomas (82)	12	14.6 Reliability 85.4
Dizner et al., 1967	500	Carcinoma epidermoid (39) Reticulosarcoma (1) Cylindroma (1)	4 1	10.3 100
Dargent et al. 1968	65	Well differentiated Carcinoma Malpighi (1)	1	7–8
Masson, Faucon, Sandler, 1966	28 2,758 (592 biopsies)	Malignant (315 of 592 biopsies)	7	7–8 2 Reliability 98

*From Shklar, G., Meyer, I., Cataldo, E., and Taylor, R.: Correlated study of oral cytology and histopathology. Oral Surg. 23(1):61–69, January, 1968.

enlargement, chromatin clumping, chromatolysis, karyorrhexis, pyknosis, and nuclear vacuoles.[58]

No correlation could be found between radiation responses and the clinical outcome. There was poor correlation between the cytology at the end of radiation and the clinical outcome up to the end of one year. There appeared to be a correlation between the pre-treatment size of the tumor and the clinical outcome at the end of the follow-up period.

These results were different from those found for predictability of radiosensitivity of carcinoma of the cervix uteri during radiation therapy, in which a significant association between good RR and good clinical results and between poor RR and poor clinical results was found.[59, 60]

Ultrastructure. Ultrastructural changes of cells exposed to radiation occasionally included nuclear and cytoplasmic damage as independent phenomena. Increases in cytoplasmic fibrils, vacuoles, and lysosomes; altered mitochondria and endoplasmic reticula; disruption of nuclear DNA; and rupture of membranes were the characteristic alterations.

Malignant cells differed from normal cells by numerous multivesicular bodies, increases in Golgi complexes and endoplasmic reticula, and a marked diminution of cytoplasmic fibrils.[61]

Aspiration Biopsy Smears. Aspiration biopsy of salivary gland lesions yields a high degree of reliability in those cases with histologically verified tumors.[2]

In 33 of 413 primary benign tumors of the salivary glands (1953–1965), no tumor cells were identified cytologically — a false negative of approximately eight per cent. The papillary cystadenoma proved to be the most difficult to identify.[62]

In one study, eight of 89 malignant salivary gland tumors (nine per cent) were denoted as cysts. In another study, of 81 malignant salivary gland tumors in which tumor cells were found, only 44 to 54 per cent were evaluated cytologically as malignant or of suspected malignancy.[62] Cytologic and histologic findings were compared in 632 cases in which surgery was performed after aspiration biopsy of suspected salivary gland tumor. In 31 of 377 cases of benign tumor, no tumor cells were found at cytologic examination — false negative rate of 8.4 per cent; reliability was 92 per cent.

In 105 histologically verified malignant tumors, 53 were identified as carcinomas and eight as suspected malignant epithelial tumors; 52 of these cases presented with no malignant tumor cells on cytologic examination. This represents a false negative rate of 49 per cent.[63]

In some studies, adenoid cystic carcinoma aspirates were characterized by cells with round or oval nuclei surrounded by a thin rim of cytoplasm. Cells were usually tightly packed in clusters, with "cylinders" of homogeneous mucoid material — spherical bodies surrounded by carcinoma cells.[63, 64]

DEEP SUCTION ABRASION. The Waldemar cytoaspirator (CA) is an instrument designed to improve oral tissue sample collection and to reduce the incidence of false negatives. In one study, the cytoaspirator (CA) produced more than twice the number of parabasal cells as did the tongue blade method (Fig. 15–6).[65]

Clinical Tests. Assay visceral function! The clinical laboratory should be utilized often for the patient suspected of having advanced or incipient cancer. Analysis of blood, urine, and bone marrow reveals much about the blood cells (immaturity, composition, and hematopoietic properties), the hormone output (17-ketosteroids and estrogen levels), liver function, and kidney function. This may help rule out leukemia, diabetes, hepatoma, and prostatic carcinoma as the cause of oral symptoms.

Consultation with obstetricians and gynecologists, proctologists, and specialists in internal medicine can help to rule out cervical, breast, and prostatic cancer as the primary site for oral tumorogeneses. The frequency with which visceral lesions metastasize to the oral tissues and the graphic changes in the maturity of hematopoietic cells would tend to impart a high level of reliability to these clinical tests, thus providing good diagnostic evidence to support the clinical impression.

Biopsy. When in doubt, take it out!

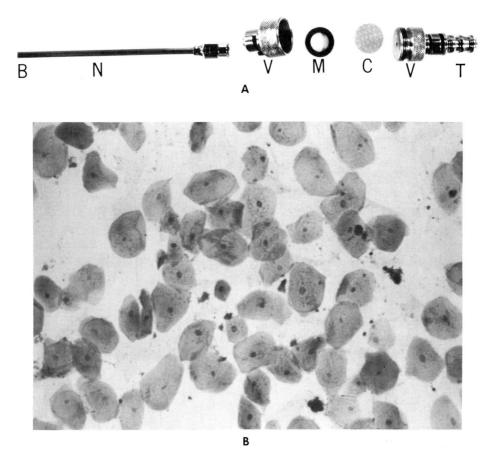

Figure 15-6 *A*, The cytoaspirator disassembled. B, abrasive, beveled end; N, 12 gauge needle; V, Ventura chamber to prevent distortion of cells; M, magnetic rubber washer; C, cell screen; V, other half of vacuum chamber; T, suction hose adapter. *B*, Specimen, typical field. (Magnification, ×100; reduced 2/5.)

The biopsy is the most important and reliable test for the definitive diagnosis of a suspicious oral lesion. The technique requires that a portion of the lesion plus a wide margin of normal tissue be removed for histologic preparation and examination.

The biopsy may be incisional or excisional. The incisional biopsy takes a part of the lesion and is especially useful when the lesion is large. The excisional biopsy provides the opportunity to remove the entire lesion and is especially useful when the lesion is small.

In either case, a wedge of tissue is removed, under local or general anesthesia, to a depth that provides a good opportunity for the oral pathologist to gauge the degree of invasion or extension of the malignancy.

What happens to the biopsy specimen? It is placed immediately into an appropriate fixative (10 per cent formalin, Helly's fluid, or formalin-alcohol-calcium acetate) and sent to the oral pathology laboratory along with a complete history, x-rays, and clinical photographs of the lesion and a clinical impression. After fixation, the specimen is processed routinely in paraffin, sectioned at six microns, stained with hematoxylin and eosin, and observed under the microscope. The final report is forwarded to the health professional who requested the studies.

Ten per cent formalin is the most widely used fixative and has the advantage that tissues can remain in it for long periods of time without harm or deterioration. Helly's fluid contains potassium dichromate and bi-

TABLE 15-26 WHAT THE DENTIST CAN DO TO DETECT CANCER

1. Listen to the patient talk
2. Observe the patient grossly
3. Examine the oral and paraoral tissues
4. Use exfoliative cytology on suspected lesions
5. Biopsy suspected lesions
6. Employ diagnostic tests routinely, i.e., x-ray, toluidine blue, sialography
7. Use the clinical laboratory for screening
8. Aspirate when convenient
9. Refer to colleagues for visceral evaluation
10. Correct oral habits and inadequacies

chloride of mercury. It provides good cytologic preservation. Formalin, alcohol, and calcium acetate (FAC) fixative is a specific fixative for the identification of mast cells in the tissue section.

Educate. Inform the laity! The battle to protect and save lives from intercurrent oral malignancy in the final analysis depends upon the existence of an alert, non-apathetic patient. The necessity for patient education cannot be overemphasized.[66] Patient education starts as a one-to-one relationship between the patient and the dentist. To be effective, the dentist has to know how to relate, how to communicate, and how to motivate the patient to get him to change his behavior and his attitudes toward his own oral health. Patient education also involves a dentist-community relationship. The dentist must not only provide education about oral cancer to the individual patient who comes to his office for services, but he must also educate the wider community.

One method of community education involves case-finding projects.[11] In these, a two- or three-man team (dentist, dental assistant, dental hygienist) visits nursing homes, prisons, low-rent housing projects, high schools, civic organizations, churches,

colleges, industrial plants, and professional health organizations. The approach is to:

1. Shock the attendees with the grotesqueness of advanced oral cancer.

2. Show how debilitating the disease is.

3. Provide assurances that the disease can be corrected, if detected early.

4. Demonstrate techniques that the dentist and the patient can use that may lead to early detection and diagnosis (Table 15-26).

5. Provide a list of danger signals that the patient can look for (Table 15-27).

6. Provide a list of things the patient can do to prevent cancer (Table 15-28).

7. Perform on-the-spot screening examinations and oral smears of those in attendance.

The public health nurse, as part of her home visitation program to shut-ins, can instruct members of the family in terms of good oral health. Film strips, rear projection screens, automatic projectors, hand-outs, throw-aways, animated film, 8 and 16 mm movies, and closed-circuit T.V. may be used to help the dentist meet this responsibility. The effectivenss of this approach hinges upon the ability of the dentist to "tell it like it is", that is, to talk about the "face" of cancer

TABLE 15-27 SIGNALS WHICH SHOULD ALERT THE PATIENT AND THE
DENTIST TO THE POSSIBILITY OF INCIPIENT OR ADVANCED ORAL CANCER

1. A persistent, scaly, white patch
2. A pigmented spot that suddenly increases in size
3. An ulcer that does not heal
4. Puffy bleeding gums in the absence of medication
5. Progressive facial asymmetry
6. Teeth that loosen suddenly, without a history of trauma or a blow to the jaw
7. Paresthesia, anesthesia, and oral numbness
8. Trismus and pain upon movement of the jaw
9. A lump in the neck, on the face, or in the oral tissues
10. An extraction wound which does not heal
11. Altered taste

TABLE 15-28 WHAT THE PATIENT CAN DO TO PREVENT CANCER

1. Don't use snuff, nasally or in the mucobuccal fold
2. Use alcohol moderately
3. Maintain balanced, adequate, nutritious diet
4. Have dental deficiencies corrected
5. Avoid excessive direct exposure to sunlight
6. Use tobacco sparingly
7. Don't pick, lance, or burn bumps or pimples
8. Keep the lighted end of the cigar or cigarette outside the mouth
9. Don't use lime and tobacco as a chew
10. See your dentist twice yearly

in the language of the population with which he is dealing. Shock, sympathy, rapport, and empathy must be established and felt!

In summary, besides the responsibility to recognize and identify suspicious oral lesions, the dentist also has the obligation of educating patients and the public so that they may be aware of lesions that may predispose to oral cancer and understand that cancer is preventable, although difficult to treat. Finally, it is the responsibility of the dentist to refer any patient suspected of having cancer to specialists who are experts in the management and treatment of oral cancer.

DIFFERENTIAL DIAGNOSIS

The prevention and early detection of oral cancer requires that the dentist be able to differentiate between the "face" of oral cancer and several of the look-alikes that appear on the oral mucosa. These include leukoedema, lichen planus, leukoplakia, moniliasis, and syphilis. The dentist also must check the oral cavity for signs of local irritation and counsel the patient about good oral hygiene procedures.

Leukoedema

Leukoedema affects the buccal mucosa (Fig. 15-7).[67] It presents as a whitish-gray lesion, which either persists or disappears when the tissue is stretched. It may involve any age group but tends to predominate in individuals around 40 years of age. In one study, the youngest subject was 14 and the oldest 89.[67] The incidence varies among population groups. It has been reported as high as 90 per cent and as low as 68 per cent in the

Negro, 43 per cent in American Caucasians,[68] and from 2.4 to 16.9 per cent in Papuans and New Guineans.[69] The entity is asymptomatic. Biopsy reveals an irregular surface without keratinization. Intracellular edema, acanthosis, and elongated and irregular epithelial ridges are also present.

Lichen Planus

Lichen planus is a subacute or chronic dermatitis that is usually extremely pruritic and tends to be generalized but may be localized. It is characterized by small, flat-topped, violaceous papules, oftentimes with minimal scaling. The lesions vary in size from two to nine mm or more. The disease appears in three principal forms: lichen planus, lichen planus hypertrophicus, and lichen planus atrophicus.

Lichen planus may occur on the cheek as white lacy lines producing a white lesion or as a red, ulcerated lesion in its erosive form. It may involve the gingiva, palate, or tongue. On the tongue, white plaques with little or no evidence of a linear pattern may be produced. Areas of oral mucosa affected by lichen planus become more pronounced upon stretching. The cause of lichen planus is unknown. The typical history of exacerbations and remissions of dermal and mucosal lesions preceding moments of stress tends to highlight psychogenic factors as causative.[70]

Lichen planus in a 29-year-old freshman dental student presented during periods of examination. Lesions on the buccal mucosa tended to follow the line of occlusion (Fig. 15-8). Lesions on the dorsal surface of the left hand were scaly and dry. The dorsal surface of the right foot contained approximately 16 flat to elevated violaceous, dry, scaly lesions varying in size form two to nine mm.[70]

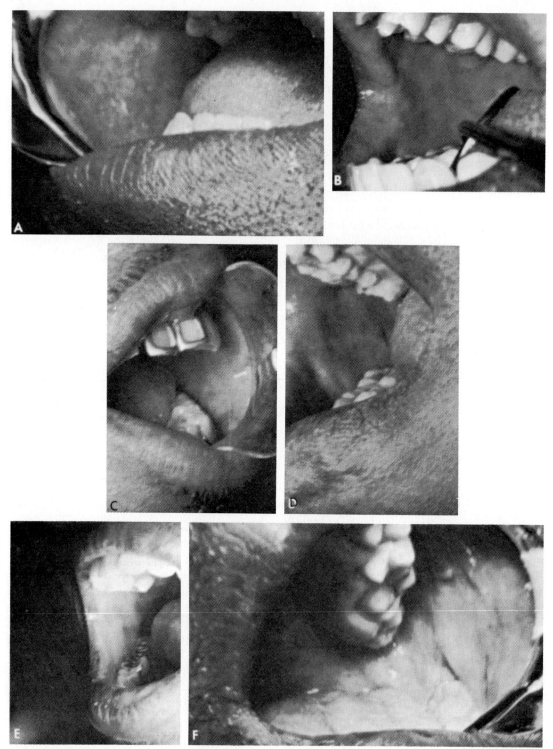

Figure 15–7 Leukoedema, buccal mucosa. *A*, None; *B*, slight; *C* and *D*, moderate; *E* and *F*, severe. (From Martin, J. L., Buenahora, A. M., and Bolden, T. E.: Leukoedema of the buccal mucosa. Meharri-Dent. *24*(3):7–9, June 1970.)

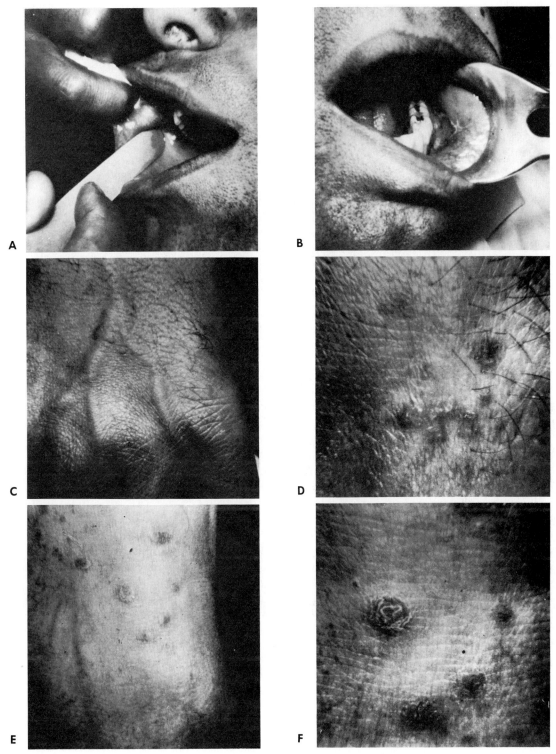

Figure 15–8   Lichen planus. *A*, Buccal mucosa; *B*, mandibular mucobuccal fold; *C*, left hand, dorsal surface; *D*, left hand, closer view; *E*, right foot, dorsal surface; *F*, right foot, closer view. (From Massey, R. M., and Bolden, T. E.: Chronic lichen planus: A case report. The Meharri-Dent. *28*(2):12–13, March 1969.)

Leukoplakia

Leukoplakia, a precancerous lesion, may present as a developmental defect, be associated with syphilis, be invaded by Candida organisms,[71] be associated with the use of various forms of tobacco,[72, 73] or result from chronic irritation or friction. An incidence of leukoplakia as high as 32 per cent[74, 75] may rise to 90 per cent in the presence of reverse smoking. The lesion presents as a white patch or plaque on the oral mucosa.

Developmental leukoplakia may appear as a widespread edematous thickening of the surface epithelium in an irregular fashion, or it may be present as a non-inflammatory, soft, well-defined, butterfly-like lesion on the ventral surface of the tongue.[71] The lesions are generally not seen until middle age.

Leukoplakia associated with chronic friction on the oral mucosa caused by abraded teeth or smoking usually reverses itself if the irritant is removed.

Moniliasis

Moniliasis produces a white patch and is usually observed in the very young and the aged without teeth. The lesion of moniliasis is a surface phenomenon caused by the mycelia of the fungus *Candida albicans*. When the lesion is scraped, the fungi are removed, leaving a raw, bleeding surface. There is evidence that the organism invades the tissue, causing hyperplasia of the epithelium. It is suggested that infective diseases such as syphilis and severe candidiasis may be more carcinogenic than tobacco.[71]

Syphilis

Syphilis, infection by *Treponema pallidum*, is the great mimic. One must always be alert to the possibility of this marauder. In addition to the mucous patches and fistula of the palate, seen in tertiary syphilis, one should be aware of ulcerations, especially of the dorsum of the tongue. The lesion may resemble the typical leukoplakia. That oral syphilitic leukoplakias may develop into cancer is seen in the evidence presented by Weisburger.[76] He reported that 100 per cent

TABLE 15–29 CARCINOMAS FOLLOWED UP POST-THERAPEUTICALLY, ENT DEPARTMENT OF THE UNIVERSITY HOSPITAL, ERLANGEN (n = 1160)

Oral cavity	86
Oropharynx	54
Larynx	627
Upper Jaw	58
Parotid	34
Others	75
"Precancerous states" (predominantly larynx)	226

(From Thumfart, W., Weidenbecher, M., Waller, G., and Pesch, H. J.: Chronic mechanical trauma in the aetiology of oro-pharyngeal carcinoma. J. Maxillofac. Surg. 6:217–221, 1978.)

of patients with serologic evidence of syphilis and leukoplakia developed carcinoma in the areas of the leukoplakias.

OTHER FACTORS IN THE DEVELOPMENT OF ORAL CANCER

Local Irritants. The case for surface-insert dentures and regular hygiene as important requirements for the prevention of oral-cavity carcinoma has been eloquently presented by Thumfart and coworkers.[77]

They examined 86 oral cavity tumors in a series of 1,160 cancer patients and correlated the site of the tumors or epithelial lesions with results of a biopsy and possible etiologic components.

The tongue was the site of 62 per cent of the oral cavity tumors (Tables 15–29 and 15–30). In this study, the population was made up predominantly of farmers and laborers. Most of these patients showed poor oral hygiene, abuse of both alcohol and tobacco (Table 15–31), and persistent mechani-

TABLE 15–30 SITE OF THE ORAL-CAVITY CARCINOMAS (n = 86)

Tongue and floor of the mouth	53 (62%)
Isolated involvement of the floor of the mouth	12 (14%)
Palate	10 (12%)
Gum	7 (8%)
Cheeks/vestibule of the mouth	4 (4%)

(From Thumfart, W., Weidenbecher, M., Waller, G., and Pesch, H. J.: Chronic mechanical trauma in the aetiology of oro-pharyngeal carcinoma. J. Maxillofac. Surg. 6:217–221, 1978.)

TABLE 15–31 FREQUENCY OF EXOGENOUS ETIOLOGIC FACTORS IN ORAL-CAVITY CARCINOMAS (n = 86)

Smokers (20 cig./day and more)	71 (83%)
Alcohol consumption	
2 liters of beer and more	42 (49%)
excessive, i.e., spirits	8 (9%)
Marked mechanical irritation factors	38 (44%)

(From Thumfart, W., Weidenbecher, M., Waller, G., and Pesch, H. J.: Chronic mechanical trauma in the aetiology of oro-pharyngeal carcinoma. J. Maxillofac. Surg. 6:217–221, 1978.)

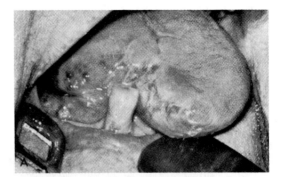

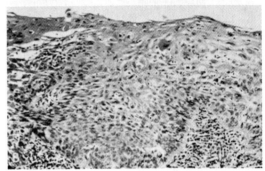

Figure 15–10 Typical injury caused by residual tooth. *A,* The right lower canine has caused damage to tissue in the anterior region of the tongue (♂, 67 years). *B,* Histology: Carcinoma in situ with transformation of the squamous cells; the basal membrane is still intact (HE, 100×). (From Thumfart, W., Weidenbecher, M., Waller, G., and Pesch, H. J.: Chronic mechanical trauma in the aetiology of oro-pharyngeal carcinoma. J. Maxillofac. Surg. *6*:217–221, 1978, Georg Thieme Verlag, Stuttgart.)

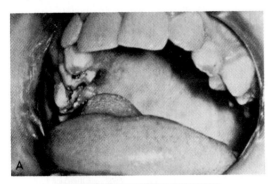

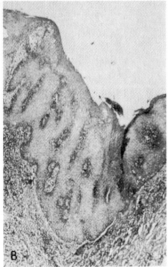

Figure 15–9 Irritation by tooth. *A,* Deep ulcer of the tongue with surrounding epithelial wall in immediate proximity to the sharp remains of a molar (♂, 10 years). *B,* Histology: Surrounding wall with chronic nonspecific inflammation and hyper-regenerative reactive acanthosis of the epithelium (HE, 40×). (From Thumfart, W., Weidenbecher, M., Waller, G., and Pesch, H. J.: Chronic mechanical trauma in the aetiology of oro-pharyngeal carcinoma. J. Maxillofac. Surg. *6*:217–221, 1978, Georg Thieme Verlag, Stuttgart.)

cal irritation at the site of cancer. The mechanical irritation was caused by sharp teeth edges (Figs. 15–9 and 15–10), or projecting fillings, ill-fitting dentures (Fig. 15–11), or deficient clasp devices or partial dentures (Fig. 15–12) (Table 15–32).

Some 83 per cent of the patients with oral cancer were smokers, and 49 per cent regularly consumed alcohol, some to excess. In 44 per cent of cases of oral-cavity carcinoma, tumor development was related to sharp remaining teeth, deficient dental fillings, badly finished edges of dentures, loose anchoring elements, and unsuitable denture-bearing tissue. In those who have pre-injured mucosa caused by alcohol and tobacco abuse and lack of oral hygiene, it is presumed that it is the chronic intermittent trauma and constant trauma with the unphysiologic effect of mechanical pressure caused

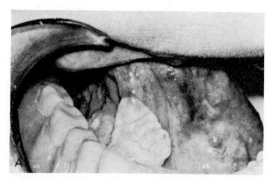
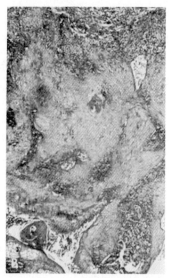

Figure 15–11 Papillomatous tumor with leukoplakic changes in the neighborhood of the sublingual edge of a complete lower denture (♀, 73 years). *A*, Clinical aspect. *B*, Histology: Papillomatous squamous-cell carcinoma, grade II (HE, 40×). (From Thumfart, W., Weidenbecher, M., Waller, G., and Pesch, H. J.: Chronic mechanical trauma in the aetiology of oro-pharyngeal carcinoma. J. Maxillofac. Surg. 6:217–221, 1978, Georg Thieme Verlag, Stuttgart.)

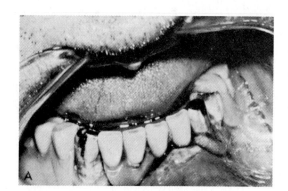
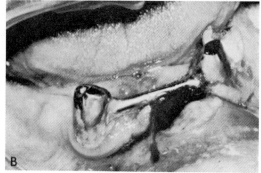

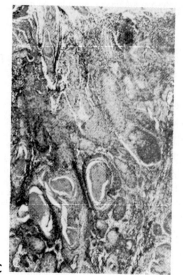

Figure 15–12 *A*, Tumor of the lower anterior gum with lower partial denture in place (♂, 67 years). *B*, Deep ulcer extending to the bone, when partial denture removed. *C*, Histology: Keratinizing squamous-cell carcinoma, grade II (HE, 40×). (From Thumfart, W., Weidenbecher, M., Waller, G., and Pesch, H. J.: Chronic mechanical trauma in the aetiology of oro-pharyngeal carcinoma. J. Maxillofac. Surg. 6:217–221, 1978, Georg Thieme Verlag, Stuttgart.)

TABLE 15–32 DENTAL STATUS OF THE PATIENTS WITH SIGNS OF MECHANICAL IRRITATION OF THE TUMOR REGION (n = 38)

Ill-fitting complete denture	10
Partial denture	8
Teeth remaining	14
Sharp teeth remaining	6

(From Thumfart, W., Weidenbecher, M., Waller, G., and Pesch, H. J.: Chronic mechanical trauma in the aetiology of oro-pharyngeal carcinoma. J. Maxillofac. Surg. 6:217–221, 1978.)

by remnants and solitary teeth that influence the development of carcinoma. The denture material itself does not seem to be the critical factor.

Chronic Habits. Prolonged exposure to an inert substance may terminate in malignant change in the oral mucosa. An 81-year-old female presented with symmetric exophytic tumors on the buccal mucosae in the absence of adenopathy, leukoplakia, or evidence of distant metastases. The patient had packed wads of plain sterile cotton daily into both posterior buccal areas for over 30 years to improve the appearance of her sunken cheeks.[78] The lesions proved to be well-differentiated intra-epithelial squamous cell carcinoma (left cheek).

REFERENCES

1. Cheek, R., and Pitcock, J. A.: Sebaceous lesions of the parotid. Arch. Path. 82:147–150, 1966.
2. Klein, A. W., Weikel, A. M., and Bingham, H. G.: Cancer of the lip. J. Fla. Med. Assoc. 62(11):31–33, 1975.
3. Keller, A. Z.: Cellular types, survival, race, nativity, occupations, habits and associated diseases in the pathogenesis of lip cancers. Am. J. Epidemiol. 91:486–499, 1970.
4. Latourette, H. B., and Meyers, M. H.: End results of treatment of oral and laryngopharyngeal cancer. Fifth National Cancer Conference Proceedings, Philadelphia, J.B. Lippincott Co., 1964, p. 281.
5. Greimer, R., and Veraguth, P.: Die Bedeutung der Strahlentherapie bei der Behandlung der Lippenkarzinome. Schweiz. Med. Wschr. 108:922–927, 1978.
6. Calhoun, J. J.: Malignant hemangioendothelioma (angiosarcoma). Oral Surg. 27:156–160, 1969.
7. Oettle, A. G.: Cancer in Africa, especially in regions south of the Sahara. J. Nat. Cancer Inst. 33:383–436, 1964.
8. Rosenfeld, L., and Calloway, J.: Snuff dipper's cancer. Am. J. Surg. 106:840–844, 1963.
9. Harrold, C. C., Jr.: Cancer of the floor of mouth and gingiva. In Chambers, R. G., et al. (ed.): Cancer of the Head and Neck. Amsterdam, Excerpta Medica, 1975. W.S. Ey89 No. 365, 1975.
10. Pindborg, J. J.: Oral cancer from an international point of view. J. Canad. Dent. Assoc. 31:219–226, 1965.
11. Mobley, E. L.: Oral Cancer Detection Program. Am. J.P.H. 53:1214, 1963.
12. Krishnamurthi, S., and Shanta, V.: Evaluation of treatment of advanced primary and secondary gingival carcinoma. Br. Med. J. 1:1201–1263, 1963.
13. Shedd, D. P., Von Essen, C. F., Ferraro, R. H., Connelly, R. R., and Eisenberg, H.: Cancer of the floor of the mouth in Connecticut, 1935–1959. Cancer 21:97–101, 1968.
14. Correa, J. N., Bosch, A., and Marcial, V. A.: Carcinoma of the floor of the mouth: Review of clinical factors and results of treatment. Am. J. Roentgenol. Rad. Therap. Nuclear Med. 99:302–312, 1967.
15. Caracciolo, P. R.: Surgical treatment of 150 cases of squamous cell carcinoma of the mouth. Int. Surg. 60:546–549, 1975.
16. Barton, R. T., and Ucmakli, A.: Treatment of squamous cell carcinoma of the floor of the mouth. Surg. Gynec. Obstet. 145:21–27, 1977.
17. Shaheen, O. H.: Malignant disease of the mouth. The Practitioner 203:23–29, 1969.
18. Flamant, R., Hayes, M., Lazar, P., and Denoix, P.: Cancer of the tongue: A study of 904 cases. Cancer 17:377–385, 1964.
19. Fisch, U.: Zur Diagnose und Therapie der Speicheldrüsentumoren. Schweiz. Med. Wschr. 108:927–932, 1978.
20. Hendrick, J. W.: Malignancy of buccal mucous membrane, gingiva, soft and hard palate. Ann. Otol. 61:1094–1113, 1952.
21. Shedd, D. P., Von Essen, C. F., Connelly, R. R., and Eisenberg, H.: Cancer of the buccal mucosa, palate and gingiva in Connecticut, 1935–59. Cancer 21:440–446, 1968.
22. Reddy, D. G., and Rao, V. K.: Cancer of the palate in coastal Andhra due to smoking cigars with the burning end inside the mouth. Indian J. Med. Sci. 11:791–797, 1957.
23. Dodge, O. G.: Tumors of the jaw, odontogenic tissues and maxillary antrum (excluding Burkitt lymphoma) in Uganda Africans. Cancer 18:205–215, 1965.
24. Bridgewater, V. R. C., and Bolden, T. E.: Cancer of the pulp — A review of the literature — 1904–1967. The Meharri-Dent. 28, March, 1969.
25. Rowe, N. H., and Kwapis, B. W.: Oral and perioral cancer detection. Dent. Clin. N. Am. pp. 189–201, March, 1968.
26. Owor, R., and Madda, J. P.: Cause of death in acute leukemia in African patients. East African Med. J. 55:453–457, 1978.
27. Sarnquist, J. L.: Oral manifestations of leukemia. J. Am. Dent. Hygienist Assoc. 43:145–150, 1969.
28. Arthur, A. L., and Salman, S. A.: Leukemia — Report of two cases.
29. Chen, Karl T.: Metastasizing pleomorphic adenoma of the salivary gland. Cancer 42:2407–2411, 1978.
30. Cobb, J. P., and Kupfer, A.: Environmental influences of the growth of Cloudman S-91 mouse melanoma in organ culture. In Bolden, T. E.:

Proceedings of an Oral Research Seminar, School of Dentistry, Meharry Medical College 3, 1971.

31. Bolden, T. E.: The "face" of oral cancer. The Meharri-Dent. 29:11–16, 1970.
32. Pomerance, W.: The cancer-screening dilemma. Postgrad. Med. 64:42–50, 1978.
33. Cawson, R. A.: The Cytological Diagnosis of Oral Cancer. Br. Dent. J. 108:294–298, 1960.
34. Shira, R. B.: Preventive oral surgery. Prev. Med. 5:360–376, 1976.
35. Rubin, P., and Hoot, J. F.: Secretory sialography in diseases of the major salivary glands. Am. J. Roentgenol. Rad. Therap. Nuclear Med. 77:575–598, 1957.
36. Shedd, D. P., Hukitt, T. B., and Bahn, S.: In vivo staining properties of oral cancer. Am. J. Surg. 110:631–634, 1965.
37. Shedd, D. P.: Further appraisal of in vivo staining properties of oral cancer. Am. J. Surg. 110:631–634, 1965.
38. Strong, M. S., Vaughn, C. W., and Incze, J. S.: Toluidine blue in the management of carcinoma of the oral cavity. Acta Otolaryngol. (Chicago) 87:527–531, 1968.
39. Myers, E. N.: The toluidine blue test in lesions of the oral cavity. Ca-A Cancer Journal for Clinicians 20:135–138, 1970.
40. Putnam, W. J.: The early detection of oral cancer through the application of exfoliative cytology. Hemispheric Conference for Better Oral Health for the Americas, 35–36, September, 1966.
41. Sandler, H. C.: Cytological screening for early mouth cancer. Interim report of the Veterans Administration Cooperative Study on Oral Exfoliative Cytology. Cancer 15:1119–1124, 1962.
42. Montgomery, P. W.: A study of exfoliative cytology of normal human oral mucosa. J. Dent. Res. 30:12–18, 1951.
43. Miller, S. C., Soberman, A., and Stahl, S. S.: A study of the cornification of the oral mucosa of young male adults. J. Dent. Res. 30:4–11, 1951.
44. Montgomery, P. W., and Von Hamm, E.: A study of the exfoliative cytology of oral leukoplakia. J. Dent. Res. 30:260–264, 1951.
45. Montgomery, P. W., and Von Hamm, E.: A study of the exfoliative cytology in patients with carcinoma of the oral mucosa. J. Dent. Res. 30:308–313, 1951.
46. Watanabe, Y.: Exfoliative cytology of maxillo-oral sarcoma. Twelfth Annual Meeting, American Society of Cytologists, Pittsburgh, November, 1964.
47. Statistics on Cancer. New York, American Cancer Society, 1967, p. 5.
48. Hunter, H. A.: Three year experience with an oral cytology service for the Ontario Dental Profession. Laval. Med. 39:8–10, 1968.
49. Watanabe, Y.: Methods for the early diagnosis of oral tumors. Int. Dent. J. 18:708–723, 1968.
50. Ross, N. M., and Gross, E.: Oral findings based on an automated multiphasic health screening program. J. Oral Med. 26:21–26, 1971.
51. Sandler, N. C.: Errors of oral cytodiagnosis. Report of follow-up of 1,801 patients. J. Am. Dent. Assoc. 72:874–888, 1966.
52. Shklar, G., and Taylor, R.: Metastasis of pulmonary carcinoma to oral mucosa: Report of case. J. Oral Surg. Anesth. Hosp. D. Serv. 23:549–552, 1965.
53. Medak, H., McGrew, E. A., Burlakow, P., and Tiecke, R. W.: Correlation of cell populations in smear from the oral cavity. Acta Cytol. (Balt.) 11:279–288, 1967.
54. Rovin, S.: Assessment of the negative oral cytologic diagnosis. J. Am. Dent. Assoc. 74:759–762, 1967.
55. Gaither, W. D.: Comparison of exfoliative cytodiagnosis and histodiagnosis of oral lesions: Review of the literature and report of 75 cases. J. Oral Surg. 25:446–453, 1967.
56. Shapiro, B. L., and Gorlin, R. J.: An analysis of oral cytodiagnosis. Cancer 17:1477–1479, 1964.
57. Cataldo, E.: Comments. J. Oral Surg. 25:464, 1967.
58. Memon, M. H., and Jafarey, N. A.: Cytologic study of radiation changes in carcinoma of the oral cavity: Prognostic value of various observations. Acta Cytol. (Balt.) 14:22–24, 1970.
59. Graham, R. M.: The effects of radiation on vaginal cells in cervical carcinoma. I. Description of cellular changes. II. Prognostic significance. Surg. Gynecol. Obstet. 84:153–173, 1947.
60. Graham, R. M., and Graham, J. B.: Cytologic prognosis in cancer of uterine cervix treated radiologically. Cancer 8:59–70, 1955.
61. Silver, H., and Goldstein, M. A.: Sebaceous cell carcinoma of the parotid region. Cancer 19:1773–1779, 1966.
62. Eneroth, C. M., Franzen, S., and Zajicek, J.: Cytologic diagnosis on aspirate from 1000 salivary gland tumors. Acta Otolaryng. (Suppl.) 224:168–172, 1966.
63. Eneroth, C. M., Franzen, S., and Zajicek, J.: Aspiration biopsy of salivary gland tumors: A critical review of 910 biopsies. Acta Cytol. (Balt.) 11:470–472, 1967.
64. Zajicek, J., and Eneroth, C. M.: Cytological diagnosis of salivary gland carcinomata from aspiration biopsy smears. Acta Otolaryngol. 263:183–185, 1970.
65. Englert, R. J., and Pasqual, H. N.: Metastatic chorionepithelioma of gingival tissue: Report of a case. Oral Surg. 10:813–818, 1957.
66. Lemeh, D.: Personal Communication.
67. Martin, J. L., Buenahora, A. M., and Bolden, T. E.: Leukoedema of the buccal mucosa. The Meharri-Dent. 29:7–9, 1970.
68. Sandstead, H., and Lowe, J. W.: Leukoedema and keratosis in relation to leukoplakia of the buccal mucosa in man. J. Natl. Cancer Inst. 14:423–433, 1953.
69. Pindborg, J. J., Barnes, O., and Roed-Petersen, B.: Epidemiology and histology of oral leukoplakia and leukoedema among Papuans and New Guineans. Cancer 22:379–384, 1968.
70. Massey, K. M., and Bolden, T. E.: Chronic lichen planus — A case report. The Meharri-Dent. 28:12–13, 1969.
71. Cawson, R. A.: Leukoplakia and oral cancer. Proc. Roy. Soc. Med. 62:610–615, 1969.
72. Borota, A.: Tobacco and the oral mucosa. J. Am. Geriat. Soc. 9:774, 1961.
73. Moertal, C., and Foss, E.: Multicentric carcinomas of the oral cavity. Surg. Gynecol. Obstet. 106:642–654, 1958.
74. Paymaster, J. C.: Oral and pharyngeal cancer in India. In Cancer of the Head and Neck. International Workshop on Cancer of the Head and Neck, New York, May 10–14, pp. 308–316.
75. Yashar, J. S., Guralnick, E., and McHuby, R. L.:

Multiple malignant tumors of the oral cavity, respiratory system and upper digestive system. Experience at the Pondville State Hospital from 1949–1959. Am. J. Surg. *112*:70, 1966.

76. Weisburger, D.: Precancerous lesions. J. Am. Dent. Assoc. *54*:507–513, 1957.

77. Thumfart, W., Weidenbecher, M., Waller, G., and Pesch, H. J.: Chronic mechanical trauma in the aetiology of oro-pharyngeal carcinoma. J. Maxillofac. Surg. *6*:217–221, 1978.

78. Li, F. P., Miller, R. W., and Levene, M. B.: Cotton as a cause of cancer. Lancet *1*:1014, 1972.

CHAPTER SIXTEEN
Pit and Fissure Sealant

Richard J. Simonsen, D.D.S., M.S.

The term pit and fissure sealant is used to describe a resin material that is introduced into the occlusal pits and fissures of caries-susceptible teeth, forming a mechanical physical protective layer against the action of acid-producing bacteria and substrates.

The introduction of such materials has provided the missing link for the theoretical complete prevention of dental caries. In the past, despite diligent oral hygiene, optimal fluoride environment, and adequate diet, occlusal caries was unavoidable for most people. Pit and fissure sealant provides the means to virtually eliminate this previously inescapable scourge of dental adolescence. It remains to be seen whether or not the dental profession will accept and utilize the concept of primary prevention of dental caries with pit and fissure sealant.

The problems with pit and fissure caries were recognized long ago. Marshall-Day and Sedwick[1] and Knutson and coworkers[2] published studies documenting that 43 to 57 per cent of all carious lesions in children were found on the occlusal surfaces.

In 1923, Hyatt[3] proposed a solution to the problem in which cavities were prepared and filled with amalgam in all pits and fissures — the prophylactic odontotomy. There are still practitioners active today who utilize the prophylactic odontotomy in lieu of pit and fissure sealants.

There were other methods attempted to forestall the almost inevitable carious occlusal lesions, including enamel fissure eradication[4,5] and chemical action on enamel.[6,7] Since none of these methods gained wide acceptance, prevention of occlusal lesions had been impossible until the advent of acid etched occlusal resins.[8,9,10]

The incorporation of fluoride into the drinking water supplies of cities has, over the years, had a tremendous effect on reducing the incidence of caries. Studies, such as the one of Ast and coworkers[11] have reported significant decreases of 50 to 60 per cent in the caries rates of children of various ages.

It is generally accepted that the primary effect of either ingested or topically applied fluoride is in prevention and control of smooth-surface caries. With ideal fluoride environment, it is suspected that pit and fissure caries is delayed one or two years, but it is apparently not prevented on the scale of smooth-surface caries reduction. Pit and fissure sealing, therefore, can have a tremendous impact on caries incidence.

TECHNIQUE FOR FISSURE SEALING

The basic technique for fissure sealing follows. Variations do occur, particularly in methods of isolation, but the step-by-step procedure for etching and sealing is a simple process that can be quickly learned by dentist, hygienist, or assistant. The important point to be remembered is that the success of sealant retention is virtually completely technique-dependent. As soon as the operator has mastered the technique and adheres strictly to the principles of sealant application, sealant retention can be almost 100 per cent. Only in cases in which the technique has broken down (such as with salivary

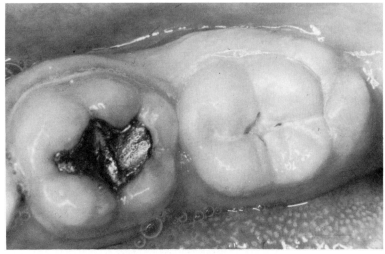

Figure 16–1 An occlusal fissure defect such as in this second permanent molar, along with evidence of caries having been present in other teeth (first permanent molar), indicates almost certainly that caries will attack this tooth unless it is sealed.

contamination of the etched surface) will there be sealant loss. It cannot be emphasized enough that meticulous attention to the details of the technique will lead to rewarding experiences when recalling patients for checking sealant retention.

Step 1. Selection of Patients and Teeth

As with any technique, pit and fissure sealing is not indicated for every child. In cases in which rampant or moderate decay exists and the chances for rapidly developing interproximal caries are high, one does not save very much by placing sealant on occlusal pits and fissures (neither, however, does one do any harm). Similarly, there are those

patients with no clinical caries and coalesced fissures (shallow, rounded grooves) where caries is extremely unlikely. Again, in such cases, applying sealant is a waste of the operator's and the patient's time.

Many children, however, have occlusal anatomy that an experienced operator can accurately predict will become carious within six months or one year. If they have sharp, deep pits and fissures, possibly with evidence of previous occlusal caries (Fig. 16–1) they are prime candidates for sealant application. It is physically impossible to clean out the deep fissure anatomy on most children's teeth. The toothbrush bristle is much too wide to penetrate into the base of the average occlusal groove. Thus, even though the child may have a good diet,

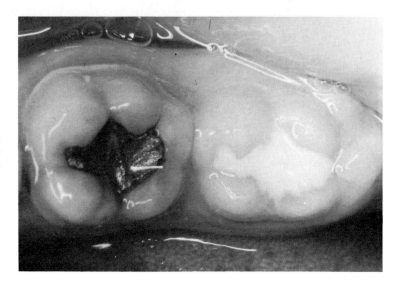

Figure 16–2 After etching for 60 seconds with phosphoric acid (37 per cent) the occlusal pits and fissures are sealed. In this case, 3M White Sealant was used.

excellent oral hygiene, regular dental visits, and optimal fluoride environment, occlusal caries is still inevitable in the majority of children unless pit and fissure sealant is applied (Fig. 16–2).

Step 2. Cleaning the Teeth

The tooth surface to be etched and sealed must be thoroughly cleaned. A pointed bristle brush, in a slow-speed contra-angle handpiece, is excellent for gross plaque removal. It can be used with a pumice/water slurry, or it can be used dry. Oil-based mixtures of pumice should be avoided, as the oils may stick to the enamel surface and interfere with etching. After cleaning the occlusal pits and fissures with a pointed brush, it is frequently beneficial to pull an explorer tine through all the grooves. This will remove some of the deeper plaque that the brush cannot reach. The tooth should then be washed with water, and dried carefully prior to acid application.

Step 3. Isolation

Isolation is extremely important and is probably the most critical step with regard to the success or failure of the sealant. Rubber dam is ideal for isolation. Cotton rolls, however, are more practical and more frequently used. It is perfectly possible, with good technique, to get excellent isolation with cotton rolls, and this method is recommended from a practical and cost-effective standpoint. It is estimated from the 500 patients who had their teeth sealed during a clinical study by the author[12] that isolation would have been significantly improved with use of the rubber dam in less than 5 per cent of the cases. In such cases, however, rubber dam is essential for complete retention of the sealant.

The use of cotton rolls for isolation requires a special technique that, once mastered, provides for a rapid and effective means of moisture control. The technique is described for a right-handed operator.

Mandibular Right Quadrant. Two cotton rolls are used initially, one lingually, held down by the thumb of the operator's left hand, and one buccally, held down by the operator's index finger. In this way, the operator has far better control over the patient's tongue than if a cotton roll holder was used. After etching and washing, the cotton rolls will be saturated, and the critical moment in the technique is reached. Before drying the etched tooth, a new cotton roll is placed on top of the lingual saturated roll which is then removed from under the fresh cotton roll by the assistant (Fig. 16–3). Sometimes the saturated roll can be left in place

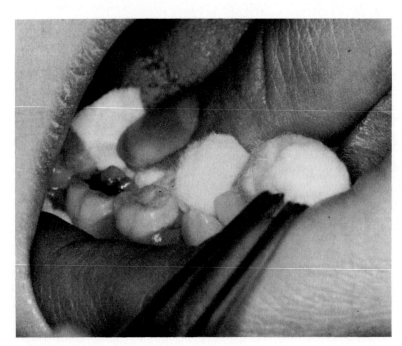

Figure 16–3 After etching, cotton rolls will need to be changed. By placing the dry cotton roll on top of the saturated roll and then removing the wet roll from underneath the dry one, the exchange can take place without contamination of the etched tooth.

underneath the fresh cotton roll. The assistant removes the buccal cotton roll, and the operator replaces it with a fresh one. In this way, the operator's thumb and index finger are always in complete control of the patient's tongue and cheek. If cotton roll holders are used, there is a far greater chance of contamination during removal and exchange of the cotton rolls and holder. Care must be taken at all times to avoid salivary contamination of etched enamel.

One area that is frequently neglected is the buccal groove on mandibular first permanent molars. It is easy, during exchange of cotton rolls, to let the cheek collapse onto the buccal surface of the tooth, thus contaminating this surface. Special care must be taken when replacing the buccal cotton roll. This is even more important for the second permanent molar where the posterior position of the teeth frequently complicates cotton roll isolation.

Two fresh cotton rolls, one on top of the other, are sometimes required lingually for patients with a heavy salivary flow. After exchange of cotton rolls, the tooth can be dried thoroughly and the sealant applied.

Mandibular Left Quadrant. From personal preference, it is recommended to operate in this quadrant with the left hand. This means the operator's right thumb is used on the lingual cotton roll and right index finger on the buccal cotton roll. One can easily adapt to completing the etching, washing, and sealant application by working left-handed. The operator has far better control of the cotton rolls (and it is much less strain on the wrist) using one's right hand when sitting in the normal position for a right-handed operator, with the patient in the supine position.

Maxillary Right Quadrant. The operator's left index finger holds the buccal cotton roll in place, while the second finger is used as a guard to prevent the tongue from contaminating the lingual surfaces.

Maxillary Left Quadrant. The operator's second finger controls the buccal cotton roll while the index finger controls the tongue. Some operators prefer to use Iso-Shields* for

_____
*3M Company, St. Paul, Minnesota, U.S.A.

isolation, particularly in the maxillary quadrant. These Iso-Shields block the parotid duct, and they are an effective substitute for buccal cotton rolls.

Step 4. Etching

After isolation, the teeth are thoroughly dried to remove any remaining saliva that may hinder acid coverage of the enamel.

Phosphoric acid, in the range of 30 to 40 per cent, is the best etching solution.[13] It is best applied using a small mini-sponge, but a cotton pellet or a brush may also be used. A lockable pliers is helpful to hold the pellet or sponge.

Acid should be applied approximately two-thirds of the way up cuspal slopes or even further if any supplemental grooves extend beyond this area. It is important to etch approximately 2 mm on either side of an exposed groove (such as the buccal groove on mandibular molars or the lingual groove on maxillary molars) in order that there be a sufficient area of etched enamel for sealant application. If too little sealant is applied on exposed grooves, it will be more easily lost. Also, if sealant is applied to unetched enamel it will not bond and will eventually either lift off the surface or fracture away from the main body of sealant. As soon as the complete area to be etched is covered with acid, the time is noted, and the tooth enamel is etched for 60 seconds. Fresh acid should be continually dabbed on the surface at all times. Care must be taken, as the etching time progresses, to treat the enamel surface very carefully and not to rub the cotton pellet or sponge on the surface during acid application, because this may damage the fragile enamel latticework being formed. It was Rock's impression that "bond strength was more related to the nature of the adhered surface than to the resin used."[14] Thus the enamel surface environment after etching and prior to resin application is of critical importance.

Step 5. Washing

Another important step in the success or failure of the technique is the washing of the tooth after etching. All too frequently this step is completed in a very cursory manner. It is imperative to remove all the phosphoric acid and the reaction precipitates produced during etching. To accomplish this, water under pressure and a water-air spray is essential, along with high power evacuation.

Initially, pure water is used to remove most of the acid. The evacuator tip should be placed adjacent to or slightly above the tooth and the water directed towards the tip. In this way, one retards saturation of the cotton rolls, thereby minimizing the chances for the overflow of saliva onto the etched surface. After approximately 5 seconds of pure water, the air button is also pressed forming a strong water-air spray, which should be played over the etched surface for approximately 15 seconds. It is difficult to satisfactorily wash an etched tooth over all surfaces in just 5 to 10 seconds. A minimum of 15 seconds per tooth or 20 seconds per quadrant is recommended. The operator should be especially careful to point the spray directly at surfaces that may be behind cusps, or otherwise out of the path of the spray (for example, buccal and lingual surfaces).

After completion of the washing phase, the assistant removes all the excess water and saliva with the aspirator. It has been suggested by Ibsen and Neville[15] that after etching the patient should rinse, although in the same book the authors stress "isolation to prevent contamination." How these factors (that is, rinsing and non-contamination) are compatible is hard to understand. Most authors presently agree that rinsing by the patient after etching should definitely not be allowed, and that the sealant should be applied as soon as possible after etching, washing, and drying with air that is not contaminated by oil or water.

Step 6. Re-isolation

After washing of the etched surfaces, the cotton rolls will need replacing, as described previously in Step 3. If there is any salivary contamination of the etched enamel at this time, the area should be re-etched for about 10 seconds before washing again. Meurman[16] has shown, with the use of scanning electronmicroscopy, that salivary contamina-

tion of acid-etched enamel decreased retention of resin by deposition of material that blocks resin penetration. Meurman suggests postponing sealant application until a later visit if contamination occurs, since re-etching will not demineralize the absorbed external matrix. Clinically, however, this appears neither practical nor necessary.

Step 7. Drying the Etched Enamel and Mixing the Resin

As soon as fresh cotton rolls are in place, compressed air is directed over all etched surfaces. The drying phase is also most important, since moisture on the etched surface hinders penetration of the resin into the enamel. While the assistant is mixing or preparing the resin according to the manufacturer's instructions, air is continually directed over the etched enamel until the sealant is ready for application. A minimum of 15 seconds drying time is recommended for a single tooth and 20 seconds for a quadrant.

The air hose used for drying etched surfaces should be periodically checked, to be certain it is free of contaminants such as oil and water. Water leaking into the air hose will render the drying phase, and thus also the complete procedure, a failure.

When mixing the resin, care should be taken not to spatulate the mix too vigorously, since this will lead to incorporation of air bubbles in the resin.[17] These bubbles can be removed (with some difficulty) prior to sealant polymerization. Sometimes, however, bubbles that come to the surface after some wear of the material can be mistaken for caries, since plaque will accumulate in these areas (Figures 16–4 and 16–5). The use of a colored sealant is beneficial because it makes bubbles more visible during application.

Step 8. Sealant Application

A brush is the preferred method of applying sealant to an etched surface. It is possible to pick up sealant with certain small metal instruments, but touching the fragile etched surface may result in damage to the etched enamel prisms. In the ultraviolet cur-

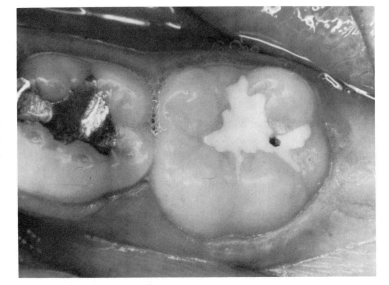

Figure 16–4 Bubbles in sealant (as in this two-year recall) may collect plaque and be mistakenly diagnosed as caries under the sealant. Additional sealant should be applied if bubbles are seen at application.

ing systems, a brush can be used many times over, since the unpolymerized resin can be easily cleaned from the brush. The autopolymerizing systems, however, should use disposable brushes, as it is not possible to completely remove all the resin from the bristles prior to polymerization, and after one or two applications, the brush becomes clogged with resin and is unusable.

An excellent disposable brush, specifically designed for pit and fissure sealant application, comes with 3M White Sealant Kits.* Most other manufacturers similarly recommend brush application of sealant.

---

*3M Company, St. Paul, Minnesota, U.S.A.

The 3M Applicator Brush comes with disposable brush tips (black pointed bristles). The brush tips are excellent for use as a soft carrier of the sealant from the mixing pad to the tooth. In other words, the main function of the bristle tip is to carry and apply the sealant to the tooth, providing a soft applicator that will not damage the delicate enamel latticework surface. A hard carrier of any kind may damage the enamel surface as sealant is deposited on the tooth.

The opposite end to the bristle brush on the 3M Applicator Brush is designed to be used to apply very small drops of sealant in delicate areas where precise application is very important. This unique feature makes

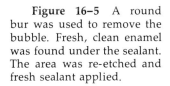

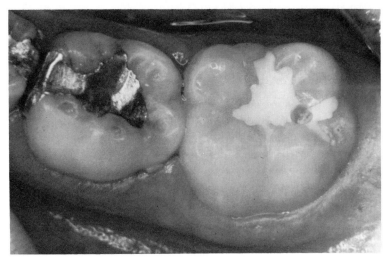

Figure 16–5 A round bur was used to remove the bubble. Fresh, clean enamel was found under the sealant. The area was re-etched and fresh sealant applied.

this particular applicator very useful. The pointed tip is used particularly on partially erupted buccal and lingual grooves. It makes accurate placement of small (or large) drops of resin very easy, thus eliminating or minimizing the amount of excess sealant flowing onto the tissue. Other manufacturers have similar applicator brushes available. For example, the L. D. Caulk Co.* supplies an applicator brush with their Nuva-Cote sealant. This is an excellent applicator, but the 3M applicator is preferred for two reasons:

1. The disposable brushes come to a point. In the Caulk version, they are flattened.

2. The angle and point of the minimal drop end are much more amenable to delicate sealant application.

Delton Pit and Fissure Sealant† has a unique applicator, consisting of disposable plastic tubes into which sealant is drawn up by suction. The end of the tube is then placed on the tooth and the sealant expelled. The idea behind this principle is excellent, but the size of the tube makes delicate application in difficult areas (close to gingiva or areas of restricted access) a problem.

Whichever sealant one uses, the 3M Applicator can be recommended. The minisponges supplied with the 3M White Sealant kits and originally intended for sealant application are not recommended for this purpose. The sponges rapidly become saturated with resin, which cannot then be extracted from the sponge without compressing the sponge on the delicate enamel surface. This is definitely not desirable. In addition to possibly damaging the fragile enamel surface, the use of sponges tends to increase the number of bubbles within the sealant. The mini-sponges, therefore, should be used for acid application only.

Sealant should be applied in a relatively thick layer. It is better to apply too much sealant, which may cause a temporary occlusal interference until the high-spot is rapidly abraded away by the forces of mastication (probably within 2 to 3 days), than to apply too little. The thicker the sealant, the longer it will last. A thin layer of sealant may not have the strength to resist fracture.

When applying autopolymerizing sealant to a whole quadrant, it is best to cover all the etched areas on each tooth as soon as possible with a layer of sealant, and then go back to each tooth and add bulk as necessary. This is done to ensure that the resin used to cover the etched enamel is in the early stages of polymerization, thus obtaining optimal "tag" penetration. Should insufficient sealant have been mixed initially, fresh resin can always be mixed and added to the polymerized material, provided isolation has been maintained.

Most sealants polymerize in 1 to 3 minutes. The outer surface layer of any sealant will not polymerize, because of inhibiting effect of the oxygen in the atmosphere on the chemical reaction. Thus the sealant will always appear to have a greasy film after polymerization. This film should be wiped off, in order to minimize the unpleasant taste of resin remaining in the patient's mouth.

The complete procedure from Step 3 (after isolation of a quadrant) to polymerization of the sealant should take approximately 3½ minutes. Assuming one applies sealant to only one quadrant at a time, a patient should be able to have four quadrants sealed in less than 20 minutes from seating to dismissal. The average time for four quadrant application in the author's study is 19 minutes and four single tooth (first permanent molars) quadrants is 15 minutes. The breakdown of one quadrant occurs as follows:

Etch	60 seconds
Wash	30 seconds
Change cotton rolls	
Dry tooth	30 seconds
Mix sealant	
Apply sealant	30 seconds
Polymerization	60 seconds
Total Time	3½ minutes

INDICATIONS FOR THE USE OF SEALANT

1. Deep pits and fissures on molars (or bicuspids) that are likely to become carious.

---

*L.D. Caulk Company, Milford, Delaware
†Johnson and Johnson, East Windsor, New Jersey

2. Minimal or questionable fissure caries. A small exploratory preparation may be desirable in some cases (see Chapter 18). However, with the research results now available,[18, 19] an experienced user of sealants should have no qualms about covering incipient carious lesions with sealant, thus effectively using sealants in a therapeutic as well as preventive manner.

3. Patient unable to maintain ideal oral hygiene (for example, handicapped child).

CONTRAINDICATIONS TO THE USE OF SEALANTS

1. Rampant or moderate decay where interproximal caries is probable in the near future.

2. Rounded, shallow fissures where decay is unlikely.

QUESTIONS FREQUENTLY RAISED CONCERNING SEALANTS AND THE ACID ETCH TECHNIQUE

1. *What happens to etched areas that are not covered by sealant?* The areas of etched enamel not covered by resin return to their original appearance and approach the same levels of acid resistance as adjacent unetched enamel within 24 hours.[20] Remineralization by deposition of the organic and mineral components of saliva and from fluoride (from drinking water or other sources) is thought to account for this rapid return to normal macroscopic appearance. Even if unsealed etched areas do not histologically or microscopically return to normal for a long period of time, there is no evidence in any published study that these areas are more susceptible to caries.

2. *Why does a stronger solution of phosphoric acid create a less desirable etching pattern than a weaker solution?* This question is still unanswered. Silverstone[21] has suggested that it "may be related to the degree of ionization of the acid. The weaker the acid the greater effect of diffusion into the tissue. In addition, one must consider the formation of other phases, in this way soluble or

insoluble precipitates will affect further the dissolution rate."

3. *Does spillage of phosphoric acid onto soft tissue create any undesirable effect?* It is a frequent occurrence for the etching agent to contact soft tissue during etching for sealant application, particularly in areas adjacent to buccal and lingual grooves. No adverse reaction has been seen or documented from phosphoric acid acting on the gingiva or oral mucosa for short periods of time.

4. *What happens if a carious lesion is inadvertently sealed over?* Studies by Handelman and coworkers[18] indicate that sealing-over diagnosed carious lesions results in a decrease in the viable bacteria count (a 2000-fold decrease after 2 years). Preliminary clinical and radiographic findings suggest that there is no progression of the carious lesions.

Going and coworkers,[19] in a five-year study, found similar results, concluding that "sealant treatment resulted in an apparent 89 per cent reversal from a caries-active to caries-inactive state."

As stated earlier, these studies may well pave the way for a therapeutic use of pit and fissure sealant, in addition to eliminating the fear of the potential problems from the inadvertent sealing-over of carious lesions in the preventive use of sealants.

5. *A related question is, Can caries be initiated under a sealant?* Properly applied sealants do not leak and thus the initiation of decay is not possible. The previously discussed studies of Handelman and of Going confirm this.

It is feasible that caries can initiate below a margin that has "lifted" and is allowing the penetration of oral fluids. This is not the fault of the material, however. Some error in technique (Possibly a groove was subgingival at application and did not etch properly, or the etched enamel was contaminated by the capillary action of adjacent gingival crevicular fluids) was responsible for the margin leaking. The question of whether the sealant, in such a case, can contribute to caries initiation becomes academic when one considers that only the most caries-susceptible teeth are sealed in the first place.

6. *What happens to the maturation of enamel after sealant application immediately post-eruption?* If maturation of enamel is defined as the acquisition of organic and inorganic material by immature enamel, then the application of resin would stop maturation of sealed enamel. The basic question is, however, at just what stage after eruption can maturation be said to have reached an optimal level? *In vitro* studies by Silverstone,[22] simulating post-eruptive maturation of enamel, show no additional benefit to the surface enamel after 48 hours of exposure to the oral fluids. If maturation is a protective process that continues for some time after eruption, it apparently does little to protect against pit and fissure caries, which can frequently be diagnosed before a tooth is even fully erupted. Thus, application of a sealant to a caries-susceptible fissure can certainly not have a deleterious effect on the tooth if it prevents caries at the expense of the hypothesized maturation of the sub-sealant enamel.

7. *How long will sealants last?* This probably is the question most frequently asked by parents, and it is the hardest to answer. Buonocore[23] expects properly applied sealants to show a half-life of approximately four years. Horowitz and coworkers[24] has presented the five-year results of the Kalispell study, which showed that 42 per cent of the teeth examined after five years still retained all the sealant, 14 per cent had sealant partially missing and 44 per cent had no visibly retained sealant. With improvements in materials and techniques, it is hoped that the five-year retention figures will be dramatically improved. Simonsen has shown retention rates of 96 per cent for permanent teeth and 98.8 per cent for deciduous teeth at two years[25] and approximately 94 per cent retention at three years.[26] Preliminary retention results at five years indicate that more than 80 per cent of the material was retained.

8. *Can partially lost sealants increase the chance of caries developing?* Horowitz and

coworkers[24] reported in his five-year Kalispell results that 7 per cent of the teeth with sealant partially missing became carious, whereas comparison with that group's paired, unsealed controls, showed a 41 per cent caries incidence. One cannot preclude the possibility that in the group of 7 per cent with sealant partially missing that became carious, there are some teeth that decayed as a result of the partially missing sealant creating a cariogenic situation. However, it is clear from Horowitz's results that, in general, partially sealed teeth are less susceptible to decay than unsealed teeth.

Charbeneau and coworkers[27] also studied partially sealed teeth. The following is their conclusion: "Sealant loss from a surface did not appear to initiate pit and fissure caries on maxillary teeth. Such loss may have been a contributing factor in 6 of 38 mandibular tooth surfaces."

9. *Can amalgams be covered with sealant?* There is no adhesion or bonding between silver amalgam and sealant resin. However, in the case of small, single-surface amalgams, marginal leakage of the amalgam can be eliminated (and thus secondary caries potential eliminated) if the amalgam is covered with a layer of sealant.

If, during a routine sealant appointment, small amalgams are seen, it certainly will not do any harm to seal over them. It is assumed that there is no clinically or radiographically diagnosable caries associated with the amalgam. The life of the amalgam will be extended for as long as the sealant is covering all the amalgam margins. Even when the sealant wears down to the amalgam surface, the marginal leakage of the amalgam will still be less than it would be with no sealant present, since sealant is probably present to some degree between amalgam and enamel walls.

It must be remembered when sealing-over amalgams that, as the amalgam increases in size, so the sealant retentive area decreases. Thus, it would not be recommended to seal-over large amalgams with little surrounding area for enamel bonding.

10. *Can dental auxiliaries apply sealant?* Each state in the United States legis-

lates the scope of practice of dentists and auxiliaries alike. A properly trained auxiliary can be just as successful at sealant application as a dentist. In a study by Stiles and coworkers,[28] it was observed that there was "no difference in the retention of the sealant when applied by a dentist or a trained dental auxiliary. . . ."

Increasing use of dental auxiliaries should enable more children's teeth to be sealed at a lower cost. Provided proper training and supervision are given, there is no reason why dentists should object to expanding the role of dental auxiliaries to the application of pit and fissure sealant.

11. *When should sealant be applied?* At the initial dental examination after eruption of the primary second molars, it should be determined whether these teeth require sealant application. Rarely do first primary molars require sealant application. After eruption of first permanent molars, sealant will in most cases be considered a benefit. Similarly, after eruption of the second permanent molars and bicuspids, sealants should be considered. Thus, the ages when sealants are most frequently applied would be around 3 to 4 years, 6 to 7 years, and 12 to 13 years. Annual (or bi-annual) examination of sealant retention at routine dental visits is desirable.

PROBLEMS ENCOUNTERED DURING SEALANT APPLICATION

The tremendous benefits of adding color to sealants, (the first colored sealant on the market was the 3M Concise Brand White Sealant System, March, 1977) are clearly seen in the illustrations within this chapter. In January, 1980, a yellow tint was added to Delton* pit and fissure sealant, and another sealant, Nuva-Cote† is somewhat colored, although more as the result of adding a filler than as a specific result of adding a color. In early studies by this author yellow and pale white sealants were used, both of which exhibited excellent retentive properties. The white color was considered to be more esthetic than yellow.

Advantages of colored sealant over clear sealant:
1. It is easier to apply.
2. It is easier to check for complete coverage and polymerization.
3. It is easier and quicker to check for retention at recall.
4. It allows more accurate tabulation of retention progress.
5. It is a helpful motivational agent in the overall preventive dental health program.

Color addition also has positive side effects inasmuch as problems with sealant handling can also be documented, but these are by no means unique to colored sealant. They frequently may have gone unnoticed with the clear sealants. These problems include the following:

Excess Sealant Spillage onto Gingival Tissues

Figure 16–6 shows what can occur distal to upper molars during sealant application with the patient in the supine position. The material flows distally, and once it touches the gingiva, it may flow in excess onto an adjacent area. Similarly, in the buccal groove of lower molars, one frequently has to apply sealant very close to gingival tissue. Contact with the tissue will result in an excessive amount of sealant accumulating at the gingival margin. Use of the 3M Applicator Brush will minimize the amount of sealant flowing in excess onto the adjacent gingiva, since the amount of sealant applied in a specific area can be easily controlled.

Once contact is made with the gingiva prior to sealant polymerization, it is best to simply let the material polymerize before trimming the material down. Trying to remove the material prior to polymerization, or attempting to flick off the excess after polymerization, may weaken the sealant bond. A 7901 FG Midwest American carbide composite finishing bur* is excellent for high-speed

---

*Johnson and Johnson, East Windsor, New Jersey
†L. D. Caulk Company, Milford, Delaware

*Beavers Dental Products Ltd., Morrisburg, Ontario; distributed by Midwest American, Melrose Park, Illinois

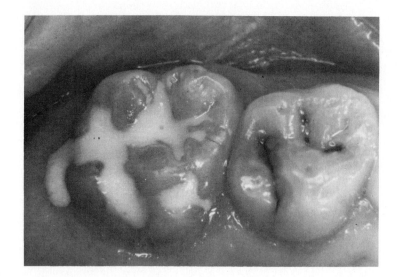

Figure 16–6 Sometimes sealant will flow in excess onto adjacent gingival tissues. The best remedy is to cut off the excess after polymerization with a twelve-fluted composite resin finishing bur.

removal of sealant flash, leaving a relatively smooth resin surface after removal. The bur is thin enough to be able to enter the gingival sulcus without damaging the tissue.

Resin Bubbles

Air bubbles within resins have always been a problem. With the introduction of colored sealant, bubbles have been more easily observed (see Fig. 16–4). Most small bubbles are not of concern, but obviously it is not desirable to have sealant surfaces full of bubbles. If the bubble penetrates to the depth of the fissure or is seen to be in a potentially weak area of the sealant, another mix of sealant should be made and the bubble filled in. Careful instruction of the dental assistant in slow, deliberate mixing together of the resin drops, rather than using a rapid stirring action will almost completely eliminate bubbles of any consequence. The 3M minisponges also have a tendency to increase the incidence of bubbles if used for resin application. As stated previously, these sponges are contraindicated for sealant application.

Sealant Loss

Sealant loss, if the operator follows the technique meticulously, is rare and usually confined to the following areas:

1. Areas of difficult access (Cause: improper cleaning, etching, and washing).
2. Areas adjacent to gingival margins (Cause: contamination by capillary action of tissue and crevicular fluids).
3. Areas of saliva contamination after etching (Cause: moisture control problems).

Most sealant loss, as a result of the problems just noted, will occur within the first 12 months after application. In the author's study,[25] 69 per cent of sealant loss was confined to the lingual side of maxillary molars and the buccal side of mandibular molars.

Before reapplying the sealant, the reason for loss should first be established, so that the error is not repeated. In the case of sealant loss soon after application, it is unlikely that the sealant penetrated the enamel to form "tags," and the enamel, after cleaning, should be just as easily etched as fresh enamel. The adjacent sealant, to which the new sealant will also bond, should have the surface layer removed with a bur to expose uncontaminated resin. Apart from possible plaque accumulation, the old surface resin layer contains absorbed moisture that will interfere with bonding unless it is removed.

In the case of sealant loss as a result of gradual abrasion, the enamel surface is probably impregnated with resin and may require a slightly increased etching time, before adding fresh resin.

CONCLUSIONS

The two major concerns expressed by 400 dentists in the State of Minnesota who

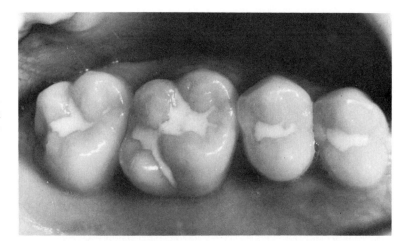

Figure 16–7 The six-month recall photograph of a patient with 3M White Sealant.

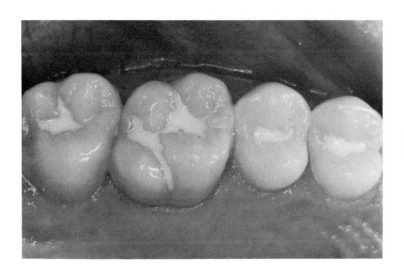

Figure 16–8 The 12-month recall photograph of a patient with sealant present.

Figure 16–9 The 24-month recall photograph.

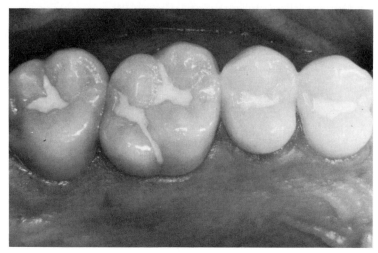

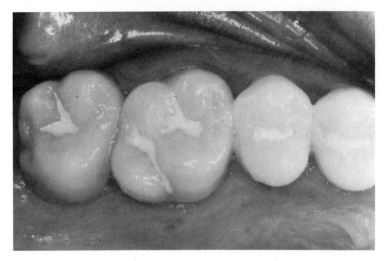

Figure 16–10 The 48-month recall photograph showing excellent retention and virtually no wear of the sealant since the six-month recall photograph.

were surveyed[29] on their attitudes towards the use of pit and fissure sealants were:

1. Sealants do not last long in the mouth.

2. Decay can be initiated or progress under sealants.

Based on the available scientific literature, it would appear that the concern of clinicians regarding poor longevity of sealant and problems associated with the inadvertant sealing of undetected carious lesions is not justified.

Furthermore, there appears to be general agreement in the published literature that there exists a positive relationship between sealant retention and occlusal caries protection. It is, therefore, most unfortunate that such a large number of practitioners (61.7 per cent of those surveyed in Minnesota[29]) do not use pit and fissure sealants.

It is certainly to be hoped that with accurate documentation of clinical trial results (Figs. 16–7 to 16–10) and education of the general practitioner the use of pit and fissure sealants will be increased for the dental health benefit of the general public.

REFERENCES

1. Marshall-Day, C. D., and Sedwick, H. J.: Studies on the incidence of dental caries. Dent. Cosmos 77:442, 1935.
2. Knutson, J. W., Klein, H., and Palmer, C. E.: Dental needs of grade school children of Hagerstown, Maryland. J. Am. Dent. Assoc. 27:579, 1940.
3. Hyatt, T. P.: Prophylactic odontotomy: The cutting into the tooth for the prevention of disease. Dent. Cosmos 65:234, 1923.
4. Bodecker, C. F.: Enamel fissure eradication. N.Y. J. Dent. 30:149, 1964.
5. Bodecker, C. F.: Dental caries immunization without filling. N.Y. J. Dent. 30:337, 1964.
6. Ast, D. B., Bushel, A., and Chase, H. C.: Clinical study of caries prophylaxis with zinc chloride and potassium ferrocyanide. J. Am. Dent. Assoc. 41:437, 1950.
7. Klein, H., and Knutson, J. W.: Studies on dental caries. XIII. Effect of ammoniacal silver nitrate on caries in first permanent molars. J. Am. Dent. Assoc. 29:1420, 1942.
8. Buonocore, M. G.: A simple method of increasing the adhesion of acrylic filling materials to enamel surfaces. J. Dent. Res. 34:849–853, 1955.
9. Ripa, L. W., Buonocore, M., and Cueto, E.: Adhesive sealing of pits and fissures for caries prevention: Report of a two-year study. IADR Abstr. No. 247, March, 1966.
10. Cueto, E. I., and Buonocore, M. G.: Sealing of pits and fissures with an adhesive resin: Its use in caries prevention. J. Am. Dent Assoc. 75:121, 1967.
11. Ast, D. B., Smith, D. J., Wachs, B., and Cantwell, K. T.: Newburgh-Kingston caries-fluorine study XIV. Combined clinical and roentgenographic dental findings after ten years of fluoride experience. J. Am. Dent. Assoc. 52:314–325, 1956.
12. Simonsen, R. J.: Clinical Applications of the Acid Etch Technique. Chicago, Ill., Quintessence Publishing Company, 1978, pp. 19–42.
13. Silverstone, L. M.: Fissure sealants: Laboratory studies. Caries Res. 8:2–26, 1974.
14. Rock, W. P.: The effect of etching of human enamel upon bond strengths with fissure sealant resins. Arch. Oral Biol. 19:873–877, 1974.
15. Ibsen, R. L., and Neville, K.: Adhesive Restorative Dentistry. Philadelphia, W. B. Saunders Co., 1974.
16. Meurman, J. H.: Detrimental effect of in vitro salivary contamination on acid-etched enamel. Proc. Finn. Dent. Soc. 72:30, 1976.
17. Stombaugh, E. F., and Simonsen, R. J.: Vierhändiges Versiegeln von Fissuren und Grübchen. Quintessenz Journal 6:19–26, 1980.
18. Handelman, S. L., Washburn, F., and Wopperer, P.: Two-year report of sealant effect on bacteria in

dental caries. J. Am. Dent. Assoc. *93*:967, 1976.

19. Going, R. E., Loesche, W. J., and Grainger, D. A.: The viability of microorganisms in carious lesions five years after covering with a fissure sealant. J. Am. Dent. Assoc. *97*:455, 1978.

20. Silverstone, L. M.: Fissure sealants: The susceptibility to dissolution of acid-etched and subsequently abraded enamel. Caries Res. *11*:46–51, 1977.

21. Silverstone, L. M., and Dogon, I. L. (eds.): Proceedings of an International Symposium on the Acid Etch Technique. St. Paul, Minnesota, North Central Publishing Co., 1975, p. 82.

22. Silverstone, L. M.: Personal Communication.

23. Buonocore, M. G.: The Use of Adhesives in Dentistry. Springfield, Illinois, Charles C Thomas, 1975.

24. Horowitz, H. S., Heifetz, S. B., and Poulsen, S.: Retention and effectiveness of an adhesive sealant after five years. AADR abstract no. 72, J. Dent. Res., June, 1977.

25. Simonsen, R. J.: The clinical effectiveness of colored pit and fissure sealant at 24 months. Pediatric Dent., *2*:1, 10–16, 1980.

26. Simonsen, R. J.: The clinical effectiveness of a colored sealant at 36 months. J. Dent. Res. *59*:560, 1980.

27. Charbeneau, G. T., Dennison, J. B., and Ryge, G.: A filled pit and fissure sealant: 18-month results. J. Am. Dent. Assoc. *95*:299–306, 1977.

28. Stiles, H. M., Ward, G. T., Woolridge, E. D., and Meyers, R.: Adhesive sealant clinical trial: Comparative results of application by a dentist or dental auxiliaries. J. Prev. Dent. *3*:8–11, 1976.

29. Simonsen, R. J.: Pit and fissure sealants: Attitudes toward and use by dentists in Minnesota. Unpublished data.

CHAPTER SEVENTEEN
The Acid Etch Technique and Preventive Resin Restorations

Richard J. Simonsen, D.D.S., M.S.

One of the most far-reaching recent improvements in the practice of dentistry has been the development of the acid etch technique.

The significance of the work by Buonocore,[1] in which he reported that the bonding of acrylic restorative material to enamel could be greatly enhanced with use of an acid conditioning agent, has not even today been fully appreciated by many dentists. Undoubtedly, Buonocore's work will be recognized in the years to come as the pioneering essay on the development of one of the most widely used techniques in dentistry. Even today improvements in the method are being made continually as the result of new research. The technique had a long and sometimes painful birth, but it can now be said to be past its infancy stage and maturing rapidly.

Buonocore was the first to apply the industrial use of phosphoric acid to resin retention in dentistry. It took many years for others to adopt the technique, and it was not until the late 1960's and early 1970's that articles concerning various *in vivo* and *in vitro* studies were published. Today, along with its widespread use in fissure sealing for caries prevention, we see the acid etch principle widely used in many clinical disciplines. Some uses of the acid etch principles are outlined in the following paragraphs.

PREVENTIVE DENTISTRY

Fissure Sealants. Fissure sealing is the primary preventive use of the acid etch technique. This technique also has secondary preventive uses, for instance, in very conservative tooth preparation.

RESTORATIVE DENTISTRY

1. Restoration of fractured incisors.
2. Class III and V restoration.
3. Restoration of teeth with developmental defects, for example, peg-shaped laterals, hypocalcification marks, fluorosis, and iatrogenic defects such as tetracycline stains.
4. Splinting of teeth that have become mobile as a result of trauma or periodontal disease.
5. Construction of temporary bridges and space maintainers. (The acid etch principle may well have a more than temporary effect on crown and bridge dentistry in the future).
6. Preventive resin restorations.
7. Esthetic adjustment of tooth anatomy.

A more detailed description of the preventive resin restoration follows later in this chapter.*

ORTHODONTICS

1. Bonding of brackets directly onto teeth.
2. Attachment of space maintainers and retainers.

---

*See also reference 12.

ETCHING AGENTS

Buonocore[1] initially used 85 per cent phosphoric acid for his etch of enamel. This strength was chosen apparently in deference to the industrial use of phosphoric acid in treating metal surfaces to obtain better adhesion of paint and resin coatings.

Gwinnett and Buonocore[2] tested several etching agents and reported that "with the solutions of phosphoric acid, it was noted that with increasing concentrations progressively less change was produced on the enamel surface." In 1972, the same authors[3] described the effect of etching on enamel as "an increase in porosity, with the prism cores being preferentially dissolved." The most recent significant work on acid strength has been done by Silverstone[4] and by Silverstone and coworkers.[5] In his studies, Silverstone confirmed an inverse relationship between acid strength and change in surface topography on the enamel surface when using the acid of choice, orthophosphoric acid.

Additionally, and more importantly, he found that the depth of histologic change was greatest at weaker acid concentrations. This area of histologically changed enamel allows the resin to the form the "tags that are the foundation for the mechanical retention of the resin within the enamel." At weaker acid solutions, however, the loss in surface contour is greatest, and the ideal acid for etching combines the least loss in surface contour with the greatest depth of histologic

TABLE 17–1 DEPTH OF ETCH AND HISTOLOGIC CHANGE IN ENAMEL (TO NEAREST μM) FOLLOWING A ONE MINUTE EXPOSURE TO VARIOUS CONCENTRATIONS OF PHOSPHORIC ACID

ONE MINUTE EXPOSURE	CONCENTRATION OF PHOSPHORIC ACID, %						
	20	30	40	50	50 ZnO	60	70
Depth of etch	14	10	9	7	6	2	2
Depth of histologic change	20	20	15	12	10	4	2
Total depth of enamel affected	34	30	24	19	16	6	4

50 ZnO = 50% phosphoric acid + 7% zinc oxide by weight

(From Silverstone, L. M.: Caries Res. 8:2–26, 1974.)

TABLE 17–2 LOSS IN DEPTH OF SURFACE CONTOUR (TO NEAREST μM) AFTER EXPOSURE TO VARIOUS CONCENTRATIONS OF PHOSPHORIC ACID

EXPOSURE TIME IN MINUTES	CONCENTRATION OF PHOSPHORIC ACID, %						
	20	30	40	50	50 ZnO	60	70
1		14	10	9	7	6	2	2
2		17	15	14	9	7	5	2
3		40	34	27	14	11	5	2

50 ZnO = 50% phosphoric acid + 7% zinc oxide by weight

(From Silverstone, L. M.: Caries Res. 8:2–26, 1974.)

change. As can be seen from Table 17–1, 30 per cent phosphoric acid (H_3PO_4) produced a surface loss of 10 microns and a depth of histologic change of 20 microns, for a total depth effect of 30 microns. Silverstone's conclusion was that "unbuffered 30 per cent phosphoric acid proved to be the most satisfactory conditioning fluid. . . ." Silverstone also found the ideal etching time to be 1 minute (Table 17–2).

Silverstone's later studies confirmed his earlier results, and it has become generally accepted that etching with 30 to 40 per cent H_3PO_4 will provide the ideal surface contour for resin retention. Rock[6] compared the bond strength of Silverstone's recommended 30 per cent H_3PO_4 solution with the more commonly used 50 per cent H_3PO_4 buffered with 7 per cent zinc oxide (as used in Nuva System, L. D. Caulk Company, Milford, Delaware). He found an increase of over 50 per cent in the tensile strength of a sealant bond when 30 per cent H_3PO_4 was used to etch the enamel.

Enamel is predominantly hydroxyapatite, $Ca_{10}(PO_4)_6(OH)_2$. The hydroxyapatite crystals are packed together to form prisms, which, in the mature tissue, are flattened hexagons in transverse section. The prisms are oriented at right angles to the enamel surface, thus providing a latticework surface that when selectively etched produces an ideal base for the mechanical attachment of resins.

Silverstone[5] described three basic types of surface characteristics in etched enamel.

In the most common, called type 1 etching pattern, prism core material was preferentially removed, leaving the prism peripheries relatively intact. In the second, type 2 etching pattern, the reverse pattern was observed. The peripheral regions of prisms were removed preferentially, leaving prism cores remaining relatively unaffected. In the type 3 etching pattern, there was a more random pattern, areas of which corresponded to types 1 and 2 damage together with regions in which the pattern of etching could not be related to prism morphology.

All three etching types were found in single samples of etched enamel, suggesting that "there is no one specific etching pattern produced in human dental enamel by the actions of acid solution."[5] Gwinnett,[7] another knowledgeable author who has done much work on the subject, reported similar findings. "Summarily the most common appearance of the conditioned enameled surface is that of rods showing a preferred loss of material from the rod cores. Less frequently, the preferred loss is from the peripheries. Such losses are not clinically predictable and preferred loss at cores and peripheries may occur at adjacent sites in the same tooth."

The etched surface is of critical importance to the strength of the bond, for it is into this roughened surface that the resin flows, forming the "tags" that are the basis for resin retention. The surface not only must be etched for the correct time with the ideal strength of the best acid; it also must be dry and free of contaminants when the resin is applied.

Primary enamel has been described as prismless by Gwinnett[7] and by Ibsen and Neville.[8] Silverstone and coworkers[5] formed the impression that primary enamel was not significantly prismless, but that it did require an increase in etching time to two minutes to produce an etch comparable to adult enamel, using H_3PO_4 in a concentration range of 20 to 50 per cent. Correctly etched enamel, whether permanent or primary, has a characteristic chalky or frosty appearance. The luster is removed, and if the enamel does not appear frosty after the correct etching time, the etch should be repeated. Intrinsic factors such as the age of the tooth or the fluoride content of the enamel can prevent a satisfactory etch. The incidence of prismless enamel and its effect on etching in both deciduous and permanent teeth is

still an area of disagreement among authors. In a clinical study, Simonsen[10] found that etching occlusal primary surfaces for one or two minutes resulted in no significant differences in the retentive properties of a colored pit and fissure sealant.

RESIN MATERIAL

There are two basic types of resin material on the market today: those that contain an ultraviolet catalyst and are polymerized by exposure to ultraviolet light and those that are autopolymerizing.

The main advantage of the ultraviolet systems (and the recently introduced visible light curing systems) is that the operator has complete control over the polymerization time. However, problems with depth of polymerization (about 1.5 mm) and uniformity of light output have caused some concern.

In the autopolymerizing systems, one has some control over setting time by regulating the amount of accelerator used in the liquid or paste resin systems. In addition there is no concern over depth of polymerization, and no investment in a costly and sometimes less than reliable light system is necessary. If a light system can be developed to give a consistent light output and wavelength with a rapid resin polymerization time (say 5 seconds), it may well prove to be advantageous. At the present time, however, the autopolyermizing systems appear to be preferable.

All the resin-based materials available consist mainly of dimethacrylates or a mixture of mono- and dimethacrylate resins. Inorganic fillers, such as quartz or silica, are used in the filled (composite) resin to increase strength and hardness, reduce polymerization shrinkage, and increase wear resistance.

THE PREVENTIVE RESIN RESTORATION

A technique for caries restoration and simultaneous caries prevention without extension of the preparation for prevention had been impossible before the introduction of the acid etch technique. It is now feasible to lay aside the time-worm techniques of the prophylactic odontotomy, of fissure eradication, and of extension for prevention. Instead, filled or unfilled resins can be used with the acid etch technique in restoring minimal carious pit and fissure lesions.

The prophylactic odontotomy, first used by Hyatt[10] in the 1920's, is still in use today. This technique undoubtedly has served the purpose of reducing the size of the preparation in some teeth by restoring potentially carious areas prior to caries attack taking hold. Just as certainly, however, many teeth that never would have decayed were subjected to a restorative procedure.

Smoothing the cuspal slopes to flatten out the sharp pits and fissures, thus making them easier to keep clean rather than restoring them, was another frequently used method of caries prevention.[12] This technique also is still used today, although rarely. The improvement in and increasing use of pit and fissure sealants and composite resins have rendered these techniques obsolete.

After diagnosis of caries in pits and fissures, amalgam is presently accepted by most practitioners as the restorative material of choice. Many questionably carious or "sticky" fissures are restored with amalgam. Several disadvantages relating to the use of amalgam as a restorative material have caused composite resins, used with the acid etch technique, to move to the forefront of clinical dental research. The recent variability in the cost of silver and concerns over the toxicity of mercury will also have an effect on the choice of material for restorative dentistry in the future.

The primary goal of restorative dentistry should be to seek out the most conservative approach possible to any restorative procedure. If this approach fails, it is then always possible to go one step further with a more radical technique. Thus, the old and still much-used adage of "extension for prevention" sometimes brought serious doubts to mind when an occlusal surface riddled with supplemental grooves and having just one small spot of decay was observed. Inevitably, no matter how conservative the tooth preparation, healthy tooth substance is removed in order to prevent caries from attacking at another site on the same tooth (this is an extension of Hyatt's principle).

The challenge, then, is to develop a technique whereby minimal carious lesions (usually in young permanent teeth) are restored with the minimum of tooth removal while concurrently preventing caries from attacking other pits and fissures on the same surface without mechanical removal of these areas.

Patients not suitable for pit and fissure sealant application as a result of small carious lesions in young permanent molars (or primary molars) are ideal candidates for a restorative technique utilizing a filled or unfilled resin and the acid etch technique.

Occlusal surfaces are thoroughly examined using a sharp probe or explorer. Bitewing radiographs are used to eliminate any teeth with interproximal caries. In deciding whether to use only unfilled resin or a combination of unfilled and filled resin, the graded teeth are split into three groups, A, B, or C, depending on the size of preparation necessary. Preparations are kept to a minimum, but all caries is removed. Anesthesia and rubber dam are used where caries is definitely present. Exploratory preparations (very small preparations to see if caries is present) can be made without anesthesia and with cotton roll isolation.

Group A consists of teeth with single or multiple preparations, none of which exceed the approximate size of a #1 round bur. Group B consists of teeth with single or multiple preparations greater than a size #1 round bur but less than a size #2 round bur. Group C consists of teeth with single or multiple preparations greater than a size #2 round bur.

Group A Treatment

All non-prepared pits and fissures, minimal exploratory preparations (size #1/4 or #1/2), or minimal carious restoration (size #1 or smaller) are sealed with a pit and fissure sealant. The technique followed has been described in Chapter 16 and in other references.[13] Sealant is introduced initially into the minimal preparations with an explorer.

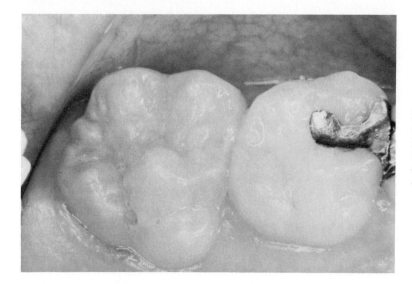

Figure 17–1 Group B. If the preparation size exceeds the size of a no. 1 round bur or if multiple preparations are necessary, addition of filler to the unfilled resin is desirable.

In this way, no air is trapped in the preparations before the bulk of the sealant is applied with a disposable brush.

Research has established the safety of sealing-over carious lesions.[14-16]. Thus, exploratory preparation may not be necessary as frequently in the future. No detrimental effect from sealing-over questionably carious areas has been observed.

Group B Treatment

Starting with round bur #¼ and going up in size as necessary, it is decided whether the tooth can be treated as in Group A, or if a partially filled preventive resin restoration is indicated. The size of the preparation and its position (susceptibility to wear), determine whether filler should be added to the unfilled resin (Fig. 17–1).

Very careful clinical examination of the preparation is necessary at this time to ensure that all carious tissue has been removed. A stained pit is not always completely removed unless softness is detected with an explorer. If caries is found and further exploration is necessary (up to size #2 round bur) until an area of sound tooth structure is reached, a dilute resin restoration is indicated. Any commercially available unfilled resin/filled resin combination can be used for this technique. A description follows utilizing the 3M Enamel Bond and Concise System.*

---

*3M Company, St. Paul, Minnesota

Any exposed dentin is covered with a calcium hydroxide base wherever possible. The dilute Concise is prepared while the tooth is being etched for 60 seconds with 37 per cent orthophosphoric acid under cotton roll isolation. The etchant is applied using a small sponge held in a self-locking cotton pliers. Care is taken to etch approximately 2 mm beyond the margins of the exploratory preparation, as well as over all other exposed pits and fissures.

The diluted filled resin mix is prepared by diluting a small amount of one side of the filled system (for example, Concise paste B) with an approximately equal amount of the other side of the unfilled system (for example, Enamel Bond resin A).

After etching, thorough washing, and drying, with great care being taken to avoid contamination of the etched surface, an unfilled resin layer (enamel Bond) is first applied with a disposable brush. The presence of the unfilled resin layer is clinically beneficial, since it allows the dilute Concise to flow better into small preparations. However, the necessity of an intermediate resin layer for better "tag" formation or reduction of microleakage is disputed in the literature.[17-23]

The dilute Concise is applied into small preparations with an explorer and applied over remaining pits and fissures (to the same degree that they would be covered with a pit and fissure sealant) with either a disposable brush or carefully (in order not to touch and damage the etched enamel surface) with an explorer or other instrument (Fig. 17–2).

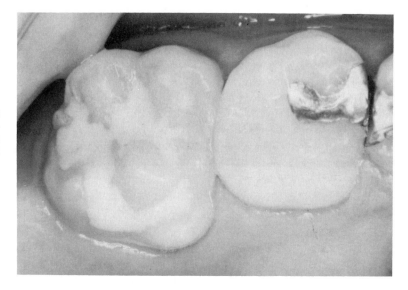

Figure 17–2 The tooth has been restored and the adjacent pits and fissures sealed with a mixture of sealant and filled resin.

All cases are checked after polymerization for occlusal interferences and adjusted as necessary using a #7408* composite finishing bur.

Group C Treatment

The same principles of minimal cavity preparation apply to Group C. No extension for prevention is attempted, and only carious enamel or dentin is removed. The slightly larger size of preparation encountered with Group C cases (round bur size #2 or larger) facilitates the application of a calcium hydroxide base to all exposed dentin.

*Beavers Dental Products Ltd., Morrisburg, Ontario; distributed by Midwest American, Melrose Park, Illinois

A small bevel is placed at the cavity margins. The enamel margins and all remaining pits and fissures are etched as previously described. After application of the unfilled resin layer, pure filled resin (Concise) is injected into the preparation(s) using the Centrix C-R syringe.* This resin is also carried over the unfilled resin layer covering other exposed pits and fissures, thus sealing these areas with a filled resin. Occlusal adjustment is carried out after rubber dam removal, as in Group B cases.

The results of a three-year study utilizing the technique described has been published[24] (Fig. 17–3). The results of this study

*Clev-Dent Division, Cavitron Corp., Brook Park, Ohio

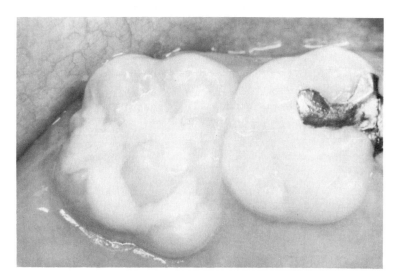

Figure 17–3 The same case seen three years after the preventive resin restoration was placed.

and others using diluted filled composite resin as a pit and fissure sealant[25-27] and as a partial restorative[28, 29] are most encouraging.

With further developments in the area of more wear-resistant composite resins, it is anticipated that this technique will become an even more valuable alternative to conventional amalgam restorations in young permanent molar teeth. The advantage of the preventive resin restoration in the saving of healthy tooth structure is a major consideration for the selection of a restorative technique.

REFERENCES

1. Buonocore, M. G.: A simple method of increasing the adhesion of acrylic filling materials to enamel surfaces. J. Dent. Res. 34:849–853, 1955.
2. Gwinnett, A. J., and Buonocore, M. G.: Adhesives and caries prevention: A preliminary report. Br. Dent. J. 119:77–80, 1965.
3. Gwinnett, A. J., and Buonocore, M. G.: A scanning electron microscope study of pit and fissure surfaces conditioned for adhesive sealing. Arch. Oral Biol. 17:415–423, 1972.
4. Silverstone, L. M.: Fissure sealants: Laboratory studies. Caries Res. 8:2–26, 1974.
5. Silverstone, L. M., Saxton, C. A., Dogon, I. L., and Fejerskov, O.: Variation in the pattern of acid etching of human dental enamel examined by scanning electronmicroscopy. Caries Res. 9:373–387, 1975.
6. Rock, W. P.: The effect of etching on human enamel upon bond strengths with fissure sealant resins. Arch. Oral Biol. 19:873–877, 1974.
7. Gwinnett, A. J.: The bonding of sealants to enamel. J. Am. Soc. Prev. Dent. 1:21–29, 1973.
8. Ibsen, R. L., and Neville, K.: Adhesive Restorative Dentistry. Philadelphia, W. B. Saunders Company, 1974.
9. Silverstone, L. M., and Dogon, I. L. (eds.): Proceedings of an International Symposium on the Acid Etch Technique. St. Paul, Minnesota, North Central Publishing Company, 1975.
10. Hyatt, T. P.: Prophylactic odontotomy: The cutting into the tooth for the prevention of disease. Dent. Cosmos 5:234, 1923.
11. Simonsen, R. J.: The clinical effectiveness of colored pit and fissure sealant at 24 months. Pediatric Dent. 2:10–16, 1980.
12. Bodecker, C. F.: Eradication of enamel fissures. Dent. Items 51:859–866, 1926.
13. Simonsen, R. J.: Clinical Applications of the Acid Etch Technique. Chicago, Quintessence Publishing Company, 1978, pp. 19–31.
14. Handelman, S. L.: Microbiologic aspects of sealing carious lesions. J. Prev. Dent. 3:29–32, 1976.
15. Handelman, S. L., Washburn, F., and Wopperer, P.: Two year report of sealant effect on bacteria in dental caries. J. Am. Dent. Assoc. 92:967–970, 1976.
16. Going, R. E., et al.: The viability of microorganisms in carious lesions five years after covering with a fissure sealant. J. Am. Dent. Assoc. 97:455–462, 1978.
17. Dreyer Jorgensen, K.: The adaptation of composite and noncomposite resins to acid etched enamel surfaces. In Silverstone, L. M. and Dogon, I. L. (eds.): Proceedings of an International Symposium on the Acid Etch Technique. St. Paul, MN, North Central Publishing Company, 1975, pp. 93–99.
18. Raadal, M.: Mikroretensjon av plastfyllingsmaterialer paa syreetset emalje. Den Norske Tannlaegeforenings Tidende. 10:404–413, 1975.
19. Asmussen, E.: Penetration of restorative resins into acid etched enamel. IADR abstract no. 349, February, 1977.
20. Buonocore, M. G.: The Use of Adhesives in Dentistry. Springfield, Illinois, Charles C Thomas, Publisher, 1975, p. 257.
21. Mohammed, H., Schoen, F. J., and Burrell, E. R.: A simple comparative adhesion test method for composite resins. IADR abstract no. 350, February, 1977.
22. Dogon, I. L.: Studies demonstrating the need for an intermediary resin of low viscosity for the acid etch technique. In Silverstone, L. M., and Dogon, I. L. (eds.): Proceedings of an International Symposium on the Acid Etch Technique. St. Paul, MN, North Central Publishing Company, 1975, pp. 100–118.
23. Forsten, L.: Effect of different factors on the marginal seal of composites. IADR abstract no. 427, February, 1977.
24. Simonsen, R. J.: Preventive resin restorations: Three year results. J. Am. Dent. Assoc. 100:535–539, 1980.
25. Ulvestad, H.: Clinical trials with fissure sealant materials in Scandinavia. In Silverstone, L. M. and Dogon, I. L. (eds.): Proceedings of an International Symposium on the Acid Etch Technique. St. Paul, MN, 1975, pp. 165–174.
26. Ulvestad, H.: A 24-month evaluation of fissure sealing with a diluted composite material. Scand. J. Dent. Res. 84:41–44, 1976a.
27. Ulvestad, H.: Evaluation of fissure sealing with a diluted composite sealant and an UV-light polymerized sealant after 36 months observation. Scand. J. Dent. Res. 84:401–403, 1976b.
28. Raadal, M.: Microleakage around preventive composite fillings in occlusal fissures. Scand. J. Dent. Res. 86:495–499, 1978.
29. Azhdori, S., Sveen, O. B., and Buonocore, M. G.: Evaluation of a restorative preventive technique for localized occlusal caries. IADR abstract no. 952, January, 1979.

CHAPTER EIGHTEEN

The Composite Resin: A Preventive Operative Procedure

C. H. Pameijer, D.M.D., M.Sc.D., D.Sc.

Dental operative procedures have been carried out since the turn of the century basically in accordance with the principles advocated by G. V. Black. Black's investigations were thorough and impressive and carried out in a time when dental research was in its early stages. His knowledge of clinical dentistry and research has influenced every aspect of dentistry. Improvement of research facilities and an increased knowledge in the areas of physics, microstructure, and biological science have stimulated interest and challenged many established techniques that were practiced for years. During recent decades, the refining of existing research equipment and the invention of new equipment have enabled investigators to obtain more accurate and detailed data. High magnifications with better resolution may now be obtained. All these have contributed greatly to a better understanding of the many problems encountered in dental research.

Extensive research by numerous people has resulted in the production of dental restorative materials with improved mechanical and esthetic properties. This is important, since the major objectives in restoring teeth are (1) the restoration of function and (2) the creation of or improvement in esthetics. Ironically, most materials have been developed to satisfy the need to restore carious lesions. Prevention of these lesions would serve the patient more effectively and allow time and effort to be devoted toward other areas in dentistry that have not received the proper attention. Prevention does not receive the attention it deserves, and the profession should be concerned with the existing situation. There are, however, many positive aspects involving unusual and often demanding situations, for instance, the repair of a fractured incisor. Esthetically and functionally, this type of restoration (depending on the severity of the case) has usually been a compromise. With the new materials and techniques, the final results can sometimes be so sophisticated that one wonders how these problems could have been solved in the past.

Another example is the treatment of enamel hypoplasia. Today, with the development of adhesive restorative materials, these lesions can be treated so that the esthetic value is remarkable. More attention to the actual operative procedures will be given later in this chapter.

For many years, anterior teeth were restored with silicate cements, which were developed in Europe around the turn of the century. They were noted for their esthetic value but criticized for the irritative effects caused by their release of phosphoric acid. Improvements in the composition of the material and the use of cavity liners to protect the pulp have lessened the chances of jeopardizing the intercoronal structure. The esthe-

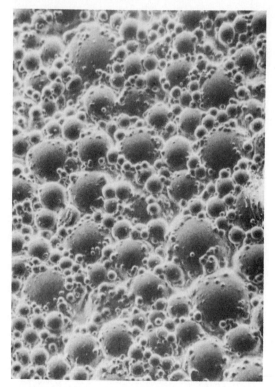

Figure 18–1   A scanning electron micrograph of an unfilled resin. Note the variety in size of the spherical polymer particles (× 200).

tic results, when the materials are properly handled, are unequalled by any other restorative material. The advantage of incorporating fluoride in silicates[14] to reduce secondary decay is attributed to the solubility of the filling material, thus resulting in release of the fluoride. Since this is a long-term process, a continuous topical application protects the surrounding enamel by increasing its resistance to acid solubility.

In the early 1940's, a group of filling materials were introduced that were completely different from the silicate cements. For all practical purposes, these materials can be classified as unfilled resins to distinguish them from composite resins, which were developed later. The particle shape of these resins is usually spherical, and their diameter varies individually (Fig. 18–1). They are chemically accelerated and can be polished to a smooth surface. Immediately after placement and for a short period thereafter the esthetic value is high; however, marginal discoloration due to percolation and darken-

ing over a period of time yield an inferior restoration. This is because of the porous nature of the material coupled with other factors, such as a high coefficient of thermal expansion, which causes the resin to shrink and expand seven or more times as much as tooth structure for every degree of temperature change.[17]

The introduction of composite resins brought us to a new era in restorative dentistry. They have gained tremendous popularity over existing filling materials. Initially, composites were utilized only in Classes III and V restorations. The physical properties were so favorable, however, that other possibilities were readily recognized.

Components of composite resins include monomers, polymerization and color stabilizers, polymerization initiators and accelerators, inorganic filler, and silane coupling agents.

Filler particles of early composite resin systems included glass beads and rods, synthetic calcium phosphates, and fused silica. Some of the currently available composites contain lithium-alumino silicate crystalline compositions, quartz, pyrogenic silica, and barium alumino-borate silica.

In order to improve the physical properties of composites, organo-functional silane coupling agents are applied to the filler during manufacturing. The most used silane at the present time is 3-methacryloxy-propyltrimethoxy silane. Proper application during manufacturing may give some degree of covalent bonding between the polymer and filler. It is this interface, however, that represents the weakest link in a composite resin system.

Of the dimethacrylate monomers, BIS-GMA is the most extensively used and is an addition reaction product of Bisphenol A and glycidyl methacrylate.[19, 20]

In recent years, a considerable number of radiopaque formulations have been marketed. Most of these formulations are probably composed of SiO_2, 66 per cent; BaO, 17 per cent; B_2O_2, 11 per cent; and Al_2O_3, 6 per cent.[13] Clinically, the barium compounds are a problem in that they cause an alkaline reaction in water because of the soluble barium compound.

One of the most widely used inhibitors is of the phenolic type, monomethyl ether of hydroquinone.

The hardening of composite resins begins with reactions generating free radicals, which initiate polymerization. Usually benzoyl peroxide is used. Heat and light can accelerate breakdown of the initiator. Therefore, storage in a cool, dark environment is recommended by the manufacturer.

In order to accomplish rapid hardening at mouth temperature, polymerization accelerators are used. Currently, N, N-di-hydroxyethyl-p-toluidine is being used, which interacts with benzoyl peroxide, thus generating free radicals.[13]

Some composite resins polymerize after exposure to ultraviolet light. These photo initiators, such as methyl ether of benzoin, generate free radicals after ultraviolet light absorption. The tendency of composite resins to turn darker over a period of time is prevented by the addition of ultraviolet stabilizers, with the exception of those materials that utilize photo initiators for hardening.

Thus, these materials are, with reference to mechanical properties, superior to the conventional resins. Factors that are improved include (1) greater compressive and tensile strength, (2) higher modulus of elasticity, (3) superior hardness and resistance to abrasion, (4) lower polymerization shrinkage, and (5) a reduced coefficient of thermal expansion.[17]

The first composite resin commercially introduced was Addent 35. Its filler consisted of glass balls and glass rods. After the introduction of Addent 35, other brands appeared on the market. The main difference consisted of the type of filler particles. Wetting properties were improved. The convenience was enhanced in that the composites do not have to be stirred prior to use. In the past, particles precipitated over a period of time, causing the filler concentration of the bottom layers to increase. It can easily be understood that when small quantities were taken from the top without stirring the contents of the jar, the final mixture was low in particle concentration and, therefore, did not produce the optimal physical properties, while the bottom layers were saturated with particles.

The marginal adaptability of commercially available composite resins has been investigated by means of microleakage techniques and scanning electron microscopy. In addition, specimens have been subjected to thermal cycling.[12] Although the composite resins are definitely superior to the conventional filling materials, one should bear in mind that several so-called "improved" properties, such as increased hardness and abrasion resistance, have never been proven to be of clinical significance. Like many new materials, there are many inherent problems associated with composite resins. The presence of the filler, for instance, determines the surface characteristics and always produces a rough surface, regardless of the type of filler that is used. A study conducted by Johnson and coworkers[9] to investigate the effect of different finishing burs on the surface of composite resins revealed that, in the opinion of the writers, the 12-fluted bur produced the smoothest surface. Another study evaluating 15 different finishing procedures[5] concluded that the smoothest surface was obtained when the material polymerized in contact with a Mylar matrix strip. Any finishing method subsequently employed caused a deterioration of the surface smoothness, rather than improving it. According to the authors, a white stone produces the best finished surface characteristics. A special diamond disc was developed by Chandler and coworkers,[4] which, according to their findings with a scanning electron microscope, produced a smoother surface than commercially available composite finishing burs.

A first concern when using a new restorative material should be its irritative potential to the underlying pulp. As discussed previously, the release of phosphoric acid from silicate cements may cause symptoms that range from mild inflammation to pulp death. Several investigators have histologically studied the effects of composite resins on pulp tissue.[2, 8] Among other findings, it was observed that the amount of thickness of the remaining dentin was important. In these cases, the pulp inflammation caused by most of the resins appeared to be reversible. The inflammatory reaction was attributed to (1) chemical irritation from the material and (2) poor adaptation of the restorative material. The space between the material and pulpal wall allows percolation of microorganisms from the oral cavity to the pulp chamber. A significant improvement was accomplished when cavity liners were applied to the walls of the cavity preparation. Therefore, it is generally recommended that these cavity sealers be used beneath composite resins.

Another matter of concern is the reaction of the gingival tissues to the filling material. Several studies reported a favorable reaction.[3, 18] The presence of marginal gingivitis was observed by Larato[11] and was attributed to the fact that the resin was under the gingival surface. It was felt, however, that the main cause of the inflammation was the ready collection of plaque on the rough surface of the composite resins rather than the roughness of the material and retention per se. It is, therefore, advisable to place the gingival margin of a composite restoration 1 millimeter away from the gingival margin. In practice, however, this may not always be possible. Careful finishing of the restoration, blending the contour with the natural anatomy of the tooth, enables the patient to clean the restoration adequately, which will prevent the accumulation of plaque. The application of a thin layer of pit and fissure sealant to prevent microleakage[10] may be beneficial.

The principle of sealing composites is based on the following technique. After placement and contouring of the restoration, the surface of the restoration and approximately 1 to 2 mm of the surrounding enamel are prepared with the conditioner. Sixty seconds after the acid has been applied, the preparation is thoroughly washed and air dried. With a fine camel's-hair brush, a thin layer of sealant is painted over the restoration and the conditioned enamel; by means of ultraviolet light this material hardens, and a protective shell of plastic covers the tooth. For as long as this protective layer is present, microorganisms from the oral environment will not have access to the interface filling material and enamel, thus preventing microleakage. An *in vitro* study by the afore-

mentioned authors, in which bovine teeth were boiled for 24 hours after application of the sealant, revealed that no microleakage had occurred. One must bear in mind, however, that the circumstances to which these specimens were exposed, and *in vitro* experiments in general, differ totally from the *in vivo* situation. Factors such as saliva, bacteria, pH, plaque, and masticatory forces may all together or individually determine the longevity of the applied principle. An *in vivo* and *in vitro* study of this sealing principle was conducted by Kun and Pameijer.[10] After 12 months, a clinical evaluation of 57 teeth indicated that 78.4 per cent of the experimental teeth were still completely covered with the protective layer. In 21.6 per cent the sealant was either completely or partially absent. Additional *in vitro* experiments revealed that no leakage of basic fuchsin dye was observed in cross sections of the experimentally treated teeth. In other words, the material provided a perfect seal against microleakage. Scanning electron micrographs demonstrated the intimate relationships between adhesive and sealant, as well as between sealant and restorative material.

The clinical manipulation of composites is sometimes complicated by their tendency to adhere to the instruments. This may result in voids in the material or poor adaptation of the material to the cavity walls. Without any question, the use of a matrix band is recommended during insertion of the composites. A very valuable adjunct in inserting composite resins is a specially designed syringe. The instrument has proved to be ideally suited for poorly accessible areas. The fabrication of a composite core when pins are used for retention is a clear example for the use of the syringe. The tip of the nozzle can be inserted into the matrix to the floor of the cavity. Injection of the material is quick and usually guarantees a perfect adaptation. Overfilling with subsequent finger pressure thus yields a well condensed composite restoration. After removal of the matrix, the cylindrical tooth is immediately ready to be cut to a crown preparation. The composite is mixed as directed and packed in a disposable plastic nozzle. A self-lubricating rubber plug is inserted in the nozzle, and this assembly is

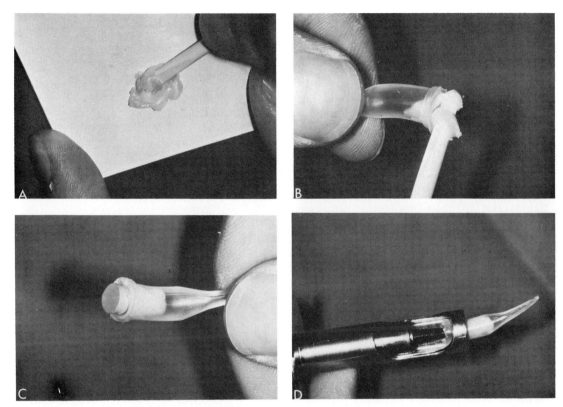

Figure 18–2 *A*, The composite restorative material is mixed as recommended in the manufacturer's instructions and subsequently packed into a plastic nozzle (*B*). *C*, A rubber self-lubricating plunger is inserted in the nozzle, and this assembly is mounted in the syringe (*D*). Practical experience has demonstrated that the opening of the nozzle should be trimmed at the end to widen its orifice, allowing for the low viscosity of some composite materials, which may cause too much tension in the nozzle. The result is that the nozzle may "pop," and the material escapes through other openings.

placed into the syringe. The plunger of the syringe will push the plug, and the material can then be ejected into the cavity (Fig. 18–2). The working time is limited but adequate. No maintenance is required, since the plastic nozzle with the rubber plug is disposable.

The instructions for handling composite resins vary considerably among manufacturers. A majority of composites consist of two pastes that are mixed in equal portions. Another brand had to be mixed on a special, catalyst-impregnanted mixing pad in order to set. Also available was a paste-liquid combination.

In general, it is recommended that composite resins be allowed to polymerize against a matrix band of Mylar. Findings in this laboratory confirm the results of Dennison and Craig[5] that the matrix band in close contact with the composite resin produces

the smoothest surface. Our studies were carried out utilizing a scanning electron microscope, which, because of its great depth of field and excellent contrast, together with the three-dimensional image, provides detailed information about surface texture. In contrast to the excellent results obtained under laboratory conditions, the clinical picture demonstrated other features. In order to study the behavior of composite resins *in vivo*, a replica technique was developed for use with scanning electron microscopy.[15]

Under the stated ideal laboratory conditions, composite resins exhibited a smooth surface where intimate contact had been present with the matrix band. Occasionally, however, surface defects in the form of voids could be observed (Fig. 18–3). The surface defects were attributed to the trapping of air during the mixing of materials. Clinically, however, the results differed considerably.

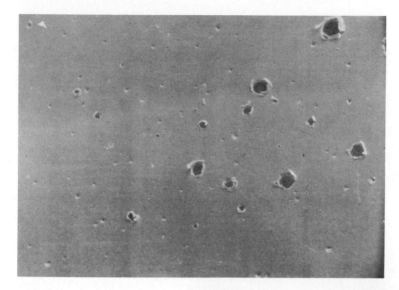

Figure 18–3 Surface texture of a composite resin cured against a matrix band under laboratory conditions. Note the smooth surface and several small and large voids (× 50).

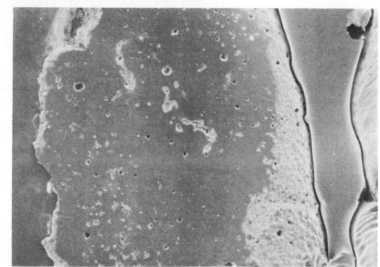

Figure 18–4 A low power micrograph (× 25) of a replica of an *in vivo* duplicated restoration (Cl. III). Note the overhang, the void at the margin and the multiple surface defects.

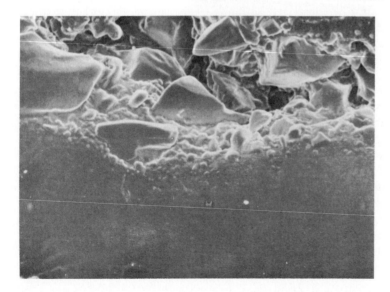

Figure 18–5 This is a high-power magnification (× 1000) of one of the surface defects shown in Figure 18–4. The filler particles are immediately below the smooth surface.

Working time, type and size of restoration, use of rubber dam, and patient cooperation were all factors that greatly influenced the ultimate success and quality of the restoration.

A clinical experiment to study marginal adaptation and surface characteristics of composite resins was conducted by Pameijer and Stallard in 1973.[16] Several commercially available composite resins were tested. The preparations were standard, and rubber dam was used. The restorative materials were inserted with a plastic instrument and allowed to cure against a Mylar matrix band. Upon removal of the matrix band it was noticed that flash was present and extended over the enamel surface. This could easily be removed with a sharp instrument. No attempt was made to correct the contour or the margins of the restoration. Prior to removing the rubber dam, the restorations were duplicated, utilizing a replica technique reported previously. By means of this technique an exact copy of the restoration was obtained, which was prepared for scanning electron microscope investigation. The results appeared to be rather uniform, and regardless of the composite restorative material used, the following could be observed: Upon clinical examination all restorations appeared to be clinically acceptable and were considered successful; the smooth, shiny appearance, which was characteristic for the *in vitro* prepared samples, was not always observed, however. On a microscopic level, pits and voids and surface irregularities were usually present and were attributed to the fact that the matrix band cannot be completely immobilized during the polymerization process (Fig. 18–4). On areas where no contact with the matrix band was accomplished, or where movement had occurred, filler particles could clearly be seen penetrating the resin matrix (Fig. 18–5).

Most disconcerting, however, was the presence of either partial or total overhanging margins, with a surface that was elevated in relation to the enamel surface. No attempt was made to correct these margins, since it was of interest to observe this situation again after periods of weeks and months. Therefore, the replicating procedure was repeated at intervals ranging from weeks to months, with no special home care instructions given to the patient. These replicas provided a series of samples that permitted analysis of the surface changes on a sequential basis. Figure 18–6 shows a series of scanning electron micrographs obtained from replicas of a freshly placed restoration to the postinsertion appearance after a period of seven weeks. As can be seen in part A of this figure, the fact that a matrix band was utilized provided no guarantee that a smooth surface would be produced. Overhanging margins and voids mar the surface of the restoration. A replica made one week after insertion demonstrated a completely different surface appearance. In the areas where a smooth surface was present immediately after operation, filler particles could now be observed penetrating the resin matrix. In other words, after one week, all superficial resin matrix had disappeared, presumably by abrasion. The results after seven weeks were essentially not different from those after one week.

It is of interest to note that after the initial disappearance of the resin matrix, the materials demonstrate a much higher resistance to abrasion. For example, in Figure 18–6B a specific filler particle was observed that could be replicated in the same detail after a period of seven weeks. Another example is presented in Figure 18–7. This time a different composite resin was utilized, and clinically the restoration demonstrated an acceptable result. Part A depicts the enamel-composite interface. It is of particular interest to note that this time, although a matrix band was utilized, no smooth surface was created whatsoever. At a higher magnification (× 150), a surface saturated with quartz filler was shown. Note the detail of enamel rods in the damaged margin of the cavity wall. Part C shows the surface after a period of seven weeks. Plaque has now accumulated at the margins (see arrow) and has filled the enamel defect of the cavity wall (part D). Only a small amount of the superficially present quartz filler was retained; the majority has been washed away by saliva.

A fractured sample of a composite material (Fig. 18–8) demonstrates the smooth,

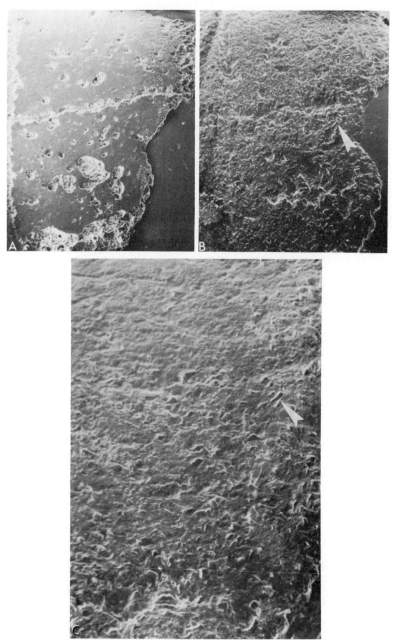

Figure 18–6 *A*, This replica of a Class V restoration demonstrates the surface characteristics of an *in vivo* placed restoration. Numerous surface defects can be seen along with smoother areas, together with overhanging margins. Note the crossed grooves that serve as reference lines between the different replicas (× 50). *B*, Appearance of the same restoration of *A* after one week. Over the entire surface, exposure of filler particles has occurred, owing to abrasion of the superficial resin matrix (× 50). *C*, After seven weeks the appearance is similar to that demonstrated after one week. The arrow shows a particular filler, among others, which also could be observed after one week. This proves that initial abrasion of the resin matrix is a rapid process, but that once the filler is exposed composite resins exhibit a high resistance to abrasion.

Figure 18–7 *A*, A replica of a composite resin immediately after placement. Although a matrix band was utilized, no smooth resin surface was obtained. *B*, A high-power view demonstrating the abundance of quartz particles at the surface. *C*, The appearance of the restoration after a period of seven weeks. Note the accumulation of plaque (see arrow), bordering the interface enamel composite resin. *D*, A high-power view of the same area of *B* after a period of seven weeks. With a few exceptions (see arrows) most superficial filler particles are washed away.

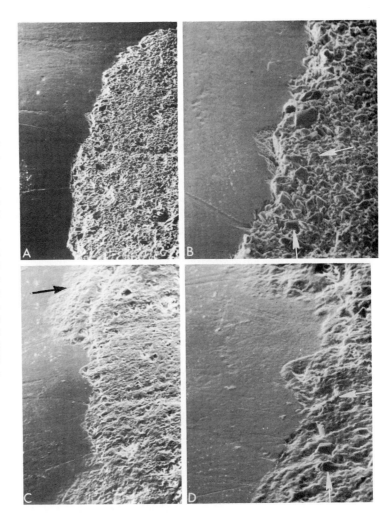

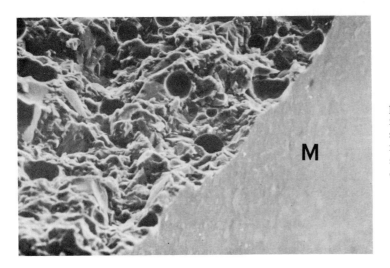

Figure 18–8 Fractured sample of Adaptic. The smooth surface of the resin matrix (M) can be seen and immediately below it numerous quartz particles and several voids, caused by trapping of air.

superficial resin material underneath which the filler can be seen. Deeper layers are composed of resin matrix surrounding the filler, and occasional voids caused by trapping of air. The pure resin of the surface layer disappears in a matter of weeks, exposing the filler, which is extremely hard and resistant to abrasion. Continuous loss of filler particles proceeds, however, owing to abrasion of the surrounding matrix or to other, as yet unknown factors.

These clinical findings confirmed the *in vitro* experiments of Eames.[6] Similar studies had been conducted by the author in which samples were prepared *in vitro* and polymerized against a matrix band. The specimens were brushed for 5, 10, and 30 minutes with an electric toothbrush. Examination with a scanning electron microscope revealed that basically no differences in surface characteristics were observable. The results of five minutes of brushing caused abrasion of the surface resin layers and protruding of filler particles (Fig. 18–9). In other words, brushing for five minutes is sufficient to abrade the superficial layer of resin, thus exposing the underlying filler. Even if clinically a smooth, shiny surface could be obtained, it would be of very short duration once the restoration is exposed to the oral environment.

It can be concluded from the foregoing that the overhanging margins are undesirable, as they create food traps (see Fig. 18–4). What, then, are the alternatives to finish these surfaces? A variety of finishing burs and stones were designed, among which were special paper discs, white stones, and superfine high-speed diamond finishing burs. The most efficient bur in finishing and contouring resins was found to be the diamond bur. However, the devastating effect on the surrounding enamel, causing grooves and scratches, should be considered highly undesirable. A similar effect, although perhaps to a lesser extent, was observed with all finishing burs. Figure 18–10 is a scanning

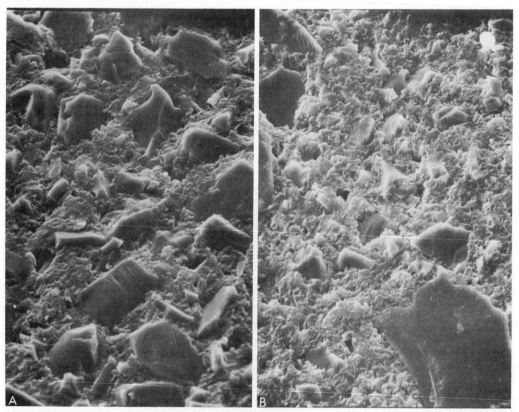

Figure 18–9 *A,* Example of a specimen of Concise, cured against a matrix band and brushed for five minutes with an electric toothbrush (× 1000). *B,* The same resin but now brushed for 30 minutes with an electric toothbrush. Essentially, no difference can be noted as the only change occurs after the resin matrix is worn out (× 1000).

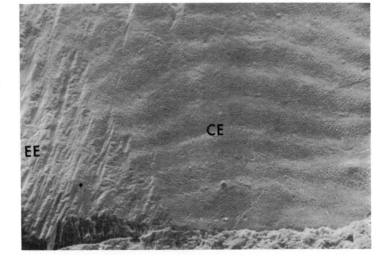

Figure 18–10 The result of the use of a superfine finishing bur on the surrounding enamel. Note the grooves and scratches on the experimental side (EE) compared to the smooth appearance of the control side (CE) (× 127).

electron micrograph of a composite resin finished with a superfine diamond bur. Note the roughening of the enamel surface (EE) compared to the other half of the tooth, which was not touched (CE).

Ironically, no improvement of surface smoothness of the composite resins was accomplished. It is, therefore, of importance to always finish the contoured restoration with pumice or polishing paste. This will polish the grooves and scratches in the enamel caused by finishing burs or discs, but is not intended to polish the composite. It is essential that these grooves be eliminated, since their retention of plaque will promote microleakage, which may subsequently cause a discoloration of the margins and finally result in failure of the restoration.

New methods have recently been introduced that by-pass the problems encountered with the rough surface of composite resins. One method utilizes the principles of pit and fissure sealants. After the restoration is contoured and finished to the operator's satisfaction, 1½ to 2 mm of surrounding enamel is conditioned with phosphoric acid. The conditioner will etch the enamel and clean the composite resin. The 50 per cent phosphoric acid is commercially termed "conditioner," since this term sounds less alarming than 50 per cent acid. After one minute the acid is thoroughly washed away and the preparation air dried. Using a fine camel's-hair brush, a thin layer of sealant is painted on the restorative material and the 1½ to 2 mm of surrounding enamel. By

means of ultraviolet light the material is polymerized, and the excess monomer is wiped off with a wet cotton roll. An esthetically superior restoration is obtained, and chances that microleakage will occur are diminished if not eliminated for as long as the sealant is present. Figure 18–11 represents a clinical case of two Class V restorations. It can be observed that the dull appearance of the surfaces has disappeared upon application of the sealant. The composite restoration on the canine shows the "highlight," which is so characteristic of wet enamel and determines esthetics of natural teeth.

It should be clear from the foregoing that the numerous advantages that accrue with the addition of filler particles become drawbacks when it comes to finishing the restorations to a smooth surface. That diamond particles could polish fillers such as glass balls or quartz appeared to be clinically impossible. Diamond can polish glass, but not the combination filler and resin, since the resin is significantly softer.

Recently, new polishing stones and pastes have been developed that are capable of polishing filler particles. It requires only minutes to smooth the particles at the surface. This can be illustrated by scanning electron micrographs made from the following samples. A representative sample was replicated by means of the hard replica technique[15] and subsequently polished for 30 seconds. At this time another replica was made, followed by a second period of 60-second polishing. A third replica was then

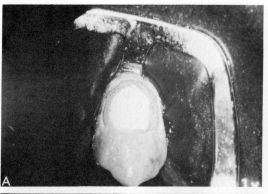
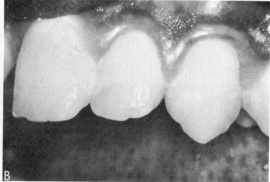
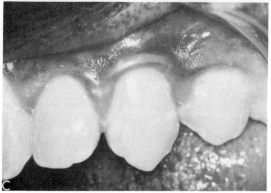

Figure 18–11 *A*, Clinical view of an extensive Class V cavity preparation with a cavity liner covering the pulpal floor. *B* depicts the completed restorations in both the lateral incisor and canine. Note the dull appearance of the composite restorations. *C*, A thin layer of adhesive sealant has been painted on the restoration and 1½ to 2 mm of surrounding enamel after previous conditioning. Protection of the integrity of the margins and improved esthetics were thus accomplished.

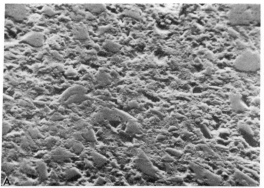
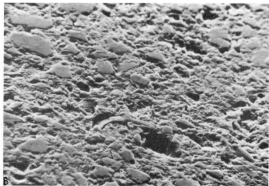
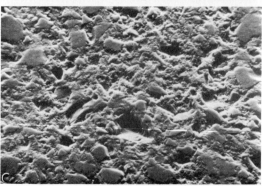

Figure 18–12 A sequence of replicas representing the effect of a composite finishing stone. *A* demonstrates the effect of polishing during 30 seconds. The filler particles appear to be definitely flattened and polished. The effect of another 30 seconds (*B*) caused the release of several fillers, and the same occurred with an additional 30 seconds (*C*) (× 220), without significantly improving the surface smoothness.

made, representing the total surface changes after 90 seconds. The original and two replicas were compared and can be seen in Figure 18–12 *A*, *B*, and *C*. The scanning electron micrographs show that only a short time is required to polish the filler particles. That particles are actually polished is demonstrated by the flat appearance. With this type of surface, essentially composed of filler, a considerable resistance against abrasion can be anticipated. Whether in the long run this surface will prove to be satisfactory depends on the rate of abrasion of the interparticle resin matrix. Wear will eventually cause the release of polished particles, thus exposing new ones which have their original sharp and pointed appearance. Over how long a period of time this will happen remains to be seen and needs further investigation.

In conclusion, it can be said that (1) from a clinical point of view, the use of a matrix strip with composite resins to produce a smooth surface is not realistic. The matrix band keeps the restorative material within the basic contours of the preparation, yet rarely produces a clinically microscopically smooth surface. (2) Routinely, overhanging margins and an elevated resin surface to the enamel level exist in what appears to be a clinically acceptable restoration. Theoretically, even if an ideal, smooth surface could be obtained with perfect marginal adaptation, utilizing a matrix strip, exposure to the oral environment would still cause the surface resin layer to wear in a short period of time, thus exposing the deeper filler particles and resulting in a rough surface. (3) Diamond finishing burs or discs do not polish composite resins, but rather are effective in contouring restorations; at the same time they cause damage to the surrounding enamel. (4) The rough enamel surface thus created retains plaque better, and promotes marginal leakage and discoloration. (5) Subsequent polishing with pumice or polishing pastes creates a smoother enamel surface, which can be maintained more easily and is less prone to plaque retention. (6) The application of a thin layer of pit and fissure sealant not only improves the esthetics but also prevents microleakage as the porte d'entree is sealed off. Thus the composite resin restoration must be considered a tremendous addition to the armamentarium of the dentist in preserving and restoring natural teeth.

NEW DEVELOPMENTS IN COMPOSITE RESINS

It was recognized by the dentists and manufacturers of composite resins that one of the inherent problems of the material was surface roughness. It is quite obvious from the preceding pages that the size and the shape of filler particles are the cause of this problem. Lately, new types of composite resin have appeared on the market that are based on a microfine filler composition. A typical composition of such a material is as follows: BIS-GMA resin, triethylene glycol dimethacrylate, bisphenol A dimethacrylate, silanated silica filler, silanated barium glass filler, polymerization initiator, polymerization accelerator, light stabilizer, polymerization inhibitor, and polymerization regulator. This new family of composites can, in contrast to the conventional material, be polished to a smooth surface, resembling the surface morphology of enamel.

Figure 18–13 *A*, *B*, and *C* represents a low power view of a microfine composite restoration 8 months post-operatively. At a higher magnification of $\times 1000$, a comparison can be made between the surface smoothness of the enamel (part *B*) and the microfine composite resin (part *C*).

The physical properties of these microfilled composite resins are somewhat different from the conventional formulas. For instance, the size of the filler is of the order of 0.04 μm, whereas conventional composite resins contain particles of a size ranging from 8 to 15 μm. Also the per cent filler by weight has been reduced from 75 per cent in conventional resins to 50 per cent in the microfilled formulas. This has a bearing on the compressive strength, which, in conventional composites, is in the neighborhood of 38,000 p.s.i. vs. 33,000 p.s.i. for the microfilled resins. On the other hand, tensile strength increased slightly for the newer formulas. A drawback in the changed formula could be the increase in thermal expansion, which in

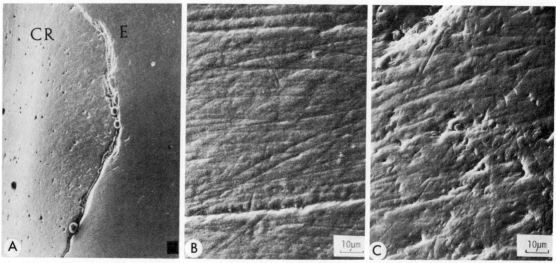

Figure 18–13 *A, B, C.* This series of micrographs was obtained from a replica of an eight-month old microfilled composite resin. The preparation is of the conventional butt joint type. The confluence of composite resin (CR) and enamel (E) is in sharp contrast to that in Figure 18–7B. At higher magnification hardly any difference in surface smoothness between enamel (*B*) and restorative material (*C*) can be observed.

some cases may be 50 per cent higher than the conventional formula. Clinical data will have to be accumulated in order to determine whether these newer formulas in the long run will be as successful as conventional composites. One conclusion that can be made at this point in time is the fact that these materials can definitely be polished to a smooth surface, thus enhancing physiologic cleaning and making it easier for the patient to maintain the restoration. From the point of view of preventive dentistry, this is a tremendous improvement.

The Use of an Intermediary Bonding Agent

A major goal in restorative dentistry is to place restorations in teeth in such a way that an effective seal between enamel and restoration is accomplished, thus eliminating the possibility of bacteria penetrating the space between enamel and restorative material, which may result in secondary decay. Brännström and Nyborg have conclusively demonstrated that bacteria are present in cavities filled with composite resin.[33] Various studies have demonstrated the usefulness of an intermediary resin of relatively low viscosity when utilized in combination with etched enamel.[21-25] The resin acts as an

effective seal and prevents penetration of isotopes when thermally stressed. The seal obtained has been demonstrated to be more effective with a modified cavity preparation. A feather edge extending into the enamel surface surrounding the margins of a restoration instead of the conventional butt joint improved the quality of the restoration.[26-29] The penetration of resin into etched enamel depends on several factors including wettability and contact angle of the resin on the etched enamel surface, viscosity of the resin, and the available time for penetration. The reader is referred to Chapter 17 for more detail with regard to the effect of acid treatment of enamel. This chapter will focus only on the combination of composite resins and an intermediary bonding agent. The use of these intermediary resins has changed the cavity preparation concept as established by Black. It saves sound hard tooth structure and takes advantage of the benefits of enamel conditioning. Modified techniques have been described by Lutz and Burkart.[30] This technique has been successfully used in Classes III, IV, and V cavities for several years. The marginal adaptation and microleakage in conventional and modified cavity preparations has been described in detail by Luescher and coworkers.[31, 32] The authors point out that the physical properties of composite materials demand that the volume of the restoration be kept minimal if marginal integrity is to be maintained. This means that for Class II restorations the treatment is limited. Their description of the design of Class II restorations is an extension of the measures of preventive dentistry. In the presence of initial proximal carious enamel lesions in children, this treatment may be indicated. In that way, healthy tooth structure is conserved, the peripheral area is restored, etched, and sealed, and an "extension for prevention" treatment is accomplished. The ideal modifications of cavities suitable for this type of treatment will have to be investigated further before a definite change can be advocated. The success of this method, however, and the serious implications of microleakage as described by Brännström and Nyborg,[33] strongly support the usefulness of this new approach in preventive restorative dentistry.

Clinical studies conducted by the author and coworkers at Boston University[34] have demonstrated the advantage of using an intermediary bonding agent in combination with a modified cavity preparation. These studies evaluated the discussed principles *in vitro* and *in vivo*. For the laboratory study, 180 teeth were prepared according to various cavity preparation concepts. The 180 teeth were subdivided into 3 major groups of 60 teeth each. Table 18–1 shows the materials from various manufacturers that were used for each particular group. The preparations were all Class III. In each of the three major subgroups I, II, and III, there were six subgroups, A through F, which had the following characteristics: Group A teeth were prepared conventionally with a moderate bevel. This group received an acid etch treatment

TABLE 18–1 MATERIALS USED IN A STUDY OF 180 TOOTH RESTORATIONS

GROUP	NUMBER OF TEETH	ETCHANT MATERIAL	BONDING AGENT	COMPOSITE RESIN
I	60	3 M°	3 M	J&J
II	60	J&J†	J&J	J&J
III	60	Caulk‡	Caulk	Caulk

°3 M Co., St. Paul, Minnesota
†Johnson & Johnson, E. Windsor, N.J.
‡Caulk, Milford, Delaware

followed by a bonding agent and composite resin. The cavity design for group B was slightly different. It was similar to group A with the exception that the bevel was long rather than short. This group also was treated by means of the acid etch technique followed by a bonding agent and composite resin. Group C received a conventional preparation without bevel in combination with the use of acid etch and a bonding agent. The teeth of Group D received a conventional preparation. The preparations were etched, but no bonding agent was utilized. The composite resin was inserted over the etched surface. In Group E, a modified preparation, that is, a preparation with no undercut, was prepared with a moderate bevel. The teeth in this group were treated with acid and received a bonding agent followed by composite resin. The specimens of Group F were somewhat similar to Group E; however, a long bevel was prepared. All teeth were exposed to thermal cycling (1000 cycles) at temperature changes of 5° C to 60° C. Following cycling, sections were made and the leakage assessed according to scores ranging from 0 to III, depending on the extent of leakage. (0 = no leakage, I = leakage restricted to enamel, II = leakage extending to dentine, III = leakage extending to the floor of the cavity.)

The results of the leakage scores for groups I to III can be seen in Tables 18–2 to 18–4. It can be concluded from these tables that the role of an intermediary bonding agent is of great significance. It prevents dye penetration and does so more effectively, depending on the amount of surrounding enamel that is available. Groups A and B clearly demonstrate that a long bevel is more effective in rendering a seal than a short one. Group B scored the highest number of 0 leakage patterns in the conventional preparation group. It should also be noted from the tables that the use of acid etch without a bonding agent and a composite resin does not prevent microleakage, as is often believed. Apparently the resin matrix is incapable of tag formation in comparison to the low viscosity resins that are used as intermediary bonding agents. Groups E and F are of particular importance. Both groups consti-

TABLE 18–2 LEAKAGE SCORES FOR GROUP 1

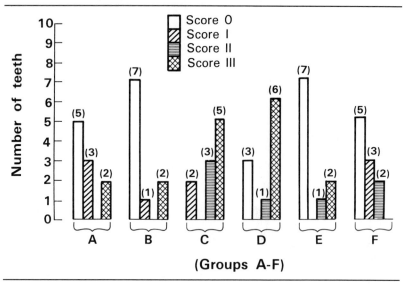

(Groups A–F)

tute experimental modified cavity preparations that require a minimum amount of enamel reduction. These cavity preparations are unsuitable for a conventional technique, since they lack undercuts for retention. Retention is solely derived from the bonding of the intermediary bonding agent, which in turn bonds to the composite resin. Groups E and F also demonstrate that when more enamel is available for adhesion, a more effective seal will be accomplished.

Comparison between the three groups also supports the evidence that bonding agents and composite resin of the same manufacturer should be used. Mixing different brands does not produce optimal properties. Compare group I with groups II and III.

The results of this study coincide with the clinical data from a similar study on a smaller scale. The same principles as applied to the *in vitro* study were carried out in patients on bicuspids requiring extraction for orthodontic reasons. Butt joint preparations were compared to the acid etch-bonding agent technique. A total of 19 adhesive restorations were compared to 20 teeth

TABLE 18–3 LEAKAGE SCORES FOR GROUP 2

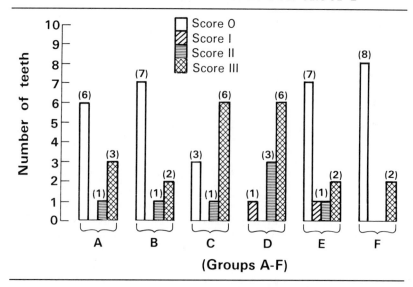

(Groups A–F)

TABLE 18–4   LEAKAGE SCORES FOR GROUP 3

that were restored according to the conventional method without a bonding agent. The teeth were extracted after periods of time and immersed in ethylene blue. Then they were sectioned and assessed for microleakage as

TABLE 18–5   LEAKAGE SCORES IN A STUDY OF 39 TOOTH RESTORATIONS

OBSERVED VALUES

Rating	Acid Etch	Butt Joint	Total
0	11	2	13
1	4	7	11
2	2	3	5
3	0	5	5
Total	19	20	39

The proportion of teeth with the acid etch bonding technique is $\frac{19}{39} = 0.48$. The proportion of teeth with butt joint restorations is $\frac{20}{39} = 0.51$. The expected values are listed below.

EXPECTED VALUES

Rating	Acid Etch	Butt Joint	Total
0	$13 \times 0.48 = 6.24$	$13 \times 0.51 = 6.63$	13
1	$11 \times 0.48 = 5.28$	$11 \times 0.51 = 5.61$	11
2	$5 \times 0.48 = 2.4$	$5 \times 0.51 = 2.55$	5
3	$5 \times 0.48 = 2.4$	$5 \times 0.51 = 2.55$	5
4	$5 \times 0.48 = 2.4$	$5 \times 0.51 = 2.55$	5
Total	18.72 / 19	19.89 / 20	

was described earlier. The observed values can be seen in Table 18–5.

Further statistical analysis leads to the calculation of the contribution to χ^2. The value for χ^2 is 12.44 with one degree of freedom (df).

Since in the row and column totals of the observed and expected values the counts are identical, some of the expected counts may be derived by subtraction from the fixed row and column totals. It may be seen that one determines the expected counts of acid etch in rating 0, 1, 2, and 3; all remaining expected counts result by subtraction. Therefore, the χ^2 calculation will entail 4 df. The difference is statistically significant at the .05 level (<0.55). In other words, the use of an intermediary bonding agent effectively seals the port of entry, thus preventing marginal percolation and penetration of microorganisms. More clinical data will have to be collected in order to make this method a standardized technique for the dental profession.

REFERENCES

1. Buonocore, M. G., and Sheykoleslam, Z.: Effect of enamel adhesives on marginal leakage. I.A.D.R. Abstracts No. 711, March, 1972.
2. Brännström, M., and Nyborg, H.: Pulpal reactions to composite resin restorations. J. Prosthet. Dent. 27:181–189, 1972.

3. Chan, K. C., Soni, N. N., and Khowassah, M. A. F.: Fissure reactions to two composite resins. J. Prosthet. Dent. 27:176–180, 1972.
4. Chandler, H. H., Bowen, R. L., and Paffenbarger, G. C.: Method for finishing composite restorative materials. J. Am. Dent. Assoc. 83:344–349, 1971.
5. Dennison, J. B., and Craig, R. G.: Physical properties and finished surface texture of composite restorative resins. J. Am. Dent. Assoc. 85:101–108, 1972.
6. Eames, W. B.: Finishing and polishing restoratives. J. Tenn. Dent. Assoc. 51:(No. 1) Jan., 1971.
7. Eames, W. B., et al.: The effect of brushing on the surfaces of filled resins. J. Alabama Dent. Assoc. 55:22–25, 1971.
8. Goto, G., and Jordan, R. E.: Pulpal response to composite resin materials. J. Prosthet. Dent. 28:601–608, 1972.
9. Johnson, L. N., Jordan, R. E., and Lynn, J. A.: Effects of various finishing devices on resin surfaces. J. Am. Dent. Assoc. 83:321–332, 1971.
10. Kun, W. B., and Pameijer, C. M.: An adhesive for sealing composite resins. J. Dent. Child., pp. 25–31, March-April, 1975.
11. Larato, D. C.: Influence of a composite resin restoration on the gingiva. J. Prosthet. Dent. 28:402–404, 1972.
12. Lee, H. L., and Swartz, M. L.: Scanning electron microscope study of composite restorative materials. J. Dent. Res. 49:149–158, 1970.
13. Bowen, R. L.: Compatibility of various materials with oral tissues. I. The components in composite restorations. J. Dent. Res. 58:1493–503, 1979.
14. Norman, R. D., Phillips, R. W., and Swartz, M. L.: Fluoride uptake by enamel from certain dental materials. J. Dent. Res. 39:11–16, 1960.
15. Pameijer, C. H., and Stallard, R. E.: Application of replica techniques for use with scanning electron microscopes in dental research. J. Dent. Res. 51:672, 1972.
16. Pameijer, C. H., and Stallard, R. E.: The fallacy of polishing composite restorations. Dent. Surv. 33–37 April, 1973.
17. Phillips, R W.: Science of Dental Materials. 7th ed., Philadelphia, W. B. Saunders Co., 1973, p. 228.
18. Trivedi, S. C., and Talim, S. T.: The response of human gingiva to restorative materials. J. Prosthet. Dent. 29:73–80, 1973.
19. Bowen, R. L.: Properties of a silica-reinforced polymer for dental restorations. J. Am. Dent. Assoc., 66:57–64, 1963.
20. Bowen, R. L., and Rodriguez, J. S.: Tensile strength and modulus of elasticity of tooth structure and several restorative materials. J. Am. Dent. Assoc., 64:378–387, 1962.
21. Dogon, I. L., and Henry, P.: Calcium 45 penetration and scanning electron microscopy — study of the acid etch system. (Abstract) J. Dent. Res. 54:19, 49, 1975.
22. Dogon, I. L.: Studies demonstrating the need for an intermediary resin of low viscosity for the acid etch technique. In Silverstone, L. M ., and Dogon, I. L. (eds.): Proceedings of the International Symposium on the Acid Etch Technique. St. Paul MN, North Central Publishing Co., 1975, pp. 110–118.
23. Eriksen, H. M., and Buonocore, M. G.: Marginal leakage with different composite restorative materials in vitro. Effect of cavity design. J. Oral Rehab. 3:315–322, 1976.
24. Hembree, J. H., Jr., and Andrews, J. T.: In situ evaluation of marginal leakage using an ultraviolet light activated resin system. J. Am. Dent. Assoc. 92:412–418, 1976.
25. Galan, J., Jr., Mondelli, J., and Coradazzi, J.: Marginal leakage of two composite restorative systems. J. Dent. Res., 55:74–76, 1976.
26. Kopel, H. M., Grenoble, D. E., and Kaplan, C.: The effect of cavo surface treatment on marginal leakage of composites. J. Cal. Dent. Assoc. 3(6):56–63, 1975.
27. Rafei, S. A., and Moore, D. L.: Marginal penetration of composite resin restorations as indicated by a tracer dye. J. Prosthet. Dent. 34:435–439, 1975.
28. Baharloo, D., and Moore, D. L.: Effect of acid etching on marginal penetration of composite resin restorations. J. Prosthet. Dent. 32:152–155, 1974.
29. Jorgensen, K. D.: The adaptation of composite and non-composite resins to acid etched enamel surfaces. In Silverstone, L. M., and Dogon, I. L. (eds.): Proceedings of the International Symposium on the Acid Etch Technique. St. Paul, MN, North Central Publishing Co., 1975, pp. 93–99.
30. Lutz, F., and Burkart, R.: Das Concise-Enamel-Bond System, eine Alternative? Schweiz. Monatsschr. Zahnheilkd. 84:1113–1129, 1974.
31. Luescher, B., et al.: Microleakage and marginal adaptation in conventional and adhesive Class II restorations. J. Prosthet. Dent. 37:300–309, 1977.
32. Luescher, B., et al.: The prevention of microleakage and achievement of optimal marginal adaptation. J. Prevent. Dent. 4:16–20, 1977.
33. Brännström, M., and Nyborg, H.: The presence of bacteria in cavities filled with silicate cement and composite resin materials. Sven. Tandlak. Tidskr. 64:149–155, 1971.
34. Ashayeri, N.: Evaluation of microleakage in vitro of conventional and modified Class III restorations with and without the use of an intermediary bonding agent. Thesis, Boston University Goldman School of Graduate Dentistry, May, 1980.

SUGGESTED ADDITIONAL READING

Ast, D., Bushel, A., and Chase, H.: A clinical study of caries prevention with zinc chloride and potassium ferrocyanide. J. Am. Dent. Assoc. 41:437–442, 1950.
Bodecker, C.: Enamel fissure eradication. N.Y. State Dent. J. 30:149–154, 1964.
Buonocore, M. G.: Caries prevention in pits and fissures sealed with an adhesive resin polymerized by ultra-violet light: A two year study of a single adhesive application. J. Am. Dent. Assoc. 82:1090–1093, 1971.
Hyatt, T. P.: Prophylactic odontotomy. Dent. Cosmos 65:234–241, 1923.
Klein, H., and Knutson, J.: Effect of ammoniacal silver nitrate on caries in first permanent molars. J. Am. Dent. Assoc. 29:1420–1426, 1942.
Walter, O., and Moreira, B.: Effectiveness of acetic acid and chromic anhydride in prevention of dental caries. J. Dent. Child. 38:70–72, 1971.

CHAPTER NINETEEN

Preventive Orthodontics

Thomas K. Barber, D.D.S., M.S.
Larry S. Luke, D.D.S., M.S.

Twenty years ago the general dentist asked, "How do you bend a labial wire for a Hawley retainer?" or "How do you use rapid cure acrylic?" We were technique-oriented, and what appeared important to the practitioner was his learning to use materials and instruments, and appliance construction.

Manual skill technique is still important, but today's graduate and today's general dentist more frequently ask questions related to what, why, and when. What is the status of this child's occlusion? What can be expected to occur if I do not treat it? Why are these teeth crowded? Why has the deciduous cuspid space closed? When can I expect to see a growth change? When is it necessary to open the bite? These and many similar questions point out the desire on the part of the busy practitioner to gain greater insight into the dynamics of growth and dental development of the child. In addition, he seeks practicality — How do I apply this knowledge to everyday use in my practice?

Equally important are the frustrations of the practitioner who feels insecure in the great desire to include minor orthodontic service in his dental practice, yet lacks confidence in his ability to discriminate between those types of problems he can treat and those with which he needs help or which he should refer to a specialist. It all depends upon his individual diagnostic skill.

Prevention of malocclusion and the success of minor or major orthodontic interven-

tion of a developing malocclusion depend almost entirely upon diagnostic skill and the ability of the dentist to recognize his capability to reverse the process of dentition maldevelopment. Thus, the objectives of this chapter are to:

1. Define the needs for participation in preventive orthodontics.

2. Provide an overview of the types of common problems encountered in mixed dentition development.

3. Present and discuss diagnostic aids, their uses, and their application by the dentist.

4. Suggest treatment needs for a sample of the most common problems.

THE SCOPE OF PREVENTABLE MALOCCLUSION

Undoubtedly, the major reason parents desire orthodontic care for their children is aesthetic — a pretty smile on a pleasant face. However, this is not the only reason. Parental concern for caries prevention and periodontal disease prevention extends beyond the aesthetics of a good occlusion to the recognition that an acceptable occlusion relates to these other disease entities. Not all minor malocclusions should or even could be treated. The dentist can be expected to discriminate between acceptable and unacceptable occlusion and advise the parent on the child's needs for treatment.

What Is Malocclusion?

Normal occlusion generally implies an acceptable relationship of the teeth in one jaw to each other and to those of the opposing jaw. Stated in another way, malocclusion is broadly of two types:

1. The relationship of the upper and lower jaws to each other is quite acceptable, but *within* the jaws the teeth are in malrelation. This is a *dental malocclusion*.

2. The teeth may or may not be in acceptable relation within each jaw, but the jaws are in malrelation. The malocclusion is thus the fault of the skeletal malrelation. This is a *skeletal malocclusion*.

The generally accepted key to occlusion and means of classification lies in the rela-

tionship to each other of the first permanent molars in occlusion. As the lower molar relates to the upper, Dr. Angle described occlusion as (1) normal, (2) Class I malocclusion, (3) distal or Class II malocclusion, and (4) mesial, or Class III malocclusion.[1]

There is an important discrimination to be noted in the above classifications that often goes unnoticed and is graphically illustrated in Figure 19–1. "Normal" means that both the jaw relations to each other and the occlusion of the teeth within these jaws are normal (or desirable). A "Class I malocclusion" means that the jaws relate to each other desirably, but the teeth within these jaws are in malrelation. Thus, a Class I malocclusion is a *dental malocclusion*. It must be recognized that molar relations to each other can be

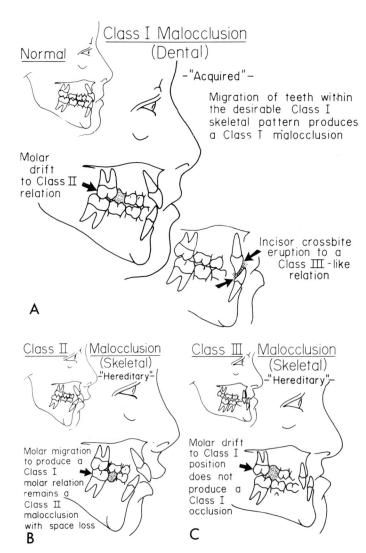

Figure 19–1 Discrimination between "dental" malocclusion of teeth alone on a normal skeletal relationship (*A*) and that of retrognathism, Class II (*B*), and prognathism, Class III (*C*), commonly termed "skeletal" malocclusion. Note that individual teeth may drift to alter the molar or incisor relation without changing the basis for the type of malocclusion.

altered locally through migration of one or both of the permanent molars. Thus, the molars could relate to each other in a Class II position but still be a Class I malocclusion skeletally.

Both Class II and Class III malocclusions are the result of jaw malrelation. They are the *skeletal malocclusions*. As in the former example, the molars in a Class II or Class III skeletal relation can migrate to a Class I molar relation, but the malocclusion still has as its basis a skeletal malrelation and classification (Figs. 19–1*B* and 19–1*C*).

Etiologic Considerations

To relate the malocclusion to its etiologic factors is a step toward reaching our objective of discrimination, that is, the development of diagnostic skill. Our knowledge and understanding of the etiology of malocclusion have a strong bearing on treatment. The point has been made that malocclusion is either the result of tooth migrations within the jaw base (dental malocclusion) or a malrelation of the jaw bases themselves (skeletal malocclusion). The latter is strongly related to jaw growth and anatomy.

Class II Malocclusion. It can be seen by referring to Figure 19–1 that the child with a true Class II malocclusion pattern gives the impression that the mandibular anatomy is one of a lengthened ramus and shortened body. At least, when compared with the maxillae and the profile, a mandible of this shape would produce a facial profile showing a retruded (retrognathic) chin. The result is the distoclusion of the molar relation and a wide variety of incisor relations, the most common being an apparent maxillary protrusion.

Class III Malocclusion. In contrast, the reverse anatomic variation is seen in the true Class III malocclusion; that is, the characteristic mandibular anatomy is one of shortened ramal height and a lengthened body. The result is mesioclusion of the molars with a protrusive chin profile (prognathic). The common incisor relation in a Class III case is one of crossbite. Quite frequently the entire maxillary dental arch is contained (crossbite) within the mandibular arch and almost gives the impression of an underdeveloped maxilla

(see Fig. 19–1*C*). Both true Class II and Class III malocclusions are related to skeletal jaw growth patterns and are regarded as having a *hereditary* etiology.

Let us emphasize once again the teeth *within* the Class II and Class III jaw relations can migrate to produce a Class I molar relation, but the occlusion remains a Class II or a Class III malocclusion. It is not a Class I malocclusion, and the practitioner must learn this discrimination (see Figs. 19–1*B* and 19–1*C*).

Class I Malocclusion. The Class I malocclusion has been labeled the "dental malocclusion," although some Class I problems such as bimaxillary protrusion and tooth size–arch length discrepancies are considered to be more hereditary than environmental in etiology. However, if the skeletal relations of maxilla to mandible and of both of these to the cranial base are normal (desirable), the teeth may still migrate to malrelationships as a result of dental developmental disturbances. The child "acquires" his malocclusion as distinguished from an inherited malocclusion (see Fig. 19–1*A*).

Dental development from birth to adulthood depends upon a finely integrated and balanced oral environment. The normal growth process must continue unencumbered by traumatic accidents or other undesirable internal or external environmental influences. The oral environment includes a muscular influence as teeth erupt. When the oral musculature is imbalanced, the teeth migrate to undesirable positions in response to the abnormal muscular pressures or lack of pressure. Actively erupting teeth exert a force upon the already erupted teeth that is sufficiently strong to alter their dental arch position, should the environment permit. Unopposed, the erupting tooth will migrate to a malposition in the arch. Once in place and in occlusion, each tooth is subject to forces of occlusion sufficient to drive teeth into positions of malrelation, should they be unopposed or out of contact or rotated.

The practitioner must be able to recognize those molar teeth that have migrated to a Class II or Class III *molar relation* in a Class I skeletal case. It is still a Class I case, and because the teeth have migrated, it becomes a "Class I malocclusion," not a Class II or III malocclusion.

In summary, excluding tooth-jaw discrepancies and bimaxillary protrusion, Class I (dental malocclusion)is a desirable jaw relation on top of which the teeth have *acquired* a malocclusion as the result of disturbances in the timing, pattern, or sequence in (1) normal growth, (2) muscular balance, (3) eruption forces, or (4) occlusion forces.

The Frequency of Malocclusion

Our attention is drawn to statistical surveys of the types of malocclusion and their frequency in the child population, since they have bearing on a program of preventive or minor orthodontic care. The non-specialist, or general practitioner, may be expected to render a significant dental service to that segment of the child population whose developing malocclusion is the result of developmental disturbances in timing, sequence, or pattern. Thus, the Class I malocclusion may be prevented or may respond favorably to early minor orthodontic guidance for correction.

The dental literature contains numerous reports of isolated surveys tabulating the variability of normal and abnormal occlusion of the child population.[2-14] The data from the older literature are difficult to compare because of the wide diversity of criteria used, the wide range of ages examined, and the irregular intermixing of data from both deciduous and permanent dentitions. The more recent data tend to identify the incidence of malocclusion based upon Angle's classification.[1]

In general, the prevalence of Class I, or dental malocclusion types, in the United States will vary between 50 and 60 per cent of the child population at almost any age. At the same time, Class II malocclusion will range from 30 to 45 per cent, while Class III malocclusions are seen from 0 to 10 per cent in the child population. Both Classes II and III arise as the result of skeletal growth patterns and are strongly based on heredity.

The Importance of Diagnosis

Treatment of the preventable or minor orthodontic problem by the general dentist depends upon his ability to distinguish between the Class I, II, and III malocclusions. He must be able to reasonably distinguish a skeletal pattern from a dental pattern of malocclusion. In addition, his diagnosis will depend upon the ability to identify the acquired pattern and to determine what, when, and how he can intervene to reverse the aberrations of normal dental development.

An experienced diagnostician can usually distinguish between skeletal and dental malocclusions in some percentage of cases by his clinical examination alone. In some additional percentage, he will call upon diagnostic aids for further information to help him make his decisions. In another percentage of cases, he will still not be certain of his diagnosis even with the use of diagnostic aids, but he will speculate. He will repeat the diagnostic tests at yearly intervals to help him determine more accurately the value of his speculations. And in some percentage of cases, he will never be sure of his diagnosis.

CLINICAL EXAMINATION OF THE PATIENT

The clinical examination of the child patient is probably the most essential element of diagnosis. Dental study casts, or models, intraoral or cephalometric radiographs, and photographs are aids to the diagnosis made clinically. Generally, these aids are used to confirm the impressions gained by the clinical examination. They add information not observed clinically by allowing a better or more complete view of the clinical material as it relates to occlusion. In any event, a systematic clinical examination of the state of occlusion should be performed so that important signs will not be overlooked. A suggested order of examination is discussed in the following paragraphs.

Examination of the Face

The facial characteristics of the child reveal information relative to his dental occlusion, and quite frequently the examiner is able to gain a solid impression of the skeletal growth pattern by this examination alone.

The dentist should examine the facial morphology carefully, and by employing a few simple procedures, he can identify quite accurately the facial type, the symmetry, and the facial proportions of vertical dimension.

Facial Type

One of our major objectives is to distinguish between Class I, II, and III skeletal patterns. Begin by examining the full face from in front. It generally holds true that a narrow face will contain narrow dental arches and a broad face, broad arches. Frequently, one is able to view a broad face that contains narrow dental arches and would lead the examiner to be suspicious of dental crowding possibly caused by muscle patterns or habits.

Frontal View. Of particular interest is the symmetry of the right and left sides of the face. Are they equal in size? Do they display similar contours? If not, explore the possibilities. Perhaps there has been unequal growth, traumatic accident, or other factors, all of which may be reflected in the shape or size of the dental arches. Examine the midline of the face and its relation to the incisor dental midline.

Figure 19–2 illustrates how the examiner may take any straight-sided card or paper and, standing directly in front of the patient, hold the edge of the card in front of the face so that it coincides with the center of the bridge of the nose and filtrum of the upper lip. Now ask the patient to close on the back teeth. Part the lips and note whether the edge of the card coincides with the interproximal line between the upper incisors. Let us suppose it does not. Ask the patient to relax, that is, to part the teeth slightly, and note the relation of the card to the lower incisor midline. If it coincides with the card, the upper dental arch is not symmetrical with the face. If the upper dental arch has been found to be correct and the lower midline coincides with it, both are correct. If the upper dental arch is correct, but the lower one does not coincide with it, the lower dental arch is not symmetrical. Be sure to note all relations exactly, because all manner of variations are possible; that is, both dental arches may deviate to the same side, or the

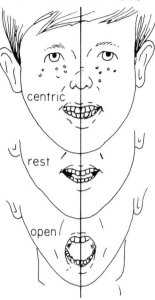

Figure 19–2 Identification of the facial midline and examination of right and left facial symmetry. Note the relation of upper and lower dental midline in centric, rest and wide open positions.

upper and lower ones may deviate to opposite sides. The information has considerable value when related to the dental examination and the need for minor corrective orthodontics.

Other factors of facial symmetry that should be looked for in the frontal view include the parallelism of the eyes, the ears and the dental occlusal plane. Figure 19–3A illustrates the transporionic, transorbital, and occlusal plane axes. Examine to determine if the ears and eyes are level with one another. Use the midplane of the face for reference and determine if the horizontal plane of the iris of the eye is at right angles to the mid-facial plane. Ask the child to place one of his fingers in each ear and examine to determine if the external auditory canals are similarly horizontal and perpendicular to the midplane of the face (transporionic axis).

One can expect symmetry of the face to display symmetry in the dental arches. Conversely, asymmetry of the face may display asymmetry in the dental arches. Next, examine the horizontal relation of the occlusal plane. Ask the child to bite on a straight edge such as a heavy card or small ruler in such a

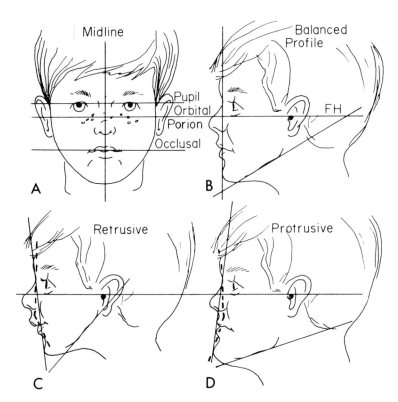

Midline — Pupil / Orbital / Porion / Occlusal — A — Balanced Profile — FH — B — Retrusive — C — Protrusive — D

Figure 19–3 Parallelism of the transverse pupillar, orbital, porionic, and occlusal plane axes with each other and their perpendicular relation to facial midline (*A*). Lateral profile view in *B* shows orthognathic or balanced features of Class I, while *C* illustrates the steep mandible, convex and retrognathic face of the Class II, and *D* the concave and prognathic face of the Class III skeletal patterns.

way as to allow for observation of the horizontal parallelism of the occlusal plane in relation to the eyes and ears and vertical to the mid-facial plane. Do they all coincide? Are they in symmetrical relation to each other? Let us, as an example, find that they do not. The possible reasons cannot be explored fully, but these side-by-side asymmetries relate to maxillary and mandibular growth and development and very frequently display relations to dental findings.

The Lateral Profile. With the patient sitting upright in the chair, examine the lateral profile by visualizing two planes: the Frankfort horizontal plane and the facial plane. The lateral profiles in Figure 19–3 illustrate these. The Frankfort horizontal plane extends horizontally from the upper border of the external ear canal forward to the palpated lower border of the bony orbit. The facial plane is visualized vertically as a plane from the bridge of the nose to the chin.

Does the patient show a balanced (Class I) pattern as in Figure 19–3*B*, where the facial and Frankfort planes form nearly a right angle? Or does the profile appear retrog-

nathic as in Figure 19–3*C*, where the maxillae look protrusive and the mandible retrusive with a receding chin (Class II)? The reverse may be seen as in Figure 9–3*D* with the maxillae straight or retrusive and the mandible protrusive (Class III). It is often helpful to hold a right-angle card, such as the patient's record folder, next to the face to aid in this visualization.

Note that in Figures 19–3*B*, *C*, and *D* the profile examination includes an assessment of the facial convexity. Note the relation of the angulation formed from the bridge of the nose to the upper lip and from the lip to the chin. A straight line or plane is part of the balanced Class I skeletal pattern (see Fig. 19–3*B*), while the Class II pattern (see Fig. 19–3*C*) displays convexity, and the Class III pattern (see Fig. 19–3*D*) is concave or shows an excessively long face.

Vertical Dimension. The lateral profile examination should also include an assessment of the angulation of the lower border of the mandible. Using a straight edge, such as a card, placed along the lower border of the mandible, examine this mandibular plane in relation to the Frankfort horizontal (ear-eye) plane. A steep (excessively angled) mandibular plane, as seen in Figure 19–3C, usually relates to the downward and less forward-growing mandible of the Class II patient.

The lower anterior face height can also be visualized by relating the vertical distance from the base of the nose to the base of the chin (lower face height) as a proportion of the distance from the bridge of the nose to the base of the chin (total face height). The lower face height should be about 55 per cent of the total face height.

A steep mandibular plane and a long lower face in a patient may signal a potential open bite with a poor prognosis for treatment. In such patients, correction of Class II skeletal problems and crowded dentition is also more difficult. On the other hand, a flat mandibular plane and a short lower face height in a patient may indicate a potential deep bite, which also has a poor prognosis for treatment.

Clinical data of this type can usually be correlated quite well with cephalometric data obtained from careful measurement of oriented lateral radiographs, which will be discussed later. However, the clinician is frequently able to identify the skeletal pattern of Class I, II, or III on the basis of the clinical examination alone.

Functional Examination

The purpose of this phase of the examination is to determine the symmetrical function of right and left temporomandibular joints (TMJ) and their functional relation to the dental occlusion. Stand in front of the patient and lightly palpate each TMJ. While doing this, have the patient open his mouth wide and slowly close to centric occlusion as seen in Figure 19–2. You should palpate a bilaterally symmetrical initial hinge action on opening to rest position, followed by a forward glide of the mandibular condyle. Carefully observe the behavior of the upper and lower dental midlines during this functional test. They should continue to coincide from occlusion to a wide-open position and return to a symmetrical pattern.

Occasionally, a child demonstrates asymmetry of mandibular function either upon opening or upon closing his mouth. In Figure 19–4A, the child deviates his mandi-

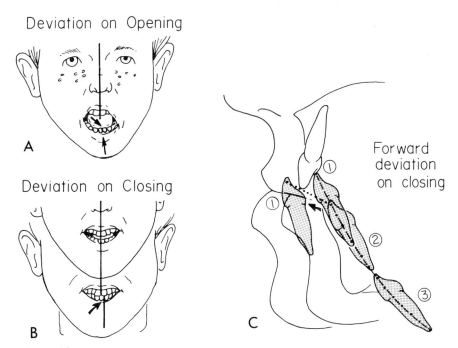

Figure 19–4 Alterations in occlusion pattern during function as in *A* where the mandible skews to the left upon opening and *B* where the skewing occurs upon closure. In *C* the pattern is one where the child closes in a forward pattern. In each, the dental pattern may affect function.

ble to the left upon opening. This may occur as the result of asymmetrical mandibular growth with related dental findings. In Figure 19–4B the child shows a deviation of mandibular closure from rest position to centric occlusion. This is a fairly common occurrence and most frequently relates to dental findings wherein the dental occlusion shows a deviate midline and a unilateral crossbite. It can be speculated that at some early time during dental development the young child experienced a dental cuspal interference and developed a "convenience" bite, closing his mandible to one side. Clinically, the picture is one of crossbite, whereas in reality the fault is not dental; it is a functional deviation of the mandible. Dental treatment usually consists of maxillary expansion to allow the mandible to close into centric occlusion.

Another example of functional crossbite is seen in Figure 19–4C. In this example, the child appears to show a Class III pattern in centric occlusion. Dentally, he may exhibit a crossbite of the total maxillary-mandibular occlusion. As in the previous example, his pattern of mandibular closure might be quite smooth from a wide-open position to rest position; but from there to full occlusion, he can be seen to thrust the mandible forward to produce an anterior crossbite. The TMJ may be palpated to exhibit a forward thrust of the mandible. Here, too, the child may be demonstrating a forward "convenience" bite, and, while resembling a Class III occlusion pattern, it may not be one at all. As in the

laterally displaced mandible, dental treatment of the forward displaced mandible usually consists of maxillary expansion to accommodate the mandible in occlusion.

Facial (Soft Tissue)
Physiology

The clinical examination of the face includes an assessment of muscle tone, particularly of the lips and tongue, and of the patient's facial habits, breathing, swallowing, and speech. Since each constitutes a part of the muscular environment of the teeth and dental arches, several points should be noted during the initial examination to distinguish between an acceptable pattern and one which may affect the dental occlusion.

Lips. The level of the lip line, lip size, tonus, and any evidence of abnormal function should be noted.

Figure 19–5 illustrates the usual anatomic variations observed in lip level. It may vary from the edge of the upper incisor teeth (Fig. 19–5A) to a level well up on the labial surface of the alveolar process above the incisors (Fig. 19–5C). The average lip level is about one third up from the maxillary incisal edge (Fig. 19–5A). A shortened upper lip, as seen in Figure 19–5D), will often require the patient to close the lips with difficulty. Frequently, such patients have an "open-mouth" habit and are mouth breathers. The occlusion may demonstrate protrusive incisors with spacing caused by the migration of

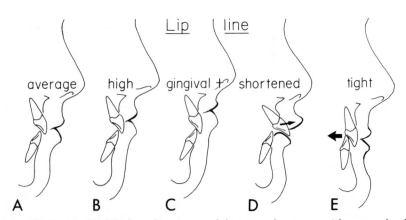

Figure 19–5   The level of the lipline, lip size, and functional tone provide muscular force to retain tooth position. In *D*, the incisors are protrusive because of muscular imbalance typical of thumb and tongue habits. *E* illustrates the upright incisor position attending excessive labial pressures.

the teeth unopposed by a normal lip musculature.

Lip *tonus* relates to tension and is usually described as flaccid (loose), rigid, or average. Through experience, the dentist may develop an impression of tonus by gently pinching the lip with thumb and forefinger and gently pulling the lip forward. If there is a definite feeling of a loose and rather fatty lip with little tone, the incisors will often protrude, evincing deficient muscle tone (Fig. 19–5D). Others will show crowded and lingually positioned lower incisors with hyperactive lips (Fig. 19–5E).

In a relaxed oral posture (in the rest position), a child may have his lips apart (open-mouth habit), thus producing a lack of *lip seal*. In such cases the lips are usually flaccid and produce no external pressure forces on the upper anterior teeth. The upper anterior teeth may then tend to protrude as a result of the lack of lip pressure. Occasionally, a child may develop habits of chronic breathing through the mouth. The gingivae may then become dried and inflamed because of constant exposure to air.

A lack of lip seal may also occur in severe Class II malocclusions and in digit suckers where the lower lip fits beneath the maxillary incisors at rest. During swallowing, the lower lip produces an anterior oral seal by closing with the tongue, the lingual side of the maxillary incisors or the palate instead of the upper lip. This may accentuate the protrusion of maxillary incisors.

Another cause for lack of lip seal can be a disproportionately long lower face height relative to lip length. As a result, the lips are unable to touch without tension in the muscles and thus they are habitually parted. As patients mature from 9 to 12 years of age, the lips tend to lengthen and patients are more conscious of their appearance. Thus, a lack of lip seal becomes less frequent.

The mentalis habit is that of chronic puckering of the chin muscle (golf-ball chin). It is quite strong and capable of producing a severely crushed and crowded lower dental arch. Usually, the habit is formed by forcing the lower lip to reach for a shortened upper lip because of a lack of lip seal. Such an abnormal and constant pressure may collapse the lower anterior teeth lingually and prevent full eruption of the upper anteriors. The dental effects are profound, and a suggested treatment consists of applying a "lip bumper" to reduce the labial pressures on the teeth (see Figure 19–21).

Tongue. Little is known of the physiologic-neuromuscular synergism between the lips and tongue, although a great deal of clinical importance is attached to their muscular balance and related tooth position. Examination of the face should include an examination of the tongue, since dental findings often reflect tongue pressures and their influence on tooth position.

The absolute *size* of the tongue is not as important as its size relative to the oral cavity. While true macroglossia is rare, relative macroglossia is not infrequently encountered in children, especially those with Down's syndrome. An overly large tongue will almost invariably be accompanied by spacing of the teeth. This may be seen in both arches or only in the lower one. If spacing of the teeth occurs in the lower arch alone, it may indicate that the tongue habitually lies low in the floor of the mouth. If both upper and lower teeth, and particularly the anterior ones, are spaced, it indicates a tongue that completely fills the mouth.

The so-called physiologic spacing that occurs in many children coincident with or just prior to the eruption of the permanent successors can usually be distinguished quite easily from the spacing caused by an oversized tongue. In the former, the arch will be typical in form and only the anterior teeth will exhibit the spacing, whereas in the latter the arch will be rounded out in the buccal areas and the buccal teeth will also show spacing.

The tongue may also function in such a way as to alter the position of the teeth. One of the most frequently encountered tongue habits is that in which the tip of the tongue is habitually held between the roof of the mouth and edges of the lower incisor teeth. The incisor teeth will be prevented from fully erupting, and a significant space will be noted with the teeth in occlusion (Figs. 19–6A and 19–6B). This tongue position results in a perfectly even mandibular incisal

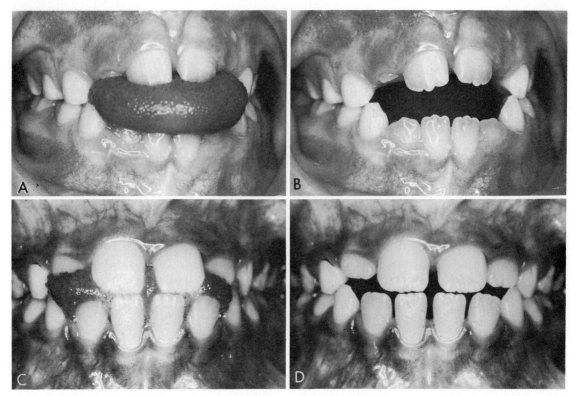

Figure 19–6 Dental effects of abnormal tongue habits. *A* and *B* illustrate tongue "resting," while *C* and *D* show incisor protrusion from tongue "thrusting" associated with the visceral swallowing pattern of the young child.

line but one which is below the occlusal plane of the other lower teeth. The upper arch may show no deviation from the normal, or the upper incisors may also be prevented from erupting or be protrusive.

Occasionally, a child will be seen in whom both upper and lower incisors have been pushed forward either by an excessively large tongue or by a habit of thrusting the tongue against these teeth while swallowing (Figs. 19–6C and 19–6D). These conditions can usually be differentiated by noting the form of the dental arch. The large tongue is usually found in an arch that is wide as well as spaced; the thrusting habit is frequently associated with an abnormally narrowed arch.

Tongue thrusting during swallowing is considered normal in the infant, and he may not change to an adult swallow pattern until puberty. This may be related to the fact that the tongue matures earlier than the rest of the oral space and thus is relatively large until puberty. Also, lymphoid tissues, such as large tonsils, may cause a forward posi-

tioning of the tongue to allow an adequate airway. Thus, treatment of tongue thrust is usually delayed until puberty, and then, if it persists, myofunctional therapy in conjunction with orthodontic therapy may be indicated.

Speech. The only speech deviation that has ever been shown to be caused by disarrangement of the anterior teeth is lisping. Lisping results from the inability of the patient to bring the front teeth together when pronouncing *S*, *Sh*, or related sounds. Spaces between the teeth of the two arches permit air leakage and cause the lisp. Parents frequently ask the dentist for his opinion regarding the speech of their children, particularly those under the age of six. Spacing of teeth that produces a minor effect on speech patterns is common but not abnormal. Part of a thorough clinical examination should relate aural observations with dental patterns to identify the presence or absence of a relationship. Usually no dental treatment is necessary.

Airway Obstruction. The role of airway obstruction in the causation of malocclusion is still controversial although there are studies that suggest a definite relationship.[16, 17] The nose should be examined for deviated septum, large turbinates, polyps, or allergic rhinitis. The walls of the pharynx should be observed for enlarged adenoids or tonsils. A history of mouthbreathing, especially at night, or frequent allergies or middle ear infections should alert the dentist to examine for airway obstruction as a cause for a developing malocclusion.

INTRAORAL EXAMINATION OF OCCLUSION AND DENTAL DEVELOPMENT

The clinical examination of the child to determine the relationships of the teeth to each other within each arch and to the arches together should be systematized so as to minimize the chance of overlooking any one factor of importance. Many details are observed more thoroughly through study of a set of dental casts, or models. This technique will be discussed separately.

First, count the teeth in each arch. This seems like an unnecessary step, especially to a trained examiner. Yet it is remarkable how frequently supernumerary teeth will occupy space in an arch, often adversely affecting the positions of adjacent teeth and the occlusion, and go unnoticed. Most often the supernumerary tooth should be removed. Teeth that are absent, either for congenital reasons or because they were lost through normal exfoliation or through extraction, will also adversely affect the spacing of the dental arch. Usually, space loss and crowding result. Frequently, the need to open or regain lost space is identified through the simple process of counting the teeth.

Secondly, examine each arch, upper and lower, to identify the deciduous and permanent components. Try to establish the dental age of the child as compared with his chronologic age. Occasionally, the dental age will be advanced; that is, permanent teeth are erupting earlier than normally expected. Occasionally, some crowding will be present. What is the relation of tooth size to the growth status? Large teeth in small jaws lead to crowding, while smaller, even peg-shaped,

teeth will result in generalized interdental spacing. Do the arches look symmetrical in shape from right to left side? Do they appear collapsed, too narrow, too wide? Do they appear to correspond to the wide or narrow face?

An important part of this preliminary observation of the arches is to examine the mid-palatine suture or median raphe of the palate. It should coincide with the middle of the face. The later examination of the dental study casts uses this raphe as a plane of reference. Any skewing of the raphe to one side should be noted for future reference.

The Arches and Teeth in Occlusion

Each arch is examined independently. The state of oral hygiene, periodontal condition, and the presence or absence of dental caries should be noted. The presence of rotated, displaced, or tipped teeth is noted in each quadrant. With the teeth in occlusion, the occlusion is observed in the three planes of space.

Transverse Plane. Figure 19–7 illustrates the *buccolingual* relation of teeth. Ordinarily, the upper teeth overhang the lower throughout the entire extent of the arch from molar to molar. The upper incisors pass in front of the lowers, and the buccal cusps of the upper posterior teeth overhang the buccal cusps of the lower. The lingual cusps of the upper posterior teeth thus drop into the fossae between the buccal and lingual rows of lower cusps.

Crossbite is the term given to any departure from the normal buccolingual relation of the upper to the lower teeth. In the buccal segment, one or more teeth of the upper arch may be so positioned that the buccal cusp of the upper is caught between the buccal and lingual cusps of the lower teeth (molar or bicuspid crossbite, Fig. 19–7A). The crossbite may be so marked that the upper molars are completely buccal to the lower, as in Figure 19–7B (or lowers in complete lingual relation to the uppers, as in Figure 19–7C).

Most frequently, the crossbite is the manifestation of an ectopic or deviate eruption pattern and is easily correctable by the general dentist. On some occasions, the

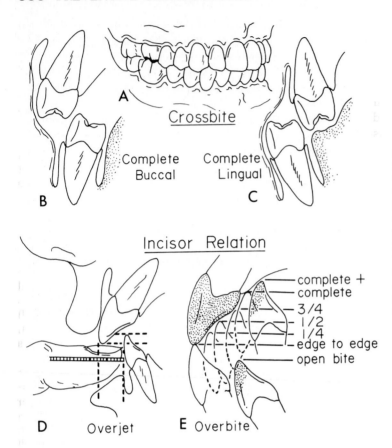

Figure 19-7 A crossbite is evidenced when opposing teeth meet so that the buccal cusp of the upper tooth occludes with the central fossa of the lower as in *A*. In *B* and *C*, the crossbite is either completely buccal or completely lingual when the teeth fail to occlude centrally. *D* illustrates incisor overjet measurement using a millimeter scale, and *E* provides a means of defining the amount of overbite or closed bite.

crossbite is produced by a deviation of the mandible during function (see previous section). Suggestions for treatment follow in a later section.

In the anterior segments, the transverse plane is recorded by observing the relationship of the maxillary and mandibular midlines. Discrepancies may be the result of functional shifts of the mandible to accommodate occlusal interferences (see previous section), or they may be the result of shifts of the mandibular or maxillary teeth. This may occur because of premature loss of primary cuspids, supernumeraries, crowding, or other causes.

Lateral Plane. The occlusion in the lateral plane is observed by noting the molar, bicuspid, and cuspid relations and the incisor overjet.

The child should be instructed to close his back teeth together and hold them tight. Occasionally, the young child will close on the incisors, and no attempt by the dentist to move his mandible back is successful. The

operator may find it difficult to gain the child's understanding and cooperation.

Place a small piece of paper on the lower molar on each side, asking the child to bite on the paper. He will usually accomplish centric occlusion with the aid of the tactile sensation provided by the presence of the paper. Retract the corners of the mouth and examine the molar relation directly from a side view. At the same time, examine the relation of the deciduous second molars and the deciduous cuspid teeth.

Figure 19-1 illustrates three of the four anteroposterior molar relationships. In the small diagram labelled "normal," the tip of the mesiobuccal cusp of the upper molar and the buccal groove of the lower molar coincide. The examination of the second primary molars is the same as for the permanent molars. A Class I relation finds the mesiobuccal cusp of the upper molar falling into the buccal groove of the lower molar. In a Class II relation the distobuccal cusp of the upper first permanent molar (or second primary molar) drops into the buccal groove of the corresponding lower molar. In Class III, the mesiobuccal cusp of the upper may occlude anywhere from the distobuccal groove of its normal antagonist back to complete lack of contact with it. The fourth possibility is termed "cusp to cusp" or "edge to edge" (not illustrated). The cusp-to-cusp relation is halfway between Class I and Class II; that is, the tips of the mesial buccal cusp of the upper molar coincide with the mesial buccal cusp of the lower molar. Remember, the molar relationship can be "true" or "false" owing to migration. As an example, the molar relation could be Class I in a Class II skeletal pattern because of space loss in the mandibular arch and forward migration of the lower molar into a Class I position.

Bicuspids and cuspids in the maxilla are one-half cusp distal to their antagonists when in Class I occlusion.

Overjet relates to the distance by which the upper teeth fail to contact the lowers in a horizontal or posteroanterior direction (Fig. 19–7D). To measure the overjet, insert a millimeter rule scale horizontally at the incisal edge of the anterior tooth. The overjet can be measured more accurately from study models, but satisfactory approximations can be made directly on the patient. Overjet will frequently be excessive when the child exhibits an oral habit, such as finger sucking.

Vertical Plane. The overbite or open bite of the incisors and posterior segments indicate the vertical component of the occlusion. Overbites are measured as illustrated in Figure 19–7E.

Anterior overbite relates to the distance by which the upper incisors overhang the lower, vertically or in a superoinferior direction. It may range from a condition of no contact (open bite) to one in which the upper teeth completely obscure the lower when the jaws are together. To arrive at a judgment of the overbite of the anterior teeth while in occlusion, mark the position of the incisal edge of the upper right central incisor on the lower central with a pencil. Note the degree of overbite in estimated fractions of the amount of the lower incisor crown that was covered, as follows: open bite, edge to edge: 1/4; 1/2; 3/4; complete; complete +. If the

incisal edge of the upper closes to a position below the gingival margin of the lower, this is considered complete ++. The open bite that exists during the early stages of incisor eruption persists as a consequence of several oral habits and muscle imbalances. The closed bite is seen after eruption is complete and is normal during the early stages of growth and dental development. The closed bite of the young child is reduced through mandibular growth. It persists as a treatable phenomenon, usually because of supra eruption of the incisors and as a consequence of arch collapse. Treatment suggestions follow in a later section.

In summary, the objectives of the clinical examination are to:

1. Attempt to identify the skeletal pattern from the observation of the frontal and lateral profile of the face.

2. Identify the occlusion and its relation to the clinical assessment of the facial variants.

3. Develop a preliminary appraisal of the need for minor orthodontic correction and the feasibility of its treatment by the dentist.

RADIOGRAPHIC CEPHALOMETRY

Growth and development of children are difficult to predict. Physical growth of young children is usually a continuous process, but between children there exists manifold variation in patterns and rates of growth.

The dentist must appreciate the changes that occur during jaw growth and the changes that occur during dental development. The ultimate occlusion of the grown child is the result of these two factors, and since each has an effect on the other, their influence is difficult to separate.

Radiographic cephalometry provides an additional tool whereby we may continuously appraise the growing jaws in several ways.

Cross-sectional cephalometry is the comparison of the data obtained from a child's head film with like data obtained from a population of children at the same age. Stated another way, how does this child's skeletal pattern differ from that of other children, particularly those who exhibit a normal, desirable jaw growth and relationship? *Longitudinal* or *serial* cephalometry allows the comparison of a given child's skeletal pattern from one year to the next. Stated another way, how is he growing when you compare his data from year to year? Cephalometry provides a means for evaluating the pattern of jaw growth, the roles and direction of jaw growth, and some related facets of dental development. Superimposed tracings of radiographic head films permit an analysis of the changes occurring in jaw relation and give evidence of accompanying dentitional change.

Cephalometric Technique

There are a variety of cephalometric "analyses" utilized to appraise skeletal and dental growth patterns from a lateral head film. Each employs measurement of planes and angles determined from anatomic landmarks of the skull and facial structures. The reader will find a fairly comprehensive presentation of cephalometric technique in Graber's text of orthodontics[17] and is referred to individual reports and studies[18-42] for more detailed information.

In general, desirable skeletal patterns fall within a range of acceptable "norm values." These are regarded as Class I skeletal patterns. Class II and Class III skeletal malocclusions demonstrate various deviations in growth pattern from the normal, desirable range. Thus, the skeletal analysis provides a means to appraise the facial type and the anteroposterior relationships of the denture base. Examination of the opposing incisor teeth in relation to each other and to their individual bony bases provides information on tooth position and its relation to dental arch space availability.

Skeletal Pattern

In general, "norm standard values" for cephalometric data are available for a young adult age range,[19, 27, 29, 47] but there are limited data for the younger childhood ages.[18, 20, 22, 23, 26, 31, 32, 34]

Lateral Plane. There are many angles and measurements for relating the maxilla and mandible to the cranial base and to each other. Probably the most frequently used are the Sella-Nasion-A point (SNA), the Sella-Nasion-B point (SNB), and the A point-Nasion-B point (ANB) angles.

Figure 19–8 depicts a generalized gross differentiation between the skeletal profiles of Class I, II, and III types. In Figure 19–8A the normal pattern of skeletal jaw growth illustrates that the slightly convex face of the young child grows to become a straight profile. The mandible grows downward and forward faster than the maxillae, bringing the profile of the young child to the balanced profile of the adult. This is seen as the angles SNA (maxillae) and SNB (mandible) increase with time, and the mandibular SNB often increases more than the maxillary SNA. The chin follows a downward and forward pattern depicted by the "Y" axis within acceptable range (59°). In the Class I pattern, the face "swings out from under" the cranium. The steep mandibular plane and occlusal plane flatten or become less acute. The face develops at a right angle to the Frankfort plane, and facial convexity is reduced.

In Figure 19–8B, the growth pattern is that of a Class II. The original profile shows factors wherein the mandible is retrognathic and the maxilla is protrusive. The growth vector of the mandible continues more downward than forward. The "Y" axis angle (64°) is less acute than the Class I case in Figure 19–8A. The facial profile becomes more convex, and the angulation of the mandibular and occlusal planes becomes more steeply angled.

Figure 19–8C represents a converse picture for the typical Class III growth pattern. The straighter or concave face of the young child becomes more concave with growth. In this case, the mandible grows more forward than downward. The chin point and "Y" axis are generally more acute than the Class I profile; the mandibular and occlusal planes are flattened.

Limited cephalometric values for the young child[18, 22, 26, 31] make early skeletal comparisons difficult. However, the age range from three to seven years will generally appear to have some Class II skeletal characteristics when compared with cephalometric data of the young adult. The child grows to

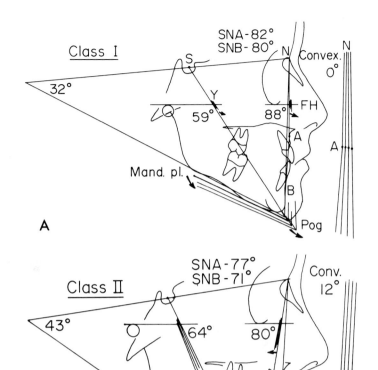

Class I

SNA-82°
SNB-80°

Convex.
0°

32°

59°

88°

FH

Mand. pl.

Pog

A

Figure 19–8 The fundamental differences between Class I (*A*), Class II (*B*), and Class III (*C*) skeletal patterns as viewed via cephalometric tracings. In *A*, the Class I pattern shows a straight profile, which grows to reduce the slight convexity. In *B*, the Class II pattern increases convexity during growth, while in *C*, the Class III pattern is one of increasing concavity and prognathism.

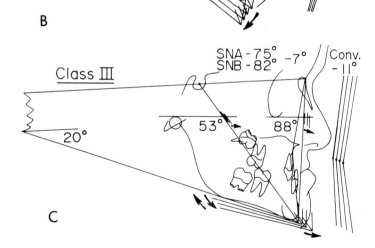

Class II

SNA-77°
SNB-71°

Conv.
12°

43°

64°

80°

B

Class III

SNA-75°
SNB-82°

-7°

Conv.
-11°

20°

53°

88°

C

become the young adult. Thus, only the marked Class II and III patterns are identified with some ease at the younger ages. The Class I skeletal pattern of the young child has some Class II–like elements. The skeletal pattern becomes more clearly identified through longitudinal study, that is, as films of the child are compared with earlier data. The skeletal change from one year to the next (serial study) begins to show that he is "becoming a Class I" or that he is growing like a Class II (more downward than forward) or like a Class III (markedly more forward than downward, beyond the range of Class I).

Vertical Plane. Measurements that provide information relative to the vertical growth include the Frankfort-mandibular plane angle, the maxillary-mandibular plane angle, and the lower facial height (proportion of lower face height [maxillary plane to menton] to the total face height [nasion to menton] approximately 55 per cent).

Patients with steep mandibular plane angles and long lower face heights have a tendency toward vertical growth with open bite tendencies. They frequently have crowding of the dentition that is unstable when treated by extractions, but especially when treated by arch expansion.

Patients with flat mandibular plane angles and short lower face heights have a tendency toward round or square faces with deep bite tendencies. Crowding in these patients when treated by extraction or expansion seems to have more stable results, although correction of the deep bite is frequently very difficult and time consuming.

Patients who are outside normal vertical values are usually best treated by specialists or dentists with experience in handling their special problems.

Transverse Plane. Posterior-anterior radiographs to visualize the transverse plane have not been heavily utilized. Landmarks are difficult to visualize and their importance in treatment planning has yet to be confirmed. These films are very useful to check for airway obstruction in the nose caused by a deviated septum, large turbinates, or a narrow nasal passage.

Soft Tissue Pattern

The soft tissues may be visualized on the lateral radiograph. Various measures that have been suggested include the Holdaway Line, the esthetic plane, the upper lip length, and the lip embrasure to the occlusal plane. The size of the adenoids and sometimes the tonsils may also be noted.

Dental Pattern

The cephalometric analysis of dental pattern refers mainly to the incisors. Figure 19–9 illustrates a common method of appraising incisor relations and represents the combination of the work of Steiner[41, 42] and Downs.[27, 28] The standard norm values represent average values of desirable relations at maturity for the young adult and bear little

relation to the unknown values for the deciduous teeth of the child. In Figure 19–9*A*, the incisors are in balance with good overjet and overbite; the lower incisor stands relatively upright on the mandibular base, as represented by the mandibular plane angle.

Graber[17] points out that it is unwise to attach too much significance to any one criterion, such as the axial inclination of the lower incisor, since a wide range of acceptable inclinations have been reported. However, in the individual case, the incisor angulations present give useful information when some form of desirable treatment is contemplated. For example, in Figure 19–9*B* the upper incisors are found to be quite protrusive, and the lower incisors are inclined lingually in the thumbsucking child. In Figure 19–9*C*, the incisors are upright and inclined lingually in an overbite (closed bite) example. With the knowledge of where these teeth would more desirably be positioned in a normal relation, the dentist is often able to determine how far he may adjust these labiolingual relations and still remain within normal limits. Frequently, the analysis of incisor position provides considerable data in determining the adequacy or inadequacy of available arch space and its regulation.

Another measure of incisor position that is used extensively is the lower incisor to the A point-Pogonion plane. This indicates the position of the incisor between the jaws, which seems to be useful in predicting the stability of treating crowding by anterior expansion. Positioning the incisor more than 3 mm anterior to the A-Po line is unlikely to be stable, even with long retention.

In summary, the use of cephalometric data to determine skeletal pattern and appraise dental relations in order to support the data obtained from the clinical examination will aid the practitioner in deciding whether he should involve himself in the treatment of the existing developing malocclusion and how it may be best treated.

ANALYSIS OF DENTAL STUDY CASTS

One of the most important diagnostic aids is a set of accurate dental study casts, or models. They provide a view of the occlusion not readily obtained from clinical examina-

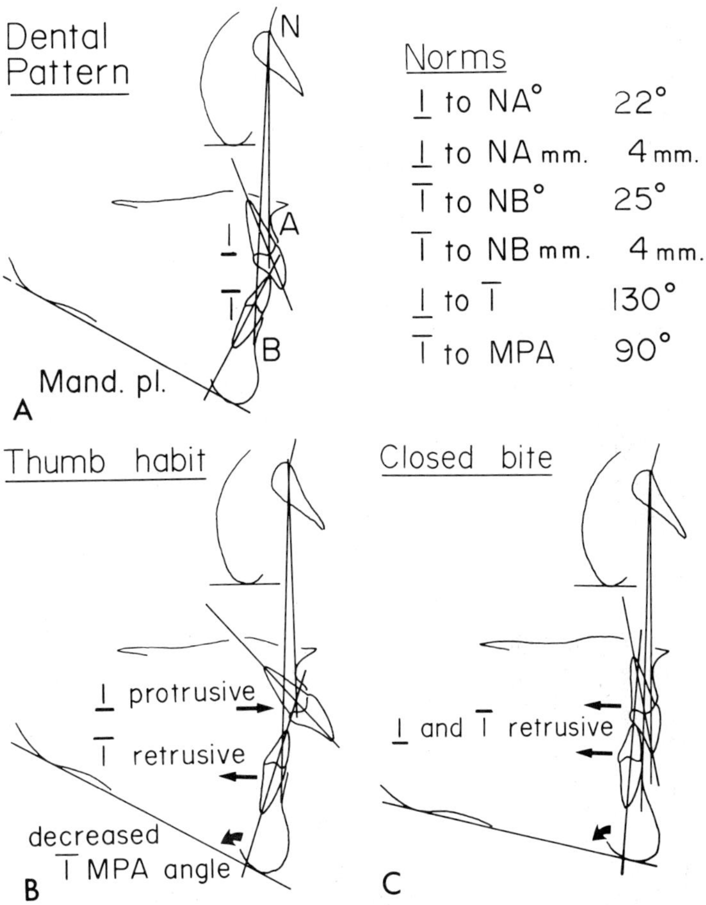

Dental Pattern

Norms

1 to NA°	22°
1 to NA mm.	4 mm.
1̄ to NB°	25°
1̄ to NB mm.	4 mm.
1 to 1̄	130°
1̄ to MPA	90°

Mand. pl.

A

Thumb habit

1 protrusive

1̄ retrusive

decreased 1̄ MPA angle

B

Closed bite

1 and 1̄ retrusive

C

Figure 19–9 *A* depicts the generally acceptable dental pattern of incisal relation along with the norm values of angular and linear measurement. *B* illustrates a typical angular change coincident with the thumb habit, while *C* depicts the incisor angulation frequently associated with a closed bite or an excessively active lip musculature.

tion alone and enhance the data obtained through cranial radiographs. Unfortunately, the average dental practitioner has neglected to appreciate the importance of diligently obtained dental study casts as a form of dental record and as a source of useful and detailed information. Any consideration for minor tooth guidance during dental development requires repetitive record-taking on study models. Dental casts, when taken at periodic intervals, provide a basis for comparison from period to period and allow the appraisal of such problems as space loss, diastemata, tooth size differences, malpositions, arch shape and symmetry, the relation of one arch to the other, and many other conditions.

Symmetrical Analysis

The technique is to examine the dentoalveolar complex, comparing dental arches and antimere teeth positions for symmetry. It is a

technique of "seeing." Once an asymmetry is seen, the examiner can apply his knowledge of the possible causes of the asymmetry and add to his diagnostic data. When he can see what is wrong, his plans for treatment become more valid.

In addition to a properly trimmed set of dental casts, the materials used are a pair of double-pointed dividers with the points adjustable for length and a Boley gauge. Dividers of this type are available at most drawing supply and art stores.

Overview. To begin the study cast analysis, examine the overall appearance of the models in occlusion, as illustrated in Figure 19–10*A* to *C*. Take note of any crossbite, an open bite, or the presence of malposed teeth and the general appearance of occlusal symmetry. From the frontal view, as in Figure 19–10*B*, draw a vertical line between the maxillary and mandibular central incisors. This is the *dental midline*. Compare how the upper and lower dental midlines

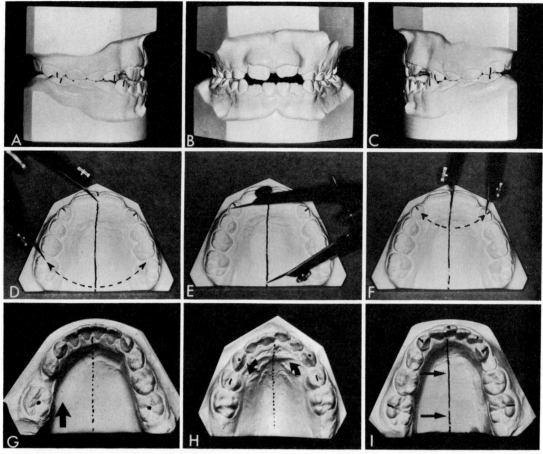

Figure 19–10 Study cast (model) analysis. *A* through *C* depict the preliminary examination of the casts from frontal (*B*) and lateral (*A* and *C*) aspects noting molar and cuspid relationships in occlusion. *D* through *F* illustrate the method of comparing right and left tooth positions for symmetry using a double pointed divider. Molar position (*D*) is tested for anteroposterior symmetry, and the cuspid teeth (*E*) are similarly examined. In *F*, the lateral position of opposite teeth may be estimated. An example of anterior molar asymmetry is seen in *G*. In *H*, an asymmetry in cuspid position can be noted. In *I*, the left buccal segment is seen to be closer to the midline than the right side.

relate to one another. When they do not coincide, it suggests that either one or the other deviates to one side, or there may be a combination of both.

Rotate the casts to view the right side, as seen in Figure 19–10*A*. Draw a vertical line through the mesial buccal cusp of the upper first molar and another line through the central groove of the lower molar. Note the molar relationship as Class I, II, III, or cusp to cusp. While viewing each side, examine the relationship of the upper and lower cuspid teeth. In a balanced occlusion, the maxillary cuspid occludes with the interproximal space distal to the mandibular cuspid. This is a Class I cuspid relation. Compare cuspid and

molar relations on the same side. Are they the same? If they differ, is there a readily explainable reason such as the loss of a tooth between the cuspid and molar on either arch with evidence of tooth migration to close the space?

Rotate the casts to view the opposite side, as seen in Figure 19–10*C* and repeat the examination of the molar and cuspid relationships. The profile examination of incisor overbite and overjet can also be performed to support the information gained during the clinical examination of the patient.

The cast overview provides a general impression of the occlusion. We generally ask ourselves, were the two buccal sides symmetrical? If not, was there an impression of space loss, a right and left discrepancy suggestive of a skeletal or dental shift in the arches? How did right and left buccal segments relate to any shift in dental midline? A deviation in one often is reflected in the other two.

Examination of Separate Casts. The study models are examined separately from a view of the occlusal surfaces beginning with the maxillary cast. First, do the arches appear symmetrical from side to side or is there evidence of a skewed shape in the outline of the circumference? The midpalatine suture, or raphe, serves as the skeletal midplane for reference. The suture is the base for comparing right and left arch symmetry and individual tooth position both bucally and anteroposteriorly. When transferred to the mandibular arch, the midpalatine suture serves the same purpose for the mandibular teeth and provides a clue to the way the mandible relates to the maxilla in occlusion. The line serves as a skeletal reference. For example, a right-angle square could be placed along the midpalatal suture with the intersecting right-angle plane placed to correspond to the mesial surface of antimere molar teeth. If the molars are equidistant anteroposteriorly, their mesial surfaces could be expected to lie in the same plane at right angles to the midpalatal suture.

The principles of simple geometry can be applied to examine tooth and arch symmetry using an adjustable double-pointed divider for measurement. Figure 19–10D illustrates how one leg of the divider is placed on the midline at an anterior point, and the divider is adjusted to correspond to an easily identifiable anatomic landmark on one first permanent molar. While maintaining the anterior divider position, the divider is rotated to compare the position of the molar on the other side (antimere) using the same anatomic landmark. Thus, the anteroposterior molar positions can be compared. Figure 19–10E illustrates the comparison of cuspid teeth for anteroposterior position using a point distally on the midline for reference. In the same fashion, a buccolingual symmetrical determination of antimere teeth can be made as seen in Figure 19–10F.

Examples of the kinds of information revealed from the symmetrical appraisal are illustrated in the remainder of Figure 19–10. In 19–10G, one of the molar teeth has migrated mesially and is identified through the asymmetry. In 19–10H the cuspid asymmetry identified indicates a space loss due to distal migration of one cuspid and similarly shows collapse of the anterior segment with a midline deviation. Figure 19–10I shows the type of buccolingual asymmetry that might accompany a crossbite on one side.

When the casts are placed in occlusion, it is relatively easy to transfer the median raphe line to the lower cast. The anterior point will be most accurate. The symmetrical appraisal can then be repeated for the mandibular cast, revealing similar information for that dental arch.

Another useful aid is to draw a line on the occlusal surfaces and incisal edges of each tooth, extending from one contact point to the other. As the "contact line" for each arch is viewed, any minor rotations of individual teeth become readily apparent.

Review. The final step in symmetrical cast analysis is to compile the information into usable form. The technique is to "see" the differences, after which we need to assess the findings with the following questions in mind:

1. *What* asymmetries were observed that can be considered normal for the stage of dental development?

2. Having observed what is out of the ordinary, we must next establish *why* the condition is there.

3. Bring the data together by asking *how* the irregularities occurred. Such influences as muscular imbalances, loss of space, crowding, crossbites, and others have a profound effect on the developing occlusion.

By attempting to answer what, why, and how the developing irregularities have occurred, the examiner may improve his diagnosis and approaches to dental therapy.

Mixed-Dentitional Analysis

In any examination of the child's developing occlusion, it is necessary to analyze the relation of tooth size and dental arch size.

This is especially important during the transition from the deciduous arch to the permanent arch from 6 to 12 years of age. These measurements are most accurately made on the plaster dental study casts. The purpose is to determine if each dental arch contains enough space (arch length) to accommodate the yet unerupted remaining permanent teeth. Usually, the need to do an arch-length analysis arises following eruption of the first permanent molars and at the time when the permanent incisors have erupted in their most common crowded position. The dentist would like to determine at that point if there will be sufficient room (arch length) later to allow for straightening of the incisors with enough remaining space for the unerupted cuspid and bicuspid teeth.

There are several popular methods for determining the space needs of the arch, namely the Nance,[43] Hixon-Oldfather,[44] and Moyers-Michigan[45] analyses. The Moyers

Mixed Dentition Analysis is the most commonly used technique, offering a high degree of accuracy and reliability. Based upon the concept that the sizes of one group of teeth bear relation to the sizes of another group of teeth in the same mouth, Moyers has supplied a table of prediction measurements based upon the mesiodistal widths of the lower permanent incisors.

Technique

1. Measure the mesiodistal widths of the lower central and lateral incisors, as in Figure 19–11A. The sums of these four measurements represent the arch length (space) needed to properly align the four permanent incisors.

2. One half of this total sum is the space needed in each incisor quadrant on either side of the midline. Note that in some cases the "dental midline" does not coincide with

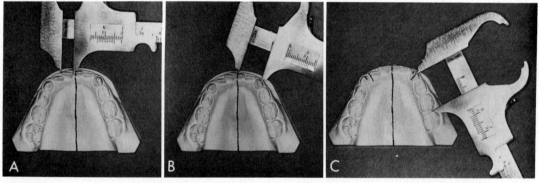

Σ 21⃒12	19.5	20.0	20.5	21.0	21.5	22.0	22.5	23.0	23.5	24.0
Max. 75%	20.6	20.9	21.2	21.5	21.8	22.0	22.3	22.6	22.9	23.1
Mand. 75%	20.1	20.4	20.7	21.0	21.3	21.6	21.9	22.2	22.5	22.8

Figure 19–11 Mixed Dentition Analysis (Michigan-Moyers) is utilized to estimate the space available in the deciduous arch to accommodate the unerupted permanent cuspid and bicuspid teeth. In *A,* the four lower permanent incisors are measured. In *B,* the illustration indicates the space needed to accommodate one half the sum of the incisors. Note that a portion of the cuspid space is needed, and this is called "incisor liability." *C* shows the space available from the point of incisor liability to the permanent molar for the cuspid and bicuspids. The chart below the figure provides an estimate of the unerupted cuspid and bicuspid size. Find the sum of the four measured lower incisors in the top row labeled Σ 2,1,1,2. Next, locate the maxillary or mandibular "predicted" size for the unerupted teeth in the column beneath the sum of the incisors measured. Comparison of "space needed" (predicted tooth size) with "space available" (measured on the cast) materially aids space management.

the "skeletal midline." Thus, one half of the sum is the space needed on either side of the *corrected* midline to properly position the central and lateral incisors.

3. When the incisors are normally crowded, some of the space necessary to align the incisors is occupied by the deciduous cuspid. Thus, the Boley gauge is adjusted for one half the total sum of the incisors, and with one point of the gauge placed at the *corrected* midline, the other is held along the arch circumference to make a mark on the deciduous cuspid (Fig. 19–11*B*). This represents the space needed for the incisors, and the amount of cuspid space used is termed the *incisor liability*.

4. The space remaining between the mark on the deciduous cuspid and the mesial surface of the permanent molar is the *space available* for the unerupted permanent cuspid and bicuspid teeth (Fig. 19–11*C*).

5. Having determined the space available in each arch, the next step is to determine the space needed or to predict the sum of the sizes of the unerupted teeth. Moyers has provided a probability chart for each maxillary and mandibular set of teeth.[45] The purpose is to locate the predicted sizes of the unerupted teeth on the chart, based upon the total sum of the mandibular incisor widths of the case being measured. The sum of the mandibular incisor teeth is used to locate predicted cuspid and bicuspid widths for both maxillary and mandibular arches. Since the 75 per cent level of probability has been shown to be the most accurate, only that level is presented in Figure 19–11. This is the highest confidence level and is generally the only set of numbers used. Referring to Figure 19–11, locate the sum of the four mandibular incisor widths in the top line closest to the measurement in your case. The corresponding numbers beneath this sum of incisor widths are the predicted total mesiodistal widths of the cuspid and bicuspid teeth for your case. A separate value is given for the maxillary and mandibular arches.

6. By comparing the space needed (predicted tooth size) with the measured space available (Fig. 19–11*C*), you can readily determine the needs for total space in each quadrant.

At this point, it should become obvious

that space deficiencies may relate to the forward migration of molar teeth (often observed on study cast symmetry analysis) or the collapse of the anterior segment (often seen on lateral head-film incisor analysis). On other occasions lateral collapse of the arches (frequently with crossbites) will produce loss of needed space and, finally, the teeth may be too large for the arch. It would appear that minor adjustments of malposed teeth can frequently regain the needed space. On the other hand, when the adjacent teeth will not allow adjustment for space regaining, it may be necessary to consider extraction of bicuspid teeth. Determine *first* if tooth adjustment is possible before resorting to extraction to gain necessary space. This is the conservative approach.

SUMMARY OF DIAGNOSTIC TECHNIQUES

A fairly thorough examination of the patient provides a visualization of the denture in its surrounding bony and soft tissue framework. In addition to providing a gross overview of the occlusion, it allows for an examination of function and muscular environment and the relation of each to tooth position. Cephalometric analysis may be utilized to confirm the clinical appraisal. At the same time, the cephalometric appraisal provides a more finite method of assessing skeletal and dental patterns. It gives a basis for discriminating changes in skeletal growth patterns.

The critical appraisal of dental study casts for symmetry provides information about the arches as a whole and the positions of the tooth units within each arch. The mixed dentition analysis allows for the accurate description of space needs within each dental arch.

Additional data that must be considered before treatment include a medical history, a dental history, and the attitude of parents and child toward treatment. The importance of medical history, particularly as it may relate to the patient's ability to accept orthodontic care, cannot be overemphasized. Conditions such as rheumatic heart disease, bleeding disorders, or neuromuscular disorders may make treatment ill-advised or impossible.

The dental history should particularly explore oral habits that might be involved in the etiology of the malocclusion. Digit-sucking, lip-sucking, and mouthbreathing are among the more common. Also of importance is the history of dental disease, both dental caries and periodontal disease, as orthodontic treatment may exacerbate these problems. The family history of previous malocclusion may provide clues regarding hereditary tendencies, particularly toward skeletal disproportions or crowding problems.

Finally, the attitude of the child toward his present appearance, what he feels needs changing, and his willingness to wear appliances can greatly influence treatment. Likewise the attitude of the parents regarding the child's appearance, the cost of therapy, and the inconvenience of regular visits for an extended period of time must be assessed.

Having evaluated the patient, the radiographic head films, and the models, a summary in written form of the findings should be made, citing all of the significant variances from the norm and including etiologic factors when known. Using this summary, a listing of the treatment objectives can be made. These might include such objectives as regaining arch length, relief of crowding, reduction of overbite or overjet, correction of crossbite, or correction of rotations, depending on the problems noted. The planning of treatment or appropriate referral can then be based on the ability of the dentist to perform the treatment required. Too often a patient undergoes extensive treatment for a minor problem, but the dentist does not recognize a major problem. Usually, the treatment of the major problem could easily include the treatment of the minor problems, while saving the family time, money, and considerable inconvenience.

PREVENTIVE ORTHODONTICS IN PRACTICE

The terms "preventive," "interceptive," and "early" orthodontic treatment have been used interchangeably. The rationale for such therapy has been to intercept malocclusions during development and thereby reduce their consequences. Since treatment occurs early in growth, orthopedic alterations have more opportunity to be expressed. Harmful habits and their consequences can be removed or reduced. Serious esthetic problems that might lead to problems with self-image can be reduced or eliminated. Occlusal interferences that might alter function and growth at the temporomandibular joint may be removed. Ideally, preventive orthodontics would eliminate the need for future treatment, but in reality it usually only reduces the severity of the problem and thereby reduces treatment time in the permanent dentition. On the negative side, extended early treatment can be expensive and uses up the patients' cooperation and patience. Every attempt should be made to minimize the time required for treatment, especially if later care is envisioned. Common orthodontic problems that are candidates for early treatment will be discussed in the categories of skeletal, dental, and soft tissue.

Skeletal Tissue

Lateral Plane. The problems of Class II and Class III skeletal discrepancies have been the subjects of a controversy about whether or not they should be treated early. The rationale for early intervention is that by the application of orthopedic forces in the deciduous or mixed dentition, changes in the direction or magnitude of growth of the maxilla or mandible can be achieved.

Two methods that have been devised for the treatment of Class II problems are the use of extra-oral forces through the headgear to retract the maxilla and the use of functional appliances such as the Andresen and Frankel appliances to encourage growth of the mandible.

Headgears generally apply their forces through bands or splints to the teeth. The force is transmitted by the teeth to the periodontal ligament, bone, and ultimately to bone articulations. Primate experiments using heavy, constant force over extended periods have shown dramatic skeletal changes in the maxilla. However, studies on human subjects have shown less conclusive results and more investigations are required to show how the technique can be used more effectively. At present, the headgear may be attached to molars only, to molars splinted to incisors and/or bicuspids, or to splints on the full dentition. Forces are generally in the one- to two-pound range and use cervical pull, high pull, or combination pull, depending on the vertical sensitivity of the subject. The high pull is used in patients with tendencies toward vertical growth, and the cervical pull is used in patients with horizontal growth tendencies. Wearing time for the headgear varies from 14 to 24 hours by dentist preference. Much remains to be learned about the use of headgear in young children.

The headgear has been advocated for those patients with a Class II skeleton and a maxilla that is protrusive relative to the cranial base. There are, however, many patients with a Class II skeleton whose maxilla is normal or retrognathic relative to the cranial base. The use of headgear to retract the maxilla on these patients usually accentuates an already prominent nose. This patient needs mandibular growth rather than retraction of the maxilla. Functional appliances provide assistance in treating these patients. Recent primate studies in which the mandible was held in a protracted state have demonstrated an apparent acceleration in the

growth at the condyle.[46] The appliance that seems to most closely parallel the forces produced in the primate study is the Frankel appliance (Fig. 19–12A and B). This appliance is designed to be worn 24 hours a day. It works by releasing labial and buccal muscular forces from the dentition while encouraging a protracted forward position of the mandible. After two to three years of wear, the Class II relation tends to change to a Class I with a mild expansion of the dental arches. The results appear to be stable, yet additional clinical studies must be done to confirm these initial impressions before the system can be advocated with confidence. However, the Frankel appliance promises to be a very useful appliance system.

Class III skeletal problems may be intercepted in the deciduous or mixed dentition stage of tooth development. The chin cup has been in use for many years as a means of redirecting and diminishing mandibular growth. In addition, remodeling changes in the glenoid fossa have been observed. Figure 19–13 shows the formation of a chin cup and its use in conjunction with a "reverse" headgear (elastics from the maxillary molars to struts from the chin cup) to correct a developing Class III relationship in a young child. Force levels that have been used successfully range from 150 to 300 g to 3 to 4 pounds.[47, 48] The higher force values tend to produce more discomfort for the child. Treatment time is usually a few months. However, if the face

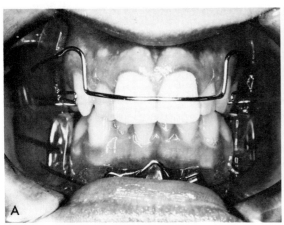 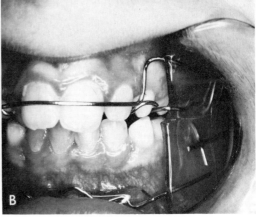

Figure 19–12 *A* and *B*. The Frankel appliance is used to encourage anterior growth of the mandible by displacing it forward. The lip bumper and buccal shields also remove muscular influences from the teeth and encourage widening of the arches. (Courtesy of Dr. J. Mulick, Canoga Park, CA.)

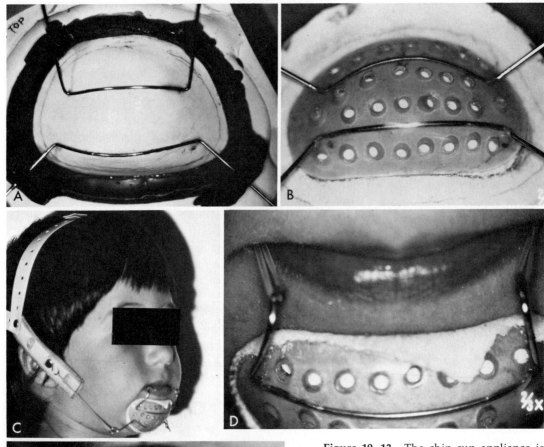

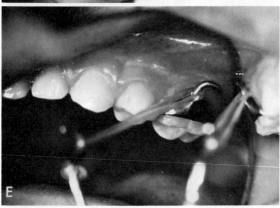

Figure 19–13 The chin-cup appliance is constructed by taking an impression of the chin and pouring it in stone. An outline of the appliance is formed with wax on the model, and the wire struts (.040 inch) are positioned with the wax (A). The acrylic is cold-cured on the model and ventilating holes are created to minimize tissue irritation (B). The chin cup is held in position by the elastic tension to the head strap (C). Elastics are also used from the anterior wire struts to hooks on the maxillary second deciduous molar bands (D and E) to produce a "reverse headgear" effect on the maxillary arch. Tissue or gauze is placed inside the chin cup to keep it comfortable.

tends to relapse toward the Class III relationship, additional episodes of chin cup wear may be required. Patients who show promise of large mandibular growth are not good candidates for this appliance. Rather mild class III tendencies in the mandible appear to respond the best.

The chin cup is useful for early treatment of mandibular prognathism, but sometimes the problem is maxillary deficiency and the mandible is normal. The use of the "reverse" headgears or "protraction" headgear has shown promise for obtaining orthopedic improvement in the maxilla. Most practitioners use elastics directly from the maxillary molars to the chin cup struts or a facial mask (Fig. 19–13E). Since development of the appliance is relatively new and rapidly changing, few clinical studies of its use have been completed. However, the reported case histories show great promise for its future use.[49, 50]

Vertical Plane. Patients with steep mandibular plane angles, long lower face heights, and open bite tendencies have traditionally been the most difficult to treat. There is evidence that these facial patterns can be related to airway obstruction with resultant mouthbreathing. Certainly the possibility of this etiology should be investigated before attempting treatment. The most common means used for early treatment has been a vertical pull chin cup with heavy force (based on the Milwaukee Brace effect). A variation of the Frankel appliance has also been used. Again insufficient documentation exists to comfortably predict the outcome of such therapies.

Correction of deep overbite in patients with a skeletal tendency for a short face is possible using cervical pull headgear, an acrylic bite plate, and/or a fixed appliance with intrusion mechanics. The problem is in maintaining the bite opening once it has been achieved. Frequently, it is wise to postpone the treatment of a deep bite patient until the inevitable anterior-posterior discrepancy can be corrected at the same time. Otherwise, retentive appliances must be maintained during the time span between the early treatment and the final treatment, and the patient's storehouse of patience and cooperation is concomitantly reduced.

Transverse Plane. The most common skeletal problem in this plane is a relatively deficient maxilla relative to the mandible, resulting in a unilateral or bilateral crossbite in the buccal segments. Haas[49, 51, 52] suggested the use of a rapid expansion appliance to orthopedically expand the maxilla by opening the midpalatal suture. Figure 19–14A to G shows the use of the appliance. The opening is greatest in the anterior region as evidenced by the spacing of the maxillary central incisors. The incisors quickly return to their normal relationship because of the pull of the interdental periodontal tissue fibers. The expansion is rapid and relatively comfortable for the patient. It is recommended where excessive tipping of the maxillary teeth would be required to correct the crossbite should light tooth-moving forces be

used. The correction must be maintained for at least three months to ensure stability.

Dental Tissue

The indications for preventive or interceptive orthodontic treatment for dental problems are many and include early loss of primary teeth, arch-length deficiencies, occlusal interferences, supernumerary or missing teeth, ankylosis, ectopic eruption, and others. Only the most frequently encountered problems will be discussed.

Arch-Length Maintenance

Arch length is a measure of the total mesiodistal diameters of the teeth. This is the total space necessary to properly align the teeth in the dental arch. The total space in a young child's deciduous arch gives way to the erupting permanent teeth to form the permanent arch. Thus, the transitional period and the space available is a combination of tooth size and jaw growth. The segment of the arch concerned during this period is from the mesial surface of the erupting first permanent molars through the arch contacts to the mesial surface of the first permanent molar on the opposite side. This dimension must provide sufficient space in which to position the unerupted permanent segment of incisors, cuspid, and bicuspids. It is the segment that gives us the greatest concern.

Mesiodistal Widths of Teeth

In 1947, Nance[43] provided the concept of *leeway space.* He found that the deciduous mandibular cuspid and molar teeth are 1.7 mm larger than their successors. The maxillary deciduous group are 0.9 mm larger than their successors. In application through the years, it meant that the permanent molars could be allowed to migrate forward 1.7 mm, and there would still be sufficient room for the permanent successors. Nance did not take into account the differences in deciduous and permanent incisor sizes.

In 1959, Moorrees[53] measured the widths of deciduous and permanent teeth in a repre-

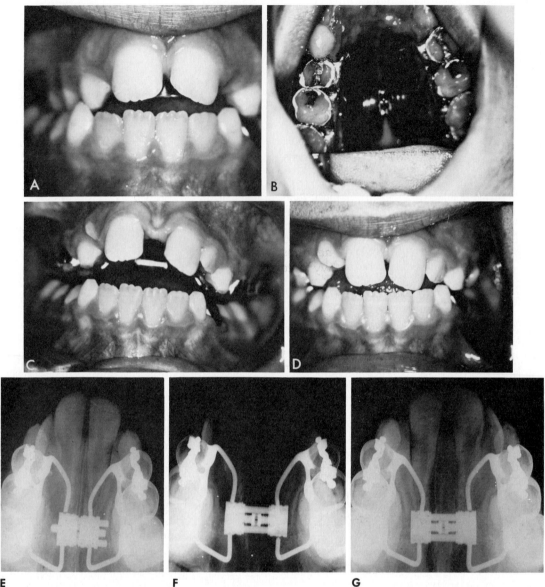

Figure 19–14 A "palate-splitting" appliance may be used to correct a unilateral or bilateral posterior crossbite. In *A*, the occlusion is seen pre-operatively. The appliance used consists of bands, cemented on the primary and permanent maxillary molars, which are soldered to a lingual bar (*B*). The bar is embedded in an acrylic palate with a screw positioned in the midline. The device can also be made without the acrylic palate, to minimize tissue trauma. The separation after two weeks can be detected by the separation produced in the maxillary central incisors (*C*). The incisors soon return to their original spacing as seen at 8 weeks (*D*). The occlusal radiographs taken preoperatively (*E*), at 3 weeks (*F*), and at 8 weeks (*G*) show the splitting effect on the mid-palatal suture and subsequent filling in of new bone.

sentative group of children, which included the incisors, and showed that the average mandibular deciduous and permanent arches are nearly the same size (< 1.0 mm total difference). The permanent tooth group was slightly larger than the deciduous group.

In this study,[53] the comparison of deciduous and succedaneous maxillary teeth showed the permanent tooth group to average 3 to 5 mm larger than the deciduous group. Thus, the credibility of the leeway-space concept must be questioned. Various factors of arch growth and change in shape contribute to ultimate space availability for the permanent teeth, but as leeway space was built on the concept of tooth size, so it must be questioned on that same basis. It appears that the 1.7 mm of leeway space described by Nance is taken up by the larger permanent anterior teeth, as seen in part *A* of Figure 19–15. Note also in part *A* that the larger permanent incisors require the eruption of the permanent cuspid tooth in a position more distal on the dental arch than was the position of the deciduous cuspid. This will allow for reduced incisor crowding. At the same time, the old leeway space is used by the more distal position of the cuspid. Part *B* illustrates that the distance from the mesial surface of the permanent molar to the tip of the deciduous cuspid on the left model is greater than the same distance to the permanent cuspid on the right model taken of the same child at a later age. Thus, the permanent cuspid is positioned more distally, using the leeway space to allow incisor alignment. In part *C*, there is a comparison of these same two casts, indicating a negligible difference

in overall molar to incisor distance. The molar has not moved forward. Instead, the cuspid is positioned more distally. Thus, any migration of the first permanent molars forward in the dental arch would reduce available necessary space.

In 1950, Baume[54] described the occlusal relation of the deciduous second molars, whereby their distal surfaces form a straight line (straight terminal plane), as in Figure 19–15D. This relation is seen particularly in the younger age ranges. He noted that the permanent molars erupted into an end-to-end or cusp-to-cusp occlusion, which he stated was corrected by the mandibular molar migrating forward in the dental arch to close any existing space or to utilize the leeway space as the second deciduous molar exfoliates.

Since this molar migration could contribute to loss of space, perhaps it would be more appropriate to expect that the permanent molar relation will normally adjust to become Class I as the result of the downward-forward growth of the mandible, which is accelerated over that of the maxilla.

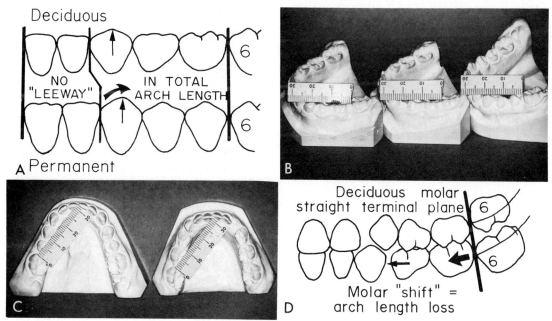

Figure 9–15 Comparison of the deciduous mandibular quadrant with the permanent replacements. In total measurement they are similar (*A*). The larger deciduous molars are counteracted by the larger permanent incisors for total arch length similarity. Note that the permanent cuspid will be further distal on the arch than was the deciduous cuspid, as seen in (*A*) and in *B* where the cast on the left is from a seven-year-old girl, and the cast on the right is from the same child at 11 years of age. In *C*, these same casts show little length difference. In *D* the deciduous terminal plane, when forming a straight line, does not automatically indicate that the lower molar should move forward. This may produce a loss in needed arch length.

That this molar relation change occurs as the result of mandibular growth has not yet been confirmed through longitudinal cephalometric study. However, the dental changes described by Baume,[54] based upon examination of dental casts alone, could have occurred as the result of jaw growth.

Arch-Length Loss

As was noted earlier, the eruptive and occlusal forces of the permanent molars tend to drive them forward in arch position. Should this occur as the result of caries in the deciduous arch, then arch length is lost, as in Figure 19–16A. Similarly, if a deciduous tooth is lost through extraction, the first permanent molars may migrate mesially a considerable amount, as in Figure 19–16B. This mesial movement of the molars is acceptable to many dentists in their belief that there is leeway (extra) space.

Total arch length is lost in other ways.

Occasionally, the incisor segment will be forced lingually because of a lip habit or a closed bite, or through the early loss of a deciduous cuspid tooth, as in Figure 19–16C. Frequently, this excessive lingual tipping of the incisor segment can be demonstrated by analyzing the position from a lateral head film. Many times it can be clearly visualized on clinical examination alone. In some cases, total arch length is decreased by the collapse, or lingual tipping, of the buccal segments, as in Figure 19–16D. This is more difficult to diagnose, since clinical judgment is applied in place of a valid diagnostic measurement technique.

Lastly, arch length can be inadequate because the erupting permanent teeth are genuinely too large by comparison to the deciduous predecessors. This is generally referred to as a "tooth size–jaw base discrepancy." Lacking a diagnostic method for measuring jaw base size, it becomes difficult to justify with assurance.

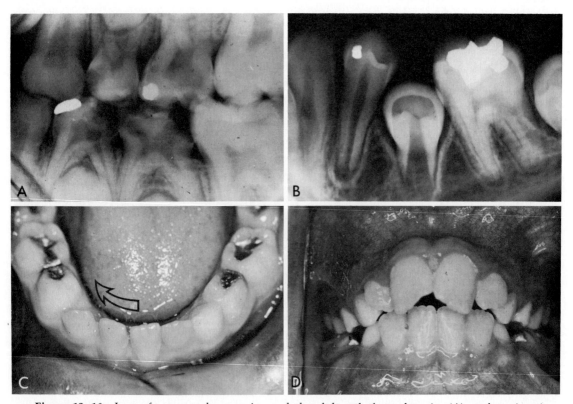

Figure 19–16 Loss of space or decrease in needed arch length through caries (A), molar migration (B), incisor segment collapse or migration (C), and buccal segment collapse (D). Each decreases space availability in the arch for the remaining unerupted permanent teeth.

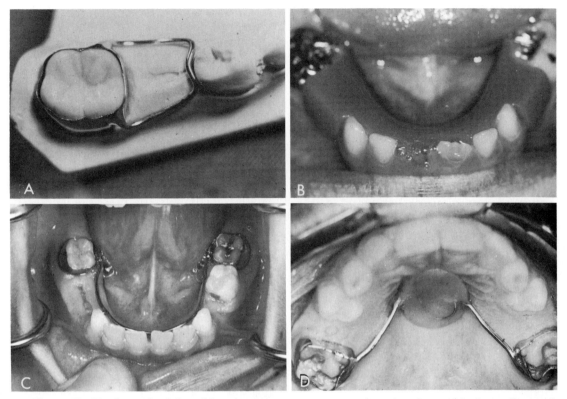

Figure 19–17 Space (arch length) maintenance to prevent molar migration and incisor collapse. *A* shows the band-loop space maintainer for single deciduous tooth loss, and *B* is the acrylic space maintainer commonly used for bilateral loss. Fixed appliances commonly employed are the lingual arch (*C*), which passively holds the entire arch in place, and the Nance holding arch (*D*), employing a "button" of acrylic adapted to the palatal vault to resist forward molar movement.

Arch-Length Management

There are two main approaches to guiding the individual arch-length needs of the child patient: conservative and sacrificial. The conservative approach has as its goals the preservation of all permanent teeth in the dental arch (if possible, recognizing that third molars may be lost), while the sacrificial approach "sacrifices," through extraction, tooth units (usually first bicuspids) to alleviate the needs for arch length. Each approach has merit, and there is overlap between them, so that management of the individual child's needs for arch length should be carefully examined. It should be our goal to preserve the permanent segment *in toto* (conservative) wherever possible and employ extraction as a means of treatment (sacrifice) only when necessary.

Moyers[45] has suggested that when space loss is slight (for example, 1 to 3 mm), it may

be recovered if treatment can be accomplished before the second permanent molar erupts. He also said that when the amount of space to be regained is excessive (for example, 5 to 7 mm), it may be necessary to consider removal of a tooth, and "when in doubt, a sound plan for the average nonspecialist is never to extract but instead to try all of the suggested procedures for regaining the length of the arch."

Space Maintenance

Space maintainers begin with restorative dentistry. The loss in arch length, pictured in Figure 19–16*A*, can be prevented by operative dentistry applied before space loss occurs. After loss of space has occurred, the problem becomes one of space regaining. Space maintainers are but one facet of arch length preservation. Our goal should be to preserve the total arch, of which one space is but a part of the whole.

When do you place a space maintainer? The answer is, before there has been any arch length loss. Any factor that leaves the arch vulnerable to diminution (for example, caries, loss of a tooth, possible incisor collapse from lip habits, and the loss of a deciduous canine tooth) should be counteracted with a holding appliance or a restoration. Figure 19–17 illustrates the most commonly employed holding appliances. The band-loop space maintainer in part A has fallen into disfavor today, for it usually has to be removed too early and replaced by a lingual arch. This is usually because of exfoliation of the deciduous abutment tooth or because the bicuspid erupts through the loop, lulling the practitioner into the belief that the job is done. The permanent molar can then begin its mesial migration with insidious space loss after the band-loop is removed.

Indications for Arch
Maintenance and Regaining

The needs for arch length are determined by the mixed dentition analysis. The study casts are further analyzed to identify asymmetry and the possibility of tooth migration. If anterior tooth collapse is suspected, we may elect to utilize cephalometric data. Mesial molar migrations are most commonly visualized by model analysis with the aid of clinical examination and intra-oral radiographs. Any potential environmental factor of the deciduous arch that may lead to space loss should be counteracted by the placement of holding appliances.

Once it has been determined that arch length has been lost, the following questions must be answered: How much has been lost? Where has the loss occurred? Why did it occur? Application of the diagnostic examinations described earlier will frequently identify how much loss has occurred and where it has occurred. Determining why the space loss has happened will require the application of basic knowledge coupled with a re-examination of the patient and his dental history.

Mesial migration of the molar teeth usually follows caries attack in the deciduous teeth, as seen in Figure 19–16A, or the loss of a deciduous molar, as in Figure 19–16B. In each instance, the task is to move the molar distally to regain the space. It is important to initiate this treatment before the second permanent molar has erupted far enough to contact the distal surface of the first molar. The contact of the second molar compounds the problem. Space regaining becomes quite difficult and may not be accomplished at all by the general practitioner. Frequently, it will be necessary to extract a bicuspid tooth if the space loss is great and the second permanent molar is fully erupted. Therefore, it is important to regain molar space as early as possible.

A common occurrence in permanent molar eruption is the ectopia associated with impaction beneath the second deciduous molar, as seen in Figure 19–18A. Occasionally, the deciduous tooth requires extraction because of pulpal involvement, in which case care should be taken to insure that the upper permanent molar is tipped distally to its desirable position. An acrylic palate with an embedded light wire (0.028 in. steel) is useful for this purpose (Fig. 19–18D and E) as is a headgear appliance when the condition is bilateral. When pulpal involvement does not require extraction of the deciduous molar, the placement of a brass separating wire (Fig. 19–18B) will exert a force against the permanent molar sufficient to tip it distally, unlock the impaction, and free it to continue its normal eruption path. Longitudinal radiographic studies have shown that the antagonistic resistance provided by the deciduous arch is quite sufficient to prevent forward movement of the deciduous teeth. A similar technique may be employed with impacted lower permanent molars, as seen in Figure 19–18C. However, this occurs in lower molars far less often than in maxillary molar eruption patterns.

When deciduous molars have been lost through extraction, after which the permanent molar tips mesially because of its eruptive path or the forces of occlusion (see Fig. 19–16B), the regaining of modest amounts of space may be accomplished with an appli-

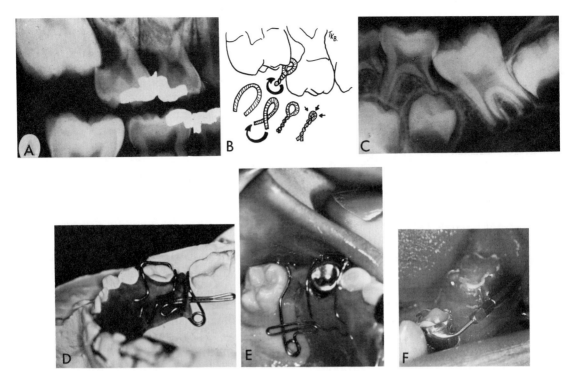

Figure 19–18 Space regaining by distal molar movement in small amounts. The molar impaction in *A* and *C* may be unlocked by employing a ligature wire passed under and tightened around the contact. *D* and *E* shows methods of applying spring pressure against a molar tooth while using the rest of the arch or palate for reciprocal resistance. The "jack-screw" in *F* is to be avoided, for the weaker anterior tooth can be expected to move forward instead of the desired molar movement being achieved.

ance similar to the maxillary appliance illustrated in Figure 19–18*D*.

The lingual arch described previously may be modified to perform the same task as the acrylic appliance, should a fixed type of appliance be desired. The lingual arch may be adapted with a coiled push spring activated against the molar tooth. In addition, the arch wire may be bent to utilize the loop principle for activation. In each case, the entire anterior segment is utilized for resistance or anchorage to insure distal molar movement and should be observed closely for proclination. If this tipping of anterior teeth is undesirable, the anchorage will need to be supplemented by other means.

The type of appliance illustrated in Figure 19–18*F*, employing a jack-screw or coiled push spring, is to be discouraged, for, unlike the acrylic appliance just described or a lingual arch that utilizes the entire anterior segment for anchorage and resistance, not enough reciprocal anchorage or resistance is present. From this illustration, it can be predicted that the "weaker" of structures will

move. In this case, the deciduous teeth anterior to the space can be expected to be driven forward instead of the desired distal movement of the molar tooth being achieved. Often the deciduous canine is driven forward to destroy the contact with the lateral incisor.

Incisor Crowding and Serial Extraction

Crowding of the incisor segments is a normal part of early dental development and must be carefully assessed in each child as to its effect on the total arch-length availability. Basically, incisor crowding must be regarded as:

1. Temporary: The arch length is adequate and will be self-correcting.

2. Artificial: The arch length has been decreased through incisor tipping or collapse, is correctable through adjustment of tooth position, and may lead to ultimate bicuspid extraction if left untreated.

3. Permanent: The incisors are in their

proper labio-lingual position, the crowding cannot be corrected, and the total arch length is inadequate.

We can expect to see some degree of crowding in almost every child's dentition during the emergence of the permanent incisor segment. The presence of this crowding should not automatically be diagnosed for bicuspid extraction without determining why the crowding exists. Graber[17] states: "When an orthodontist sees a child of five or six years of age with all the deciduous teeth present in a slightly crowded state or with no spaces between them, he can predict with a fair degree of certainty that there will not be enough space in the jaws to accommodate all the permanent teeth in their proper alignment." An additional thought on the part of many practitioners is that any crowding of the permanent incisors is an indication for bicuspid removal. Throughout these concepts is the belief in the presence of the 1.7 mm of leeway space. That is, if you believe that the permanent molars are supposed to migrate forward 1.7 mm and allow it to happen, you automatically reduce available total arch length. Then the normal crowding of the incisor segment has less room for final adjustment and self-correction. When considering the total arch length, a diagnosis of bicuspid extraction on the basis of any incisor crowding must be fallacious. It is imperative to determine why the crowding is present.

Temporary (Normal) Crowding. This is almost universal. The permanent incisors cannot fit in the same arch space as the smaller deciduous incisors did. In Figure 19–15A it can be seen that the posterior leeway space is taken up by the larger permanent incisors. Figure 19–11B shows the need to determine "incisor liability," and Figure 19–11C indicates the remaining space available for the permanent canine and premolars shown in Figure 19–15A. Should the molars be allowed to come forward, decreasing available arch length, the incisor segment will not have enough room for self-correction of its temporarily crowded state. Assuming that incisor crowding is present in a hypothetical case, and the mixed dentition analysis shows that arch length is adequate, it then follows that the crowded incisor seg-

ment will gain room for proper alignment in the future as the deciduous cuspid exfoliates and is replaced by the permanent cuspid, which erupts in a more distal position. This alignment is seen in Figure 19–16A and B. Thus, the leeway space is utilized by the more distal position of the permanent cuspid, allowing the incisors to be relieved of their crowding. Again, if the molars are allowed to come forward, the distal shift of the cuspid is prevented, and the incisor crowding remains. Mesial molar movement *in the dental arch* reduces arch length and encourages incisor crowding. Examine each case carefully. Use a lingual arch.

Artificial Incisor Crowding. This can be seen when arch length has decreased because of incisor collapse. An example is seen in Figure 19–16C. In this example, the erupting permanent lateral incisor has caused resorption of the deciduous cuspid root; the cuspid exfoliates early and the incisor segment collapses toward that side with a loss in total arch length as the result. Figure 19–19A shows a similar example of collapse. The resulting closed bite is seen in part B. Instead of diagnosing only from the occlusal view of the teeth and deciding that bicuspid teeth need to be removed, it would seem more proper to visualize the arch from all aspects. Frequently, the collapsed segment can be demonstrated by examination of the lateral head film. As in Figure 19–9C, the effect of the closed bite on incisor crowding or collapse of the arch-length availability can readily be visualized. If this is the case, the bite should be opened by means of an acrylic bite plane, as shown in Figure 19–19C, recreating the lost interincisor space and thus regaining the lost arch length through forward movement of the incisors as seen in part D. The tongue may push the incisors forward naturally. However, it may be necessary to place a lingual arch appliance, to which a lingually placed finger spring has been added, to aid the forward movement of the incisors. Another very useful appliance for this purpose is the 2 × 4 fixed banded appliance (Fig. 19–19E). Using bands with buccal tubes on the molars and straight wire brackets on the incisors, an advancing arch wire is used to tip the incisors labially and position them around the midline. Then a

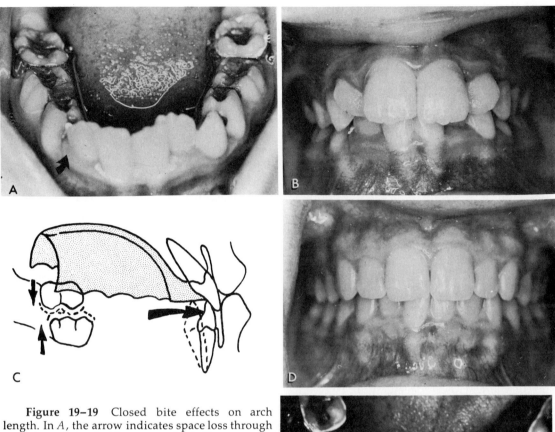

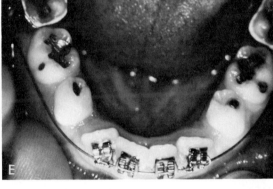

Figure 19–19 Closed bite effects on arch length. In *A*, the arrow indicates space loss through early loss of the deciduous cuspid. *B* illustrates the resultant closed bite. *C* represents the method of opening the bite with an acrylic palate, allowing the molars to erupt and the creation of interincisal space to allow forward incisor movement in the mandible, thereby recreating the cuspid space. *D* shows modest bite opening improvement compared to *B* and the successful eruption of all permanent mandibular teeth. A 2 × 4 banded appliance may also be used to upright and align the mandibular incisors (*E*).

lingual arch with stops at the distal end of the lateral incisors may be used for retention (see Fig. 19–17*C*).

Similar incisor collapse can be produced by muscular pressures from the labial side, such as is seen in lip-wetting and sucking habits and the thumb and mentalis habits. In each instance, the cause of the incisor collapse and crowding should be corrected. It is improper to resolve all crowding through bicuspid extraction on the basis that because crowding is present, extraction is necessary.

On the other hand, incisor crowding may actually be visualized in a "true arch-length discrepancy." In this instance, the

incisor crowding is *permanent,* unless extraction is performed. Here the incisors can be demonstrated to be in their proper labio-lingual positions; the molar teeth have not drifted foward, and the total arch length is shown to be inadequate. There is truly a tooth-size–arch-length discrepancy, and bicuspid extraction will be required. When in doubt, consult and seek justification for extraction in the individual case.

Serial Extraction. This was originally designed[55-58] to provide room in the arch for the erupting lateral incisors by extracting the deciduous cuspids early so that the incisors do not become crowded. Following this, sequential extraction of the deciduous molars allows for the uncrowded eruption of the remaining permanent teeth. Graber[17] provides a thorough and excellent review of the procedure. Without support, the arch will most frequently collapse, and when the molar teeth are not prevented from moving forward, loss of arch length will result. In the final stages of the serial extraction routine, it is necessary to sacrifice one of the bicuspid teeth. In some instances this is desirable, especially when it has been determined that the arch was totally inadequate to begin with. However, if the mixed dentition analysis demonstrates that the total arch length is adequate and extraction of the deciduous cuspid teeth is contemplated to alleviate incisor crowding, the arch should be prevented from collapsing following the extraction. Thus, the placement of a lingual arch appliance must *precede* the extraction.

Many practitioners desire to "shave" or reduce the mesiodistal widths of the deciduous cuspid teeth to allow the alignment of the permanent incisor teeth. This is acceptable provided caution is taken to insure that the arch will not collapse as a result. The placement of a lingual arch appliance first will insure that the total arch-length availability will not decrease as the result of the reduction of the size of the deciduous cuspid.

In summary, the presence of incisor crowding should not automatically lead to the diagnosis of a space discrepancy, requiring extraction of a tooth unit. Is the available arch length adequate for all of the teeth in the arch? Is it inadequate because of incisor malposition? Can that be corrected? Have the molars tipped forward, thus contributing to the incisor crowding? Or, if the dentist is satisfied that the arch is genuinely inadequate and that there is no possibility of adjusting tooth position, is extraction of a tooth unit the only option? The careful clinical examination of the patient, followed by the use of diagnostic aids, such as the study-cast analysis, mixed dentition analysis, and the use of a lateral radiograph, will markedly improve the plan of treatment related to incisor crowding as a clinical problem.

Crossbites

Crossbites refer to any departure from a normal buccolingual or labiolingual relation of the upper to the lower teeth (see Fig. 19–7). They occur quite commonly during the mixed dentition period and are usually related to a deviate eruption pattern of the permanent teeth. Occasionally, however, the crossbite may only be symptomatic of the child's pattern of abnormal jaw closure or mandibular function, as described in Figures 19–2 and 19–4.

The simple crossbite involving only one or two teeth has an adverse effect on arch length, serving to decrease the space available in the arch for the remainder of the teeth, and may influence growth at the temporomandibular joint if abnormal jaw closure is present. Thus, crossbites generally should be corrected as soon as they are observed. An exception to this may be a simple crossbite in the deciduous dentition, where its correction, or lack of correction, may have no relation to the permanent arch development.

The common incisor crossbite shown in Figure 19–20A usually occurs as the result of failure of the deciduous predecessor to exfoliate in time. The permanent successor is deflected lingually. The deciduous incisor should be extracted if it is still present. Measure the space to make certain it is large enough to receive the permanent incisor in a proper position before attempting to move the malposed incisor forward. Figure 19–20B illustrates an acrylic resin bite plane cemented to a number of lower incisors. The bite plane itself is contoured to present a vertically inclined extension, serving to drive the malposed incisor forward, using the patient's muscular occlusal forces as the stimulus. Part C illustrates the corrected incisor position after treatment and the removal of the bite plane. Usually, treatment can be accomplished in a period of two weeks with patient cooperation. A removable appliance may also be used to correct anterior crossbite. Part D demonstrates a common design for the spring (0.020 in steel). The key to success for this appliance is excellent reten-

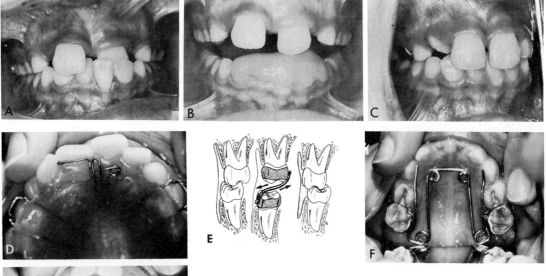

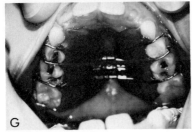

Figure 19-20 Crossbite correction using an acrylic bite plane (*B*) to correct the incisor relation in *A* to that of *C*. A removable appliance with a cantilever spring could also be used in a similar situation (*D*). Single tooth buccal crossbites are corrected with an elastic band as in *E*, while bilateral crossbite is more commonly corrected using a "quadhelix" expansion appliance (*F*) or a removable expansion appliance (*G*).

tion, usually by means of the modified arrowhead or Adams clasp.

The simple posterior crossbite, as illustrated in Figures 19–7*A, B,* and *C,* can readily be corrected with an elastic rubber band extended across the occlusal plane from the lingual surface of one affected tooth to the buccal surface of the other tooth in crossbite (Fig. 19–20*E*). The rubber band is attached to hooks soldered or welded to the banded teeth. The rubber band selected (available in sizes) should be small enough to maintain tension between the hooks at all times and is to be worn 24 hours per day. It is advisable to "overcorrect" the malposed teeth so that when the bands are removed, the teeth will "settle in" to proper position rather than revert to the previous crossbite condition.

The buccal segment crossbite involving several teeth should be carefully examined to determine if it is merely the malposition of upper or lower teeth or the manifest symptom of a deviate pattern of jaw closure. Referring to the clinical examination of the

patient and the closure pattern previously discussed and illustrated in Figures 19–2 and 19–4, it can be seen that a deviation of the mandible can produce a buccal crossbite on one or both sides. Most frequently this results from cuspal interference in the very young child and his "learning" to close his mandible to one side "for convenience." Generally, one dental arch will not fit within the other, thus requiring a modest amount of buccal expansion. The appliance seen in Figure 19–20*F* is one example in which a quadhelix expansion arch exerts a buccally expansive force against the molar segments. The appliance is constructed on a stone model and the helices in the wire (0.040 in steel) are "opened" the buccolingual width of a molar prior to intraoral cementation. Part *G* of this figure illustrates a removable appliance with an expansion screw that may also be used. Both the quadhelix and the removable appliance provide a tipping force to the teeth, although the force level of the quadhelix can be increased to the orthopedic range. As the crossbite is corrected, the child will begin to correct his path of mandibular closure, and a correction of the central incisor midline deviation (see Fig. 19–4B) can be noted.

Incisor crossbites should be examined in the same fashion. Occasionally, the child will close his mandible as shown in Figure 19–4C. In this instance, he may initially be thought to have a Class III malocclusion. Often, his narrow maxillary arch development can be attributed to a "convenience" forward bite. Buccal expansion, as for the buccal crossbite, will often bring about a similar correction in the path of mandibular closure and a correction in the incisor relation. Examine all crossbites carefully. Are they simple tooth crossbites or related to functional paths of mandibular closure?

Soft Tissue

The most common soft tissue problems that benefit from early treatment are oral habits and undesirable frenum attachments.

Oral Habits

Oral habit patterns in children are common. Some, such as thumb- or finger-sucking, are obvious and easily diagnosed. Others, such as tongue-thrusting, tongue-resting, lip-biting, the mentalis habit, and mouthbreathing, are more difficult to diagnose, but each produces a typical malocclusion.

Digit Habits. Thumb and finger habits usually space and protrude the maxillary incisors and at the same time push the lower incisors lingually, producing an open bite, as seen in Figure 19–21A. A discussion of thumb-habit correction is lengthy and the reader is directed to any standard text in pedodontics for suggestions of treatment. However, thumb-sucking can be disastrous to the occlusion if the child continues the habit beyond the age of six years. Psychological preparation, or motivation of the child to abort his habit, precedes successful management. Frequently, the mere placement of a tape bandage on the thumb will successfully serve as a reminder to the motivated child, and he will abort the habit pattern on his own. In most instances, the malposed teeth will return to more normal position as the

lip-tongue muscle balance is restored. Frequently, an acrylic retainer with activated labial wire (Fig. 19–22) will aid incisor retraction.

Tongue Habits. Tongue habits or abnormal swallowing patterns produce an occlusion in which both maxillary and mandibular incisor segments are protrusive and spaced (see Fig. 19–21B and 19–6). The patient and parents are generally unaware of the pattern, which can be demonstrated by asking the child to swallow. Immediately separate the lips, at which time the tongue is observed to be solidly thrust into the incisor spaces (see Fig. 19–6 C). The dental approach is generally mechanical; that is, a barrier against the thrusting tongue is constructed to remove the tongue pressures from the teeth. Figure 19–21C illustrates a removable acrylic palate to which has been added an extension lingual to the incisor teeth. This barrier serves to trap the thrusting tongue and directs the tip of the tongue upward and forward where the normal swallowing pattern is initiated. Some practitioners prefer a fixed type of appliance, in which case they adapt bands to the permanent canine or molar teeth. A soldered wire barrier is constructed that extends forward from the bands to occupy the space lingual to the incisors, as in Figure 19–21D, E, and F. The incisor spacing and protrusion often is self-corrective as the normal muscular balance is restored, at which time the appliance is removed.

Lip Habits. Lip habits and an overactive mentalis muscle are capable of severely crushing the lower incisor segment and are frequently the cause of incisor collapse and loss of arch length (see Figs. 19–16C and 19–19A). Lip-wetting is extremely common in young children, while the mentalis habit is uncommon. The latter is quite severe in action on the lower incisors, markedly increasing lower incisor crowding. Therapy for lip and mentalis habits consists of placing a "lip bumper" or lip guard, as illustrated in Figure 19–23. Heavy bands are adapted to the molar teeth to which are soldered 0.045 in round buccal tubes. A section of 0.045 in steel wire is adapted to surround the dental arch, free of the teeth, and is inserted into the buccal tubes. "Stops" or "rests" are sol-

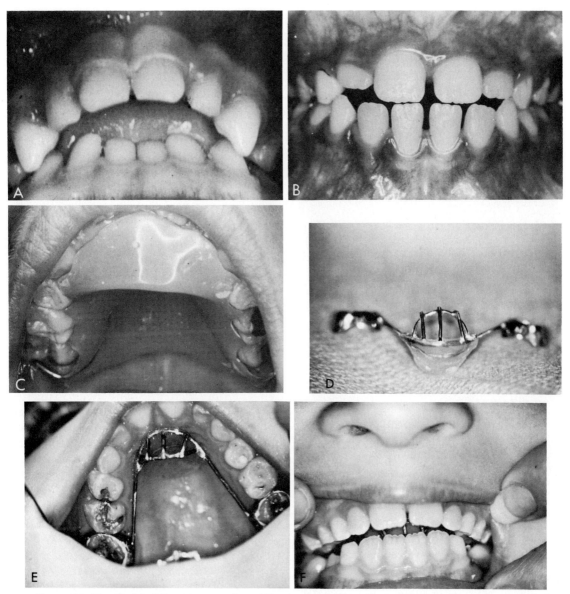

Figure 19–21 Oral habit patterns and resulting incisor malpositions. The typical pattern of a thumb-sucker is seen in *A*, while that of a tongue-thruster is seen in *B*. Tongue habits are commonly treated using the acrylic palate and tongue barrier (*C*) or the fixed wire barrier shown in *D, E,* and *F*. An acrylic button has been added to stabilize the wire crib and prevent embedding of the appliance in the palate.

Figure 19–22 An acrylic retainer with an activated labial wire may be used for incisor retraction. The spring shown is a Roberts Retractor, which uses .020 inch internal diameter tubing to support the labial bow up to the helices.[59] The light wire produces a light force ideal for tipping incisors. A biteplane is utilized to open the bite prior to incisor retraction.

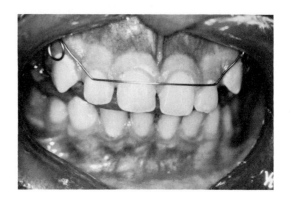

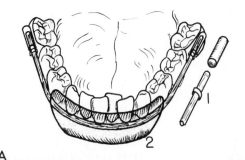

A

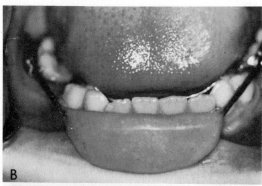

B

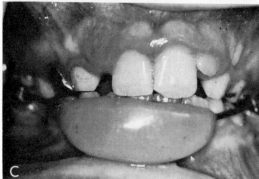

C

Figure 19–23 Excessive lip or mentalis muscle pressures are inhibited by a "lip bumper." It is constructed as a labial arch wire (*A*), to which is attached a flat ribbon-like bumper of acrylic (*A* and *B*). It causes no occlusion interference (*C*). The lip bumper transmits the muscular force to the unyielding molar teeth, thereby reducing the force as applied previously to the incisor teeth.

dered to the arch wire anterior to the tubes so that any force to the anterior position of the wire is transmitted to the molar teeth (Fig. 19–23*A*). A flat, ribbon-like, acrylic band is formed around the wire anteriorly, which presents a broad, smooth, surface of the lip without contacting the teeth or interfering with the occlusion (Figs. 19–23*B* and 19–23*C*). Habit correction is accomplished by preventing the musculature of the lip or mentalis from exerting pressure on the teeth. The musculature becomes fatigued and is

brought to the child's conscious level, whereupon he voluntarily ceases the activity. Again, normal muscle balance is restored, and the teeth return to normal position. Occasionally, it may be necessary to place an active lingual arch wire with accessory spring attachments to aid tooth position correction labially.

Mouthbreathing. In recent years, considerable attention has been directed toward the habit of mouthbreathing. Usually the habit begins because of an airway obstruction and may continue even though the obstruction has been relieved. Obstruction can occur from problems in the nose, the pharynx, the larynx, or the bronchial tree, all with the result that the patient uses the mouth to assist air intake. The effect of mouthbreathing on facial growth and development has been a long-standing controversy. However, recent evidence would seem to confirm that hypertrophic lymphoid tissue in the pharynx leads to a vertical facial growth pattern with a narrowed maxilla, posterior crossbite, and an anterior open bite tendency.[16] Treating such problems without removing the airway obstruction or correcting the breathing pattern will likely result in relapse and frustration. Patients with mouthbreathing habits and malocclusions that seem to be related should be examined by a physician for possible airway obstruction. Since the possible sequelae of treatment are serious, the decision to remove or not to remove the obstruction must rest with the physician and family after fully explaining the possible consequences of no treatment.

Frenum

Another area of long-standing controversy is the relationship of the maxillary labial frenum and the midline diastema. Since the diastema is considered a normal state in the "ugly duckling" stage prior to permanent cuspid eruption, it is generally wise to wait until after eruption of the permanent cuspids before considering treatment. However, sometimes a child presents in the mixed dentition stage with a very esthetically unpleasing diastema. They are frequently teased by their peers and lack self-esteem. In such cases with a large frenum that blanches between the incisors when tension is applied, the appropriate treatment would be to approximate the central incisors and perform a frenectomy. The frenum is removed in the later stages of space closure or following space closure. A simple procedure that permits bodily control of the incisors is to direct bond brackets onto the incisors and use an arch wire to align. When aligned, an elastic chain or elastic thread is used to close the space.

SUMMARY

As stated in the earlier sections of this chapter, prevention of malocclusion or early interception through minor orthodontics depends wholly upon diagnostic skill. Truly, no orthodontics is "minor." Apparently, the notion of minor orthodontics relates to the use of simple or uncomplicated appliances. However, what may at first glance appear to be a simple problem for correction might instead be superimposed upon a more involved or complicated problem in treatment.

The orthodontist does not frequently see young children in his practice. Unless the diagnostic skills of the generalist and pedodontist are sharp enough to differentiate normal from deviant patterns of dental development in the child patient, interdisciplinary consultation and cooperative care will not occur.

Hopefully, the generalist will further his detailed study of diagnostic technique and the use of diagnostic aids. It can be expected that the guidance of normal dental development lies within the scope of general dental care. Careful attention to the need for restorative dentistry and to problems of space management should be given within every dental office. Certainly, the general dentist must be skillful in the recognition of factors in dental development that act to reduce needed arch length. Procedures to regain small losses in arch length caused by ectopia and to correct crossbites, oral habits, spacing, and inadequate restorative dentistry are all within the scope of general dental care.

Our child population will be served better as the profession worries less about jurisdictional boundaries for treatment and enters a period of mutual education for more effective delivery of preventive and modestly corrective orthodontic care for vastly expanded numbers of young children.

REFERENCES

1. Angle, E. H.: Classification of malocclusion. Dent. Cosmos 41:248–264, 350–357, 1899.
2. Thielemann, K.: Über die Laufigkeit von Stellungsanomalien der Zähne im Kleinkindersalter. Dissertation, Leipzig, 1923.
3. Korkhaus, G.: The frequency of orthodontic anomalies at various ages. Int. J. Orthod. 14:120–135, 1928.
4. Stallard, H.: The general prevalence of gross symptoms of malocclusion. Dent. Cosmos 74:29–37, 1932.
5. Taylor, A. T.: A study of the incidence and manifestations of malocclusion and irregularity of the teeth. Aust. Dent. J. 7:650, 1935.
6. Goldstein, M. S., and Stanton, F. L.: Various types of occlusion and amounts of overbite in normal and abnormal occlusion between two and twelve years. Int. J. Orthod. Oral Surg. 22:549–569, 1936.
7. Mumblatt, M. A.: A statistical study of dental malocclusion in children. Dental Items of Interest 65:43–63, 1943.
8. Sclare, R.: Orthodontics and the school child. A survey of 680 children. Br. Dent. J. 79:278–280, 1945.
9. Huber, R., and Reynolds, J. W.: A dentofacial study of male students at the University of Michigan in the physical hardening program. Am. J. Orthod. Oral Surg. 32:1–21, 1946.
10. Massler, M., and Frankel, J. M.: Prevalence of malocclusion in children aged 14–18 years. Am J. Orthod. 37:751–768, 1951.
11. Newman, G. V.: Prevalence of malocclusion in children 6 to 14 years of age and treatment in preventable cases. J. Am. Dent. Assoc. 52:566–575, 1956.
12. Altemus, L. A.: Frequency of the incidence of malocclusion in American Negro children aged twelve to sixteen. Angle Orthod. 29:189–200, 1959.
13. Popovich, F., and Grainger, R. M.: One community's orthodontic problem. In Moyers, R. E., and Jay, P. (eds.): Orthodontics and Dentistry, Orthodontics in Mid-Century. Transactions of a workshop in orthodontics. St. Louis, C. V. Mosby Co., 1959, p. 192.
14. Ast, D. B., Allaway, N., and Draker, H. L.: The prevalence of malocclusion, related to dental caries and lost first permanent molars, in a fluoridated city and fluoride-deficient city. Am. J. Orthod. 48:106–113, 1962.
15. Harvold, E. P.: Neuromuscular and morphological adaptations in experimentally induced oral respiration. In McNamara, J. A., Jr. (ed.): Naso-

Respiratory Function and Craniofacial Growth. Monograph No. 9, Craniofacial Growth Series, Center for Human Growth and Development. Ann Arbor, University of Michigan, 1979.

16. Linder-Aronson, S.: Effects of adenoidectomy on dentition and nasopharynx. Am. J. Orthod. 65:1–15, 1974.
17. Graber, T. M.: Orthodontics, Principles and Practice. Philadelphia, W. B. Saunders Co., 1966.
18. Baum, A. T.: A cephalometric evaluation of the normal skeletal and dental pattern of children with excellent occlusions. Angle Orthod. 21:96, 1951.
19. Bjork, A.: The face in profile. Svensk Tandlak. Tidskr. Suppl. 40 No. 5B, 1947.
20. Broadbent, B. H.: The face of the normal child. Angle Orthod. 7:185, 1937.
21. Broadbent, B. H.: Ontogenic development of occlusion. Angle Orthod. 11:223, 1941.
22. Brodie, A. G.: On the growth pattern of the human head from the third month to the eighth year of life. Am. J. Anat. 68:209, 1941.
23. Brodie, A. G.: Craniometry and cephalometry as applied to the growing child. In Cohen, M. M.: Pediatric Dentistry, 2nd ed. St. Louis, C. V. Mosby Co., 1961.
24. Report on the first roentgenographic cephalometric workshop. Am. J. Orthod. 44:899, 1958.
25. Salzmann, J. A. (ed.): Roentgenographic Cephalometrics. Philadelphia, J. B. Lippincott Co., 1961.
26. Coben, S. E.: Growth concept. Angle Orthod. 31:194, 1961.
27. Downs, W. B.: Variations in facial relationships: Their significance in treatment and prognosis. Am. J. Orthod. 34:812, 1948.
28. Downs, W. B.: The role of cephalometrics in orthodontic case analysis. Am. J. Orthod. 38:162, 1952.
29. Downs, W. B.: Analysis of the dentofacial profile. Angle Orthod. 26:191, 1956.
30. Dreyer, C. J., and Joffee, B. M.: A concept of cephalometric interpretation. Angle Orthod. 33:132, 1963.
31. Higley, L. B.: Cephalometric standards for children four to eight years of age. Am. J. Orthod. 40:51, 1954.
32. Lande, M. J.: Growth behavior of the human bony facial profile as revealed by serial cephalometric roentgenology. Angle Orthod. 22:78, 1952.
33. Margolis, H. I.: The axial inclination of the lower incisors. Am. J. Orthod. Oral Surg. 29:571, 1943.
34. Moore, A. W.: Observations on facial growth and its clinical significance. Am. J. Orthod. 45:399, 1959.
35. Reidel, R. A.: The relation of maxillary structures to cranium in malocclusion and in normal occlusion. Angle Orthod. 22:142, 1952.
36. Salzmann, J. A.: Limitations of roentgenographic cephalometrics. Am. J. Orthod. 50:169, 1964.
37. Schaeffer, A.: Behavior of the axis of human incisor teeth during growth. Angle Orthod. 19:254, 1949.
38. Scott, J. H.: Growth at facial sutures. Am. J. Orthod. 42:381, 1956.
39. Scott, J. H.: The cranial base. Am. J. Phys. Anthropol. 16:319, 1958.
40. Spiedel, T. D., and Stoner, M. M.: Variation of the mandibular incisor. Axis in adult "normal occlusion." Am. J. Orthod. Surg. 30:536, 1944.
41. Steiner, C. C.: Cephalometrics for you and me. Am. J. Orthod. 39:729, 1953.
42. Steiner, C. C.: Cephalometrics in clinical practice. Angle Orthod. 29:8, 1959.
43. Nance, H. N.: The limitations of orthodontic treatment. I. Mixed dentitional diagnosis and treatment. Am. J. Orthod. 33:177–223, 1947.
44. Hixon, E. H., and Oldfather, R. E.: Estimation of the sizes of unerupted cuspid and bicuspid teeth. Angle Orthod. 28:236–240, 1958.
45. Moyers, R. E.: Handbook of Orthodontics, 2nd ed. Chicago, Yearbook Medical Publishers, 1963.
46. McNamara, J. A., Jr., Connelly, T. G., and McBride, M. C.: Histological studies of temporomandibular joint adaptations. In McNamara, J. A., Jr. (ed.): Determinants of Mandibular Form and Growth. Monograph No. 4, Craniofacial Growth Series, Center for Human Growth and Development. Ann Arbor, University of Michigan, 1975.
47. Vego, L.: Early orthopedic treatment for Class III skeletal patterns. Am. J. Orthodont. 70:59–69, 1976.
48. Graber, T. M., Chung, D. D. B., and Aoba, J. T.: Dentofacial orthopedics versus orthodontics. J. Am. Dent. Assoc. 75:1145–1166, 1967.
49. Haas, A. J.: Long-term post-treatment evaluation of rapid palatal expansion. Angle Orthod. 50:189–217, 1980.
50. Nanda, R.: Biomechanical and clinical considerations of a modified protraction headgear. Am. J. Orthod. 78:125–139, 1980.
51. Haas, A. J.: The treatment of maxillary deficiency by opening the midpalatal suture. Angle Orthod. 35:200–217, 1965.
52. Haas, A. J.: Palatal expansion: Just the beginning of dentofacial orthopedics. Am. J. Orthod. 57:219–255, 1970.
53. Moorrees, C. F. A.: The Dentition of the Growing Child. Cambridge, Harvard University Press, 1959.
54. Baume, L. J.: Physiological tooth migration and its significance for the development of occlusion. I. The biogenetic course of the deciduous dentition. J. Dent. Res. 29:123–132, 1950; 29:331–337, 1950; 29:440–447, 1950.
55. Dewel, B. F.: Serial extractions in orthodontics: Indications, objectives, and treatment procedures. Am. J. Orthod. 40:906–926, 1954.
56. Dewel, B. F.: Serial extraction: procedures and limitations. Am. J. Orthod. 43:685–687, 1957.
57. Mayne, W. R.: A concept, diagnosis and a discipline. Dent. Clin. N. Am., July, 1959, pp. 281–288.
58. Mayne, W. R.: Serial extraction as an adjunct to orthodontic treatment. Audiovisual sequence. St. Louis, American Association of Orthodontics, 1959.
59. Houston, W. J. B., and Isaacson, K. G.: Orthodontic treatment with removable appliances. Bristol, John Wright & Sons Limited, 1977, pp. 33–34.

CHAPTER TWENTY

Marketing Preventive Dentistry

Ralph A. Heiser, D.D.S., Ph.D.
Richard E. Stallard, D.D.S., Ph.D.
Karen Hess, Ph.D.

Marketing of preventive health measures has proved to be financially successful for numerous commercial enterprises. In the magazine *Prevention,* one can find ads for everything from multiple vitamins, fructose, alfalfa, bone meal, various trace (mineral) elements, garlic tablets, bee pollen, Oil of Evening Primrose, deep sea kelp, collagen placenta cream, carrot oil, RNA/DNA tablets, aloe vera, and octacosanol to instant chicken soup, all purported to "prevent" some dread disease, increase stamina, and ensure a healthy long life. The fact that these products sell clearly demonstrates desire on the part of the consumer to prevent disease; however, the practice of preventive dentistry or medicine is extremely mundane to the practitioner compared with open heart surgery, dental implants, or full mouth rehabilitation. The "newsworthiness" of prevention versus a heart transplant or other major procedures has also affected the health care provider's mental image of his/her role in society.

HISTORY

Historically, professions such as dentistry, medicine, and law have refrained from marketing. Marketing was equated with advertising and advertising simply was not to be engaged in by the "true" professional. In fact, such activities were often prohibited by professional organizations and state practice legislation.

Traditionally, practitioners worked at becoming better and more competent in their particular profession than any of their colleagues. They tried to reach a degree of distinct competence to provide the competitive edge needed to grow in the profession, increasing the size of profitability of their practice.

In today's consumer-oriented society, however, this facet of professionalism is rapidly changing. The proliferation of a "Patient's Bill of Rights" in the medical field has already spread to dentistry in such forms as the "Shopper's Guide to Dentistry" issued in the early 1970s by the Office of the Insurance Commissioner of the State of Pennyslvania. The dentist who was once held in awe and whose skills were viewed by many as almost mystic finds that his/her image has changed. Three things have happened: secularization, demystification, and demythification. Traditionally dentists were dedicated to only one thing: providing quality service. They have been anti-sales, anti-advertising, anti-marketing, and anti-change.

Society is changing, and dentistry must change with it. Changes are occurring today faster than ever before, are less predictable, and are more encompassing in their impact. The failures of numerous once-profitable industries are examples of what happens when there is an inability or refusal to use change as an opportunity. Of course, hindsight is always better than foresight; however, should "professionals" really scoff at department store dentistry, industrial dental clinics, or closed panels?

Another reason for dentistry's traditional anti-marketing stance is that marketing was not deemed necessary because the supply/demand equation did not mandate it. Until a few years ago the supply of qualified practitioners was limited relative to the demand for services. In addition, professional societies assumed the marketing function in exchange for a commitment that members would not aggressively engage in marketing activities. Marketing functions were also delegated to pharmaceutical and cosmetic industries; for example, oral hygiene and other preventive dental products emphasized that people should use Product X *and* have regular dental checkups. In the 1980s, dentistry can no longer delegate this responsibility, particularly in the area of preventive dentistry.

Yet another reason for the failure of dentists to actively market their services has been an ignorance of how to do so. Dentists in general have little working knowledge, vocabulary, or appreciation of marketing theory. Dentists and physicians are singularly unskilled in the discipline of marketing. Not so with the legal and accounting professions and, especially, the banking industry.

Dentists claim they are not businessmen but highly trained public servants who care about people rather than profits. However, consumers have responded that since they charge fees, dentists *are* business people and should be subject to the same questioning and competition as other business people. Consumers now demand as much information as possible before they contract for expensive professional services, and they are right.

A profession should not resist regulation by the market nor continue to be an insulated cartel. If resistance continues, some government entity will impose regulations that open the marketplace. This was clearly evident at least 5 years ago. The trend toward allowing "marketing" of professional services began with a young worker who moved to Fairfax, Virginia, and looked for an attor-ney to search the title of his new home. When he found that all lawyers in the area asked the same fee, he sued the Virginia Bar Association, charging violation of the anti-trust laws. In a landmark decision in 1975, the United States Supreme Court upheld the suit and prohibited professional associations from setting minimum fees. In June 1977, the Supreme Court followed up with the ruling that bar associations could not prohibit lawyers from advertising.

In December 1978, an administrative law judge ruled that the American Medical Association and several state associations had prohibited advertising in order to fix prices and inflate fees. Dr. Robert B. Hunter, AMA Board Chairman, was "appalled" by the ruling, claiming that "the very nature of professionalism is at issue." But is it? Two years ago the Federal Trade Commission sued the American Dental Association. In early February 1979, FTC staff agreed to settle the suit out of court. The resultant new Section 12 of the ADA's Principles of Ethics now provides that "a dentist may advertise the availability of his services and the fees that he charges for routine procedures. No dentist shall advertise in any form of communication in a false, misleading, deceptive, or fraudulent manner."

There are other important reasons for marketing, particularly in preventive dentistry, that have nothing to do with competition. They have to do with performing a professional service to the public, as dentistry has long claimed to do. Consider the following facts:

1. The impact of inflation on dental utilization was studied by Yankelovich, Skelly and White, a national polling firm that conducted a survey for General Mills, Inc.[1] Their sample of 1,254 families revealed the following:

- 48 per cent of all families were curtailing spending
- Cutbacks in dental work were reported by 76 per cent of the families; 13 per cent were forgoing annual health checkups and 11 per cent were reducing dental checkups
- 75 per cent said they believed annual

checkups cost too much; that as long as they felt good, they didn't need the checkup

2. Americans now save only 4.6 per cent of their after-tax income. In 1977 the consumer spent 6.2 cents out of each dollar for dentistry, compared with 8.4 cents in 1955. Adjusted for inflation, this is only 4 cents.

3. Only 48 per cent of the population receives some dental care; only 28 per cent receives regular care.

4. 46 per cent of the nation's children never see a dentist; 75 per cent of black children under 17 years never see a dentist. It is the profession's responsibility to educate the public that *preventive* dentistry is a good value for their dollar, because the greatest impact of the above facts is in the area of prevention.

This view is aptly expressed by Theodore Levitt:

> Whether the word "selling" is one that we can savour or choke upon really makes very little difference—the burden of proof—the responsibility for demonstrating that our credentials really mean something and will produce genuine benefits for the patients, constitutes a selling proposition that we must recognize. In short, if we can't sell our credentials in the sense of demonstrating that they stand for something far more substantial than the elegant initials after our name — then we are failures not only as salesmen but as professionals as well. . . . As professionals possessing professional skills, we still have not only the requirements, but the obligation of actively and energetically selling these skills. They won't sell themselves. We have to sell them. And if we have to sell them, it is better that we do so on a conscious explicit basis rather than on an unconscious implicit, hit or miss basis.[2]

PROFESSIONALISM

A professional has demonstrable knowledge and skill in a specific area of competence. Someone once said that the difference between an amateur and a professional is that the professional can do his job when he doesn't feel like it and an amateur can't do his job even when he does feel like it.

The designation "profession" has not been permanently monopolized by a few occupations. Professional status has a dynamic quality, with constant reaction to social, economic, and technological change. Architects, teachers, bankers, private security officers, and fire-fighters all call themselves professionals. Even athletes who participate in a sport for pay are called professionals.

Increasing numbers of requests from groups wishing to be certified as licensed professionals include athletic trainers, acupuncturists, shorthand reporters, masseurs, and tree surgeons. The argument for licensure is that it ensures the setting of professional standards and protects the public from charlatans. On the other hand, arguments against licensure contend that it can lead to monopolization of services, resulting in higher prices for the consumer. A working definition of a profession might be "any body of persons who use common techniques of procedures, who form an association, the purpose of which is to test competence in the technique of procedures by means of an examination."[3]

Six attributes of professionalism have been identified: intellectual bias; private practice; advisory function, with full responsibility taken by the person giving the advice; a tradition of service (the profit motive is subordinated to public service); a representative institute, association, or society to set and safeguard standards; and a code of conduct.[4] Nothing in this list precludes marketing. In fact, these characteristics can easily be maintained *if* you market professionally. It is our view that dentists who are true professionals help their patients as well as society. They *must* participate in the selling and marketing of preventive dentistry and must use special training and knowledge in marketing and selling to do so professionally.

MARKETING VS. SELLING

There is a basic difference between *selling* and *marketing*. Selling concentrates on the needs of the seller and usually relies heavily on advertising. Stephen Leacock calls advertising "the science of arresting the human intelligence long enough to get money from it."[5] In contrast, marketing concentrates on the needs of the buyer or consumer—your patients. We might paraphrase Leacock's definition by saying marketing is the science of engaging the human intelligence long enough to convince it your preventive services are of true value.

The key is to market professional services professionally. How do you focus on the needs of the buyer? The central goal of dental marketing is to develop patient satisfaction and loyalty. This is best accomplished by systematically focusing on patient needs and attitudes.

It is important to recognize that dentistry has been product and service oriented rather than consumer oriented. Most preventive dental procedures are consumer oriented, compared with restorative dentistry which is product oriented. The profession might well make the same mistake as the railroad and the movie industries if it does not become a patient-satisfying process rather than a goods-and-service-producing process. The dental delivery system should offer a cluster of value satisfactions to those patients who will want to use the services.

Your competence in dentistry is generally taken for granted by your patients. The competitive edge will come from being sensitive to their needs, particularly in the area of prevention. In fact, it is a social responsibility for you and all within your practice to be sensitive and to respond to your patients' needs.

STEPS IN THE MARKETING PROCESS

Let us now examine how to market your preventive dental services. Basically, marketing means that you must take deliberate, active steps designed to attract patient commitments. Although marketing does add costs to your practice, if you market effectively, they are very justifiable and should result in increased profit. To paraphrase Aubrey Wilson,[6] market leadership in dentistry can be obtained by doing uncommonly well that which is commonly done and/or by doing that which is uncommon. Various chapters in this text focus on the former, and

others provide information that should enable you to achieve the latter.

Market Research

Market research is gathering, organizing, and analyzing market data for use in making marketing decisions. Market research theory, principles, and applications have become increasingly sophisticated, so much so that organizations specializing in market research have proliferated.

As stated previously, the key to marketing your preventive dental services professionally is to be consumer oriented. To be so, you need to know who your consumers and potential consumers are, what services they use, what services they want, and what their expectations regarding dental services are.

A sound marketing plan is based on *accurate* data about your market. Whom are you trying to reach? To begin with, you need information about two broad populations: (1) current patients and (2) prospective patients.

CURRENT PATIENTS

Who are your current patients? Why do they come in? How efficiently are they treated? What do they expect? How satisfied are they?

The first step in determining who your current patients are is to develop a patient profile. This should include, at minimum, the total number of patients, and their ages and sexes. Other factors are also of importance in developing a marketing plan for preventive procedures: educational level, income, place of residence, whether single or married, and the like. All current patients should complete brief surveys containing questions you consider relevant. This can be done the next time they come in. Have a code on the patient's folder to indicate when the survey has been completed. After a year's time, you should have information on every patient (assuming you have an effective recall system).

You can develop your basic patient profile using existing information from patient records. You probably already have on record the age, sex, and address of your patients. This will help you determine if your practice serves primarily young or mature people, men or women, people who live close to you, or come from a distance, etc. The other information regarding income and educational level will have direct relevance as you select marketing strategies.

Services Used. Information on services used can be easily gathered if you prepare your appointment records to do so. You can also obtain this information by analyzing the billing, assuming you itemize your bills. The following key might be used to code services used:

1. Preventive dental procedures
2. Examination and x-rays
3. Fillings
4. Oral surgery
5. Crown and bridge
6. Periodontics
7. Orthodontics
8. Endodontics
9. Full and partial dentures
10. Other (specify)

It is important to know what services are most used and least used. This information will be needed in the second step of developing your marketing plan.

The more you know about who your patients are and how they are currently using your services, the better you can plan to meet their needs. However, it is not enough to know whom you are serving. Even more important is knowledge of what they expect and how satisfied they are with your services. The most important market research you do is that related to current patient expectations and satisfaction. Why? Because one of the most powerful marketing tools you have is a satisfied patient whose needs are being met. MacStravic describes a hierarchy of effects as the primary focus of marketing professional services.[7] Marketing basically seeks to reach the consumer who is unaware of a service, to make him aware, then interested, then determined, and then a patient. But the hierarchy does not stop here; effective marketing seeks to make the patient satisfied after the first exposure to the service, then a regular patient, and finally an "agent," that is, one who tells others of the service.

Patient Knowledge and Dental Habits. While you are surveying your current patients, you might also want to determine their knowledge about such things as flossing, toothbrushing techniques, fluoridation, preventive dental examinations, nutrition, gum disease, and oral cancer as well as their current dental habits — do they brush and floss regularly, and how many sweets do they eat? Such information can be valuable in designing preventive education materials.

No matter what type of information you are designing a survey to obtain, the survey will be more effective if you follow certain guidelines, as listed in Table 20–1.

TABLE 20–1 GUIDELINES FOR DEVELOPING WRITTEN SURVEYS

1. Carefully formulate the purpose of the survey and then state clearly how the results of the survey will benefit the person who is completing it.
2. Assure that the respondent's anonymity is preserved, but obtain needed descriptive data such as age, sex, income level, and the like. Include whatever descriptors you want to have in your profile of current and prospective patients.
3. Keep questions simple and easy to understand. Single-response questions are usually best.
4. Make responding easy, that is, minimize the amount of actual writing required, but *do* allow room for any comments respondents may want to make.
5. Keep the data analysis in mind. What data will result from the items, and will they be workable?
6. Keep the survey as short as possible.
7. End it with a thank you and clear instructions as to what the respondent is to do with it when finished.
8. Be certain that it is neatly and accurately typed and clearly reproduced; that is, that it looks professional. A sloppy appearance implies lack of importance and people will respond (or not respond) accordingly.
9. Test the survey by having five or six patients complete it and see if they have difficulty with any questions as to wording or what is wanted.

PROSPECTIVE PATIENTS

A second major data set provides information on potential patients. How many people live in your community? How many live within a 10-mile radius? What is their general economic status? Educational level? Are you in an established area, an area of growth, or an area of population decline? Usually such information can be obtained from the state department of education, which compiles such statistics in planning for educational needs at the state and local levels. It may also be available from your city hall or the Census Bureau. Or you can conduct your own survey based on a random sampling of your immediate area. This can be done by telephone, in-person interview, or mailed survey. The information you seek is: *What type of dental services do they now use? What factors are of most importance to them in selecting a dentist? What services do they need?* These three basic questions will allow you to determine what your potential market is and whether it is "reachable." The means you use to collect the information is up to you. Telephone interviews are one option, but people often consider such interviews to be an annoyance and refuse to answer questions. In-person interviews are a second option. These are more time-consuming but usually yield more information than telephone interviews. Mailed survey is yet another option for obtaining information about your potential market. This is the most expensive method, and it frequently does not generate as many responses as hoped for. If you decide to mail a survey to potential customers in your area, be certain to include the purpose for your survey and to enclose a return envelope with postage.

Additional data on patient needs, whether potential or current, may be found in professional journals; for example, results of surveys conducted by the American Dental Association, or in journals such as the *Journal of Marketing/Management for Professions.*

Whether you concentrate marketing efforts on current patients, potential patients, or both, two other important sets of information should be obtained: information about your staff and information about your competition. Your patient surveys can be constructed to elicit some of this needed information.

STAFF

Patient surveys can be used to indicate how courteous, efficient, and caring staff are. How do patients rate your dental assistant, hygienist, and receptionist? You may receive complaints if patients are not satisfied with the staff. However, you also need to know how your staff feel about you and their jobs. Staff satisfaction is a critical part of patient satisfaction; therefore, although it is technically not market research, you should devise a way to measure staff attitudes towards preventive dentistry. You might develop a brief survey with questions related to their satisfaction with their job responsibility, work environment, pay, benefits, and colleagues. You might also want to assess your ancillary staff's competence using some sort of checklists such as those available through the ADA; for example, the CASE (Chairside Assisting Skills Evaluation) materials.

COMPETITION

The second set of data, information about the competition, may be more difficult to obtain. It should be relatively easy to determine the number of dentists in your area and their types of services, whether small or large practice, fee for service or prepaid, open or closed panel. Determining what segment of the market they have and what their charges are may be more difficult. As marketing of preventive dental services becomes more prevalent, such information may be easier to obtain.

Information about the competition can also be obtained from that all-important current patient survey. Why did your patients start coming to you, and why did they stop going to their previous dental clinic?

Likewise, when you lose a patient, it is extremely important to find out why. A callback system whereby patients are sent a card or are phoned to arrange for a periodic dental exam not only will help assure that you provide good preventive care for current patients and keep them coming in but will also alert you to patients who have decided to obtain preventive dental services elsewhere and give you the chance to find out why.

SUMMARY

Market research consists of gathering as much information as possible about (1) your current patients, who they are, what services they are currently using, their expectations, their level of satisfaction; (2) potential patients, who they are, what their expectations are; (3) your staff; and (4) your competition. As you gather information on your market, be certain the information is accurate, or you will be working from a questionable data base when you develop your marketing plan. Once this information is gathered, you must tally, summarize, and analyze it carefully, and then come to some conclusions.

It is important to realize that preventive dental measures are basically public health oriented procedures and can be quantitated only by a population or epidemiological study. The oral hygiene index and other indices were designed to measure improvement or a reverse effect of a given preventive dental health measure on a population basis; however, it is extremely difficult to quantitate the effect on a single patient. This is where effective marketing comes into play. You must create an awareness in the patient's mind of the importance of the specific service and the anticipated results of the procedures if you are to be successful in marketing preventive dental measures to your patients. It is also essential to analyze the personality of your patient. An introvert normally responds to a fear of loss (fear of disease), and the extrovert will respond to anticipated gain. The approaches to these two groups of patients must be different if the preventive dental program is to be a success.

REFERENCES

1. Yankelovich, Skelly, and White, Inc.: Family health in an era of stress. *In* The General Mills American Family Report. Minneapolis, General Mills, Inc., 1978–79.
2. Levitt, T.: Innovations in Marketing. London, Pan Books, 1968.
3. Carr-Saunders, A. M., and Wilson, P. A.: The Professions. London, Cass, 1964.
4. Bennion, F. A. R.: Professional Ethics. London, Charles Knight, 1969.
5. Leacock, S.: Quoted in Walher, M.: Advertising and Promoting the Professional Practice. New York, Hawthorn Books, Inc., 1979.
6. Wilson, A.: The Marketing of Professional Services. New York, McGraw-Hill, 1972.
7. MacStravic, R. E.: Marketing Health Care. Germantown, Maryland, Aspen Systems Corporation, 1977.
8. Heiser, R. A., Stallard, R. E., and Hess, K.: Marketing Dental Services Professionally. Tulsa, PenWell Publishing, 1982.

Index

Page numbers in *italics* indicate illustrations; page numbers followed by t indicate tables.

395

Lip habits, and need for orthodontics, 382, 384, *384*
Lymphoma, Burkitt's, as factor in oral cancer, 86

Malnutrition, gingivae in, 105
lips in, 103, 105
oral manifestations of, 103–106, 104t
teeth in, 105
tongue in, 105–106
Malocclusion, 347–350, *348*
airway obstruction in, 356–357
as factors in periodontal disease, 54, *54, 66, 67*
classes of, *348,* 349–350
definition of, 348–349, *348*
dental vs. skeletal, *348,* 349–350
diagnostic techniques in, 367–368
etiologic considerations in, *348,* 349–350
examination for, 350–357, *351–354, 356.* See also under *Occlusion.*
facial type in, 351–353, *351–353*
frequency of, 350
importance of diagnosis of, 350
lips in, 354–356, *354, 356*
skeletal vs. dental, *348,* 349–350
speech in, 356
tongue in, 355–356
Mandibular quadrants, isolation of, for pit and fissure sealing, 310–311, *310*
Marketing, of preventive dentistry, 387–393, 391t. See also *Preventive dentistry, marketing of.*
Maxillary quadrants, isolation of, for pit and fissure sealing, 311
Mechanical irritation, and oral cancer, 302–303, 302–303t, *303–304,* 305, 305t
Melanodontia, 105
Mental stress, as factor in oral cancer, 87
Metastases, from oral cancer, 289, 289t
Microbial agents, in caries, 33–36
Microscope, discovery of, 1
Military services, epidemiology of caries in, 29–30, *30*
Milk, fluoridation of, 164–165
Moniliasis, vs. oral cancer, 302
Mouth, floor of, cancer of, 281, 281–282t, 283
in leukemia, 287, *288–289,* 289
skeletal tissues of, orthodontics and, 368–371, *369–370, 372*
soft tissues of, in examination for malocclusion, 354–356, *354, 356*
orthodontics and, 382–385, *383–384*
Mouth rinse(s), 192–198, 195t, 197t
anticaries drugs in, FDA-approved concentrations of, 205
antimicrobial-containing, 196–197, 197t
comparative effects on plaque of, *238,* 239
composition of, 192–193
cosmetic functions of, 193–194
definition of, 192
FDA-approved, update of, 204t, 205
fluoride-containing, 194, 195t, 196
and community water fluoridation, 198
use by adults of, 198
functions of, 193–194, 195t, 196–197, 197t

Mouth rinse(s) (*Continued*)
future trends in, 197
sodium fluoride-containing, clinical update on, 201, 204t, 205
FDA-approved concentrations for, 205
stannous fluoride-containing, FDA-approved concentrations for, 205
therapeutic functions of, 194, 195t, 196–197, 197t
Mouthbreathing, effect on dental development of, 384
MPD (maximum permissible dose of x-radiation), 272
Mucosa, buccal, cancer of, 286
from chronic habits, 305
leukoedema vs., 299, *300*
oral, 292–293, 292–293t
effects of dentifrices on, 191–192

Netherlands, oral cancer in, 75
Nutrition, and calcification processes, 94, *95*
and caries, 107, *108,* 108t, 109–116
epidemiologic data on, 107, *108,* 108t, 109–112
experimental studies in, 112–113
and disease, 90–93, *92*
and infection, 121
and oral cancer, 84–85, 119–120, 120t
and oral health, 93–97, *95, 97*
and periodontal disease, 116–119
and surgery, 121–123
as factor in oral cancer, 84–85
diet formulation for, 127, *128,* 129, 130–140t. See also under *Diet.*
effects of cancer treatment on, 120t
effects on cancer of, 120t
in oral tissue growth and development, 93–94
in tooth development, 94–97, *97*
oral disease and, 106–123, *108,* 108t, 120t
prevention and management in, 123–129, *128,* 130–140t, 139, 141
poor, 103–106, 104t. See also *Malnutrition.*
recommended daily dietary allowances (RDA) in, 97–98, *98,* 99t, 100
requirements, of, 97–106, *98,* 99–102t, 104t
stress and, *98*
Nutritional status, assessment of, 100–103, 100–102t, 104t

Observation, of dental caries, vs. radiographic examination, *22*
Occlusion, arches and teeth in, 357–359, *358*
as factor in periodontal disease, 66, *67*
diagnostic techniques in, 367–368
examination of, by analysis of dental study cases, 362–367, *364, 366*
by mixed-dentitional analysis, 365–367, *366*
by radiographic cephalometry, 359–362, *361, 363.* See also *Cephalometry.*
face in, 350–356, *351–354, 356*
intraoral, 357–359, *358*
lips in, 354–355, *354*